NOVEL STRATEGIES IN ISCHEMIC HEART DISEASE

Edited by **Umashankar Lakshmanadoss**

Novel Strategies in Ischemic Heart Disease
Edited by Umashankar Lakshmanadoss

Published by InTech

Janeza Trdine 9, 51000 Rijeka, Croatia

Publishing Process Manager Maja Bozicevic

Technical Editor Teodora Smiljanic

Cover Designer InTech Design Team

Additional hard copies can be obtained from orders@intechopen.com

Novel Strategies in Ischemic Heart Disease, Edited by Umashankar Lakshmanadoss
p. cm.
ISBN 978-953-51-0184-0

For EU product safety concerns:
IN TECH d.o.o., Prolaz Marije Krucifikse Kozulić 3, 51000 Rijeka, Croatia, info@intechopen.com or visit our website at intechopen.com.

Meet the editor

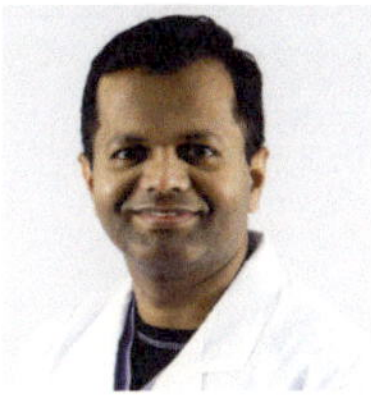

Dr Lakshmanadoss completed his residency training at Madras Medical College, India, and at Unity Hospital, an affiliate of the University of Rochester, NY, USA. He served as Director of Inpatient Medical Consult Service at Johns Hopkins University School of Medicine and then joined the Division of Cardiovascular Medicine at Guthrie Clinic, Sayre, PA, USA. He has presented his research papers multiple times in American Heart Association and American College of Cardiology conferences. He is serving as a reviewer for prestigious journals including American Journal of Cardiology, American Journal of Medicine, Journal of Hospital Medicine and Journal of Pacing and Cardiac Electrophysiology. His research interests include improving the outcome of sudden cardiac arrest survivors, reducing inappropriate shocks from ICDs and finding the appropriate pacing site for patients with heart failure. He received various awards including outstanding cardiovascular research and young cardiovascular investigator awards. He has been volunteering in Haiti after the earthquake disaster.

Contents

Preface

To study the phenomena of disease without books is to sail an uncharted sea, while to study books without patients is not to go to sea at all.

SIR WILLIAM OSLER

Ischemic heart disease continues to be the leading cause of morbidity and mortality in both developed and developing countries, and remains one of the most important public health problems. The continuous rise in the prevalence of disorders such as obesity, diabetes, dyslipidemia and hypertension is driving the ever-increasing number of incidences of ischemic heart disease. In recent years we have seen remarkable advances in the understanding of ischemic heart disease in areas such as epidemiology, risk assessment, risk factor reduction, pathophysiology, early detection, biochemical markers, imaging and in treatments. Nevertheless, the importance of prevention and personal responsibility in controlling the disease has also attracted great attention. As we all know, cardiovascular medicine is an ever-growing field; ongoing research has led to new discoveries in management, leading to improvements in the outcomes of the patients with cardiovascular diseases.

The first edition of this book will provide a comprehensive overview of ischemic heart disease, including epidemiology, risk factors, pathogenesis, clinical presentation, diagnostic tests, differential diagnosis, treatment, complications and prognosis. Also discussed are current treatment options, protocols and diagnostic procedures, as well as the latest advances in the field. The book will serve as a cutting-edge point of reference for the basic or clinical researcher, and any clinician involved in the diagnosis and management of ischemic heart disease. This book is essentially designed to fill the vital gap existing between these practices to provide a textbook that is substantial and readable, compact and reasonably comprehensive, and to provide an excellent blend of "basics to bedside and beyond" in the field of ischemic heart disease.

With increasing life expectancy and increasing prevalence of the disease, patients with ischemic heart disease are being taken care of by various health care providers. I sincerely hope that this textbook will meet the needs of nurses, healthcare providers, medical students, clinicians, physician scientists and, of course, patients. With this information easily accessible via the internet, no one is deprived of the pioneering technology and ongoing research. I am thrilled to present the various chapters like epidemiology, diagnosis of ischemic heart disease and its complications, management of ischemic heart disease and its risk factors and complications. Chapters discussing translational research and novel treatment strategies will be really exciting for those interested in basic science research.

I gratefully acknowledge the invaluable organisational skills of the publisher InTech, the timely and invaluable assistance of publishing process manager Ms Maja Bozicevic, designer, technical editors, information technology staff and finally the marketing representatives who are working constantly to promote the book on various platforms. I sincerely applaud all the contributing authors for their excellence, hard work and commitment in respect of their chapters. They have taken time from their personal and professional lives to complete this task and I thank them profusely for it.

I believe that this book will provide valuable information for all healthcare providers who are trying to make a positive difference in our fellow human beings' lives.

Let's love humanity through love of our profession.

Umashankar Lakshmanadoss MD
Formerly Director, Inpatient Medicine Consult Service,
JHBMC, Johns Hopkins University School of Medicine,
Baltimore, MD,
USA

Division of Cardiology, Guthrie Clinic,
Sayre, PA,
USA

Dedication

This book is dedicated to my mother Mrs Jana, my wife Mrs Priya for constant support, encouragement and fond memories without which this textbook would not have been possible, and to my nieces Karnika, Rithisha, Deepshika and Trisha for making my life more joyous.

Part 1

Introduction

1

Overview of Coronary Artery Disease

Umashankar Lakshmanadoss
Formerly Director, Inpatient Consult Service,
Johns Hopkins University School of Medicine, Baltimore, MD
Division of Cardiology, Guthrie Clinic, Sayre, PA
USA

1. Introduction

Coronary artery disease (CAD) is a major cause of death and disability in developed countries. Although CAD mortality rates have declined over the past four decades in the United States (and elsewhere), CAD remains responsible for about one-third of all deaths in individuals over age 35 [1,2]. It has been estimated that nearly one-half of all middle-aged men and one-third of middle-aged women in the United States will develop some manifestation of CAD.

2. Prevalence

The 2010 Heart Disease and Stroke Statistics update of the American Heart Association reported that 17.6 million persons in the United States have CAD, including 8.5 million with myocardial infarction (MI) and 10.2 million with angina pectoris [2]. The reported prevalence increases with age for both women and men. In a 2009 report that used National Health and Nutrition Examination Survey (NHANES) data, MI prevalence was compared by sex in middle-aged individuals (35 to 54 years) during the 1998 to 1994 and 1999 to 2004 time periods [3]. Although MI prevalence was significantly greater in men than women in both time periods (2.5 versus 0.7 and 2.2 versus 1.0 respectively), there were trends toward a decrease in men and an increase in women. Data from NHANES (and other databases) that rely on self-reported MI and angina from health interviews probably underestimate the actual prevalence of advanced CAD.

This is likely as advanced occlusive coronary artery disease often exists with few symptoms or overt clinical manifestations. Silent ischemia, which is thought to account for 75 percent of all ischemic episodes [4], may be brought to light by electrocardiographic changes (ST segment depression) on an exercise test, ambulatory 24 hour electrocardiographic recording, or periodic routine electrocardiogram (ECG).

3. Global trends

Heart disease mortality has been declining in the United States and in regions where economies and health care systems are relatively advanced, but the experience is often quite different around the world [5]. Coronary artery disease is the number one cause of death in adults from both low- and middle income countries as well as from high-income countries [5]. At the turn of the century, it was reported that CAD mortality was expected to increase approximately 29 percent in women and 48 percent in men in developed countries between 1990 and 2020. The corresponding estimated increases in developing countries were 120 percent in women and 137 percent in men [6].

The most dramatic increments in ischemic heart disease events on a percentage basis were forecast for the Middle East and Latin America. The experience in Asia is especially important because of the large populations involved. In India, CAD may not be largely explained by traditional risk factors [7]. In China, risk factor trends complement tracking of event rates. For example, the dramatic increase in CAD mortality in Beijing is attributable to greater cholesterol levels. The mean cholesterol level was 4.30 mmol/L (166 mg/dL) in 1984 and 5.33 mmol/L (206 mg/dL) only 15 years later [8]. In Latin America, declines in vascular disease rates have been less favorable than in the United States; unfavorable trends in physical activity, obesity, and smoking contribute to these differences [9].

International leaders have called for action plans to avert the projected global epidemic of ischemic heart disease in developing countries [10].

4. Pathophysiology

4.1 Cellular level

Angina is caused by myocardial ischemia, which occurs whenever myocardial oxygen demand exceeds oxygen supply (Figure 1). Because oxygen delivery to the heart is closely

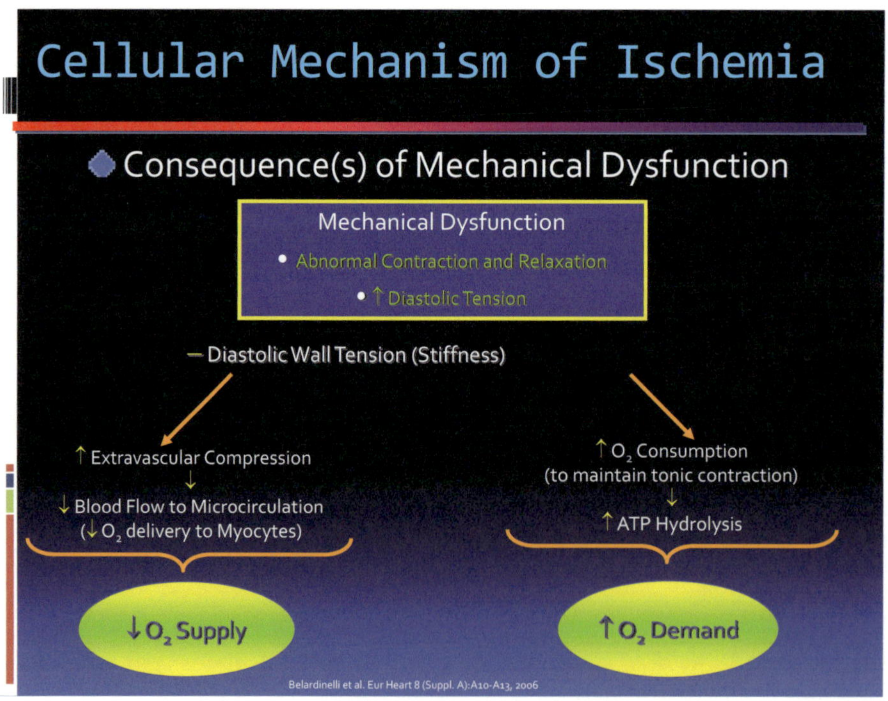

Fig. 1.

coupled to coronary blood flow, a sudden cessation of regional perfusion following a thrombotic coronary occlusion quickly leads to the cessation of aerobic metabolism, depletion of creatine phosphate, and the onset of anaerobic glycolysis. This is followed by the accumulation of tissue lactate, a progressive reduction in tissue ATP levels, and an accumulation of catabolites, including those of the adenine nucleotide pool. As ischemia continues, tissue acidosis develops and there is an efflux of potassium into the extracellular space. Subsequently, ATP levels fall below those required to maintain critical membrane function, resulting in the onset of myocyte death. Irreversible myocardial injury begins after 20 minutes of coronary occlusion in the absence of significant collaterals [11].

Irreversible injury begins in the subendocardium and progresses as a wave front over time, from the subendocardial layers to the subepicardial layers. This reflects the higher oxygen consumption in the subendocardium and the redistribution of collateral flow to the outer layers of the heart by the compressive determinants of flow at reduced coronary pressure. Factors that increase myocardial oxygen consumption (e.g., tachycardia) or reduce oxygen delivery (e.g., anemia, arterial hypotension) accelerate the progression of irreversible injury. In contrast, repetitive reversible ischemia or angina prior to an occlusion can reduce irreversible injury through preconditioning [12].

4.2 Anatomical level

Acute coronary syndrome is usually caused by an unstable atherosclerotic plaque rupture with subsequent platelet-rich thrombus overlying the culprit lesion causing severe narrowing (Figure. 2). This abrupt decrease in blood supply often results in chest pain and ECG changes indicative of ischemia, and, if prolonged, results in myocardial necrosis and

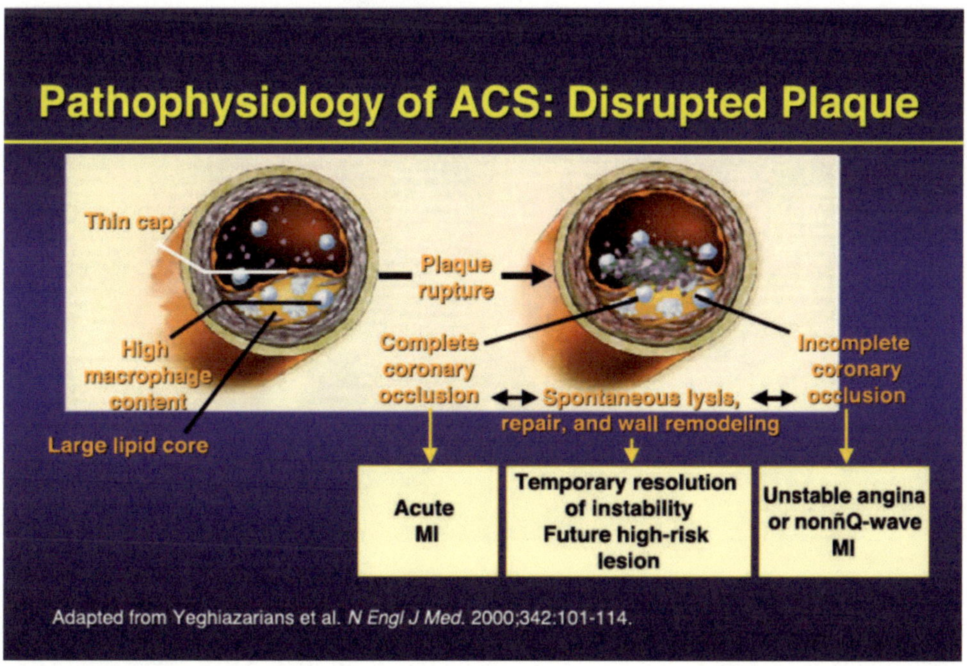

Fig. 2.

enzyme elevation. Less commonly, non ST elevation myocardial infarction is caused by diseases in which myocardial demand exceeds myocardial supply causing a similar clinical presentation. These diseases usually cause a hypermetabolic or high cardiac output state and include hyperthyroidism, anemia, fever, pheochromocytoma, hypertrophic cardiomyopathy, AV fistula and hypertensive urgency/emergency.

Whatever the mechanism of angina may be, patients usually develop the clinical manifestations in a sequence as described in Figure 3. Note that diastolic dysfunction is the earliest manifestation of ischemia, next to perfusion abnormalities which are seen in nuclear studies.

5. Clinical features

Coronary artery disease could be manifesting as a continuum from stable angina to acute coronary syndrome. Angina pectoris is a discomfort in the chest or adjacent areas caused by myocardial ischemia. It is usually brought on by exertion and is associated with a disturbance in myocardial function, without myocardial necrosis.

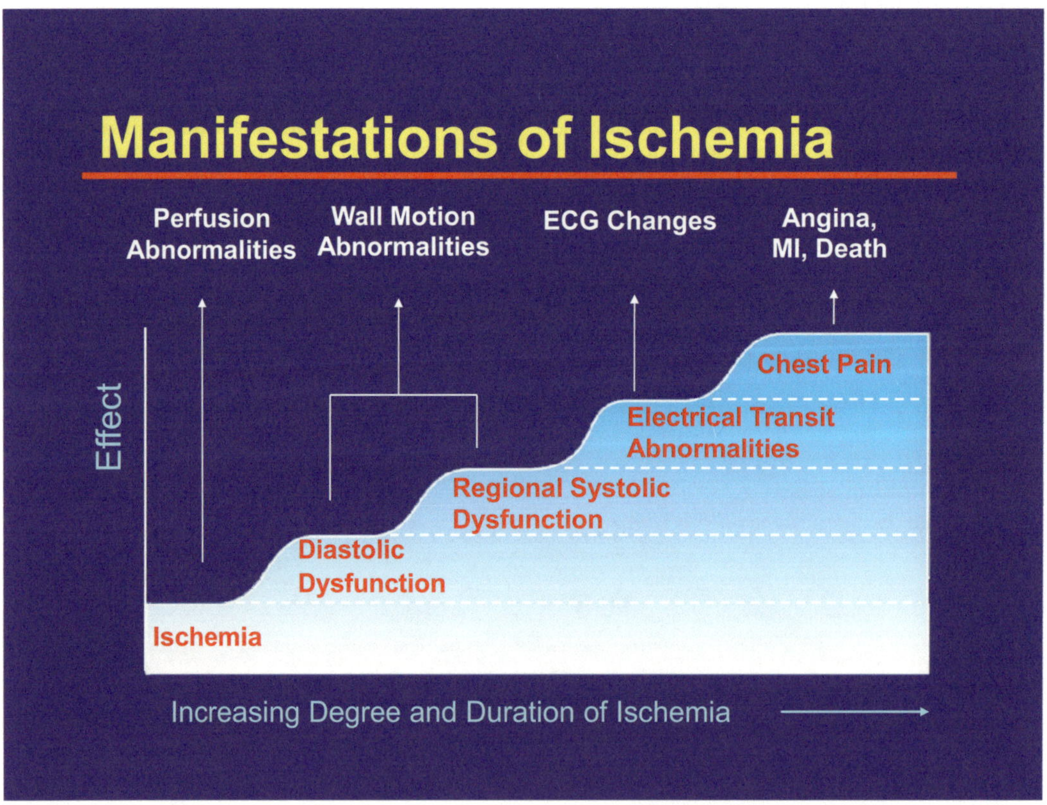

Fig. 3.

Heberden's initial description of angina as conveying a sense of "strangling and anxiety" is still remarkably pertinent. Other adjectives frequently used to describe this distress include viselike, constricting, suffocating, crushing, heavy, and squeezing. In other patients, the quality of the sensation is more vague and described as a mild pressure-like discomfort, an uncomfortable numb sensation, or a burning sensation.

The site of the discomfort is usually retrosternal, but radiation is common and usually occurs down the ulnar surface of the left arm; the right arm and the outer surfaces of both arms may also be involved. Epigastric discomfort alone or in association with chest pressure is not uncommon. Anginal discomfort above the mandible or below the epigastrium is rare. Anginal equivalents (i.e., symptoms of myocardial ischemia other than angina), such as dyspnea, faintness, fatigue, and eructations, are common, particularly in the elderly.

A history of abnormal exertional dyspnea may be an early indicator of CAD even when angina is absent or no evidence of ischemic heart disease can be found on the electrocardiogram (ECG). Dyspnea at rest or with exertion may be a manifestation of severe ischemia, leading to increases in left ventricular (LV) filling pressure. Nocturnal angina should raise the suspicion of sleep apnea.

The term acute coronary syndrome (ACS) is applied to patients in whom there is a suspicion of myocardial ischemia. There are three types of ACS: ST elevation (formerly Q-wave) MI (STEMI), non-ST elevation (formerly non-Q wave) MI (NSTEMI), and unstable angina (UA). The first two are characterized by a typical rise and/or fall in biomarkers of myocyte injury.

For many years, the diagnosis of acute MI relied on the revised criteria established by the World Health Organization (WHO) in 1979. These criteria were epidemiological and aimed at specificity. A joint European Society of Cardiology (ESC) and American College of Cardiology (ACC) committee proposed a more clinically based definition of an acute, evolving, or recent MI in 2000 (13). In 2007 the Joint Task Force of the European Society of Cardiology, American College of Cardiology Foundation, the American Heart Association, and the World Health Federation (ESC/ACCF/AHA/WHF) refined the 2000 criteria and defined acute MI as a clinical event consequent to the death of cardiac myocytes (myocardial necrosis) that is caused by ischemia (as opposed to other etiologies such as myocarditis or trauma) [14].

The criteria used to define MI differ somewhat depending upon the particular clinical circumstance of the patient: those suspected of acute MI based upon their presentation, those undergoing either coronary artery bypass graft surgery or percutaneous intervention, or those who have sustained sudden unexpected, cardiac arrest with or without death [14].

For patients who have undergone recent revascularization or who have sustained cardiac arrest or death, the criteria for the diagnosis of MI are given in detail in the Table 1.

For all other patients in whom there is a suspicion of MI, a typical rise and/or gradual fall (troponin) or more rapid rise and fall (CK-MB) of biochemical markers of myocardial necrosis, with at least one of the following is required:

- Ischemic symptoms
- Development of pathologic Q waves on the ECG
- ECG changes indicative of ischemia (ST segment elevation or depression)
- Imaging evidence of new loss of viable myocardium or a new regional wall motion abnormality.

In addition, pathologic findings (generally at autopsy) of an acute MI are accepted criteria.

The joint task force [14] further refined the definition of MI by developing a clinical classification according to the assumed proximate cause of the myocardial ischemia.

Patulous aneurysmal dilation involving most of the length of a major epicardial coronary artery is present in approximately 1 to 3 percent of patients with obstructive CAD at autopsy or angiography. This angiographic lesion does not appear to affect symptoms, survival, or incidence of MI. Most coronary artery ectasia and/or aneurysms are caused by coronary atherosclerosis (50 percent), and the rest are caused by congenital anomalies and inflammatory diseases, such as Kawasaki disease.

Type 1	Spontaneous myocardial infarction related to ischaemia due to a primary coronary event such as plaque erosion and/or rupture, fissuring, or dissection
Type 2	Myocardial infarction secondary to ischaemia due to either increased oxygen demand or decreased supply, e.g. coronary artery spasm, coronary embolism, anaemia, arrhythmias, hypertension, or hypotension
Type 3	Sudden unexpected cardiac death, including cardiac arrest, often with symptoms suggestive of myocardial ischaemia, accompanied by presumably new ST elevation, or new LBBB, or evidence of fresh thrombus in a coronary artery by angiography and/or at autopsy, but death occurring before blood samples could be obtained, or at a time before the appearance of cardiac biomarkers in the blood
Type 4a	Myocardial infarction associated with PCI
Type 4b	Myocardial infarction associated with stent thrombosis as documented by angiography or at autopsy
Type 5	Myocardial infarction associated with CABG

Table 1. Types of Myocardial Infarction

6. Diagnosis

Evaluation of new onset chest pain in stable individuals should begin with the consideration of imminently life-threatening causes (including acute coronary syndrome, pulmonary embolus, aortic dissection, pneumothorax, and esophageal rupture). This is usually accomplished using clinical judgement, along with ECG testing, and less frequently exercise testing, other noninvasive testing, or invasive angiography.

This is being discussed in detail by other authors in various chapters. nce a life-threatening etiology has been excluded, attempts should be made to identify the specific cause of symptoms and begin treatment. A diagnostic pattern will frequently emerge, based upon the patient's risk factors, description of the pain, and associated symptoms.

Standard clinical characteristics routinely obtained during the initial medical evaluation of patients with UA/NSTEMI can be used to construct a simple classification system that is predictive of risk for death and cardiac ischemic events. The TIMI (Thrombolysis in Myocardial Infarction) risk score (Table 2) includes variables that can be easily ascertained when a patient with UA/NSTEMI presents to the medical care system. The variables used to construct the score were based on observations from prior studies of risk stratification and incorporate demographic and historical features of the patient, measures of the tempo and acuity of the presenting illness, and indicators of the extent of myocardial ischemia and necrosis.

Since patients with an acute coronary syndrome are at increased risk of death and nonfatal cardiac events, clinicians must assess prognosis on an individual basis to formulate plans for evaluation and treatment. The TIMI risk score for UA/NSTEMI is a simple prognostication

TIMI Risk Score	All-Cause Mortality, New or Recurrent MI, or Severe Recurrent Ischemia Requiring Urgent Revascularization Through 14 d After Randomization, %
0–1	4.7
2	8.3
3	13.2
4	19.9
5	26.2
6–7	40.9

The TIMI risk score is determined by the sum of the presence of 7 variables at admission; 1 point is given for each of the following variables:

- age 65 y or older;
- at least 3 risk factors for CAD;
- prior coronary stenosis of 50% or more;
- ST-segment deviation on ECG presentation;
- at least 2 anginal events in prior 24 h;
- use of aspirin in prior 7 d;
- elevated serum cardiac biomarkers.

Prior coronary stenosis of 50% or more remained relatively insensitive to missing information and remained a significant predictor of events.

Table 2. TIMI Risk Score for Unstable Angina/Non-ST Elevation MI

scheme that enables a clinician to categorize a patient's risk of risk of death and ischemic events at the critical initial evaluation. A promising clinical application of this score is identification of a patient for whom new antithrombotic therapies would be especially effective.

While ECG manifestations are an important component of diagnosis, one should be aware of the pitfalls of the ECG. Tables 3, 4 and 5 describe the ECG manifestations of ischemic disease.

ST elevation

New ST elevation at the J-point in two contiguous leads with the cut-off points: $\geq$0.2 mV in men or $\geq$0.15 mV in women in leads V_2–V_3 and/or $\geq$0.1 mV in other leads

ST depression and T-wave changes

New horizontal or down-sloping ST depression $\geq$0.05 mV in two contiguous leads; and/or T inversion $\geq$0.1 mV in two contiguous leads with prominent R-wave or R/S ratio >1

Table 3. ECG manifestations of acute myocardial ischemia (in absence of LVH and LBBB)

Any Q-wave in leads V_2–V_3 $\geq$0.02 s or QS complex in leads V_2 and V_3

Q-wave $\geq$0.03 s and $\geq$0.1 mV deep or QS complex in leads I, II, aVL, aVF, or V_4–V_6 in any two leads of a contiguous lead grouping (I, aVL, V_6; V_4–V_6; II, III, and aVF)[a]

R-wave $\geq$0.04 s in V_1–V_2 and R/S $\geq$1 with a concordant positive T-wave in the absence of a conduction defect

[a]The same criteria are used for supplemental leads V_7–V_9, and for the Cabrera frontal plane lead grouping.

Table 4. ECG changes associated with prior myocardial infarction

False positives
- Benign early repolarization
- LBBB
- Pre-excitation
- Brugada syndrome
- Peri-/myocarditis
- Pulmonary embolism
- Subarachnoid haemorrhage
- Metabolic disturbances such as hyperkalaemia
- Failure to recognize normal limits for J-point displacement
- Lead transposition or use of modified Mason–Likar configuration[24]
- Cholecystitis

False negatives
- Prior myocardial infarction with Q-waves and/or persistent ST elevation
- Paced rhythm
- LBBB

Table 5. Common ECG pitfalls in diagnosing myocardial infarction

7. Management

Patients with an initial ECG reading that reveals new or presumably new ST segment depression and/or T wave inversion, although not considered candidates for fibrinolytic therapy, should be treated as though they are suffering from MI without ST elevation or unstable angina (a distinction to be made subsequently after scrutiny of serial ECGs and serum cardiac marker measurements). In patients with a clinical history suggestive of STEMI and an initial nondiagnostic ECG reading (i.e., no ST segment deviation or T wave inversion), serial tracings should be obtained while the patients are being evaluated in the emergency department.

Emergency department staff can be alerted to the sudden development of ST segment elevation by periodic visual inspection of the bedside ECG monitor, by continuous ST segment recording, or by auditory alarms when the ST segment deviation exceeds programmed limits. Decision aids such as computer-based diagnostic algorithms, identification of high-risk clinical indicators, rapid determination of cardiac serum markers, two-dimensional echocardiographic screening for regional wall motion abnormalities, and myocardial perfusion imaging have greatest clinical utility when the ECG reading is nondiagnostic. In an effort to improve the cost-effectiveness of care of patients with a chest pain syndrome, nondiagnostic ECG reading, and low suspicion of MI but in whom the diagnosis has not been entirely excluded, many medical centers have developed critical pathways that involve a coronary observation unit with a goal of ruling out MI in less than 12 hours.

Once the diagnosis of coronary artery disease is made, the management depends upon the severity of the underlying severity of the disease. The treating physician has to diagnose the clinical scenario appropriately as the treatment largely depends of the initial diagnosis. Stable coronary artery disease could be managed conservatively whereas acute coronary syndrome has to be managed very aggressively. Select patients have to be considered for early invasive strategy too.

The prehospital care of patients with suspected STEMI is a crucial element bearing directly on the likelihood of survival. Most deaths associated with STEMI occur within the first hour of its onset and are usually caused by ventricular fibrillation. Accordingly, the importance of the immediate implementation of definitive resuscitative efforts and of rapidly transporting the patient to a hospital cannot be overemphasized.

Major components of the delay from the onset of symptoms consistent with acute myocardial infarction (MI) to reperfusion include the following: (1) the time for the patient to recognize the seriousness of the problem and seek medical attention; (2) prehospital evaluation, treatment, and transportation; (3) the time for diagnostic measures and initiation of treatment in the hospital (e.g., "door-to-needle" time for patients receiving a thrombolytic agent and "door-to-balloon" time for patients undergoing a catheter-based reperfusion strategy); and (4) the time from initiation of treatment to restoration of flow (Figure 4). Thrombolytic therapy is vital for early reperfusion and this has been discussed in other chapters.

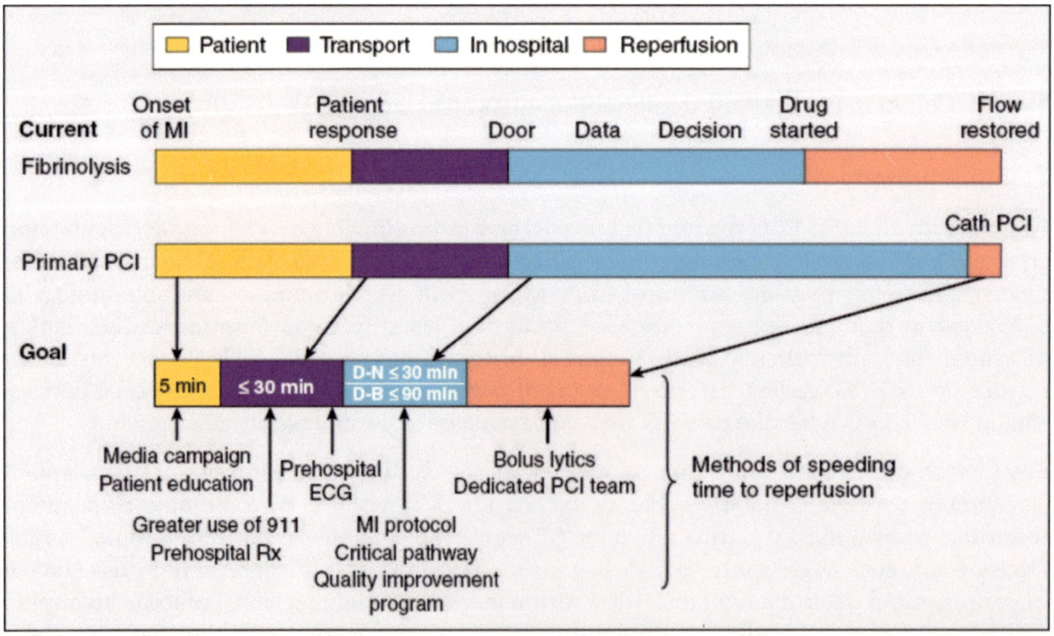

(Modified from Antman EM, Anbe DT, Armstrong PW, et al: ACC/AHA guidelines for the management of patients with ST-elevation myocardial infarction: A report of the American College of Cardiology/American Heart Association Task Force on Practice Guidelines [Committee to Revise the 1999 Guidelines for the Management of Patients with Acute Myocardial Infarction]. Circulation 110:e82, 2004.)

Fig. 4.

Adjunctive medical therapy is a critical component of therapy for STEMI and confers benefit in addition to that gained by reperfusion therapies, regardless of method of reperfusion (Table 6).

Ancillary therapy can be used to facilitate and enhance coronary reperfusion or to limit the consequences of myocardial ischemia. Early, aggressive use of antiplatelet therapies, such as aspirin, and clopidogrel, confers significant additional mortality benefit when given as adjuncts to thrombolysis or PCI. Beta-blockers, angiotensin-converting enzyme inhibitors in appropriately selected patients, and 3-hydroxy-3-methylglutaryl CoA reductase inhibitors (statins) have all been shown to reduce the risk of cardiovascular events and mortality in patients who have STEMI. Therapies such as nitroglycerin and morphine have no mortality benefit but may improve symptoms and reduce ischemic burden. Calcium-channel blockers and prophylactic anti-arrhythmic drug therapy (lidocaine) may increase mortality. The suggested benefit of metabolic modulation at the myocyte level with electrolytes, glucose, and insulin seen in small, early trials has not been reproduced in larger, randomized studies.

Mechanisms and clinical effects of adjunctive therapies for patients who have ST elevation myocardial infarction

Agent	Mechanism	Clinical Effect
Adjunctive therapies for AMI		
Aspirin	Antiplatelet	Improve survival Decrease reinfarction, CVA
Thienopyridines (clopidogrel, ticlopidine)	Antiplatelet	Recommended in aspirin-allergic patients Decrease death, MI, CVA in NSTE ACS
Glycoprotein IIb/IIIa inhibitors	Antiplatelet	Decrease MI, ischemic complications following primary PCI Decrease death or MI in high-risk NSTE ACS
Unfractionated heparin	Antithrombin	Decrease death and MI in prefibrinolytic era
Low molecular weight heparins	Antithrombin	Reduce cardiac events in NSTE ACS versus unfractionated heparin
Direct thrombin inhibitors	Antithrombin	Recommended in heparin-induced thrombocytopenia
Beta-brockers	Decrease myocardial oxygen demand (↓HR, ↓BP)	Improve survival Reduce infract size, ventricular arrhythmias, recurrent ischemia
Adjunctive therapies for AMI		
ACE Inhibitors	Vasodilator (BP) Prevent LV remodeling	Improve survival Decrease heart failure. LV dysfunction
IV nitroglycerine	Venous, arterial, coronary vasodilator (↓BP, ↓preload)	No effect on survival Decrease recurrent ischemia
HMG CoA Reductase Inhibitors	Lipid lowering Anti-inflammatory	Decrease future CV death and MI May decrease early ischemic events
Magnesium	Myocardial protective Anti-arrhythmic	Therapy for torsades depointes May improve reperfusion outcomes
Calcium-channel blocker	Decrease myocardial oxygen demand (↓HR, ↓BP)	No survival benefit Possible use in beta-blocker–intolerant patients without CHF or LV dysfunction
Warfarin	Oral anticoagulant	Reduced embolic risk with atrial fibrilliation. LV thrombus or dysfunction
Glucose-insulin potassium infusion	Metabolic modulator	May improve intracellular myocardial energy stores and outcome

Abbreviations: ACS, acute coronary syndrome; BP, blood pressure; CHF, congestive heart failure; CV, cardiovascular; CVA, cerebrovascular accident; HR, heart rate; IV, intravenous; LV, left ventricular; MI, myocardial infarction; NSTE, non–ST-segment elevation; PCI, percutaneous coronary intervention.

Adapted from Sura AC. et al.

Table 6.

8. Conclusion

Although improvements in the management of patients who have STEMI have led to a decline in acute and long-term fatality rates, reperfusion and ancillary therapies remain underused. Several initiatives (eg. Get With the Guidelines in USA) are designed to improve adherence to guidelines and access to appropriate reperfusion therapies. To date, clinical advancement is judged on achieving and maintaining epicardial artery patency. New fibrinolytics and combination therapies will continue to evolve. There will be technological advances and improvement in operator skills for PCI. The ultimate goal for the management of STEMI remains unchanged: to open occluded arteries quickly in carefully screened patients and in a cost-effective manner.

9. References

[1] Rosamond W, Flegal K, Furie K, et al. Heart disease and stroke statistics--2008 update: a report from the American Heart Association Statistics Committee and Stroke Statistics Subcommittee. Circulation 2008; 117:e25.

[2] Lloyd-Jones D, Adams RJ, Brown TM, et al. Executive summary: heart disease and stroke statistics--2010 update: a report from the American Heart Association. Circulation 2010; 121:948.

[3] Towfighi A, Zheng L, Ovbiagele B. Sex-specific trends in midlife coronary heart disease risk and prevalence. Arch Intern Med 2009; 169:1762.

[4] Deedwania PC, Carbajal EV. Silent myocardial ischemia. A clinical perspective. Arch Intern Med 1991; 151:2373.

[5] Lopez AD, Mathers CD, Ezzati M, et al. Global and regional burden of disease and risk factors, 2001: systematic analysis of population health data. Lancet 2006; 367:1747.

[6] Yusuf S, Reddy S, Ounpuu S, Anand S. Global burden of cardiovascular diseases: part I: general considerations, the epidemiologic transition, risk factors, and impact of urbanization. Circulation 2001; 104:2746.

[7] Goyal A, Yusuf S. The burden of cardiovascular disease in the Indian subcontinent. Indian J Med Res 2006; 124:235.

[8] Critchley J, Liu J, Zhao D, et al. Explaining the increase in coronary heart disease mortality in Beijing between 1984 and 1999. Circulation 2004; 110:1236.

[9] Rodríguez T, Malvezzi M, Chatenoud L, et al. Trends in mortality from coronary heart and cerebrovascular diseases in the Americas: 1970-2000. Heart 2006; 92:453.

[10] Beaglehole R, Reddy S, Leeder SR. Poverty and human development: the global implications of cardiovascular disease. Circulation 2007; 116:1871.

[11] Kloner RA, Jennings RB: Consequences of brief ischemia: Stunning, preconditioning, and their clinical implications: Part 1. *Circulation* 2001; 104:2981.

[12] Downey JM, Cohen MV: Reducing infarct size in the setting of acute myocardial infarction. *Prog Cardiovasc Dis* 2006; 48:363.

[13] Alpert JS, Thygesen K, Antman E, Bassand JP. Myocardial infarction redefined--a consensus document of The Joint European Society of Cardiology/American College of Cardiology Committee for the redefinition of myocardial infarction. J Am Coll Cardiol 2000; 36:959.

[14] Thygesen K, Alpert JS, White HD, Joint ESC/ACCF/AHA/WHF Task Force for the Redefinition of Myocardial Infarction. Universal definition of myocardial infarction. Eur Heart J 2007; 28:2525.

Part 2

Diagnostics of Ischemic Heart Disease

2

Cardiac Biomarkers

Sadip Pant[1], Abhishek Deshmukh[1], Pritam Neupane[2], M.P. Kavin Kumar[3] and C.S. Vijayashankar[4]
[1]*University of Arkansas For Medical Sciences, Little Rock, AR*
[2]*Medical College of Georgia, Augusta, GA*
[3]*Department of Internal Medicine, Priya Hospital-Heart and Diabetic Care Tamilnadu*
[4]*Apollo Hospitals Greams Road, Chennai, Tamilnadu*
[1,2]*USA*
[3,4]*India*

1. Introduction

1950's: Clinical reports that transaminases released from dying myocytes could be detected via laboratory testing, aiding in the diagnosis of myocardial infarction. The race to define clinical markers to aid in the diagnosis, prognosis, and risk stratification of patients with potential cardiovascular disease begins. Initial serum markers included AST, LDH, total CK and α-hydroxybutyrate. These enzymes are all released in varying amounts by dying myocytes. Lack of sensitivity and specificity for cardiac muscle necrosis fuels continued research.

1960's:CK known to be released during muscle necrosis (including cardiac).Quantitative assays were cumbersome and difficult to perform. Total CK designed as a fast, reproducible spectrophotometric assay in the late 1960's.CK isoenzymes are subsequently described: MM, MB and BB fractions.

In 1970's MB fraction noted to be elevated in and highly specific for acute MI.

CKMB now measured via a highly sensitive monoclonal antibody assay. It was felt for a time that quantitative CKMB determination could be used to enzymatically measure the size of an infarct. This has been complicated by release of additional enzymes during reperfusion. As CK-MB assays become more sensitive, researchers come to the paradoxical realization that it too is not totally cardiac specific. The MB fraction is determined to be expressed in skeletal muscle, particularly during the process of muscle regeneration and the search for cardiac specificity continues.

Research turns towards isolation of and development of assays for sarcomeric proteins. Myosin light chains were originally isolated and then subsequently abandoned because of specificity issues. Troponin I first described as a biomarker specific for AMI in 1987; Troponin T in 1989. Now troponins are the biochemical "gold standard" for the diagnosis of acute myocardial infarction via consensus of ESC/ACC.

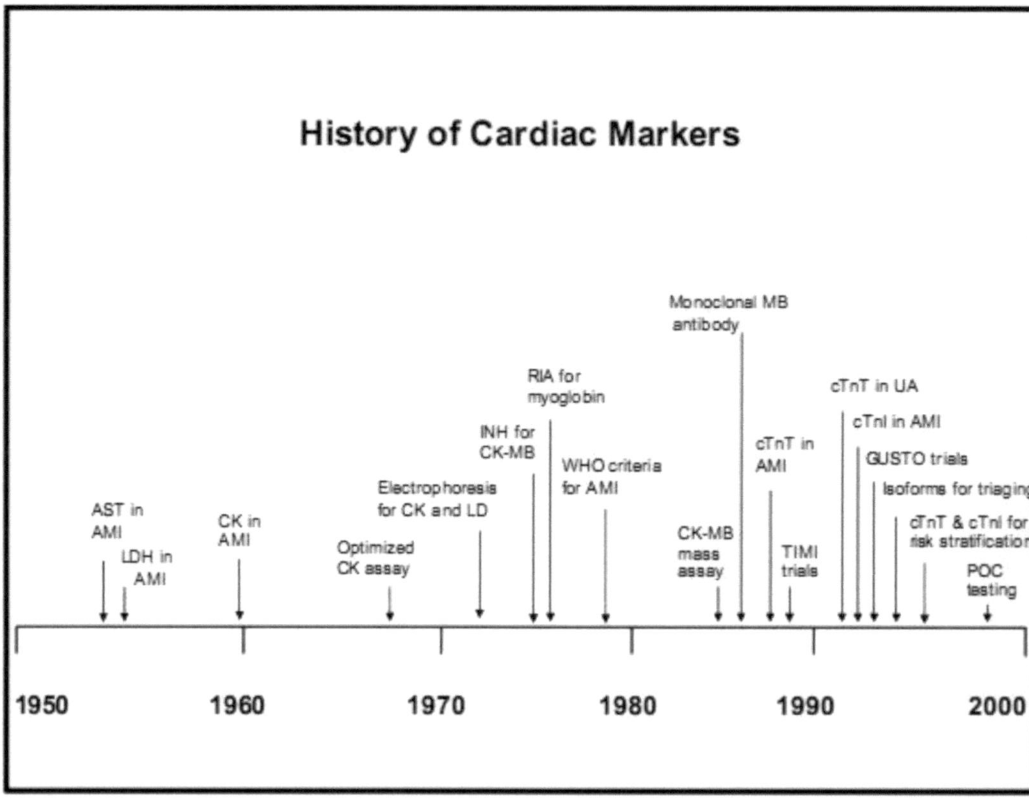

Fig. 1. Timeline showing landmark events in the development of cardiac biomarkers

1.1 Cardiac Markers: What are we looking at?

A biomarker is defined as a measurable substance or parameter that is an indicator of an underlying biological or pathological process. Therefore, depending on the underlying process that we are referring to, the cardiac markers can be classified as markers of necrosis, markers of ischemia and markers of inflammation. The features of an ideal cardiac marker would be:

- High sensitivity and specificity
- Rise and fall rapidly after ischemia
- Able to perform reliably and uniformly
- Be simple to perform
- Have turnaround time <60 min
- Not influenced by functioning of other organs, in particular, functioning of kidney.

Therefore, cardiac marker is an umbrella term which is used to define present day used necrosis markers as well as all the upstream markers of necrosis studied/under study including proinflammatory cytokines, cellular adhesion molecules, acute phase reactants, plaque destabilization biomarkers, plaque rupture biomarker and prenecrosis ischemia biomarkers. This can be simply visualized with the help of following flow diagram:

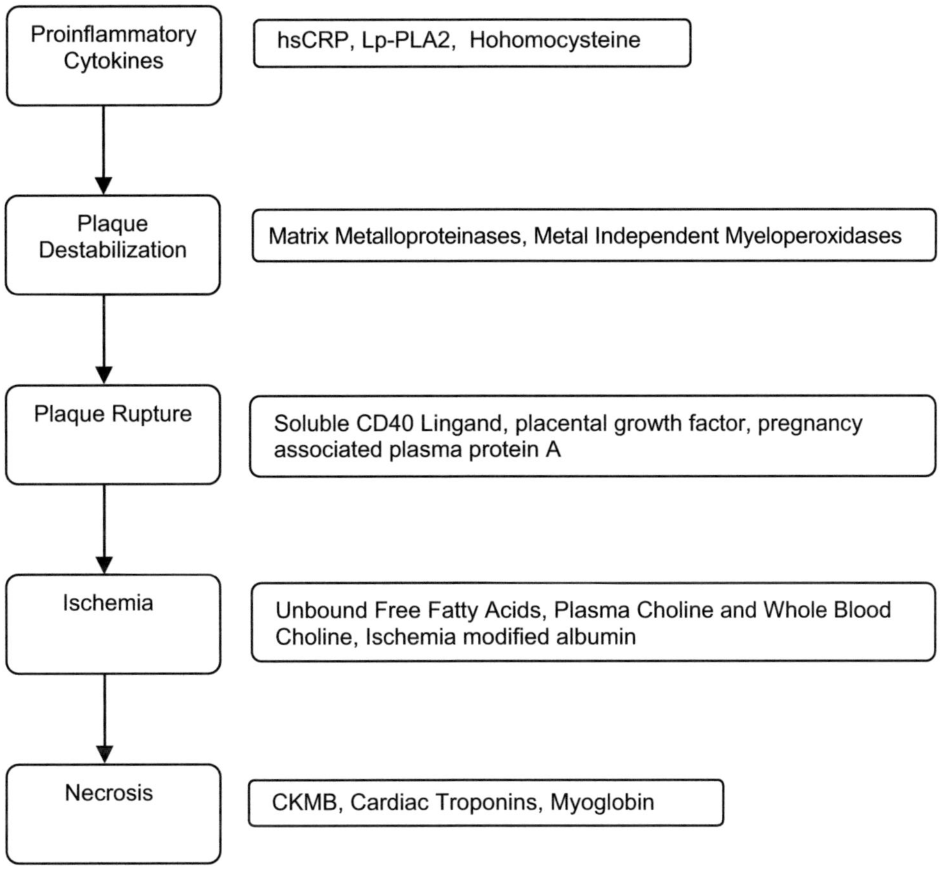

Fig. 2. Flowchart showing significance of biomarkers at various levels in the pathogenesis of acute coronary syndrome

1.2 Markers of cardiac necrosis

Cardiac markers are used in the diagnosis and risk stratification of patients with chest pain and suspected acute coronary syndrome (ACS). The cardiac troponins, in particular, have become the cardiac markers of choice for patients with ACS. Indeed, cardiac troponin is central to the definition of acute myocardial infarction (MI) in the consensus guidelines from the American College of Cardiology (ACC) and the European Society of Cardiology.

Older Definition of Myocardial Infarction- WHO 1979

1. Definite acute myocardial infarction-Definite acute myocardial infarction is diagnosed in the presence of unequivocal EKG changes and/or unequivocal enzyme changes; the history may be typical or atypical.
2. Possible acute myocardial infarction-Possible acute myocardial infarction is diagnosed when serial, equivocal ECG changes persist more than 24 hours, with or without equivocal enzyme changes; the history may be typical or atypical.
3. Old myocardial infarction-Old myocardial infarction is usually diagnosed on an unequivocal ECG in the absence of a history or enzymatic signs of acute myocardial

infarction. If there are no residual ECG changes, the diagnosis may be based on earlier, typical ECGs or on the presence of prior unequivocal serum enzyme changes.

Redefinition of Myocardial Infarction- Joint Task Force of the European Society of Cardiology, American College of Cardiology Foundation, the American Heart Association, and the World Health Federation (ESC/ACCF/AHA/WHF) 2007

A typical rise and/or gradual fall (troponin) or more rapid rise and fall (CK-MB) of biochemical markers of myocardial necrosis, with at least one of the following is required:

- Ischemic symptoms
- Development of pathologic Q waves on the ECG
- ECG changes indicative of ischemia (ST segment elevation or depression)
- Imaging evidence of new loss of viable myocardium or a new regional wall motion abnormality.

In addition, pathologic findings (generally at autopsy) of an acute MI are accepted criteria.

Markers of cardiac necrosis have come a long way since 1950s. Some of the markers used in the past are no longer in use today. Current markers and those used in the past have been outlined in the table below. Those used in the past are not discussed separately further.

Current Cardiac Markers	Cardiac Markers of the Past
• CK-MB	• Total CK Activity
• Myoglobin	• Aspartate Aminotransferase Activity
• CKMB Isoforms	• Lactate Dehydrogenase Activity
• Troponin I and T	• LD1/LD2 Ratio

Table 1. Various present day and past cardiac biomarkers

2. Creatine kinase

The enzyme creatinine kinase (formerly referred to as creatinine phosphokinase) exists as three isoenzyme forms: CK-MM, CK- MB, and CK-BB. These isoenzymes are found in the cytosol and facilitate the egress of high energy phosphates into and out of mitochondria.

CK: Dimer composed of 2 monomers: M (43,000 Da) and B (44,500 Da)---- > CK BB or CK MB or CK MM
Role: Creatine + ATP <---> ADP + Phosphocreatine + Energy (muscular contraction)
CK BB : Increased in neurological diseases ; prostatectomy; digestive cancers
CK MB : Increased with AMI
CK MM :Increased in myopathy, hypothyroidism, polymyositis, rhabdomyolysis, muscle trauma, intensive exercise, AMI

Table 2. Isoenzymes of Creatinine Kinase

Distribution of CK: Creatine Kinase (CK) isoenzyme activity is distributed in a number of tissues. The percentage of CK-MB fraction found in the heart is higher than in most other tissues. However, sensitive radioimmunoassays are able to detect small amounts of B chain protein in skeletal muscle, and some muscles have been reported to contain up to 10 percent B chain protein. Most muscles have much more CK per gram than heart tissue .As a result, despite containing only a small percent of B chain protein, skeletal muscle breakdown can lead to absolute increases in CK-MB in the plasma. Therefore, skeletal muscle damage can confound the diagnosis of an MI, as CK-MB can be released. The following are examples:

- Myocardial injury after cardiopulmonary resuscitation
- Cardioversion
- Defibrillation
- Cardiac and non-cardiac surgical procedures
- Blunt chest trauma with possible cardiac contusion
- Cocaine abuse

Total CK, CK-MB and CK-MB to Total CK ratio: Since CK is widely distributed in tissues, elevations in total serum CK lack specificity for cardiac damage, which improves with measurement of the MB fraction. The normal range of CK also varies considerably; a twofold or greater increase in the CK concentration is required for diagnosis. This criterion can be problematic in older individuals who, because of their lower muscle mass, may have low baseline serum total CK and, during MI, may have elevated serum CK-MB with values of total CK that rise but remain within the normal range. For these reasons, total CK has not been used in the diagnosis of myocardial damage for years. CK-MB has high specificity for cardiac tissue and was the preferred marker of cardiac injury for many years. An elevated CK-MB is relatively specific for myocardial injury, particularly in patients with ischemic symptoms when skeletal muscle damage is not present. Assays for CK-MB can be performed easily and rapidly. Most assays measure CK-MB mass; such measurements are more sensitive than activity assays. The relative index calculated by the ratio of CK-MB (mass) to total CK can assist in differentiating false-positive elevations of CK-MB arising from skeletal muscle. A ratio of less than 3 is consistent with a skeletal muscle source, while ratios greater than 5 are indicative of a cardiac source. Ratios between 3 and 5 represent a gray zone. No definitive diagnosis can be established without serial determinations to detect a rise. Studies to evaluate the CK-MB relative index compared with the absolute CK-MB have revealed increase in specificity but with a loss of sensitivity. The CK-MB/CK relative index is useful if patients have only an MI or only skeletal muscle injury, but not if they have both. In the combined setting of acute MI and skeletal muscle injury (rhabdomyolysis, heavy exercise, polymyositis), the fall in sensitivity is significant. It is worth noting that the diagnosis of acute MI must not be based on an elevated relative index alone, because the relative index may be elevated in clinical settings when either the total CK or the CK-MB is within normal limits. The relative index is only clinically useful when both the total CK and the CK-MB levels are increased.

Timing of Release: Creatinine Kinase starts rising in the blood 4-6 hours after the onset of chest pain. It peaks at 10-24 hours and then returns to normal after 48-72 hours. Since CK levels return to baseline 48 to 72 hours after infarction, it can be used to detect reinfarction. New elevations that occur after normalization are indicative of recurrent injury, again with the caveats in regard to sensitivity and specificity indicated above. However, for these reasons, CK-MB cannot be used for late diagnosis.

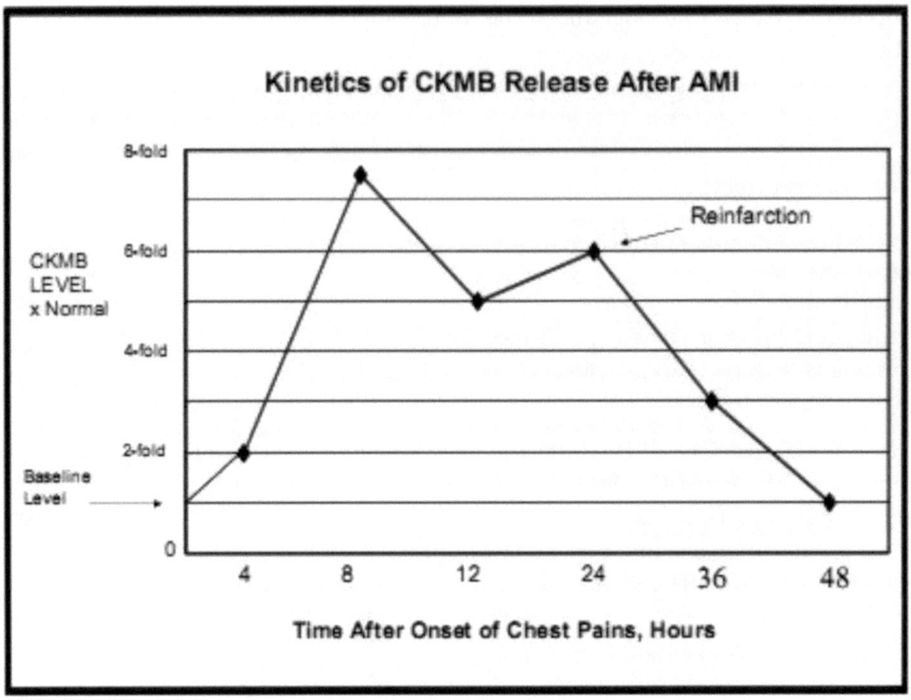

Fig. 3. Kinetics of CKMB release after AMI

Sensitivity and Specificity of CKMB: In AMI, CKMB usually is evident at 4 to 8 hours, peaks at 15 to 24 hours (mean peak=16×normal) with sensitivity and specificity >97% within the first 48 hours. By 72 hours, two thirds of patients still show some increase in CK-MB. Sampling every 6 hours is more likely to identify a peak value. False negative results may be caused by poor sample timing (e.g. only once in 24 hours or sampling <4 hours or >72 hours after AMI). Similarly, false positive may be caused by a variety of factors including but not limited to myocardial injury after cardiopulmonary resuscitation, cardioversion, defibrillation, cardiac and non-cardiac surgical procedures, blunt chest trauma with possible cardiac contusion and cocaine abuse.

CK and coronary reperfusion :The time to peak CK levels and the slope of CK-MB release can be used to assess whether reperfusion has occurred after fibrinolysis and, when used in conjunction with clinical variables, can predict whether TIMI 0 or 1 and TIMI 2 or 3 grade flow is present. The 2004 task force of the ACC/AHA concluded that serial measurements of CK-MB can be useful to provide supportive noninvasive evidence of reperfusion after fibrinolysis (class IIa recommendation). However, it should be noted that CK-MB criteria cannot identify the presence of TIMI 3 flow, which is the only level of perfusion associated with improved survival after fibrinolysis. Thus, many may elect invasive evaluation despite biomarker evidence of reperfusion. The 2004 ACC/AHA task force recommended specific guidelines for the diagnosis of reinfarction after an acute ST elevation MI. Within the first 18 hours of the initial MI, a recurrent elevation in CK-MB concentration alone should not be relied upon to diagnose reinfarction, but should be accompanied by recurrent ST segment elevation on ECG and at least one other supporting criterion (such as recurrent chest pain or hemodynamic decompensation). For patients more than 18 hours from the initial MI, a biomarker rise and at least one additional criterion is sufficient for the diagnosis. Similar criteria were established for patients presenting with possible reinfarction after percutaneous coronary intervention or coronary artery bypass grafting.

3. Cardiac Troponins

Cardiac Troponins (cTn) control the calcium-mediated interaction of actin and myosin. It exists in three isoforms: troponin C, troponin I and troponin T. Troponin C exists in all muscle tissues. cTnI is however, completely specific for the heart. cTnT released in small amounts by skeletal muscles, though clinical assays do not detect skeletal TnT. Both have cytosolic or early releasable and structural pools, with most existing in the structural pool. They are more specific compared to CKMB in detection of infarction and are the preferred biomarker for the diagnosis of acute MI (Class I recommendation from the ACC/AHA task force on diagnosis of AMI).

Characteristics	Troponin C	Troponin I	Troponin T
Weight	18 KD	26.5 KD	39 KD
Function	Calcium binding subunit	Actomyosin-ATP-inhibiting subunit	Anchors troponin complex to the tropomyosin strand
Cardiac Specificity	None	Yes	Yes

Table 3. Troponin Characteristics. KD: Kilo Dalton

3.1 Timing of release

Cardiac troponins begin rising in the blood 4-6 hours post infarction (same time as CKMB). It peaks in 12-24 hours but may take weeks to return to normal. The timing of release, peak and normal return as compared to CKMB has been presented in a graphical form below.

3.2 Sensitivity and specificity of cardiac troponins

Cardiac troponins are as sensitive as CK-MB during the first 48 hours after acute myocardial infarction. The sensitivity is 33% from 0-2 hours, 50% from 2-4 hours, 75% from 4-8 hours and approaching 100% from 8 hours after onset of chest pain. The specificity is close to 100%. Troponin elevations have been reported in a variety of clinical scenarios other than acute coronary syndromes. The following is a list of some of the causes for the elevation of troponin in the absence of a thrombotic occlusion of the coronary artery:

- Tachy- or bradyarrhythmias, or heart block
- Critically ill patients, especially with diabetes, respiratory failure or sepsis
- Hypertrophic cardiomyopathy
- Coronary vasospasm
- Acute neurological disease, including stroke or subarachnoid hemorrhage

- Cardiac contusion or other trauma including surgery, ablation, pacing, implantable cardioverter-defibrillator shocks, cardioversion, endomyocardial biopsy, cardiac surgery, following interventional closure of atrial septal defects
- Rhabdomyolysis with cardiac injury
- Congestive heart failure - acute and chronic
- Pulmonary embolism, severe pulmonary hypertension
- Renal failure
- Aortic dissection
- Aortic valve disease
- Apical ballooning syndrome - Takotsubo Cardiomyopathy
- Infiltrative diseases (ie, amyloidosis, hemochromatosis, sarcoidosis, and scleroderma)
- Inflammatory diseases (ie, myocarditis or myocardial extension of endo-/pericarditis, Kawasaki disease)
- Drug toxicity or toxins (ie, adriamycin, 5-flurouracil, herceptin, snake venom)
- Burns, especially if affecting >25 percent of body surface area
- Extreme exertion
- Transplant vasculopathy

The 2007 joint ESC/ACCF/AHA/WHF task force recommends that an elevated value of cardiac troponin, in the absence of clinical evidence of ischemia, should prompt a search for other causes of myocardial necrosis as listed above.

3.3 Troponin assays

The skeletal and cardiac isoforms of troponin T and troponin I are distinct, and skeletal isoforms are not detected by the monoclonal antibody-based assays currently in use. This specificity for cardiac isoforms is the basis for the clinical utility of cTnT and cTnI assays. Contemporary troponin assays are quite sensitive and can detect very small amounts of myocardial necrosis (<1 g). Troponin C is not used clinically because both cardiac and smooth muscle share troponin C isoforms. The ESC/ACC recommended that the diagnosis of MI be based on troponin levels in excess of the 99th percentile of a reference control group. As cTnT and cTnI levels are undetectable in most normal subjects, the 99th percentile is very low (eg, 0.04 to 0.5 micrograms/L). However, most assays are imprecise at this low level, and so it has been recommended that the definition of MI be raised to that value at which a specific assay has a coefficient of variation of 10 percent or less. New guidelines embrace 99th percentile for two reasons. This level is also low (0.1 to 1.2 micrograms/L), but higher than the 99th percentile standard. Due to variations in assay precision and individual laboratory policies, the upper limit of normal varies between laboratories, but in all cases is above the 99th percentile.

3.4 Point-of-care assays

The National Academy of Clinical Biochemistry (NACB) recommendations specify that cardiac markers be available on an immediate basis 24 h/d, 7 d/wk, with a turnaround time of 1 hour. Point-of-care (POC) devices that provide rapid results should be considered in hospitals whose laboratories cannot meet these guidelines. POC assays for CK-MB, myoglobin, and the cardiac troponins TnI and TnT are available. Only qualitative TnT assays are available as POC tests, but both quantitative and qualitative POC TnI assays are currently marketed. In a multicenter trial, the time to positivity was significantly faster for the POC device than for the local laboratory (2.5 h vs 3.4 h).In another multicenter study, which evaluated the i-STAT POC TnI assay in comparison with the central laboratory in 2000 patients with suspected ACS, POC testing reduced the length of stay by approximately 25 minutes for patients who were discharged from the ED. The sensitivity of current POC assays coupled with the benefit of rapid turnaround time make the POC assays attractive clinical tools in the ED.

3.5 Prognostic value of cardiac troponins

In addition to its use in the diagnosis of MI, an elevated troponin level can identify patients at high risk for adverse cardiac events. Specifically, data from a meta-analysis indicated that an elevated troponin level in patients without ST-segment elevation is associated with a nearly 4-fold increase in the cardiac mortality rate. In patients without ST-segment elevation who were being considered for thrombolytic therapy, initial TnI levels on admission correlated with mortality at 6 weeks, but CK-MB levels were not predictive of adverse cardiac events and had no prognostic value. Other studies revealed that an elevated troponin level at baseline was an independent predictor of mortality, even in patients with chest pain and acute MI with ST-segment elevation who were eligible for reperfusion therapy. Finally, the TIMI IIIB, GUSTO IIa, GUSTO IV ACS, and FRISC trial all demonstrated a direct correlation between the level of TnI or TnT and the mortality rate and adverse cardiac event rate in ACS.

3.6 High Sensitive Troponin (hsTroponin)

High-sensitive assay is one which has a total imprecision of less than 10% at the 99th percentile and some would propose also being able to quantitate over 50% of normal values below that 99th percentile. High-sensitive cTn assays have two differentiating features from contemporary cTn assays: 1) detection of cTn in healthy persons and 2) a precise definition of what is "normal" (= the 99th percentile). Recent multicenter studies have shown that high-sensitive cTn assays improve the early diagnosis of acute myocardial infarction (AMI). To achieve the best clinical use, cTn has to be interpreted as a quantitative variable. Rising and/or falling levels differentiate acute from chronic cardiomyocyte necrosis. The term "troponin-positive" should therefore be avoided. "Detectable" levels will become the norm and have to be clearly differentiated from "elevated" levels. The differential diagnosis of a small amount of cardiomyocyte necrosis and therefore mild elevation of cTn is broad and includes acute and chronic cardiac disorders. The differential diagnosis of a large amount of cardiomyocyte necrosis and therefore substantial elevation of cTn is much smaller and largely restricted to AMI, myocarditis and Takotsubo cardiomyopathy. Two large prospective multicenter studies showed that sensitive and high-sensitive cTn assays have a higher diagnostic accuracy compared to contemporary cTn assays at presentation, in the diagnosis of AMI. Earlier "rule in" may reduce morbidity by allowing earlier revascularization, earlier transfer to the coronary care unit, and earlier initiation of evidence-based AMI treatment. Nonetheless, the improvement in sensitivity is at the expense of specificity. There is still considerable controversy in regard to how to use these assays to detect acute events such as AMI. Hence, at this time it has not been approved for clinical use and is yet in research phase.

4. Myoglobin

Myoglobin is a heme protein found in skeletal and cardiac muscle that has attracted considerable interest as an early marker of MI. Its low molecular weight accounts for its early release profile: myoglobin typically rises 2-4 hours after onset of infarction, peaks at 6-12 hours, and returns to normal within 24-36 hours. Rapid myoglobin assays are available, but overall, they have a lack of cardiospecificity. Serial sampling every 1-2 hours can increase the sensitivity and specificity; a rise of 25-40% over 1-2 hours is strongly suggestive of acute MI. However, in most studies, myoglobin only achieved 90% sensitivity for acute MI, so the negative predictive value of myoglobin is not high enough to exclude the diagnosis of acute MI. The original studies that evaluated myoglobin used the WHO definition of acute MI that was based on a CK-MB standard. With the adoption of a troponin standard for acute MI in the ACC/ESC definition, the sensitivity of myoglobin for acute MI is substantially reduced. This significantly diminishes its utility, and a number of studies have indicated that contemporary cardiac troponin assays render the use of myoglobin measurements unnecessary.

Conditions where myoglobin increases	**Conditions where myoglobin does not increase**
Acute myocardial infarction	Non cardiac chest pain
Vigorous exercise	Mild to moderate exercise
Open heart surgery	CHF without acute myocardial infarction
Rhabdomyolysis	Cardiac catheterization
Progressive muscular dystrophy	
Shock	
Renal Failure	

Table 4. Serum myoglobin in various clinical conditions

4.1 Timing of release, peak and return to baseline of various cardiac markers

CAD is highly prevalent in patients with CKD, making interpretation of cardiac markers important. Despite this, interpretation of elevated cardiac enzymes in patients with renal failure is often confusing at best. Elevations in serum troponin often observed in asymptomatic patients with chronic kidney disease. Even using the most conservative cutoff values, a disproportionate number of patients still have elevated troponins. The mechanism for this is unclear. In a 2002 study in *Circulation*, 733 asymptomatic patients with ESRD were evaluated. Using conservative cutoff values,

- 82% had elevated cTnT
- 6% had elevated cTnI

Of those 733 asymptomatic patients on HD, 2-year mortality rates were 52% in those with cTnI ≥0.1 μg/dL .These data have been corroborated in a number of smaller studies in similar populations. Serial measurements are helpful in the setting of possible ACS. cTnI appears to be much less likely to be associated with false positives in the CKD population than cTnT, making it the preferred biomarker in this setting.

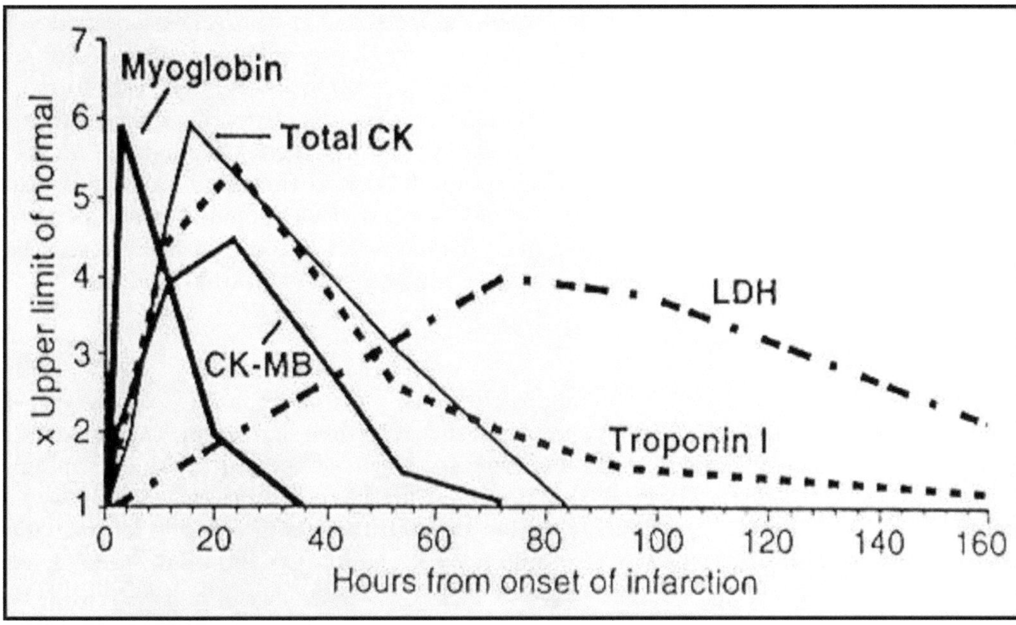

Fig. 4. A comparison of CKMB, cardiac troponins and myoglobin.

4.2 Markers of inflammation

Acute coronary syndromes are caused by vulnerable plaques. It is thought that one of the driving forces causing atheromatous plaques to rupture or erode, causing a cascade of events leading to coronary artery occlusion, is inflammation in the plaques. In this section cardiac inflammatory markers are dealt with which is at the verge of entering into clinical practice as tool for diagnosing and predicting future cardiovascular events at earlier stage and for risk stratification. Highly Sensitive Creative Protein (hsCRP), Myeloperoxidase (MPO), Matrix Metalloproteinases (MMP), Pregnancy Associated Protein A(PAPP-A),Placenta Growth Factor(PIGF) are reviewed.

4.3 C-Reactive protein (CRP)

C Reactive Protein is an acute phase reactant synthesized in liver and is elevated in inflammatory conditions. Once ligand-bound, CRP can activate the classical compliment pathway, stimulate phagocytosis and bind to immunoglobulin receptors. "High-sensitivity" only means that the concentration of CRP was determined using an assay designed to measure very low levels of CRP. The American Heart Association has defined risk groups as follows: Low risk: less than 1.0 mg/L, Average risk: 1.0 to 3.0 mg/L and High risk: above 3.0 mg/L. Two assays averaged fasting or non fasting, and optimally 2 weeks apart, provide a more stable estimate of level of this marker. If a level is greater than 10 mg/L is identified, there should be a search initiated for an obvious source of infection or inflammation, which could obscure any prediction of coronary risk that might be attributed to the elevated level. The landmark study by Liuzzo et al. showed that patients presenting with unstable angina and elevated plasma concentrations of CRP had a higher rate of death, MI and need for re-vascularisation compared with patients without elevated concentrations. In more recent trials, other investigators have confirmed the increased risk in ACS associated with higher CRP concentrations. In each of the above studies, the predictive value of CRP was independent of, and additive to, cardiac troponin. More importantly, CRP was found to have prognostic value even among patients with negative cardiac troponin and no evidence of myocyte necrosis. Methodological issues have however been highlighted and the independence between CRP and troponin release questioned. Therefore , although many studies have suggested that low-grade hsCRP elevations are independently associated with coronary risk, more complete evidence is needed to validate the use of hs-CRP as a risk assessment tool in general practice and as a target for therapy in individual patients .

4.4 Myeloperoxidase (MPO)

Myeloperoxidase (MPO) is a hemoprotein that is abundantly expressed in polymorphonuclear cells (neutrophils) and secreted during their activation. The presence of a peroxidase in the cytoplasmic granules of leukocytes was suggested at the beginning of 20th century but it was the early 1940s that it was purified for the first time. MPO plays an important role in neutrophil microbicidal action through catalyzing chloride ion oxidation to hypochlorous acid, which is a potent antimicrobial agent. On the other hand, it was demonstrated that MPO causes oxidative modification of low density lipoprotein (LDL) to a high uptake form that is considered to be a key event in the promotion of atherogenesis. Hence myeloperoxidase is believed to participate in the initiation and progression of cardiovascular diseases. MPO possesses potent proinflammatory properties and may contribute directly to tissue injury.

In a study consisted of patients diagnosed with ACS and other heart disease or unspecified chest pain, considerably higher MPO concentrations were demonstrated in the troponin-negative ACS patients on admission who became troponin-positive after 6h. This suggests that level of MPO possessed remarkably higher sensitivity than assessment of cTnI alone in all patients with ACS. MPO levels are associated with the presence of angiographically proven coronary atherosclerosis. In addition to clinical history and other tools MPO has been approved by FDA as cardiac biomarker to evaluate the patients with chest pain and at high risk for coronary artery disease.

4.5 Matrix metalloproteinases (MMP)

MMP are endogenous zinc dependent endopeptidases required for structural integrity of extracellular matrix of myocardium. TIMP (Tissue Inhibitors of Metalloproteinases) regulates MMP. MMPs may degrade myocardial ECM leading to the development of LV dilatation and heart failure and their inhibition in experimental models of AMI has been associated with reduced LV dilatation and wall stress. In a study of patients with acute myocardial infarction, TIMP-1 and MMP-9 correlated with echocardiographic parameters of LV dysfunction and remodelling after AMI and identified patients at risk of subsequent LV remodeling and associated with severe extensive CAD.

4.6 Placental Growth Factors (PGF)

Placental Growth Factor is a member of VEGF (vascular endothelial growth factor) subfamily - a key molecule in angiogenesis and vasculogenesis, in particular during the embryogenesis. Placental growth factor expression within human atherosclerotic lesions is associated with plaque inflammation and neovascular growth. Recent studies established the role of different inflammatory markers such as hsCRP, sr amyloid A, IL-6 not only gets elevated during acute coronary syndrome (ACS) but predicts its adverse outcomes. PGF was recently shown that it is upregulated in all forms of atherosclerotic lesions. PGIF induces the following

- Vascular smooth muscle cell growth.
- Recruits macrophages into atherosclerotic lesions.
- Upregulates production of TNF alpha.
- Monocyte chemotactic protein 1 by macrophages.
- Pathological angiogenesis.

Plasma PIGF levels may be an independent inflammatory biomarker of poor outcome in patients with suspected ACS. A single initial measurement of plasma PIGF appears to extend the predictive and prognostic information gained from traditional inflammatory markers.

5. Pregnancy associated plasma protein alpha (PAPP-A)

PAPP-A was originally identified in the serum of pregnant women. PAPP-A is produced by placental tissue. Circulating PAPP-A levels increase during pregnancy and they are used in the fetal diagnosis of Down syndrome. Only recently has PAPP-A been identified in nonplacental tissues. The concentrations in the sera of nonpregnant human beings being several orders of magnitude lower than during pregnancy. The physiological role of PAPP-A is only beginning to be unraveled. PAPP-A is a high-molecular-weight, zinc-binding metalloproteinase, which acts as a specific protease of IGF binding protein-4 (IGFBP-4). There is histological evidence, using specific monoclonal antibodies, that PAPP-A is abundantly expressed in both eroded and ruptured coronary plaques, but not in stable plaques, in patients who have died suddenly of cardiac causes. Furthermore, accumulating evidence suggests that PAPP-A may play a pivotal role in the development of atherosclerosis and subsequent plaque instability in ACS patients. PAPP-A is markedly elevated in the earliest hours after the onset of symptoms in patients with STEMIs treated with heparin and primary percutaneous coronary intervention, and in animal studies, heparin administration is associated with a significant increase in PAPP-A levels, presumably because of the detachment of PAPP-A from the vessel wall. If future studies confirm that concomitant heparin administration also increases PAPP-A levels in humans, the prognostic role of PAPP-A in patients with ST elevation myocardial infarction needs to be reevaluated.

5.1 Markers of ischemia

An ideal marker is one in which there is a specific easily measurable increase that clearly aligns with a predictable outcome be it evidence of ischemia, inflammation, myocardial necrosis, plaque rupture, plaque destabilization, or heart failure. Because of the underlying shared etiologies related to the process of arteriosclerosis and the complexity of the pathological processes giving rise to adverse thrombotic outcomes, a single marker that relates to each stage is unlikely. Rather more probable would be use of multiple markers with varying decision levels to either rule-in or rule-out a clinical decision. As the understanding of the niceties between ACS, inflammation, and coronary artery process develops, the ongoing search for better cardiac markers will continue.

5.2 Ischemia modified albumin (IMA)

The only ischemia marker that has been approved by the FDA is the modified albumin (IMA) using the albumin cobalt binding test (ACB) for assessment of myocardial ischemia. IMA occurs in 2 forms: 1.in which human serum albumin (HAS) binds mostly copper and 2.in which the damage to the N-terminus prevents metal binding. Patients without ischemia have more available metal binding sites on their HSA, than those from ischemic patients. This alteration is most likely due to damage caused by oxidative free radicals prevalent during ischemic events, and resulting in altered binding of trace metals resulting in IMA. As mentioned earlier, the FDA approved method for IMA (ACB Test by Ischemia Technologies) uses cobalt in its assay. Normal HSA will bind cobalt when it is added to a sample, leaving little residual cobalt. However, IMA cannot do the same due to its altered binding site. Patients having transient ischemic episodes without parallel myocyte death increases IMA which causes less cobalt binding and more residual unbound cobalt available. This can complex with chromogen (dithiothreitol) which can be measured photometrically. It is estimated that approximately 1% to 2% of the total albumin concentration in the normal population is IMA compared to 6% to 8% in patients experiencing ischemia. The clinical utility of IMA appears to be in its negative predictive value for ischemia and ACS, particularly when used in conjunction with other tests. While the optimum cutoff for IMA for ruling out ACS is 85kU/L, the manufacturer has suggested a higher value of 100 kU/L for risk stratification. Some of the limitations to be taken into consideration includes: a. there is an overlap between the normal population and that of individuals with cardiac ischemia; b. IMA is not specific for cardiac ischemia; c. false positive can occur in patients with cirrhosis, bacterial and viral infections, advanced cancers, stroke and end-stage renal disease and d. interpretation of IMA in certain populations, including those with peripheral vascular disease and in marathon runners is not yet clear. Hence IMA appears at this time as a potential marker in certain clinical situations but a number of possible interferences may limit its utility in patients with suspected ACS.

5.3 Unbound free fatty acids

Fatty acids are essential building blocks for many lipid molecules and are energy stores that can be utilized during times of fasting or increased metabolic demand. Fatty acids exist in body as esterified form (bound to glycerol or other alcohol), non-esterified form bound to albumin, and to a much smaller extent, as an unbound soluble form. Evidence exists that unbound free fatty acids increase significantly in ischemic-related events. It is not certain as of today what role the unbound free fatty acid plays in cardiac disease. It possibly partakes in the developing necrotic process and is released as a result of cell rupture or other precipitating conditions. Currently, a fluorescent probe assay is available but its clinical utility at this time is not established.

5.4 Fatty acid binding proteins (FABPs)

Fatty acid binding proteins (FABPs) are transport proteins that carry fatty acids and other lipophilic molecules like eicosanoids and retinoids across the membranes. They occur in nine different isoforms in a predictable tissue distribution and fairly long half-life of several days. The heart-type FABP (H-FABP) is released following myocardial death within 6 hours and is not specific to the heart, similar to myoglobin. It is released to a smaller extent in skeletal muscle, distal tubular cells of the kidney, specific parts of the brain, lactating mammary glands, and the placenta. It has been found that H-FABP may perform better and reach its upper reference limit sooner than either myoglobin or troponin. A number of enzyme immunoassays are available for H-FABP testing. Its relation to ischemia and prognosis for adverse events is likely to expound in near future.

5.5 Phospholipase

Phospholipase are the enzymes that release fatty acids from the second carbon group of glycerol. They are grouped into 4 major categories: A to D. Phospholipase A2 and D have drawn much attention in their role in assessing ischemia associated coronary artery disease. Lipoprotein-associated phospholipase A_2 (Lp-PLA$_2$) also known as platelet-activating factor acetylhydrolase (PAF-AH) is a phospholipase A2 enzyme that in humans is encoded by the *PLA2G7* gene. In human atherosclerotic lesions, 2 main sources of Lp-PLA$_2$ can be identified, including that which is brought into the intima bound to LDL (from the circulation), and that which is synthesized de novo by plaque inflammatory cells (macrophages, T cells, mast cells). I A meta-analysis involving a total of 79,036 participants in 32 prospective studies found that Lp-PLA$_2$ levels are positively correlated with increased risk of developing coronary heart disease and stroke. Recently, there has been a renewed interest in this molecule, not for use in cardiac assessment as it was originally approved by the FDA, but rather in stroke prediction after it was found that elevated levels of Lp-PLA2 were associated with an almost 2-fold increase in stroke in the selected population coupled with a 6-fold increase in hypertensive individuals.

Phospholipase D (PLD) is an enzyme that catalyzes the hydrolysis of membrane bound phospholipids into phosphatidic acid and choline. In addition, it is also involved in endorsement of fibrinogen binding to platelets. Increased levels of plasma (PLCHO) and whole blood choline (WBCHO) levels have been seen in tissue ischemia in patients with negative troponin values. Choline is not a marker for myocardial necrosis but indicated high-risk unstable angina in patients without acute myocardial infarction (sensitivity 86.4%, specificity 86.2%). Therefore obtaining levels of both plasma PLCHO and WBCHO may prove to be a useful aid in patients suspected of ACS.

6. Conclusion

Cardiac markers have been implicated in the diagnosis and risk stratification of patients with chest pain and suspected acute coronary syndrome (ACS). Among the markers of cardiac necrosis, troponins have become the cardiac markers of choice for patients with ACS. In fact, cardiac troponin has become central to the definition of acute myocardial infarction (MI) in the consensus guidelines from the American College of Cardiology (ACC) and the European Society of Cardiology (ESC). Current focus is on finding appropriate upstream markers which may aid in detection of myocardial ischemia and a variety of events involved in the process of pathophysiology of acute coronary syndrome especially in relation to plaque destabilization and rupture. The ideal biomarkers that offer early detection, risk stratification, selection of therapy, monitoring disease progression, and treatment efficacy remain to be elucidated.

7. References

[1] Jaffe AS, Ravkilde J, Roberts R, et al. It's time for a change to a troponin standard. Circulation 2000; 102:1216.

[2] Shave R, George KP, Atkinson G, et al. Exercise-induced cardiac troponin T release: a meta-analysis. Med Sci Sports Exerc 2007; 39:2099.

[3] Gupta S, de Lemos JA. Use and misuse of cardiac troponins in clinical practice. Prog Cardiovasc Dis 2007; 50:151.

[4] Müller-Bardorff M, Weidtmann B, Giannitsis E, et al. Release kinetics of cardiac troponin T in survivors of confirmed severe pulmonary embolism. Clin Chem 2002; 48:673.

[5] Carlson RJ, Navone A, McConnell JP, et al. Effect of myocardial ischemia on cardiac troponin I and T. Am J Cardiol 2002; 89:224.

[6] Sabatine MS, Morrow DA, de Lemos JA, et al. Detection of acute changes in circulating troponin in the setting of transient stress test-induced myocardial ischaemia using an ultrasensitive assay: results from TIMI 35. Eur Heart J 2009; 30:162.

[7] Kurz K, Giannitsis E, Zehelein J, Katus HA. Highly sensitive cardiac troponin T values remain constant after brief exercise- or pharmacologic-induced reversible myocardial ischemia. Clin Chem 2008; 54:1234.

[8] Adams JE 3rd, Abendschein DR, Jaffe AS. Biochemical markers of myocardial injury. Is MB creatine kinase the choice for the 1990s? Circulation 1993; 88:750.

[9] Katus HA, Remppis A, Scheffold T, et al. Intracellular compartmentation of cardiac troponin T and its release kinetics in patients with reperfused and nonreperfused myocardial infarction. Am J Cardiol 1991; 67:1360.

[10] Adams JE 3rd, Schechtman KB, Landt Y, et al. Comparable detection of acute myocardial infarction by creatine kinase MB isoenzyme and cardiac troponin I. Clin Chem 1994; 40:1291.

[11] Adams JE III, Bodor, GS, Davila-Roman, VG, et al. Cardiac troponin I. A marker with high specificity for cardiac injury. Circulation 1993; 88:101.

[12] Bodor GS, Porterfield D, Voss EM, et al. Cardiac troponin-I is not expressed in fetal and healthy or diseased adult human skeletal muscle tissue. Clin Chem 1995; 41:1710.

[13] Ricchiuti V, Voss EM, Ney A, et al. Cardiac troponin T isoforms expressed in renal diseased skeletal muscle will not cause false-positive results by the second generation cardiac troponin T assay by Boehringer Mannheim. Clin Chem 1998; 44:1919.

[14] Panteghini M, Pagani F, Yeo KT, et al. Evaluation of imprecision for cardiac troponin assays at low-range concentrations. Clin Chem 2004; 50:327.

[15] Apple FS, Quist HE, Doyle PJ, et al. Plasma 99th percentile reference limits for cardiac troponin and creatine kinase MB mass for use with European Society of Cardiology/American College of Cardiology consensus recommendations. Clin Chem 2003; 49:1331.
[16] Shi Q, Ling M, Zhang X, et al. Degradation of cardiac troponin I in serum complicates comparisons of cardiac troponin I assays. Clin Chem 1999; 45:1018.
[17] Labugger R, Organ L, Collier C, et al. Extensive troponin I and T modification detected in serum from patients with acute myocardial infarction. Circulation 2000; 102:1221.
[18] Heeschen C, Goldmann BU, Langenbrink L, et al. Evaluation of a rapid whole blood ELISA for quantification of troponin I in patients with acute chest pain. Clin Chem 1999; 45:1789.
[19] Katrukha AG, Bereznikova AV, Esakova TV, et al. Troponin I is released in bloodstream of patients with acute myocardial infarction not in free form but as complex. Clin Chem 1997; 43:1379.
[20] Wu AH, Feng YJ, Moore R, et al. Characterization of cardiac troponin subunit release into serum after acute myocardial infarction and comparison of assays for troponin T and I. American Association for Clinical Chemistry Subcommittee on cTnI Standardization. Clin Chem 1998; 44:1198.
[21] Thygesen K, Alpert JS, White HD, Joint ESC/ACCF/AHA/WHF Task Force for the Redefinition of Myocardial Infarction. Universal definition of myocardial infarction. Eur Heart J 2007; 28:2525.
[22] Panteghini M, Gerhardt W, Apple FS, et al. Quality specifications for cardiac troponin assays. Clin Chem Lab Med 2001; 39:175.
[23] Lee TH, Thomas EJ, Ludwig LE, et al. Troponin T as a marker for myocardial ischemia in patients undergoing major noncardiac surgery. Am J Cardiol 1996; 77:1031.
[24] Baum H, Braun S, Gerhardt W, et al. Multicenter evaluation of a second-generation assay for cardiac troponin T. Clin Chem 1997; 43:1877.
[25] Apple FS, Parvin CA, Buechler KF, et al. Validation of the 99th percentile cutoff independent of assay imprecision (CV) for cardiac troponin monitoring for ruling out myocardial infarction. Clin Chem 2005; 51:2198.
[26] Wu AH, Jaffe AS. The clinical need for high-sensitivity cardiac troponin assays for acute coronary syndromes and the role for serial testing. Am Heart J 2008; 155:208.
[27] Zethelius B, Johnston N, Venge P. Troponin I as a predictor of coronary heart disease and mortality in 70-year-old men: a community-based cohort study. Circulation 2006; 113:1071.
[28] Kavsak PA, Newman AM, Lustig V, et al. Long-term health outcomes associated with detectable troponin I concentrations. Clin Chem 2007; 53:220.
[29] Waxman DA, Hecht S, Schappert J, Husk G. A model for troponin I as a quantitative predictor of in-hospital mortality. J Am Coll Cardiol 2006; 48:1755.
[30] Schulz O, Kirpal K, Stein J, et al. Importance of low concentrations of cardiac troponins. Clin Chem 2006; 52:1614.

[31] Wu AH, Fukushima N, Puskas R, et al. Development and preliminary clinical validation of a high sensitivity assay for cardiac troponin using a capillary flow (single molecule) fluorescence detector. Clin Chem 2006; 52:2157.
[32] Kavsak PA, MacRae AR, Yerna MJ, Jaffe AS. Analytic and clinical utility of a next-generation, highly sensitive cardiac troponin I assay for early detection of myocardial injury. Clin Chem 2009; 55:573.
[33] Wilson SR, Sabatine MS, Braunwald E, et al. Detection of myocardial injury in patients with unstable angina using a novel nanoparticle cardiac troponin I assay: observations from the PROTECT-TIMI 30 Trial. Am Heart J 2009; 158:386.
[34] Venge P, Johnston N, Lindahl B, James S. Normal plasma levels of cardiac troponin I measured by the high-sensitivity cardiac troponin I access prototype assay and the impact on the diagnosis of myocardial ischemia. J Am Coll Cardiol 2009; 54:1165.
[35] Giannitsis E, Kurz K, Hallermayer K, et al. Analytical validation of a high-sensitivity cardiac troponin T assay. Clin Chem 2010; 56:254.
[36] Latini R, Masson S, Anand IS, et al. Prognostic value of very low plasma concentrations of troponin T in patients with stable chronic heart failure. Circulation 2007; 116:1242.
[37] Januzzi JL Jr, Bamberg F, Lee H, et al. High-sensitivity troponin T concentrations in acute chest pain patients evaluated with cardiac computed tomography. Circulation 2010; 121:1227.
[38] Diamond GA, Kaul S. How would the Reverend Bayes interpret high-sensitivity troponin? Circulation 2010; 121:1172.
[39] Kavsak PA, Wang X, Ko DT, et al. Short- and long-term risk stratification using a next-generation, high-sensitivity research cardiac troponin I (hs-cTnI) assay in an emergency department chest pain population. Clin Chem 2009; 55:1809.
[40] Derdeyn CP. Moyamoya disease and moyamoya syndrome. N Engl J Med 2009; 361:97; author reply 98.
[41] de Lemos JA, Drazner MH, Omland T, et al. Association of troponin T detected with a highly sensitive assay and cardiac structure and mortality risk in the general population. JAMA 2010; 304:2503.
[42] deFilippi CR, de Lemos JA, Christenson RH, et al. Association of serial measures of cardiac troponin T using a sensitive assay with incident heart failure and cardiovascular mortality in older adults. JAMA 2010; 304:2494.
[43] Katus HA, Giannitsis E, Jaffe AS, Thygesen K. Higher sensitivity troponin assays: Quo vadis? Eur Heart J 2009; 30:127.
[44] Wallace TW, Abdullah SM, Drazner MH, et al. Prevalence and determinants of troponin T elevation in the general population. Circulation 2006; 113:1958.
[45] Daniels LB, Laughlin GA, Clopton P, et al. Minimally elevated cardiac troponin T and elevated N-terminal pro-B-type natriuretic peptide predict mortality in older adults: results from the Rancho Bernardo Study. J Am Coll Cardiol 2008; 52:450.
[46] Jaffe AS. Chasing troponin: how low can you go if you can see the rise? J Am Coll Cardiol 2006; 48:1763.

[47] Mills NL, Churchhouse AM, Lee KK, et al. Implementation of a sensitive troponin I assay and risk of recurrent myocardial infarction and death in patients with suspected acute coronary syndrome. JAMA 2011; 305:1210.
[48] Saenger AK, Jaffe AS. Requiem for a heavyweight: the demise of creatine kinase-MB. Circulation 2008; 118:2200.
[49] Antman, EM, Anbe, DT, Armstrong, PW, et al. ACC/AHA guidelines for the management of patients with ST-elevation myocardial infarction. www.acc.org/qualityandscience/clinical/statements.htm (Accessed on August 24, 2006).
[50] Macrae AR, Kavsak PA, Lustig V, et al. Assessing the requirement for the 6-hour interval between specimens in the American Heart Association Classification of Myocardial Infarction in Epidemiology and Clinical Research Studies. Clin Chem 2006; 52:812.
[51] Eggers KM, Oldgren J, Nordenskjöld A, Lindahl B. Diagnostic value of serial measurement of cardiac markers in patients with chest pain: limited value of adding myoglobin to troponin I for exclusion of myocardial infarction. Am Heart J 2004; 148:574.
[52] Hollander JE, Levitt MA, Young GP, et al. Effect of recent cocaine use on the specificity of cardiac markers for diagnosis of acute myocardial infarction. Am Heart J 1998; 135:245.
[53] Reichlin T, Hochholzer W, Bassetti S, et al. Early diagnosis of myocardial infarction with sensitive cardiac troponin assays. N Engl J Med 2009; 361:858.
[54] Keller T, Zeller T, Peetz D, et al. Sensitive troponin I assay in early diagnosis of acute myocardial infarction. N Engl J Med 2009; 361:868.
[55] Jaffe, AS and Apple FS. High-sensitivity cardiac troponin: Hype, help, and reality. Clinical chemistry 2009; Dec 30. [E pub ahead of print].
[56] Antman, EM, Hand, M, Armstrong, PW, et al. 2007 focused update of the ACC/AHA 2004 Guidelines for the Management of Patients With ST-Elevation Myocardial Infarction: a report of the American College of Cardiology/American Heart Association Task Force on Practice Guidelines (Writing Group to Review New Evidence and Update the ACC/AHA 2004 Guidelines for the Management of Patients With ST-Elevation Myocardial Infarction). J Am Coll Cardiol 2008; 51:XXX. Available at: www.acc.org/qualityandscience/clinical/statements.htm (accessed September 18, 2007).
[57] deFilippi CR, Tocchi M, Parmar RJ, et al. Cardiac troponin T in chest pain unit patients without ischemic electrocardiographic changes: angiographic correlates and long-term clinical outcomes. J Am Coll Cardiol 2000; 35:1827.
[58] Ohman EM, Christenson RH, Califf RM, et al. Noninvasive detection of reperfusion after thrombolysis based on serum creatine kinase MB changes and clinical variables. TAMI 7 Study Group. Thrombolysis and Angioplasty in Myocardial Infarction. Am Heart J 1993; 126:819.
[59] Christenson RH, Ohman EM, Topol EJ, et al. Assessment of coronary reperfusion after thrombolysis with a model combining myoglobin, creatine kinase-MB, and clinical

variables. TAMI-7 Study Group. Thrombolysis and Angioplasty in Myocardial Infarction-7. Circulation 1997; 96:1776.

[60] Apple FS, Murakami MM. Cardiac troponin and creatine kinase MB monitoring during in-hospital myocardial reinfarction. Clin Chem 2005; 51:460.

[61] Babuin L, Vasile VC, Rio Perez JA, et al. Elevated cardiac troponin is an independent risk factor for short- and long-term mortality in medical intensive care unit patients. Crit Care Med 2008; 36:759.

[62] Allan JJ, Feld RD, Russell AA, et al. Cardiac troponin I levels are normal or minimally elevated after transthoracic cardioversion. J Am Coll Cardiol 1997; 30:1052.

[63] Licka M, Zimmermann R, Zehelein J, et al. Troponin T concentrations 72 hours after myocardial infarction as a serological estimate of infarct size. Heart 2002; 87:520.

[64] Panteghini M, Cuccia C, Bonetti G, et al. Single-point cardiac troponin T at coronary care unit discharge after myocardial infarction correlates with infarct size and ejection fraction. Clin Chem 2002; 48:1432.

[65] Steen H, Giannitsis E, Futterer S, et al. Cardiac troponin T at 96 hours after acute myocardial infarction correlates with infarct size and cardiac function. J Am Coll Cardiol 2006; 48:2192.

[66] Giannitsis E, Steen H, Kurz K, et al. Cardiac magnetic resonance imaging study for quantification of infarct size comparing directly serial versus single time-point measurements of cardiac troponin T. J Am Coll Cardiol 2008; 51:307.

[67] Vasile VC, Babuin L, Giannitsis E, et al. Relationship of MRI-determined infarct size and cTnI measurements in patients with ST-elevation myocardial infarction. Clin Chem 2008; 54:617.

[68] Olatidoye AG, Wu AH, Feng YJ, Waters D. Prognostic role of troponin T versus troponin I in unstable angina pectoris for cardiac events with meta-analysis comparing published studies. Am J Cardiol 1998; 81:1405.

[69] Heidenreich PA, Alloggiamento T, Melsop K, et al. The prognostic value of troponin in patients with non-ST elevation acute coronary syndromes: a meta-analysis. J Am Coll Cardiol 2001; 38:478.

[70] Heeschen C, Hamm CW, Goldmann B, et al. Troponin concentrations for stratification of patients with acute coronary syndromes in relation to therapeutic efficacy of tirofiban. PRISM Study Investigators. Platelet Receptor Inhibition in Ischemic Syndrome Management. Lancet 1999; 354:1757.

[71] James S, Armstrong P, Califf R, et al. Troponin T levels and risk of 30-day outcomes in patients with the acute coronary syndrome: prospective verification in the GUSTO-IV trial. Am J Med 2003; 115:178.

[72] Ohman EM, Armstrong PW, White HD, et al. Risk stratification with a point-of-care cardiac troponin T test in acute myocardial infarction. GUSTOIII Investigators. Global Use of Strategies To Open Occluded Coronary Arteries. Am J Cardiol 1999; 84:1281.

[73] Giannitsis E, Müller-Bardorff M, Lehrke S, et al. Admission troponin T level predicts clinical outcomes, TIMI flow, and myocardial tissue perfusion after primary percutaneous intervention for acute ST-segment elevation myocardial infarction. Circulation 2001; 104:630.

[74] Ottani F, Galvani M, Nicolini FA, et al. Elevated cardiac troponin levels predict the risk of adverse outcome in patients with acute coronary syndromes. Am Heart J 2000; 140:917.

[75] Morrow DA, Antman EM, Tanasijevic M, et al. Cardiac troponin I for stratification of early outcomes and the efficacy of enoxaparin in unstable angina: a TIMI-11B substudy. J Am Coll Cardiol 2000; 36:1812.

[76] Lindahl B, Venge P, Wallentin L. Relation between troponin T and the risk of subsequent cardiac events in unstable coronary artery disease. The FRISC study group. Circulation 1996; 93:1651.

[77] Antman EM, Tanasijevic MJ, Thompson B, et al. Cardiac-specific troponin I levels to predict the risk of mortality in patients with acute coronary syndromes. N Engl J Med 1996; 335:1342.

[78] Ohman EM, Armstrong PW, Christenson RH, et al. Cardiac troponin T levels for risk stratification in acute myocardial ischemia. GUSTO IIA Investigators. N Engl J Med 1996; 335:1333.

[79] Hamm CW, Goldmann BU, Heeschen C, et al. Emergency room triage of patients with acute chest pain by means of rapid testing for cardiac troponin T or troponin I. N Engl J Med 1997; 337:1648.

[80] Lindahl B, Diderholm E, Lagerqvist B, et al. Mechanisms behind the prognostic value of troponin T in unstable coronary artery disease: a FRISC II substudy. J Am Coll Cardiol 2001; 38:979.

[81] Heeschen C, Hamm CW, Bruemmer J, Simoons ML. Predictive value of C-reactive protein and troponin T in patients with unstable angina: a comparative analysis. CAPTURE Investigators. Chimeric c7E3 AntiPlatelet Therapy in Unstable angina REfractory to standard treatment trial. J Am Coll Cardiol 2000; 35:1535.

[82] Lindahl B, Toss H, Siegbahn A, et al. Markers of myocardial damage and inflammation in relation to long-term mortality in unstable coronary artery disease. FRISC Study Group. Fragmin during Instability in Coronary Artery Disease. N Engl J Med 2000; 343:1139.

[83] Antman EM, Cohen M, Bernink PJ, et al. The TIMI risk score for unstable angina/non-ST elevation MI: A method for prognostication and therapeutic decision making. JAMA 2000; 284:835.

[84] Morrow DA, Cannon CP, Rifai N, et al. Ability of minor elevations of troponins I and T to predict benefit from an early invasive strategy in patients with unstable angina and non-ST elevation myocardial infarction: results from a randomized trial. JAMA 2001; 286:2405.

[85] Kleiman NS, Lakkis N, Cannon CP, et al. Prospective analysis of creatine kinase muscle-brain fraction and comparison with troponin T to predict cardiac risk and benefit of an invasive strategy in patients with non-ST-elevation acute coronary syndromes. J Am Coll Cardiol 2002; 40:1044.

[86] Diderholm E, Andrén B, Frostfeldt G, et al. The prognostic and therapeutic implications of increased troponin T levels and ST depression in unstable coronary artery disease: the FRISC II invasive troponin T electrocardiogram substudy. Am Heart J 2002; 143:760.

[87] Heeschen C, van Den Brand MJ, Hamm CW, Simoons ML. Angiographic findings in patients with refractory unstable angina according to troponin T status. Circulation 1999; 100:1509.
[88] Martinez MW, Babuin L, Syed IS, et al. Myocardial infarction with normal coronary arteries: a role for MRI? Clin Chem 2007; 53:995.
[89] Christiansen JP, Edwards C, Sinclair T, et al. Detection of myocardial scar by contrast-enhanced cardiac magnetic resonance imaging in patients with troponin-positive chest pain and minimal angiographic coronary artery disease. Am J Cardiol 2006; 97:768.
[90] Dokainish H, Pillai M, Murphy SA, et al. Prognostic implications of elevated troponin in patients with suspected acute coronary syndrome but no critical epicardial coronary disease: a TACTICS-TIMI-18 substudy. J Am Coll Cardiol 2005; 45:19.
[91] James SK, Armstrong P, Barnathan E, et al. Troponin and C-reactive protein have different relations to subsequent mortality and myocardial infarction after acute coronary syndrome: a GUSTO-IV substudy. J Am Coll Cardiol 2003; 41:916.
[92] Kontos MC, Shah R, Fritz LM, et al. Implication of different cardiac troponin I levels for clinical outcomes and prognosis of acute chest pain patients. J Am Coll Cardiol 2004; 43:958.
[93] Mueller C, Neumann FJ, Perruchoud AP, et al. Prognostic value of quantitative troponin T measurements in unstable angina/non-ST-segment elevation acute myocardial infarction treated early and predominantly with percutaneous coronary intervention. Am J Med 2004; 117:897.
[94] Newby LK, Christenson RH, Ohman EM, et al. Value of serial troponin T measures for early and late risk stratification in patients with acute coronary syndromes. The GUSTO-IIa Investigators. Circulation 1998; 98:1853.
[95] Antman EM. Troponin measurements in ischemic heart disease: more than just a black and white picture. J Am Coll Cardiol 2001; 38:987.
[96] Bessman SP, Carpenter CL. The creatine-creatine phosphate energy shuttle. Annu Rev Biochem 1985; 54:831.
[97] Roberts R, Gowda KS, Ludbrook PA, Sobel BE. Specificity of elevated serum MB creatine phosphokinase activity in the diagnosis of acute myocardial infarction. Am J Cardiol 1975; 36:433.
[98] Tsung JS, Tsung SS. Creatine kinase isoenzymes in extracts of various human skeletal muscles. Clin Chem 1986; 32:1568.
[99] Neumeier, D. Tissue specific and subcellular distribution of creatine kinase isoenzymes. In: Creatine Kinase Isoenzymes, Lang, H (Ed), Springer-Verlag, Berlin/Heidelberg 1981. p.85.
[100] Trask RV, Billadello JJ. Tissue-specific distribution and developmental regulation of M and B creatine kinase mRNAs. Biochim Biophys Acta 1990; 1049:182.
[101] Fontanet HL, Trask RV, Haas RC, et al. Regulation of expression of M, B, and mitochondrial creatine kinase mRNAs in the left ventricle after pressure overload in rats. Circ Res 1991; 68:1007.
[102] Wolf PL. Abnormalities in serum enzymes in skeletal muscle diseases. Am J Clin Pathol 1991; 95:293.

[103] Siegel AJ, Silverman LM, Evans WJ. Elevated skeletal muscle creatine kinase MB isoenzyme levels in marathon runners. JAMA 1983; 250:2835.
[104] Clark GL, Robison AK, Gnepp DR, et al. Effects of lymphatic transport of enzyme on plasma creatine kinase time-activity curves after myocardial infarction in dogs. Circ Res 1978; 43:162.
[105] Vatner SF, Baig H, Manders WT, Maroko PR. Effects of coronary artery reperfusion on myocardial infarct size calculated from creatine kinase. J Clin Invest 1978; 61:1048.
[106] Dillon MC, Calbreath DF, Dixon AM, et al. Diagnostic problem in acute myocardial infarction: CK-MB in the absence of abnormally elevated total creatine kinase levels. Arch Intern Med 1982; 142:33.
[107] Heller GV, Blaustein AS, Wei JY. Implications of increased myocardial isoenzyme level in the presence of normal serum creatine kinase activity. Am J Cardiol 1983; 51:24.
[108] Yusuf S, Collins R, Lin L, et al. Significance of elevated MB isoenzyme with normal creatine kinase in acute myocardial infarction. Am J Cardiol 1987; 59:245.
[109] Puleo PR, Guadagno PA, Roberts R, et al. Early diagnosis of acute myocardial infarction based on assay for subforms of creatine kinase-MB. Circulation 1990; 82:759.
[110] Puleo PR, Meyer D, Wathen C, et al. Use of a rapid assay of subforms of creatine kinase-MB to diagnose or rule out acute myocardial infarction. N Engl J Med 1994; 331:561.
[111] Jaffe AS, Landt Y, Parvin CA, et al. Comparative sensitivity of cardiac troponin I and lactate dehydrogenase isoenzymes for diagnosing acute myocardial infarction. Clin Chem 1996; 42:1770.
[112] Adams JE 3rd, Dávila-Román VG, Bessey PQ, et al. Improved detection of cardiac contusion with cardiac troponin I. Am Heart J 1996; 131:308.
[113] Adams JE 3rd, Sicard GA, Allen BT, et al. Diagnosis of perioperative myocardial infarction with measurement of cardiac troponin I. N Engl J Med 1994; 330:670.
[114] Larca LJ, Coppola JT, Honig S. Creatine kinase MB isoenzyme in dermatomyositis: a noncardiac source. Ann Intern Med 1981; 94:341.
[115] Lenke LG, Bridwell KH, Jaffe AS. Increase in creatine kinase MB isoenzyme levels after spinal surgery. J Spinal Disord 1994; 7:70.
[116] Badsha H, Gunes B, Grossman J, Brahn E. Troponin I Assessment of Cardiac Involvement in Patients With Connective Tissue Disease and an Elevated Creatine Kinase MB Isoform Report of Four Cases and Review of the Literature. J Clin Rheumatol 1997; 3:131.
[117] Hochberg MC, Koppes GM, Edwards CQ, et al. Hypothyroidism presenting as a polymyositis-like syndrome. Report of two cases. Arthritis Rheum 1976; 19:1363.
[118] Jaffe AS, Ritter C, Meltzer V, et al. Unmasking artifactual increases in creatine kinase isoenzymes in patients with renal failure. J Lab Clin Med 1984; 104:193.
[119] Gutovitz AL, Sobel BE, Roberts R. Progressive nature of myocardial injury in selected patients with cardiogenic shock. Am J Cardiol 1978; 41:469.

[120] Alexander JH, Sparapani RA, Mahaffey KW, et al. Association between minor elevations of creatine kinase-MB level and mortality in patients with acute coronary syndromes without ST-segment elevation. PURSUIT Steering Committee. Platelet Glycoprotein IIb/IIIa in Unstable Angina: Receptor Suppression Using Integrilin Therapy. JAMA 2000; 283:347.

[121] Savonitto S, Granger CB, Ardissino D, et al. The prognostic value of creatine kinase elevations extends across the whole spectrum of acute coronary syndromes. J Am Coll Cardiol 2002; 39:22.

[122] Halkin A, Stone GW, Grines CL, et al. Prognostic implications of creatine kinase elevation after primary percutaneous coronary intervention for acute myocardial infarction. J Am Coll Cardiol 2006; 47:951.

[123] Galla JM, Mahaffey KW, Sapp SK, et al. Elevated creatine kinase-MB with normal creatine kinase predicts worse outcomes in patients with acute coronary syndromes: results from 4 large clinical trials. Am Heart J 2006; 151:16.

[124] Lloyd-Jones DM, Camargo CA Jr, Giugliano RP, et al. Characteristics and prognosis of patients with suspected acute myocardial infarction and elevated MB relative index but normal total creatine kinase. Am J Cardiol 1999; 84:957.

[125] Newby LK, Roe MT, Chen AY, et al. Frequency and clinical implications of discordant creatine kinase-MB and troponin measurements in acute coronary syndromes. J Am Coll Cardiol 2006; 47:312.

[126] Rao SV, Ohman EM, Granger CB, et al. Prognostic value of isolated troponin elevation across the spectrum of chest pain syndromes. Am J Cardiol 2003; 91:936.

[127] Goodman SG, Steg PG, Eagle KA, et al. The diagnostic and prognostic impact of the redefinition of acute myocardial infarction: lessons from the Global Registry of Acute Coronary Events (GRACE). Am Heart J 2006; 151:654.

[128] Califf RM, Abdelmeguid AE, Kuntz RE, et al. Myonecrosis after revascularization procedures. J Am Coll Cardiol 1998; 31:241.

[129] Tardiff BE, Califf RM, Tcheng JE, et al. Clinical outcomes after detection of elevated cardiac enzymes in patients undergoing percutaneous intervention. IMPACT-II Investigators. Integrilin (eptifibatide) to Minimize Platelet Aggregation and Coronary Thrombosis-II. J Am Coll Cardiol 1999; 33:88.

[130] Simoons ML, van den Brand M, Lincoff M, et al. Minimal myocardial damage during coronary intervention is associated with impaired outcome. Eur Heart J 1999; 20:1112.

[131] Cavallini C, Savonitto S, Violini R, et al. Impact of the elevation of biochemical markers of myocardial damage on long-term mortality after percutaneous coronary intervention: results of the CK-MB and PCI study. Eur Heart J 2005; 26:1494.

[132] Cantor WJ, Newby LK, Christenson RH, et al. Prognostic significance of elevated troponin I after percutaneous coronary intervention. J Am Coll Cardiol 2002; 39:1738.

[133] Kizer JR, Muttrej MR, Matthai WH, et al. Role of cardiac troponin T in the long-term risk stratification of patients undergoing percutaneous coronary intervention. Eur Heart J 2003; 24:1314.

[134] Nageh T, Sherwood RA, Harris BM, et al. Cardiac troponin T and I and creatine kinase-MB as markers of myocardial injury and predictors of outcome following percutaneous coronary intervention. Int J Cardiol 2003; 92:285.
[135] Kini AS, Lee P, Marmur JD, et al. Correlation of postpercutaneous coronary intervention creatine kinase-MB and troponin I elevation in predicting mid-term mortality. Am J Cardiol 2004; 93:18.
[136] Wu AH, Boden WE, McKay RG. Long-term follow-up of patients with increased cardiac troponin concentrations following percutaneous coronary intervention. Am J Cardiol 2002; 89:1300.
[137] Miller WL, Garratt KN, Burritt MF, et al. Baseline troponin level: key to understanding the importance of post-PCI troponin elevations. Eur Heart J 2006; 27:1061.
[138] Prasad A, Rihal CS, Lennon RJ, et al. Significance of periprocedural myonecrosis on outcomes following Percutaneous coronary intervention. Circ Cardiovasc Intervent 2008; 1:9.
[139] Pierpont GL, McFalls EO. Interpreting troponin elevations: do we need multiple diagnoses? Eur Heart J 2009; 30:135.
[140] Prasad A, Singh M, Lerman A, et al. Isolated elevation in troponin T after percutaneous coronary intervention is associated with higher long-term mortality. J Am Coll Cardiol 2006; 48:1765.
[141] Nienhuis MB, Ottervanger JP, Dikkeschei B, et al. Prognostic importance of troponin T and creatine kinase after elective angioplasty. Int J Cardiol 2007; 120:242.
[142] Kleiman NS. Measuring troponin elevation after percutaneous coronary intervention: ready for prime time? J Am Coll Cardiol 2006; 48:1771.
[143] Costa MA, Carere RG, Lichtenstein SV, et al. Incidence, predictors, and significance of abnormal cardiac enzyme rise in patients treated with bypass surgery in the arterial revascularization therapies study (ARTS). Circulation 2001; 104:2689.
[144] Brener SJ, Lytle BW, Schneider JP, et al. Association between CK-MB elevation after percutaneous or surgical revascularization and three-year mortality. J Am Coll Cardiol 2002; 40:1961.
[145] Januzzi JL, Lewandrowski K, MacGillivray TE, et al. A comparison of cardiac troponin T and creatine kinase-MB for patient evaluation after cardiac surgery. J Am Coll Cardiol 2002; 39:1518.
[146] Steuer J, Bjerner T, Duvernoy O, et al. Visualisation and quantification of peri-operative myocardial infarction after coronary artery bypass surgery with contrast-enhanced magnetic resonance imaging. Eur Heart J 2004; 25:1293.
[147] Carrier M, Pellerin M, Perrault LP, et al. Troponin levels in patients with myocardial infarction after coronary artery bypass grafting. Ann Thorac Surg 2000; 69:435.
[148] Croal BL, Hillis GS, Gibson PH, et al. Relationship between postoperative cardiac troponin I levels and outcome of cardiac surgery. Circulation 2006; 114:1468.
[149] Thielmann M, Massoudy P, Jaeger BR, et al. Emergency re-revascularization with percutaneous coronary intervention, reoperation, or conservative treatment in patients with acute perioperative graft failure following coronary artery bypass surgery. Eur J Cardiothorac Surg 2006; 30:117.

[150] Morrow DA, Cannon CP, Jesse RL, et al. National Academy of Clinical Biochemistry Laboratory Medicine Practice Guidelines: clinical characteristics and utilization of biochemical markers in acute coronary syndromes. Clin Chem 2007; 53:552.

3

Inflammatory Biomarkers in Ischemic Heart Disease

Mette Bjerre
The Medical Research Laboratories, Institute of Clinical Medicine, Faculty of Health Sciences, Aarhus University Denmark

1. Introduction

Ischemic heart disease (IHD) is one of the main groups within the class of cardiovascular diseases (CVD), and IHD is the most common single cause of morbidity and mortality in the Western world (Gaziano et al., 2006). According to the American Heart Association Statistics Committee one in three individuals has one or more forms of CVD (Rosamond et al., 2007).

The importance of inflammation in the pathogenesis of IHD, such as, acute myocardial infarct (AMI) and coronary artery disease (CAD), has long been established. A large body of evidence suggests that inflammation plays a key role in CVD, however, the mechanisms in the various stages of the pathological process is not completely understood (Carden and Granger, 2000). Inflammation is a complex of defensive mechanisms reacting to the entry of harmful agents into the organism or cells, in order to eliminate or repair damaged cells or tissue and to restore homeostasis. This broad definition indicates that inflammation does not only accompany infectious diseases, but also other conditions causing cell, tissue or organ damage.

The identified risk factors for IHD include both lifestyle and biological factors, such as smoking, high blood pressure, high cholesterol levels, obesity, and diabetes that all appear to exaggerate many of the vascular alterations elicited by ischemia and reperfusion. Diabetes and CVD often appear as two sides of a coin: on one side, diabetes has been rated as an equivalent of CVD, and conversely, many patients with established CVD suffer from overt or incipient diabetes (Ryden et al., 2007). The mortality from AMI is almost increased five-fold in diabetic patients compared with non-diabetics (Hansen et al., 2007) and diabetes and low-grade inflammation is closely related (Flyvbjerg, 2010). Obesity is seen at epidemic proportions all over the world, and is a significant risk factor for, and contributing factor to increased morbidity and mortality, most importantly from CVD and diabetes (Lavie et al., 2009a). Likewise, obesity is also associated with low-grade inflammation and CVD (Yudkin et al., 1999; Bastard et al., 2006).

Although the combination of traditional risk factors such as age, gender, lifestyle, dyslipidemia, hypertension and diabetes are well established for the prediction of cardiovascular mortality (e.g. the Framingham coronary risk score), these algorithms do not adequately differentiate individuals at moderate risk. Indeed, not all patients with CVD will have conventional risk factors and not all patients with risk factors will develop CVD (Khot et al., 2003). Both biomarkers of early disease and plaque instability have therefore been sought, and the development of new markers to diagnose and prevent CVD is an important public health goal worldwide. However, a recent report showed that the addition of a multi-marker score including 10 new markers to conventional risk factors added only a moderate increase in the ability to grade the risk in the general population (Wang et al., 2006).

Several inflammatory biomarkers have been shown to represent important cardiovascular risk factors, and this review will primarily focus on the complement system, the acute-phase reactant C-reactive protein (CRP), and the antimicrobial peptides: α-defensins. Whether these inflammatory proteins mediate IHD themselves or solely serve as markers of systemic inflammation and cardiovascular risk stratification is still intensely studied.

2. Inflammation and IHD

Growing evidence indicates that IHD is a broad syndrome with multiple pathogenetic and aetiological components, which may not be the same in all patients. Extensive literature supports the role of inflammation in IHD (Mehta and Li, 1999; Ross, 1999). Inflammatory cells, inflammatory proteins and inflammatory responses from vascular cells are all reported to play crucial roles in various stages of a number of CVD (Carden and Granger, 2000). Some of the inflammatory mechanisms of IHD include, among others, endothelial dysfunction, oxidative stress and vascular calcification, that all seems to play an important role for the development of cardiovascular disease.

Although timely restoration of blood-flow after a myocardial ischemic event is essential to prevent irreversible cellular injury, it is widely recognized that the outcome of tissue injury not only depends on the duration of the ischemic event, but also on reperfusion as a critical factor (Khalil et al., 2006). Paradoxically, the reperfusion exacerbates severe tissue damage, especially after longer periods of ischemia. The intensity of the inflammatory reaction in post-ischemic tissue can be so strong that the injury response to reperfusion can be manifested in distant organs (Carden and Granger, 2000).

The ischemia-reperfusion injury (IRI) results in a local and systemic inflammatory response characterized by the production of reactive oxygen species (ROS), leucocyte-endothelial cell adhesion, complement activation, endothelial leucocyte migration, increased micro-vascular permeability and decreased endothelial-dependent relaxation (Carden and Granger, 2000). Within minutes of reperfusion ROS are generated (Cannon, 2005), stimulating the release of cytokines and expression of adhesion molecules on damaged cells in reperfused tissue. Several hours after onset of reperfusion, neutrophils and other inflammatory cells are activated (Frangogiannis et al., 2002; Frangogiannis, 2007) and adhere to the damaged cell membranes (Zimmerman et al., 1990; Vinten-Johansen, 2004) for further enhancement of the inflammatory response. Thus, IRI poses major problems in the clinic, and effective therapies are required.

3. Inflammatory biomarkers

Recent research has been focused on identifying biomarkers, which alone or in combination with other risk markers could be useful in monitoring the treatment and as prognostic markers for future coronary syndromes and cardiac death in patients with IHD.

In 2001, a National Institute of Health working group defined a biomarker as "a characteristic that is objectively measured and evaluated as an indicator of normal biological processes, pathogenic processes or pharmacological responses to a therapeutic intervention (BiomarkersDefinitionsWorkingGroup, 2001). Biomarkers are traditionally specific proteins circulating in the body fluids that become altered as a consequence of disease progression or the effect of a therapeutic intervention and can be divided into different categories:

- Disease-predictive
- Diagnostic
- Prognostic
- Disease-associated
- Therapeutic efficacy.

A number of inflammatory biomarkers have been associated with cardiovascular diseases. Biomarker measurements can help explain empirical results of clinical trials by relating the effects of interventions on molecular and cellular pathways to clinical responses, thus providing an opportunity for researchers to gain a mechanistic understanding.

3.1 The complement system

The complement system is an innate, cytotoxic host defence that normally functions to eliminate pathogens and facilitates the clearance of damaged tissue and apoptotic cells. However, excessive activation of the system may lead to uncontrolled tissue damage. The relevance of complement activation in myocardial ischemia was already proposed more than four decades ago (Hill and Ward, 1971). The inflammatory mechanisms by which tissue injury after an AMI occurs has not been fully elucidated, but strong evidence obtained from animal models, as well as clinical studies, support the hypothesis of a role for the complement system in IHD (Bjerre et al., 2008).

The complement system is a biochemical cascade, which helps clear pathogens from an organism, and is thus one part of a larger immune system. Three pathways of complement activation have been identified (Figure 1), known as the classical, the alternative and the lectin pathway. The classical pathway is initiated by C1q binding to antibody complexes (Cooper, 1985) whereas the alternative pathway is initiated by spontaneous and direct activation of C3 (Muller-Eberhard, 1988). The lectin pathway is initiated either through ficolin (M-, L- or H-ficolin) (Matsushita et al., 2001; Frederiksen et al., 2005), by pattern recognition of N-acetyl-glucosamine-rich polysaccharides or through mannan-binding lectin (MBL) binding to certain carbohydrate structures (Ikeda et al., 1987; Thiel et al., 1997; Holmskov et al., 2003).

Activation of the complement system promotes three main biological activities (Walport, 2001): I) recruitment of inflammatory cells by anaphylatoxins (C3a, C4a, and C5a), leading to accumulation of activated polymorph nuclear leukocytes directly involved in tissue destruction, II) opsonisation of pathogens for phagocytosis by the generation of C3b, and III) lysis of the pathogen by the generation of a membrane attack complex (MAC, C5b-9) penetrating the cell membrane. The loss of membrane integrity destroys the ability to control the concentration of salt within the cell and the cell is killed due to this osmotic instability. MAC formed in the absence of target membranes binds to S-protein, which inhibits the membrane-damaging effect, and creates a stable non-lytic soluble C5b-9 form (sMAC, sC5b-9) (Fosbrink et al., 2005).

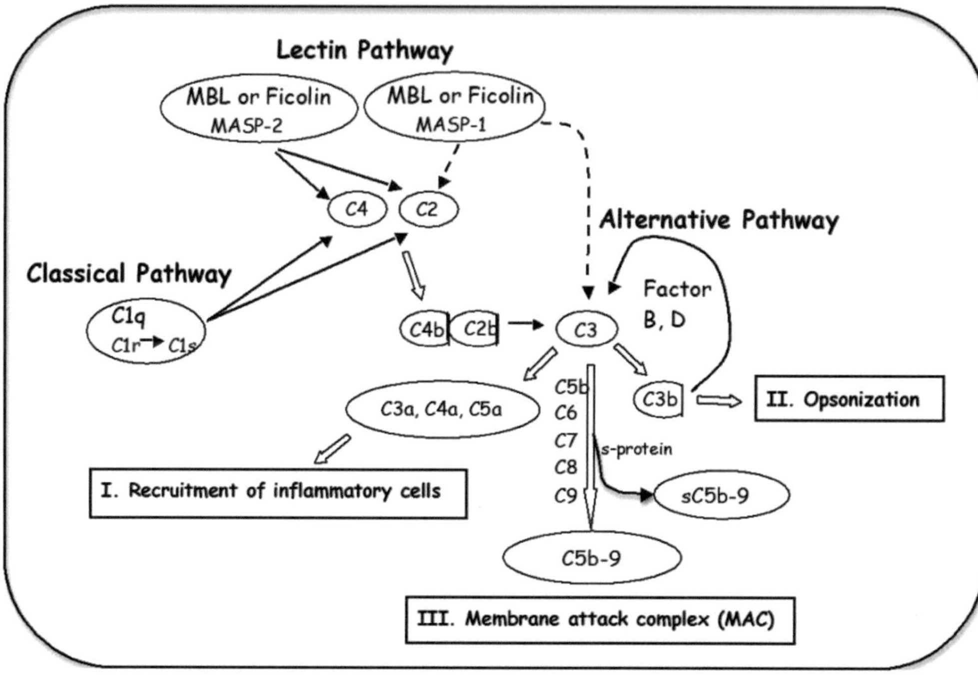

Fig. 1. The complement system can be activated through three pathways, which merge at the cleavage of C3, leading to the effector mechanisms: **I.** recruitment of inflammatory cells, **II.** opsonisation and **III.** the generation of the membrane attack complex (MAC, C5b-9) for cell lysis.

3.1.1 Role of complement in endothelial function

Ischemia and reperfusion are potent activators of the complement system and both clinical and experimental studies in different organs have shown local deposition of complement (Riedemann and Ward, 2003; Arumugam et al., 2004). It has traditionally been assumed that the liver is the source of complement proteins that participate in these events, but complement proteins are produced in several organs of the body, including the heart and the endothelium.

The human heart expresses mRNAs, translated into proteins, for all of the components of the classical complement pathway (Yasojima et al., 1998b). This production is up-regulated in areas of myocardial infarct, and the classical complement pathway was found to be fully activated on injured myocardial tissue. In addition, production of C3 and C9 mRNAs and their protein products was significantly increased in isolated rabbit heart after reperfusion injury, and the production by heart in this circumstance substantially exceeds that of the normal liver (Yasojima et al., 1998a).

Endothelial cells also represent one of the extrahepatic sources of complement components and regulators. Due to the strategic position along the surface of the vessel wall, they may supply both the circulating blood and the extravascular fluids with these proteins. Most of the information on the production of complement components by endothelial cells has been obtained using human umbilical vein endothelial cells (HUVECs). HUVECs cultured in serum free media were reported to synthesize functional C3, C5, C6, C8, and C9 and assembling of the MAC complex was found, indicating that C7 was produced as well (Johnson and Hetland, 1991). The C7 production was later confirmed (Langeggen et al., 2000) and a small production of C5, C6, C8, and C9 demonstrated by RT-PCR and Northern blot was reported (Langeggen et al., 2001). Activation of the complement cascade leads to the formation of the C5b-9 complex on the cell surface that can cause cell death. However, when the numbers of C5b-9 molecules are limited on host cell membranes, it can activate signalling pathways leading to cell cycle activation and cell survival (Niculescu and Rus, 2001).

The reduction in the capacity of the endothelium to maintain the homeostasis leads to the development of pathological inflammatory processes and vascular diseases. An intact endothelium is a fully biocompatible surface that is not recognized by the complement system. However, blood contact with a damaged endothelium will lead to a certain degree of activation of the defence system. Complement activation results in the formation of several biological active components including C3a, C5a, iC3b, and C5b-9. In addition, to stimulate inflammatory response C5a have been reported to induce production of chemokines and cytokines (Czermak et al., 1999).

3.1.2 Mechanism of complement in IHD

Cardiovascular risk factors (e.g., hypercholesterolemia, hypertension, smoking, diabetes, stress) cause oxidative stress that alters the endothelial cell capacity (Esper et al., 2006; Kyrou and Tsigos, 2007), and thus dysfunction of the endothelium has been implicated in the pathophysiology of different forms of CVD (reviewed by (Endemann and Schiffrin, 2004)). Human endothelial cells have been shown to generate reactive oxygen intermediates in response to hyperglycaemia and lead to dysfunction in type 2 diabetic patients (Bellin et al., 2006). Endothelial dysfunction has been shown to have a prognostic value in patients with chest pain (Neunteufl et al., 2000) and both C-reactive protein (CRP) and C3a were found to be elevated in patients with unstable angina pectoris (Kostner et al., 2006). Elevated plasma levels of C3 was independently associated with MI after accounting for traditional cardiovascular risk factors and CRP in patients with MI, whereas the association of CRP was dependent of C3 (Carter et al., 2009).

A number of *in vitro* studies using HUVECs have shown that under anoxic conditions the endothelial cells become activators of the complement system. Collard and co-workers showed increased MBL, C3, and iC3b deposition after hypoxia/reoxygenation (Collard et al., 2000; Collard et al., 2001). MBL deposition was attenuated in the presence of MBL ligands indicating the presence of MBL neo-epitopes on the surface of the endothelial cells. Apoptotic endothelial cells deposited C1 and C3d, thus activating the complement system (Mold and Morris, 2001). Experimental studies in porcine and rabbits reported that complement activation attenuates endothelium-dependent relaxation (Stahl et al., 1995; Lennon et al., 1996). The role of complement was mediated by the formation of C5b-9, but not through the generation of the anaphylatoxin C3a and C5a.

Hill et al. were the first to report a role for the complement system after an ischemic event in a rat model of AMI (Hill and Ward, 1971). The association between AMI and complement activation was later confirmed in baboons showing deposition of complement factors in the infarcted tissue (Pinckard et al., 1980; McManus et al., 1983). Later, several studies of experimental myocardial I/R showed deposition of complement; C1 (Vakeva et al., 1994), MBL and C3 (Walsh et al., 2005), C4, C5 (McManus et al., 1983; Crawford et al., 1988), C6 (Ito et al., 1996), and C5b-9 (Vakeva et al., 1994). MBL knock-out (KO) mice were protected from heart I/R injury, but when reconstituted with human recombinant MBL, I/R injury similar to that in wild type mice was found. Mice deficient in C2 and factor B (C2/B KO) were also protected form heart I/R injury but no protection was found in C1q or factor D KO mice (Walsh et al., 2005). In a murine model of coronary artery ischemia the involvement of natural IgM antibodies has been linked to both the classical and the lectin pathways (Zhang et al., 2006a; Zhang et al., 2006b). Mice bearing an altered natural IgM repertoire were significantly protected based on the reduced infarct size, limited apoptosis of cardiomyocytes, and decreased neutrophil infiltration.

In addition to direct lytic activity, C5b-9 also directly attenuates endothelium-dependent (i.e., NO-mediated) relaxation (Stahl et al., 1995). Furthermore, C5b-9 is found to play a role in leucocyte activation, adherence and chemotaxis by induction of different cytokines (Kilgore et al., 1996; Vakeva et al., 1998). Also, activation of endothelial NF-kB and the stimulation of expression of endothelial adhesion molecules have been observed. Furthermore, a role for C5b-9 in mediating myocardial apoptosis after ischemia-reperfusion was demonstrated in a model of rat myocardial IRI (Vakeva et al., 1998). We have shown that increased complement activity as indicated by MBL and sC5b-9 levels, was associated with increased risk of cardiac dysfunction in STEMI patients treated with pPCI (Haahr-Pedersen et al., 2009). High plasma MBL and low plasma sC5b-9 was independently associated with increased risk of cardiac dysfunction, likely due to increased complement activity during the ischemic and reperfusion process. The predictive value of low peripheral plasma sC5b-9 may be explained by an accumulation and activation of sC5b-9 in the infarcted myocardium. Furthermore, an elevated plasma sC5b-9 level was found in patients with chronic heart failure due to IHD (Bjerre et al., 2010). In addition, an independent association between sC5b-9, insulin resistance and endothelial dysfunction was found, which may suggest that insulin resistance leading to endothelial activation results in activation of the complement system thus damaging the heart.

3.1.3 Therapeutic inhibition of complement in IHD

Based on the studies discussed above, regulation of the complement system seems to be of great importance. Indeed, several animal studies point to a possible beneficial role of complement depletion in the treatment of post-ischemic MI; reviewed by (Bjerre et al., 2008; Diepenhorst et al., 2009). Unfortunately, clinical studies focused on complement depletion in humans, especially the use of anti-C5 antibodies, primarily Pexelizumab, have largely been disappointing and not proven effective in the setting of CVD, discussed in details elsewhere: (Bjerre et al., 2008; Diepenhorst et al., 2009; Banz and Rieben, 2011).

Although much of the preclinical work and data accumulated in the past years have been positive, the problem with complement-mediated damage in IR-injury was not "easy to fix". Thus conclusions drawn from animal studies should be extrapolated to the human settings with caution. It may lie in the fact that complement activation represents only a part of the cascade of attack directed against the vasculature. An exaggerated blockade of the immune system may increase the susceptibility to infections, thus a well-balanced inhibition of the complement activation is required in order to avoid side effects of pharmaceutically induced modification of the immune system. Direct targeting may be the key to future treatment strategies, including targeting of the complement inhibitor to the site of injury by localized intravascular application.

3.2 C-reactive protein

C-reactive protein (CRP), an acute-phase reactant mainly produced by hepatocytes in response to interleukin (IL) 6, is a nonspecific marker of systemic inflammation, and is the most intensively studied inflammatory biomarker in CVD. In addition, a large number of reports have shown that CRP may be implicated in the pathogenesis of many chronic diseases, including diabetes, cancer and alzheimer dementia, and major CVDs, such as, coronary heart disease (CHD), AMI and IHD (Clyne and Olshaker, 1999; Hirschfield and Pepys, 2003; Lavie et al., 2009b). Of note, CRP levels has been associated with the size of the infarct (de Beer et al., 1982).

The concentration of CRP increases rapidly; it may raise hundreds-fold after acute tissue injury or inflammation, and declines rapidly with resolution of the injurious process. In healthy persons, normal CRP levels are generally considered to be < 3 mg/L (Shine et al., 1981).

3.2.1 High sensitive CRP and IHD

In the 1990s, rapid and more precise methods of quantifying CRP was established and CRP levels measured as low as 0.04 mg/L were possible, referred to as high sensitive (hs) CRP (Jaye and Waites, 1997). Low-grade inflammation is found in IHD, and CRP levels are not as increased as compared to other inflammatory conditions. Therefore, a cardiovascular risk scale according to hsCRP levels is recommended by the American Heart Association and Centers for Disease Control and Prevention (Pearson et al., 2003).

Individuals with hsCRP levels;

- <1 mg/L are at lower relative risk for cardiovascular events,
- 1 to 3 mg/L are at intermediate risk,
- >3 mg/L are at higher relative risk.

In the Copenhagen City Heart study, investigating more than 10,000 apparently healthy participants, elevated hsCRP levels were found to be associated with increased risk of IHD. In fact, the risk of IHD was more than doubled (HR=2.2, 1.6-2.9) in individuals with CRP levels above 3 mg/L as compared to individuals with CRP levels below 1 mg/L (Zacho et al., 2008).

3.2.2 Possible links between hsCRP and IHD

Inflammation clearly plays a clinically significant role in the development of CVD. Consequently, as a marker of inflammation, hsCRP has been studied extensively in patients with CVD. The predictive value of hsCRP has been widely investigated but the results are contradictive. More than 20 large prospective trials have shown that hsCRP is an independent predictor of future cardiovascular events (Ridker, 2007). In the most recent comprehensive meta-analysis studies of cardiovascular risk factors (more than 50 prospective studies with over 160,000 participants, none of them with a history of coronary heart disease or stroke) (Kaptoge et al., 2010), hsCRP was consistently found to be an independent predictor of CVD. However, the association with ischemic vascular disease depends considerably on conventional risk factors and other markers of inflammation. A critical review by Levinson and colleagues argues that hsCRP is poor discrimination over a wide range of values when used in conjunction with risk factors for lipoprotein lipids, hypertension, metabolic syndrome, and diabetes (Levinson et al., 2004). Danesh and colleagues published a study, performed in a high-risk population with nonfatal myocardial infarct, which questioned the role of CRP in the assessment of cardiovascular risk. However, hsCRP maintained a predictive value after adjustments for smoking and hypertension (Danesh et al., 2004).

A panel of multiple biomarkers, 10 biomarkers in total including hsCRP, was used for prediction of death and major cardiovascular event in more than 3000 participants of the Framingham Off-spring study followed for 10 years (Wang et al., 2006). As a single marker, hsCRP predicted risk of death but no major cardiovascular events after adjusting for other biomarkers, and individuals with high multimarker scores had almost 4 times as great a risk of death. Nonetheless, the authors concluded that the use of contemporary biomarkers adds only moderately to standard risk factors. In the Women's Health Study, CRP was found to be additive to LDL-cholesterol in predicting future CVD in healthy American women (n=28,263 apparently healthy postmenopausal women) (Ridker et al., 2000a). Of the 12 markers measured (including hsCRP and IL-6), hs-CRP was the strongest uni-variant predictor of cardiovascular events, and the only plasma marker predicting risk after adjustment in a multi-variant analysis. This was confirmed in a large meta-analysis of hsCRP as a single biomarker in patients with stable CAD, but the authors concluded that a routine measurement of CRP should not be recommended as a single prognostic biomarker (Hemingway et al., 2010). However, in combination with other biomarkers, hsCRP seems to add significant information to traditional risk factors for CVD, and the value of adding hsCRP to standard risk equations was noted in separate cohorts of asymptomatic (middle-aged or elderly) men and women (Lavie et al., 2009b).

In the Caerphilly Prospective Heart Disease Study, Mendall and colleagues, showed a significant and positive association between CRP and incidents of IHD, not affected by ischemia history (Mendall et al., 2000). However, after adjustment of lifestyle risk factors (such as smoking and obesity) only the association with all-cause mortality remained significant. Plasma hsCRP was not found as an independent predictor of long-term IHD risk in a 13-year-follow-up study of men with no previous history of IHD (n=1982) (St-Pierre et al., 2005). The authors thus concluded that neither CRP nor the systemic inflammation appeared to have a direct role in the development of IHD. But the association of hsCRP with IHD may be that CRP levels are raised non-specifically by a variety of exposures that are themselves implicated in the pathogenesis of IHD (Figure 2).

A connection between CRP and activation of the complement system was proposed more than 35 years ago, after the discovery of aggregated or ligand-complexed human CRP was able to bind to C1q and activate the classical pathway (Kaplan and Volanakis, 1974; Siegel et al., 1974; Jiang et al., 1991), thus mediating the functions summarized in Figure 1. CRP was later found to co-localize with activated complement fragments in atherosclerotic lesions (Bhakdi et al., 1999; Yasojima et al., 2001) and CRP-mediated complement activation in the arterial wall may be considered as an important pathogenic feature in CVD.

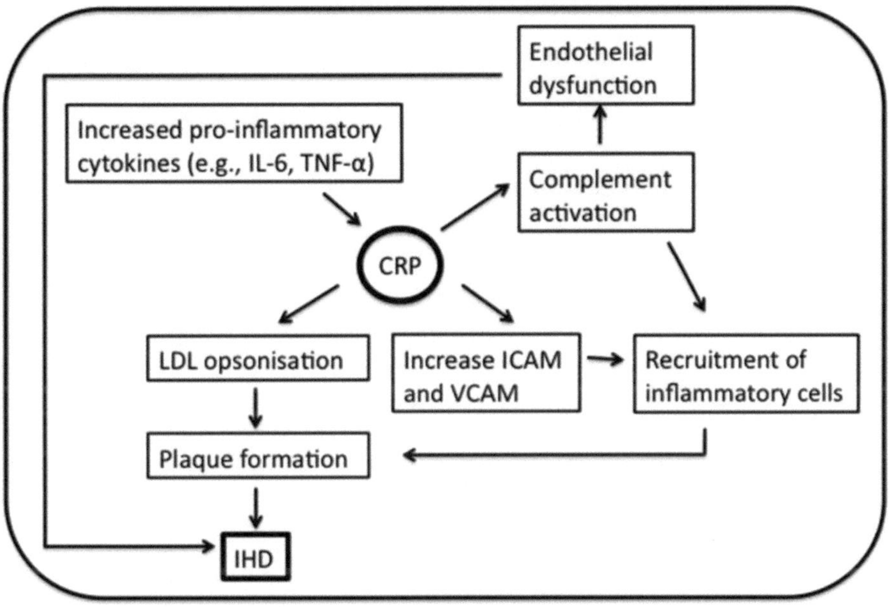

Fig. 2. Schematic depiction of potential mechanisms of CRP involvement in the pathogenesis of IHD.

A number of pro-inflammatory cytokines have been shown to play roles in the process leading to IHD, but IL-6, in particular, appears to have a central role, e.g. by stimulating the liver to increase the CRP production. However, even with a strong correlation between IL-6 and CRP, IL-6 was found to predict future AMI in a group of apparently healthy men (Ridker et al., 2000b).

CRP binds to apolipoprotein-containing lipoproteins like LDL (de Beer et al., 1982) and very low-density lipoprotein (VLDL) (Rowe et al., 1984), which may be of considerable importance in the pathogenesis of CVD. More recent studies revealed that CRP preferentially binds to modified forms of LDL; enzymatically modified LDL (Bhakdi et al., 1999) and oxidized LDL (Chang et al., 2002), and CRP was reported to mediate LDL uptake by macrophages (Zwaka et al., 2001). Opsonisation of LDL lead to monocyte infiltration and the formation of foam cells resulting in plaque formation and eventually IHD.

CRP was found to cause expression of cell adhesion molecules with a significant dose-dependent expression of ICAM-1, VCAM-1 and E-selectin in human umbilical vein endothelial cells (HUVEC) following CRP stimulation (Pasceri et al., 2000). Furthermore, production of chemokines monocyte chemoattractant protein-1 (MCP-1), which plays an important role in recruitment of monocytes into the vessel wall and thus the formation of plaques, was directly induced by CRP (Pasceri et al., 2001).

3.2.3 Is CRP a potential therapeutic in prevention of IHD?

As described in the previous section, CRP is reported to be associated with a wide range of biomarkers and risk factors of IHD. Thus, overestimating of the true effect of hsCRP on CVD risk, because of confounding effects, constitute a challenge. Support for a role of CRP in the pathogenesis of CVD comes primary from epidemiologic studies, which in general have observed an association between elevated plasma CRP and cardiovascular events.

Although hsCRP may not be the ideal marker of IHD, it seems to be very reliable, and hsCRP is a simple, non-invasive, commercially available, inexpensive and reproducible biomarker. CRP measurement has a lot of advantages; the protein is stable and the concentration is not subjected to time-of-the day variations (Meier-Ewert et al., 2001). Thus, determination of baseline hsCRP for cardiovascular risk prediction may be performed without concern for diurnal variation.

Availability of drugs to block CRP binding and its effects *in vivo* would provide a powerful tool for determining whether CRP is just a marker or does indeed participate in the pathogenesis of CVD complications. Griselli and colleagues (Griselli et al., 1999) showed that injection of human CRP in a rat model of AMI enhanced the infarct size, of note rat CRP does not activate rat complement, whereas human CRP activate both rat and human complement. However, in vivo complement depletion, by cobra venom factor, completely abrogated this. A similar effect was later found by administration of a specific synthetic CRP-inhibitor, 1,6-bis(phosphocholine)-hexane, which reduced the infarct size and thus provided promising results for therapeutic inhibition of CRP (Pepys et al., 2006).

Statins lower the levels of LDL-cholesterol and CRP. Ridker and colleagues showed, in a sub-population (n= 3745) derived from the Pravastatin or Atorvastatin Evaluation and Infection Therapy–Thrombolysis in Myocardial Infarction 22 (PROVE IT–TIMI 22) study, that patients with low hsCRP levels after statin treatment had improved cardiovascular outcome (Ridker et al., 2005). Patients in whom statin therapy resulted in hsCRP levels below 2 mg/L overall had better clinical outcomes regardless of the LDL-cholesterol level achieved. Recently, a study JUPITER: Justification for the Use of Statins in Prevention: an Intervention Trial Evaluating Rosuvastatin (n=17802), of healthy individuals without history of CVD but hsCRP > 2 mg/L and low LDL concentration, showed beneficial effect of Rosuvastatin (Ridker et al., 2007; Kones, 2010; Ridker et al., 2010). The study was terminated due to a great risk-reduction in AMI, CVD and death from cardiovascular causes, indicating that part of the statin effect may be mediated through lowering CRP.

Aside from whether measurement of CRP is useful in assessments of CVD, studies are needed to help determine if CRP is a mediator or a marker of CVD. Zacho et al. showed that genetic variants that are associated with a lifelong increased plasma CRP level are not associated with increased risk of IHD (Zacho et al., 2008), indicating CRP as a marker but not as an actual contributor.

3.3 Anti-microbial peptides

The involvement of polymorphonuclear neutrophils (PMNs) in the pathogenesis of CVD has received relatively little attention, despite their presence in the atherosclerotic plaques (Quinn et al., 2008). PMN counts have been reported as independent risk factors for cardiovascular outcome (Madjid et al., 2004) and during inflammation PMNs are activated in order to enhance the inflammatory response and releases antimicrobial peptides into circulation.

Anti-microbial peptides are polypeptides of fewer than 100 amino acids. The human innate immune system includes two main families; defensins and cathelicidins. Defensins, also termed human neutrophil peptides (HNP) as they are found in large amounts in neutrophils, are secreted during phagocytosis as a first line of defence against invading organisms (Ganz, 2003).

3.3.1 α-defensins

Three different classes of defensin are identified in mammals, two of which are found in humans; α- and β-defensin (Ganz, 1987). The human family of α-defensins are composed of 3 closely related gene products, also referred to as human neutrophil peptides 1-3 (HNPs-1-3) and HNP4, HNP5 and HNP6. The α-defensins are cationic peptides, cysteine-rich peptides of approximately 3 kDa and are normally sequestered in the granules of neutrophils, where they constitute 5% of the total cellular protein and are involved in the intracellular killing of prokaryotic organisms (Ganz, 1987). Under normal conditions, only small amounts of α-defensins (nanomolar range) are found in plasma. However, during inflammatory reactions, α-defensins are released extracellularly, which could exert harmful effects on host cells. Increased plasma concentrations of α-defensins have been described in several inflammatory diseases (Ganz, 2003; Klotman and Chang, 2006; de Leeuw and Lu, 2007).

3.3.2 Possible link between α-defensins and IHD

The cationic nature of the α-defensins prefers the negatively charged phospholipids of the bacterial membrane as target and avoids the more neutral charged mammalian cell membrane. However, both a direct and an indirect chemoattracting role of α-defensins has been reported for a number of cells (Oppenheim et al., 2003). In addition, α-defensin was found to promote oxidative stress and induces endothelial dysfunction by reducing the endothelium-dependent relaxation in porcine coronary arteries (Kougias et al., 2006). This effect is associated with increased superoxide radical production and decreased eNOS expression. Also, α-defensins is capable of forming complexes with C1q and MBL, thus playing a role in the regulation of both the classical and the lectin pathway of complement activation (Groeneveld et al., 2007).

Localization of α-defensins were analysed by the use of immunohistochemical staining of coronary arteries from patients with severe CVD or normal donor heart tissue (Barnathan et al., 1997). Of interest, α-defensin was found most prominently in association with intima smooth muscle cells of both normal or atherosclerotic vessels. α-defensins has been reported as an atherogenic agent by enhancing and promoting stable complexes with LDL particles, thus stimulating the binding to endothelial and smooth muscle cells (Higazi et al., 1997). In addition, in human cerebral vessels obtained during autopsy, α-defensin and LDL co-localized primary within the atherosclerotic areas, and the staining intensity correlated with the severity of the disease. The authors hypothesize that the small α-defensins may rapidly cross the endothelial barrier and gain access to sub-endothelial matrix and affording the binding of LDL and a complex relative resistant to degradation. Retention of LDL in the arteries may predispose to pro-atherogenic modifications, such as, oxidation and internalization by foam cells. In addition, an independent negative relationship between high-density lipoprotein (HDL) has later been described (Saraheimo et al., 2008). Furthermore, α-defensins were found to inhibit the fibrionolytic activity by binding to tissue plasminogen activator molecule (Kougias et al., 2005). In a small study of patients undergoing elective coronary artery catheterization, an accumulation of α-defensin in the human skin was described and the accumulated amount correlated with the severity of coronary artery disease (Nassar et al., 2007). Of note, no correlation between CRP and α-defensin was found in this study.

Chronic low-grade inflammation is a hallmark of obesity and diabetes, and has been causally linked to the development of premature CVD. In a group of type-1 diabetic patients, with a 10-year-follow-up-period of cardiovascular end-points, elevated baseline plasma α-defensin levels were an independent predictor for cardiovascular morbidity and mortality (Joseph et al., 2008). In a recent study, the risk of cardiovascular mortality was significantly increased with elevated plasma α-defensin levels in patients admitted for elective lower extremity artery surgery (Urbonaviciene et al., 2011). Surprisingly, patients with high α-defensin levels combined with high hs-CRP levels had a five time increased risk of cardiovascular death compared to patients in whom only one or none of the peptides was elevated.

4. Perspectives

Inflammatory biomarkers may have prognostic value for future cardiovascular risk stratification among individuals with high risk or a history of IHD, but they may also in particular be useful in apparently healthy individuals who might be at higher risk than estimated by the traditional risk factor scores. Using a biomarker profile that covers various aspects of the complex pathophysiology of IHD may increase the rational basis for cardiovascular risk assessment. As decribed above, a multiple inflammatory role of the combination of complement activation, CRP, LDL and α-defensins may participate in the pathogenesis of IHD and other CVD.

With the emergence of novel biomarkers for inflammation and vascular damage it may be possible to characterize different contributions of each of these major mechanisms to short- and long-term prognosis following CVD. Hopefully, patients may benefit from different therapeutic strategies depending on their personal biomarker profile in the future. So far, however, results about which biomarkers are the most suitable for diagnosis or prognosis of IHD remain conflicting, and further research within this field is needed.

5. References

Arumugam, T.V., Shiels, I.A., Woodruff, T.M., Granger, D.N. and Taylor, S.M. (2004) The role of the complement system in ischemia-reperfusion injury. Shock 21, 401-9.

Banz, Y. and Rieben, R. (2011) Role of complement and perspectives for intervention in ischemia-reperfusion damage. Ann Med.

Barnathan, E.S., Raghunath, P.N., Tomaszewski, J.E., Ganz, T., Cines, D.B. and Higazi, A.a.-R. (1997) Immunohistochemical localization of defensin in human coronary vessels. Am J Pathol 150, 1009-20.

Bastard, J.P., Maachi, M., Lagathu, C., Kim, M.J., Caron, M., Vidal, H., Capeau, J. and Feve, B. (2006) Recent advances in the relationship between obesity, inflammation, and insulin resistance. Eur Cytokine Netw 17, 4-12.

Bellin, C., de Wiza, D.H., Wiernsperger, N.F. and Rosen, P. (2006) Generation of reactive oxygen species by endothelial and smooth muscle cells: influence of hyperglycemia and metformin. Horm Metab Res 38, 732-9.

Bhakdi, S., Torzewski, M., Klouche, M. and Hemmes, M. (1999) Complement and atherogenesis: binding of CRP to degraded, nonoxidized LDL enhances complement activation. Arterioscler Thromb Vasc Biol 19, 2348-54.

BiomarkersDefinitionsWorkingGroup. (2001) Biomarkers and surrogate endpoints: preferred definitions and conceptual framework. Clin Pharmacol Ther 69, 89-95.

Bjerre, M., Hansen, T.K. and Flyvbjerg, A. (2008) Complement activation and cardiovascular disease. Horm Metab Res 40, 626-34.

Bjerre, M., Kistorp, C., Hansen, T.K., Faber, J., Lip, G.Y., Hildebrandt, P. and Flyvbjerg, A. (2010) Complement activation, endothelial dysfunction, insulin resistance and chronic heart failure. Scand Cardiovasc J 44, 260-6.

Cannon, R.O., 3rd. (2005) Mechanisms, management and future directions for reperfusion injury after acute myocardial infarction. Nat Clin Pract Cardiovasc Med 2, 88-94.

Carden, D.L. and Granger, D.N. (2000) Pathophysiology of ischaemia-reperfusion injury. J Pathol 190, 255-66.

Carter, A.M., Prasad, U.K. and Grant, P.J. (2009) Complement C3 and C-reactive protein in male survivors of myocardial infarction. Atherosclerosis 203, 538-43.

Chang, M.K., Binder, C.J., Torzewski, M. and Witztum, J.L. (2002) C-reactive protein binds to both oxidized LDL and apoptotic cells through recognition of a common ligand: Phosphorylcholine of oxidized phospholipids. Proc Natl Acad Sci U S A 99, 13043-8.

Clyne, B. and Olshaker, J.S. (1999) The C-reactive protein. J Emerg Med 17, 1019-25.

Collard, C.D., Montalto, M.C., Reenstra, W.R., Buras, J.A. and Stahl, G.L. (2001) Endothelial oxidative stress activates the lectin complement pathway: role of cytokeratin 1. Am J Pathol 159, 1045-54.

Collard, C.D., Vakeva, A., Morrissey, M.A., Agah, A., Rollins, S.A., Reenstra, W.R., Buras, J.A., Meri, S. and Stahl, G.L. (2000) Complement activation after oxidative stress: role of the lectin complement pathway. Am J Pathol 156, 1549-56.

Cooper, N.R. (1985) The classical complement pathway: activation and regulation of the first complement component. Adv Immunol 37, 151-216.

Crawford, M.H., Grover, F.L., Kolb, W.P., McMahan, C.A., O'Rourke, R.A., McManus, L.M. and Pinckard, R.N. (1988) Complement and neutrophil activation in the pathogenesis of ischemic myocardial injury. Circulation 78, 1449-58.

Czermak, B.J., Sarma, V., Bless, N.M., Schmal, H., Friedl, H.P. and Ward, P.A. (1999) In vitro and in vivo dependency of chemokine generation on C5a and TNF-alpha. J Immunol 162, 2321-5.

Danesh, J., Wheeler, J.G., Hirschfield, G.M., Eda, S., Eiriksdottir, G., Rumley, A., Lowe, G.D., Pepys, M.B. and Gudnason, V. (2004) C-reactive protein and other circulating markers of inflammation in the prediction of coronary heart disease. N Engl J Med 350, 1387-97.

de Beer, F.C., Soutar, A.K., Baltz, M.L., Trayner, I.M., Feinstein, A. and Pepys, M.B. (1982) Low density lipoprotein and very low density lipoprotein are selectively bound by aggregated C-reactive protein. J Exp Med 156, 230-42.

de Leeuw, E. and Lu, W. (2007) Human defensins: turning defense into offense? Infect Disord Drug Targets 7, 67-70.

Diepenhorst, G.M., van Gulik, T.M. and Hack, C.E. (2009) Complement-mediated ischemia-reperfusion injury: lessons learned from animal and clinical studies. Ann Surg 249, 889-99.

Endemann, D.H. and Schiffrin, E.L. (2004) Endothelial dysfunction. J Am Soc Nephrol 15, 1983-92.

Esper, R.J., Nordaby, R.A., Vilarino, J.O., Paragano, A., Cacharron, J.L. and Machado, R.A. (2006) Endothelial dysfunction: a comprehensive appraisal. Cardiovasc Diabetol 5, 4.

Flyvbjerg, A. (2010) Diabetic angiopathy, the complement system and the tumor necrosis factor superfamily. Nat Rev Endocrinol 6, 94-101.

Fosbrink, M., Niculescu, F. and Rus, H. (2005) The role of c5b-9 terminal complement complex in activation of the cell cycle and transcription. Immunol Res 31, 37-46.

Frangogiannis, N.G. (2007) Chemokines in ischemia and reperfusion. Thromb Haemost 97, 738-47.

Frangogiannis, N.G., Smith, C.W. and Entman, M.L. (2002) The inflammatory response in myocardial infarction. Cardiovasc Res 53, 31-47.

Frederiksen, P.D., Thiel, S., Larsen, C.B. and Jensenius, J.C. (2005) M-ficolin, an Innate Immune Defence Molecule, Binds Patterns of Acetyl Groups and Activates Complement. Scand J Immunol 62, 462-73.

Ganz, T. (1987) Extracellular release of antimicrobial defensins by human polymorphonuclear leukocytes. Infect Immun 55, 568-71.

Ganz, T. (2003) Defensins: antimicrobial peptides of innate immunity. Nat Rev Immunol 3, 710-20.

Gaziano, T., Reddy, K.S., Paccaud, F., Horton, S. and Chaturvedi, V. (2006) Cardiovascular Disease.

Griselli, M., Herbert, J., Hutchinson, W.L., Taylor, K.M., Sohail, M., Krausz, T. and Pepys, M.B. (1999) C-reactive protein and complement are important mediators of tissue damage in acute myocardial infarction. J Exp Med 190, 1733-40.

Groeneveld, T.W., Ramwadhdoebe, T.H., Trouw, L.A., van den Ham, D.L., van der Borden, V., Drijfhout, J.W., Hiemstra, P.S., Daha, M.R. and Roos, A. (2007) Human neutrophil peptide-1 inhibits both the classical and the lectin pathway of complement activation. Mol Immunol 44, 3608-14.

Hansen, H.H., Joensen, A.M., Riahi, S., Malczynski, J., Molenberg, D. and Ravkilde, J. (2007) Short and long-term outcome in diabetic patients with acute myocardial infarction in the invasive era. Scand Cardiovasc J 41, 19-24.

Hemingway, H., Philipson, P., Chen, R., Fitzpatrick, N.K., Damant, J., Shipley, M., Abrams, K.R., Moreno, S., McAllister, K.S., Palmer, S., Kaski, J.C., Timmis, A.D. and Hingorani, A.D. (2010) Evaluating the quality of research into a single prognostic biomarker: a systematic review and meta-analysis of 83 studies of C-reactive protein in stable coronary artery disease. PLoS Med 7, e1000286.

Higazi, A.A., Lavi, E., Bdeir, K., Ulrich, A.M., Jamieson, D.G., Rader, D.J., Usher, D.C., Kane, W., Ganz, T. and Cines, D.B. (1997) Defensin stimulates the binding of lipoprotein (a) to human vascular endothelial and smooth muscle cells. Blood 89, 4290-8.

Hill, J.H. and Ward, P.A. (1971) The phlogistic role of C3 leukotactic fragments in myocardial infarcts of rats. J Exp Med 133, 885-900.

Hirschfield, G.M. and Pepys, M.B. (2003) C-reactive protein and cardiovascular disease: new insights from an old molecule. QJM 96, 793-807.

Holmskov, U., Thiel, S. and Jensenius, J.C. (2003) Collectins and ficolins: Humoral Lectins of the Innate Immune Defense. Annu Rev Immunol 21, 547-78.

Haahr-Pedersen, S., Bjerre, M., Flyvbjerg, A., Mogelvang, R., Dominquez, H., Hansen, T.K., Galatius, S., Bech, J., Madsen, J.K., Sogaard, P. and Jensen, J.S. (2009) Level of complement activity predicts cardiac dysfunction after acute myocardial infarction treated with primary percutaneous coronary intervention. J Invasive Cardiol 21, 13-9.

Ikeda, K., Sannoh, T., Kawasaki, N., Kawasaki, T. and Yamashina, I. (1987) Serum lectin with known structure activates complement through the classical pathway. J Biol Chem 262, 7451-4.

Ito, W., Schafer, H.J., Bhakdi, S., Klask, R., Hansen, S., Schaarschmidt, S., Schofer, J., Hugo, F., Hamdoch, T. and Mathey, D. (1996) Influence of the terminal complement-complex on reperfusion injury, no-reflow and arrhythmias: a comparison between C6-competent and C6-deficient rabbits. Cardiovasc Res 32, 294-305.

Jaye, D.L. and Waites, K.B. (1997) Clinical applications of C-reactive protein in pediatrics. Pediatr Infect Dis J 16, 735-46; quiz 746-7.

Jiang, H.X., Siegel, J.N. and Gewurz, H. (1991) Binding and complement activation by C-reactive protein via the collagen-like region of C1q and inhibition of these reactions by monoclonal antibodies to C-reactive protein and C1q. J Immunol 146, 2324-30.

Johnson, E. and Hetland, G. (1991) Human umbilical vein endothelial cells synthesize functional C3, C5, C6, C8 and C9 in vitro. Scand J Immunol 33, 667-71.

Joseph, G., Tarnow, L., Astrup, A.S., Hansen, T.K., Parving, H.H., Flyvbjerg, A. and Frystyk, J. (2008) Plasma alpha-defensin is associated with cardiovascular morbidity and mortality in type 1 diabetic patients. J Clin Endocrinol Metab 93, 1470-5.

Kaplan, M.H. and Volanakis, J.E. (1974) Interaction of C-reactive protein complexes with the complement system. I. Consumption of human complement associated with the reaction of C-reactive protein with pneumococcal C-polysaccharide and with the choline phosphatides, lecithin and sphingomyelin. J Immunol 112, 2135-47.

Kaptoge, S., Di Angelantonio, E., Lowe, G., Pepys, M.B., Thompson, S.G., Collins, R. and Danesh, J. (2010) C-reactive protein concentration and risk of coronary heart disease, stroke, and mortality: an individual participant meta-analysis. Lancet 375, 132-40.

Khalil, A.A., Aziz, F.A. and Hall, J.C. (2006) Reperfusion injury. Plast Reconstr Surg 117, 1024-33.

Khot, U.N., Khot, M.B., Bajzer, C.T., Sapp, S.K., Ohman, E.M., Brener, S.J., Ellis, S.G., Lincoff, A.M. and Topol, E.J. (2003) Prevalence of conventional risk factors in patients with coronary heart disease. JAMA 290, 898-904.

Kilgore, K.S., Flory, C.M., Miller, B.F., Evans, V.M. and Warren, J.S. (1996) The membrane attack complex of complement induces interleukin-8 and monocyte chemoattractant protein-1 secretion from human umbilical vein endothelial cells. Am J Pathol 149, 953-61.

Klotman, M.E. and Chang, T.L. (2006) Defensins in innate antiviral immunity. Nat Rev Immunol 6, 447-56.

Kones, R. (2010) Rosuvastatin, inflammation, C-reactive protein, JUPITER, and primary prevention of cardiovascular disease--a perspective. Drug Des Devel Ther 4, 383-413.

Kostner, K.M., Fahti, R.B., Case, C., Hobson, P., Tate, J. and Marwick, T.H. (2006) Inflammation, complement activation and endothelial function in stable and unstable coronary artery disease. Clin Chim Acta 365, 129-34.

Kougias, P., Chai, H., Lin, P.H., Yao, Q., Lumsden, A.B. and Chen, C. (2005) Defensins and cathelicidins: neutrophil peptides with roles in inflammation, hyperlipidemia and atherosclerosis. J Cell Mol Med 9, 3-10.

Kougias, P., Chai, H., Lin, P.H., Yao, Q., Lumsden, A.B. and Chen, C. (2006) Neutrophil antimicrobial peptide alpha-defensin causes endothelial dysfunction in porcine coronary arteries. J Vasc Surg 43, 357-63.

Kyrou, I. and Tsigos, C. (2007) Stress mechanisms and metabolic complications. Horm Metab Res 39, 430-8.

Langeggen, H., Berge, K.E., Macor, P., Fischetti, F., Tedesco, F., Hetland, G., Berg, K. and Johnson, E. (2001) Detection of mRNA for the terminal complement components C5, C6, C8 and C9 in human umbilical vein endothelial cells in vitro. APMIS 109, 73-8.

Langeggen, H., Pausa, M., Johnson, E., Casarsa, C. and Tedesco, F. (2000) The endothelium is an extrahepatic site of synthesis of the seventh component of the complement system. Clin Exp Immunol 121, 69-76.

Lavie, C.J., Milani, R.V. and Ventura, H.O. (2009a) Obesity and cardiovascular disease: risk factor, paradox, and impact of weight loss. J Am Coll Cardiol 53, 1925-32.

Lavie, C.J., Milani, R.V., Verma, A. and O'Keefe, J.H. (2009b) C-reactive protein and cardiovascular diseases--is it ready for primetime? Am J Med Sci 338, 486-92.

Lennon, P.F., Collard, C.D., Morrissey, M.A. and Stahl, G.L. (1996) Complement-induced endothelial dysfunction in rabbits: mechanisms, recovery, and gender differences. Am J Physiol 270, H1924-32.

Levinson, S.S., Miller, J.J. and Elin, R.J. (2004) Poor predictive value of high-sensitivity C-reactive protein indicates need for reassessment. Clin Chem 50, 1733-5.

Madjid, M., Awan, I., Willerson, J.T. and Casscells, S.W. (2004) Leukocyte count and coronary heart disease: implications for risk assessment. J Am Coll Cardiol 44, 1945-56.

Matsushita, M., Endo, Y., Hamasaki, N. and Fujita, T. (2001) Activation of the lectin complement pathway by ficolins. Int Immunopharmacol 1, 359-63.

McManus, L.M., Kolb, W.P., Crawford, M.H., O'Rourke, R.A., Grover, F.L. and Pinckard, R.N. (1983) Complement localization in ischemic baboon myocardium. Lab Invest 48, 436-47.

Mehta, J.L. and Li, D.Y. (1999) Inflammation in ischemic heart disease: response to tissue injury or a pathogenetic villain? Cardiovasc Res 43, 291-9.

Meier-Ewert, H.K., Ridker, P.M., Rifai, N., Price, N., Dinges, D.F. and Mullington, J.M. (2001) Absence of diurnal variation of C-reactive protein concentrations in healthy human subjects. Clin Chem 47, 426-30.

Mendall, M.A., Strachan, D.P., Butland, B.K., Ballam, L., Morris, J., Sweetnam, P.M. and Elwood, P.C. (2000) C-reactive protein: relation to total mortality, cardiovascular mortality and cardiovascular risk factors in men. Eur Heart J 21, 1584-90.

Mold, C. and Morris, C.A. (2001) Complement activation by apoptotic endothelial cells following hypoxia/reoxygenation. Immunology 102, 359-64.

Muller-Eberhard, H.J. (1988) Molecular organization and function of the complement system. Annu Rev Biochem 57, 321-47.

Nassar, H., Lavi, E., Akkawi, S., Bdeir, K., Heyman, S.N., Raghunath, P.N., Tomaszewski, J. and Higazi, A.A. (2007) alpha-Defensin: link between inflammation and atherosclerosis. Atherosclerosis 194, 452-7.

Neunteufl, T., Heher, S., Katzenschlager, R., Wolfl, G., Kostner, K., Maurer, G. and Weidinger, F. (2000) Late prognostic value of flow-mediated dilation in the brachial artery of patients with chest pain. Am J Cardiol 86, 207-10.

Niculescu, F. and Rus, H. (2001) Mechanisms of signal transduction activated by sublytic assembly of terminal complement complexes on nucleated cells. Immunol Res 24, 191-9.

Oppenheim, J.J., Biragyn, A., Kwak, L.W. and Yang, D. (2003) Roles of antimicrobial peptides such as defensins in innate and adaptive immunity. Ann Rheum Dis 62 Suppl 2, ii17-21.

Pasceri, V., Cheng, J.S., Willerson, J.T. and Yeh, E.T. (2001) Modulation of C-reactive protein-mediated monocyte chemoattractant protein-1 induction in human endothelial cells by anti-atherosclerosis drugs. Circulation 103, 2531-4.

Pasceri, V., Willerson, J.T. and Yeh, E.T. (2000) Direct proinflammatory effect of C-reactive protein on human endothelial cells. Circulation 102, 2165-8.

Pearson, T.A., Mensah, G.A., Alexander, R.W., Anderson, J.L., Cannon, R.O., 3rd, Criqui, M., Fadl, Y.Y., Fortmann, S.P., Hong, Y., Myers, G.L., Rifai, N., Smith, S.C., Jr., Taubert, K., Tracy, R.P. and Vinicor, F. (2003) Markers of inflammation and cardiovascular disease: application to clinical and public health practice: A statement for healthcare professionals from the Centers for Disease Control and Prevention and the American Heart Association. Circulation 107, 499-511.

Pepys, M.B., Hirschfield, G.M., Tennent, G.A., Gallimore, J.R., Kahan, M.C., Bellotti, V., Hawkins, P.N., Myers, R.M., Smith, M.D., Polara, A., Cobb, A.J., Ley, S.V., Aquilina, J.A., Robinson, C.V., Sharif, I., Gray, G.A., Sabin, C.A., Jenvey, M.C., Kolstoe, S.E., Thompson, D. and Wood, S.P. (2006) Targeting C-reactive protein for the treatment of cardiovascular disease. Nature 440, 1217-21.

Pinckard, R.N., O'Rourke, R.A., Crawford, M.H., Grover, F.S., McManus, L.M., Ghidoni, J.J., Storrs, S.B. and Olson, M.S. (1980) Complement localization and mediation of ischemic injury in baboon myocardium. J Clin Invest 66, 1050-6.

Quinn, K., Henriques, M., Parker, T., Slutsky, A.S. and Zhang, H. (2008) Human neutrophil peptides: a novel potential mediator of inflammatory cardiovascular diseases. Am J Physiol Heart Circ Physiol 295, H1817-24.

Ridker, P.M. (2007) C-reactive protein and the prediction of cardiovascular events among those at intermediate risk: moving an inflammatory hypothesis toward consensus. J Am Coll Cardiol 49, 2129-38.

Ridker, P.M., Cannon, C.P., Morrow, D., Rifai, N., Rose, L.M., McCabe, C.H., Pfeffer, M.A. and Braunwald, E. (2005) C-reactive protein levels and outcomes after statin therapy. N Engl J Med 352, 20-8.

Ridker, P.M., Fonseca, F.A., Genest, J., Gotto, A.M., Kastelein, J.J., Khurmi, N.S., Koenig, W., Libby, P., Lorenzatti, A.J., Nordestgaard, B.G., Shepherd, J., Willerson, J.T. and Glynn, R.J. (2007) Baseline characteristics of participants in the JUPITER trial, a randomized placebo-controlled primary prevention trial of statin therapy among individuals with low low-density lipoprotein cholesterol and elevated high-sensitivity C-reactive protein. Am J Cardiol 100, 1659-64.

Ridker, P.M., Hennekens, C.H., Buring, J.E. and Rifai, N. (2000a) C-reactive protein and other markers of inflammation in the prediction of cardiovascular disease in women. N Engl J Med 342, 836-43.

Ridker, P.M., MacFadyen, J., Libby, P. and Glynn, R.J. (2010) Relation of baseline high-sensitivity C-reactive protein level to cardiovascular outcomes with rosuvastatin in the Justification for Use of statins in Prevention: an Intervention Trial Evaluating Rosuvastatin (JUPITER). Am J Cardiol 106, 204-9.

Ridker, P.M., Rifai, N., Stampfer, M.J. and Hennekens, C.H. (2000b) Plasma concentration of interleukin-6 and the risk of future myocardial infarction among apparently healthy men. Circulation 101, 1767-72.

Riedemann, N.C. and Ward, P.A. (2003) Complement in ischemia reperfusion injury. Am J Pathol 162, 363-7.

Rosamond, W., Flegal, K., Friday, G., Furie, K., Go, A., Greenlund, K., Haase, N., Ho, M., Howard, V., Kissela, B., Kittner, S., Lloyd-Jones, D., McDermott, M., Meigs, J., Moy, C., Nichol, G., O'Donnell, C.J., Roger, V., Rumsfeld, J., Sorlie, P., Steinberger, J., Thom, T., Wasserthiel-Smoller, S. and Hong, Y. (2007) Heart disease and stroke statistics--2007 update: a report from the American Heart Association Statistics Committee and Stroke Statistics Subcommittee. Circulation 115, e69-171.

Ross, R. (1999) Atherosclerosis--an inflammatory disease. N Engl J Med 340, 115-26.

Rowe, I.F., Soutar, A.K., Trayner, I.M., Thompson, G.R. and Pepys, M.B. (1984) Circulating human C-reactive protein binds very low density lipoproteins. Clin Exp Immunol 58, 237-44.

Ryden, L., Standl, E., Bartnik, M., Van den Berghe, G., Betteridge, J., de Boer, M.J., Cosentino, F., Jonsson, B., Laakso, M., Malmberg, K., Priori, S., Ostergren, J., Tuomilehto, J., Thrainsdottir, I., Vanhorebeek, I., Stramba-Badiale, M., Lindgren, P., Qiao, Q., Priori, S.G., Blanc, J.J., Budaj, A., Camm, J., Dean, V., Deckers, J., Dickstein, K., Lekakis, J., McGregor, K., Metra, M., Morais, J., Osterspey, A., Tamargo, J., Zamorano, J.L., Deckers, J.W., Bertrand, M., Charbonnel, B., Erdmann, E., Ferrannini, E., Flyvbjerg, A., Gohlke, H., Juanatey, J.R., Graham, I., Monteiro, P.F., Parhofer, K., Pyorala, K., Raz, I., Schernthaner, G., Volpe, M. and Wood, D. (2007) Guidelines on diabetes, pre-diabetes, and cardiovascular diseases: executive summary. The Task Force on Diabetes and Cardiovascular Diseases of the European Society of Cardiology (ESC) and of the European Association for the Study of Diabetes (EASD). Eur Heart J 28, 88-136.

Saraheimo, M., Forsblom, C., Pettersson-Fernholm, K., Flyvbjerg, A., Groop, P.H. and Frystyk, J. (2008) Increased levels of alpha-defensin (-1, -2 and -3) in type 1 diabetic patients with nephropathy. Nephrol Dial Transplant 23, 914-8.

Shine, B., de Beer, F.C. and Pepys, M.B. (1981) Solid phase radioimmunoassays for human C-reactive protein. Clin Chim Acta 117, 13-23.

Siegel, J., Rent, R. and Gewurz, H. (1974) Interactions of C-reactive protein with the complement system. I. Protamine-induced consumption of complement in acute phase sera. J Exp Med 140, 631-47.

St-Pierre, A.C., Cantin, B., Bergeron, J., Pirro, M., Dagenais, G.R., Despres, J.P. and Lamarche, B. (2005) Inflammatory markers and long-term risk of ischemic heart disease in men A 13-year follow-up of the Quebec Cardiovascular Study. Atherosclerosis 182, 315-21.

Stahl, G.L., Reenstra, W.R. and Frendl, G. (1995) Complement-mediated loss of endothelium-dependent relaxation of porcine coronary arteries. Role of the terminal membrane attack complex. Circ Res 76, 575-83.

Thiel, S., Vorup-Jensen, T., Stover, C.M., Schwaeble, W., Laursen, S.B., Poulsen, K., Willis, A.C., Eggleton, P., Hansen, S., Holmskov, U., Reid, K.B. and Jensenius, J.C. (1997) A second serine protease associated with mannan-binding lectin that activates complement. Nature 386, 506-10.

Urbonaviciene, G., Frystyk, J., Flyvbjerg, A., Urbonavicius, S., Henneberg, E.W. and Lindholt, J.S. (2011) Markers of inflammation in relation to long-term cardiovascular mortality in patients with lower-extremity peripheral arterial disease. Int J Cardiol.

Vakeva, A., Morgan, B.P., Tikkanen, I., Helin, K., Laurila, P. and Meri, S. (1994) Time course of complement activation and inhibitor expression after ischemic injury of rat myocardium. Am J Pathol 144, 1357-68.

Vakeva, A.P., Agah, A., Rollins, S.A., Matis, L.A., Li, L. and Stahl, G.L. (1998) Myocardial infarction and apoptosis after myocardial ischemia and reperfusion: role of the terminal complement components and inhibition by anti-C5 therapy. Circulation 97, 2259-67.

Vinten-Johansen, J. (2004) Involvement of neutrophils in the pathogenesis of lethal myocardial reperfusion injury. Cardiovasc Res 61, 481-97.

Walport, M.J. (2001) Complement. First of two parts. N Engl J Med 344, 1058-66.

Walsh, M.C., Bourcier, T., Takahashi, K., Shi, L., Busche, M.N., Rother, R.P., Solomon, S.D., Ezekowitz, R.A. and Stahl, G.L. (2005) Mannose-binding lectin is a regulator of inflammation that accompanies myocardial ischemia and reperfusion injury. J Immunol 175, 541-6.

Wang, T.J., Gona, P., Larson, M.G., Tofler, G.H., Levy, D., Newton-Cheh, C., Jacques, P.F., Rifai, N., Selhub, J., Robins, S.J., Benjamin, E.J., D'Agostino, R.B. and Vasan, R.S. (2006) Multiple biomarkers for the prediction of first major cardiovascular events and death. N Engl J Med 355, 2631-9.

Yasojima, K., Kilgore, K.S., Washington, R.A., Lucchesi, B.R. and McGeer, P.L. (1998a) Complement gene expression by rabbit heart: upregulation by ischemia and reperfusion. Circ Res 82, 1224-30.

Yasojima, K., Schwab, C., McGeer, E.G. and McGeer, P.L. (1998b) Human heart generates complement proteins that are upregulated and activated after myocardial infarction. Circ Res 83, 860-9.

Yasojima, K., Schwab, C., McGeer, E.G. and McGeer, P.L. (2001) Generation of C-reactive protein and complement components in atherosclerotic plaques. Am J Pathol 158, 1039-51.

Yudkin, J.S., Stehouwer, C.D., Emeis, J.J. and Coppack, S.W. (1999) C-reactive protein in healthy subjects: associations with obesity, insulin resistance, and endothelial dysfunction: a potential role for cytokines originating from adipose tissue? Arterioscler Thromb Vasc Biol 19, 972-8.

Zacho, J., Tybjaerg-Hansen, A., Jensen, J.S., Grande, P., Sillesen, H. and Nordestgaard, B.G. (2008) Genetically elevated C-reactive protein and ischemic vascular disease. N Engl J Med 359, 1897-908.

Zhang, M., Michael, L.H., Grosjean, S.A., Kelly, R.A., Carroll, M.C. and Entman, M.L. (2006a) The role of natural IgM in myocardial ischemia-reperfusion injury. J Mol Cell Cardiol 41, 62-7.

Zhang, M., Takahashi, K., Alicot, E.M., Vorup-Jensen, T., Kessler, B., Thiel, S., Jensenius, J.C., Ezekowitz, R.A., Moore, F.D. and Carroll, M.C. (2006b) Activation of the lectin pathway by natural IgM in a model of ischemia/reperfusion injury. J Immunol 177, 4727-34.

Zimmerman, G.A., McIntyre, T.M., Prescott, S.M. and Otsuka, K. (1990) Brief review: molecular mechanisms of neutrophil binding to endothelium involving platelet-activating factor and cytokines. J Lipid Mediat 2 Suppl, S31-43.

Zwaka, T.P., Hombach, V. and Torzewski, J. (2001) C-reactive protein-mediated low density lipoprotein uptake by macrophages: implications for atherosclerosis. Circulation 103, 1194-7.

4

Measurement of Myocardial Contractility in the Ischemic Heart – A Disease Immanent Uncertainty

Jens Broscheit
Department of Anethesiology, University Clinics of Würzburg
Germany

1. Introduction

The present compilation of scientific publications deals with the evaluation of a parameter of myocardial contractility (E'_{es}); the parameter can be exclusively measured using ultrasound, i.e. noninvasive and can be used for a load-independent quantification of myocardial contractility.

The standard procedure for measuring left ventricular (LV) contractility is by use of a conductance catheter with which LV volume and LV pressure can be determined simultaneously. In 1973, Sagawa (1) was the first to use this catheter, which had been developed at the University Hospital Leiden, and he was able to show that an elastance curve can be determined from a series of loop diagrams which were obtained under acute preload reduction. The slope of the elastance curve (E_{es}) increased when the positive inotropic substance isoprenaline was administered (Fig. 1).

For clinical use, however, the catheter is a monitoring procedure which is too invasive and thus involves too many risks; in the past few years there have been considerations to replace this procedure with one that is less invasive.

In 1994, Gorscan (2) presented a study with which he was able to show that LV volume can be estimated by continuous echocardiographic determination of the cross-sectional LV area and in 1997 Deanault from the same working group (3) showed that LV pressure can be approximated with the pressure from the radial artery. They generated a loop diagram from these surrogate parameters with which they could estimate LV contractility. In the years 2001-2003 the mathematicians Danielsen, Ottesen and Paladino (4-6) from the University of Roskilde published a model equation from which we deduce that, with simplified assumptions, the Doppler sonographic arterial flow would have to change in proportion to pressure and we asked ourselves if contractility could also be estimated with a flow-area relationship.

2. Question

The thoughts presented here are a model for measuring LV contractility as it could be determined in the patient, i.e. exclusively based on ultrasound and thus not very invasive.

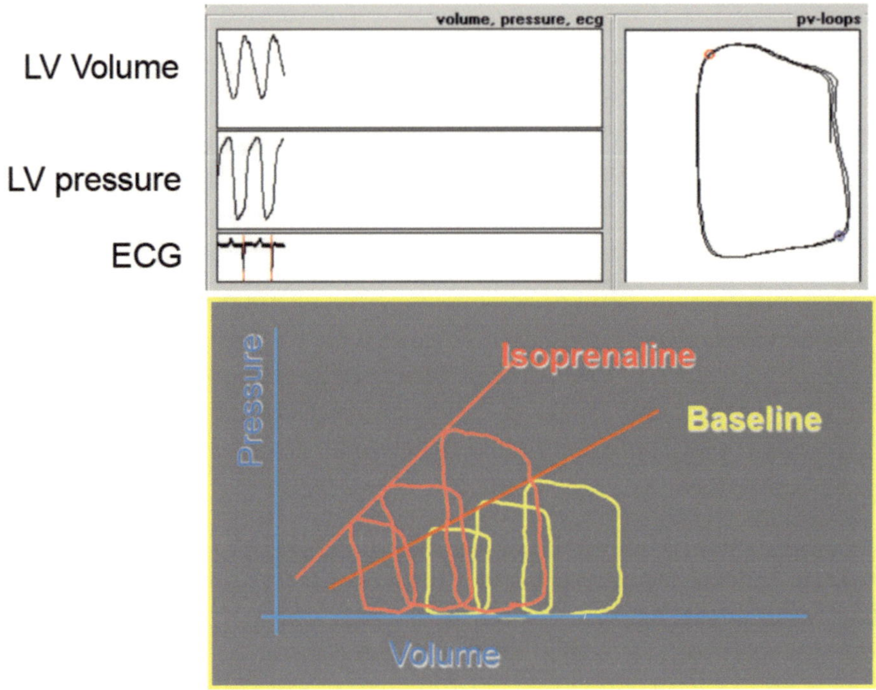

Sagawa K, et al. Am J Cardiol 1977; 40:748-753

Fig. 1. Determination of the properties of elastance curves

This raises the question of whether contractility can in fact be estimated using the index E'_{es}, which has been deduced from this theoretical model.

If the elastance of the flow-area relationship is exclusively considered as a surrogate parameter to estimate myocardial contractility in the classical sense, then E'_{es} is not a new parameter. If it is assumed, however, that the elastance of the flow-area relationship is based on a completely new mathematical model, i.e. that of the mathematicians Danielsen, Ottesen and Paladino, then we are possibly dealing with a new parameter and deviations between the classical parameter E_{es} and E'_{es} are then starting points for new examinations.

3. Background

Ultrasound-based determination of myocardial contractility: theoretical principles

The ability to actively shorten the cardiac muscle, i.e. of contractility, of the left ventricle is based on a complex process (7,8) during which individual mechanisms have to follow one another precisely. Muscle contraction is based on mechanisms and interactions associated with muscle proteins, enzymes, ions and energy sources. The large-scale structure, as well as the small-scale structure of the muscle, are involved in the contractility of the hollow muscular organ which forms the left chamber of the heart or left ventricle. Apart from power transmission towards contraction, the prevention or diversion of shearing forces is an important task which the muscle carries out through mechanisms of mechanical connections, but also through mechanisms of regulation by synchronizing the contraction of the muscle fibers.

First attempts to describe the contractility of a hollow muscular organ from a mechanical point of view date back to Otto Frank in 1985 (9). Frank determined the pressure of the individual end-diastolic volumes by conducting experiments with a single chamber frog heart as well as the maximum pressure recruitable from this relaxation period (isovolumeric maximum) and the maximum ejection fraction (isotonic or isobaric maximum). The curves established from this resulted in a pressure-volume diagram in which the maximums to be achieved from the relaxation period were connected through the contraction curve (2). Otto Frank deduced the cardiac cycle from this:

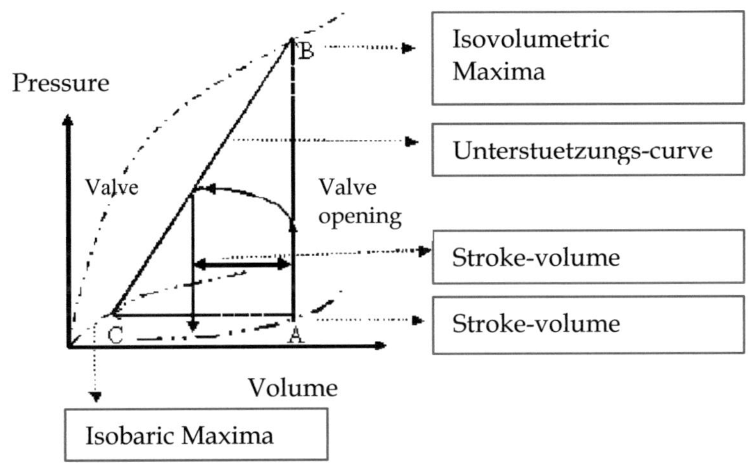

Fig. 2. LV pressure-volume diagram by Otto Frank.

The ventricle is filled with volume (preload) and during the process internal pressure in the chamber increases. Then the pressure in the chamber increases through contraction along the isometric maximum against the closed valve until the valve opens which, during the relaxation phase (diastole), prevents reflux from the aorta into the ventricle. While the heart is pumping out volume against the arterial load (afterload), it is pumping in the sense of an auxotonic contraction; this leads to a further increase of arterial pressure and to a decrease in volume through ejection in the ventricle. During the following relaxation phase the pressure in the ventricle decreases to reach its resting level and the chamber is filled again. The cardiac cycle can thus be described through a pressure-volume relationship which is known as the "work diagram" in literature.

In later experiments, Starling (10) deduced the s-shaped connection between the surface of the work diagram and the necessary preload. The two main differences between the concept described by Otto Frank and the one developed by Starling are that the contraction of the left ventricle cannot only be described as a function of filling or preload, but also as a function of time. Another difference is that when it comes to measurements, the left ventricular function is always determined in connection with the arterial vascular system behind it.

In 1959, Warner deduced the calculation of ventricular compliance C from the correlation described by Frank by relating volume V_v and the corresponding pressure P_v at the end of diastole and at the end of systole

$$C = \frac{V_v}{P_v}$$

and thus created a constant. From this formal approach, two different mathematical terms for the description of LV contraction can be concluded. In 1961, Seelen (11) described contraction through fixed capacitive reactance in series with pressure varying depending on time and in 1973, Suga (1) defined ventricular elastance *E(t)* through an inverse function of the compliance *C(t)* function.

$$E(t) = \frac{P_v(t)}{V_v(t) - V_d}$$

with the SI-unit [$m^{-4} \bullet kg \bullet s^{-2}$], while V_d represents constant, diastolic volume. The index (t) in this case means that the end-systolic point was determined using an iterative method in which the same loop is crossed by a tangent several times and with varying time (time-varying elastance). In the experimental determination of *E(t)*, the same problems arise as in the correlation already developed by Starling. The index *E(t)* cannot be determined separately from the vascular system and it is not a function of time.

To get around these problems, Beneken 1965 (12) developed a closed-loop model of the cardiovascular system, which was based on the work of Liljestrand 1938 (13) and Hill 1922 (14), and in which contraction of the heart is calculated through the contractile element described by Hill, embedded in a three-element windkessel model. Further geometrical adjustments yielded an n-element model, which was mathematically described with the finite-element method.

Based on the evaluation described by Hill, Danielsen (4) later developed a model which differentiated between an isovolumetric ventricle and an ejecting left ventricle under arterial load. In the latter model, the direct proportional correlation between arterial pressure P_a and LV outflow Q_v was deduced as follows:

$$\dot{P}_s = -\frac{1}{R_s C_s} P_s + \frac{1}{C_s} Q_v,$$

with R_s as a global peripheral resistance, R_0 as characteristic aortic impedance, C_s as total arterial compliance, P_s as systolic pressure and P_s as the change of arterial pressure with time. This equation can be transformed to This equation can be transformed to:

$$\dot{Q}_v = -\frac{1}{L_v} P_s - \frac{R_0}{L_v} Q_v + \frac{1}{L_v} P_v(t,V),$$

with L_v as inductance directly above the aortic valve and Q_v as a change of flow with time. With the simplified assumption that L_v is constant, the above equation can be simplified as follows.

$$P_a = P_s + R_0 Q_v$$

With the assumption that R_0 is constant and P_a changes in direct proportion to P_s the equation is:

$$P_a \approx Q_v$$

Olufsen (15) showed in his one-dimensional dynamic model of the systemic arteries that, corresponding to the Navier-Stokes equation, pressure changes directly proportional to flow in large vessels such as the arteria carotis communis. The model-based experimental examinations confirm that the flow generated through the left ventricle is the connecting link between the heart and vessel blood system.

Against this backdrop, our work group had the idea of developing an index E'_{es},, analogous to $E(t)$, based on the iteratively determined end-systolic points on the work diagram. This index E'_{es} was to be determined by $V_d(t)$ and blood flow $V_v(t)$ of an artery in proximity to the heart:

$$E'_{es} = \frac{V_v(t)}{V_v(t) - V_d}$$

with the SI unit [s-1]. The ventricular volume, measured during several cardiac cycles, can be determined using ultrasound technology by estimating it with the help of the surface A in the transgastral short-axis-view. Blood flow Q can be estimated through the blood flow velocity F in the arteria carotis communis measured with the Doppler technology. This then yields the following equation:

$$E'_{es} = \frac{F_v(t)}{A_v(t) - A_d}$$

The deduced index E'_{es} displays the following important differences compared to the index E_{es} :

1. By implementing blood flow velocity, the index becomes a function of time.
2. By measuring blood flow velocity in a large artery, the index becomes connected to the vascular system.
3. Through the measuring method used, the index E'_{es} can be completely determined in a noninvasive way, as both *F* and *A* are ultrasound parameters.

Measuring methods used

The measuring methods used in this context are conductance and ultrasound methods. Using these methods, myocardial contractility was measured.

Conductance catheter method

A conductance catheter was used for the simultaneous recording of LV pressure and the volume signal (16). The catheter consists of pressure-conductivity transducers. While the blood pressure signal was mechanically measured at the tip of the catheter using a pressure transducer and was subsequently transformed into electric impulses, determination of volume is carried out electromagnetically by measuring the conductivity of the surrounding compartments. The catheter consists of four electrodes and one pressure sensor. The electrodes are fitted below the pressure sensor in pairs. The measurement of cardiac blood volumes using these electrodes is based on an electric field which is established through the outer electrodes in the left ventricle. Two potential differences at the inner electrodes are continuously recorded to measure the conductance between the electrodes in the ventricle.

With the formula

$$V_i(t) = \frac{1}{\alpha} \bullet \rho L_{a^2}(G_i(t) - G_{pi})$$

intraventricular volume V(t) is calculated. With a being a volume calibration factor, *p* being the electric resistance of blood, *L* being the distance between the electrodes, G_i describing the overall conductance and G_{pi} describing the conductance of the surrounding tissue; this conductance is called "parallel conductance". This calculation makes a continuous and in vivo recording of volumes in real-time possible.

Ultrasound method

Using the ultrasound-Doppler method, the flow velocity of erythrocytes can be measured with the help of the Doppler effect. The Doppler effect arises because echoes reflected by the erythrocytes have higher or lower frequencies than the signals sent out, depending on the flow velocity and flow direction. The differences in frequency are implemented electronically in readable and recordable curves. In the continuous-wave Doppler (CW Doppler) technique, which is used for detection, one transmitter and one receiver work simultaneously and continuously in the transducer. By mixing it with suitable high frequency signals and with electronic filters, the spectrum of the Doppler frequencies or velocities and the direction can be determined from the returning wave in the evaluation electronics. The disadvantage of this method is that it is not possible to determine the base range of the Doppler echo; however, even relatively high velocities can be recorded.

With the two-dimensional, light-modulated presentation of the echoes, an immediately visible, animated picture is generated through energy and intensity proportional light points that vary according to brightness and as a result of a scan carried out in two directions and in layers. Tissue structures become visible because the points that are represented in shades of gray in relation to the intensity of the echo - as far as they originate from comparable structures - flow together to form areas and lines. The semi-automatic detection of contours serves to detect endocardial interfaces within the "region of interest" (ROI). Semi-automatic contour tracking is based on a seeded ROI algorithm which combines all adjacent pixels within a user-defined signal intensity area. The selected (seed) pixel is the starting point. In automatic segmentation, a small ROI can be positioned in the area of interest. The signal intensity area important for the growth algorithm is automatically taken from the ROI statistics (minimum to maximum value). The area defined in this way can be corrected interactively. For an ROI correction, the boundaries are activated by a click of the mouse. These boundaries can also be corrected interactively. After having selected the acoustic windows relevant for the approximation of volume - transgastral short-axis-view of the left ventricle - the window setting at an end-diastolic phase image was adjusted to achieve an ideal contrast for the detection of endocardial boundaries. This window setting as well as the curves of the ventricular area presented in the ultrasound image were then checked in all phase images of the cardiac cycle. This setting was used for the following examinations.

Measuring parameters

End-systolic elastance is derived from the end-systolic pressure-volume relation (ESPVR). The elastance model was introduced by Sagawa and Suga. (17). Using isolated rabbit hearts, they made the observation that the end-systolic pressure volume coordinates move along a straight line in the case of acute preload reduction. This could also be observed when acute preload reduction occurred at different levels of dilatation of the left ventricle (Fig. 1) is it a picture legend? A difference is made between two elastances: time-dependent elastance E_{max} and time-varying elastance E_{es}.

In this model, E_{max} describes the slope of the end-systolic linear regression curves.

In this context the time-dependent elastance E(t) from the equation

$$E(t) = \frac{P(t)}{V(t) - VL(t)}$$

is determined, with P(t) = instantaneous intraventricular pressure; V(t) = instantaneous intraventricular volume; V0 = volume, if P(t) = 0. E_{es} is elastance at the point in time when E(t) reaches its maximum, i.e. when active contraction is at its maximum. E_{es} is calculated from the slope of the linear regression curves, which is time-varying and results from the maximum of the points.

$$\frac{P}{V - V_0}$$

The calculation of maximum is repeated several times through fixed point iteration until the slope of the line is constant. E_{es} is determined if, in case of fluctuations in afterload, the time in which the end-systolic state is reached fluctuates and consequently ESPVR does not exactly meet the angle of the loop diagram and E_{max} is calculated from points which lie ahead of the end-systolic one. E_{max} is then steeper than E_{es}. While E_{max} is the basis for models concerning the mathematical adjustment of the left ventricular function, E_{es} is used for the experimental quantification of LV contractility. The calculation formula for the indices E_{max} and E_{es} is not presented in a consistent manner in literature, however. The index E'_{es} was determined analogous to the index Ees, with the difference that the flow-volume diagram was the basis for calculation

A positive inotropic effect, induced through dobutamine, can be observed through an increase of E_{es}, i.e. an increase in the slope of the linear regression curves. The opposite occurs in decreasing inotropy, when it is triggered by a β- receptor blocker like esmolol (Fig. 1) is it a picture legend?, for instance.

Hemodynamic interventions

The main goal of the studies were the controlled, targeted and pathophysiological interventions with sequential application of dobutamine, esmolol, akrinor, hydroxyethyl starch and sodium nitroprusside, with which the degree of correspondence of the two measuring methods was determined. The properties of these substances, which will be described in the following section, were the reason for them being used.

Modification of contractility through dobutamine and esmolol

Dobutamine has the effect of an α1-, β1- and β2-agonist, while β1 stimulation of the heart is the most immediate effect. The main effects of dobutamine result from this, i.e. the increase of contractility of the myocardial cells and a dosage-dependent marked increase in heart rate. This leads to increased stroke volume (SV) and cardiac output (CO). The substance has a short half-life period of approx. 2 minutes and is broken down in inactive metabolites. It is thus applied per continuitatem. needs spell check here – it is the latin spelling and ok!.

Esmolol has the effect of a β1-antagonist and is thus cardioselective at the myocardium. The main effects are a decrease in heart rate and the inhibition of contractility. This leads to a decrease in stroke volume and in cardiac output. The half-life period is only approx. 9 minutes, as esmolol, in contrast to other beta blockers, is not broken down in an organ-dependent way, but is metabolized by esterases hydrolases. For this reason, esmolol has to be administered in a continuous or repetitive way.

Modification of load through hydroxyethyl starch, akrinor and sodium nitroprusside

In statistics or kinematics, load is a unit of measurement for the force that works on a medium. Accordingly and as far as the left ventricle is concerned, preload is the force that results in the extension of fibers at the end of diastole or directly before systole and which is limited by the maximum resting length of the muscle fiber. Afterload is a force influencing the ventricle; this force counteracts ejection out of the ventricle into the cardiovascular system. In practice, preload is referred to as the end-diastolic volume in the heart. The fact that the standard index E_{es} is load-independent , i.e. that changes in preload and afterload of the left ventricle mostly do not change the contractility index over wide periods, is an important characteristic of this measurement. Changes in load induce changes in contraction force, contractility remains unchanged, however.

Hydroxyethyl starch is a synthetically produced polymer and, like dextrane, and gelatine is used for the substitution of intravascular volume. End-diastolic volume was thus increased.

Akrinor is a fixed combination of the two active ingredients cafedrin and theodrenaline. Blood pressure is primarily increased through an alpha-receptor-mediated, arterial vasoconstriction. Then contractility and heart rate are slightly increased through a less intense stimulation of beta receptors.

Apart from inhibiting guanylate cyclase and consecutively releasing nitric oxide in the smooth musculature of the vascular wall, sodium nitroprusside has a vasodilative effect on both at the resistance vessels of the arterial system and at the capacitance vessels of the venous system. Due to the short half-life period of less than 10 minutes, continuous administration is necessary.

4. Determination of preload recruitable stroke work and elastance by the relation of arterial blood flow velocity to left ventricular area

The question whether contractility can be estimated with a flow-area relationship was the starting point for this study.

In a first animal experiment, 8 Göttinger minipigs were studied in an open chest preparation. An arterial manometer was placed in the femoral artery and a microtip catheter for the measurement of LV pressure was advanced into the left ventricle from the apex. A flexible TEE probe was fixed on the myocardium to sonographically estimate volume with LV area measurement. Finally, the arteria carotis communis was dissected to fix a U-shaped 8-MHz CW Doppler probe on it. Then an inferior vena cava occlusion was performed to reduce preload. A central venous catheter was implanted for the pharmacological intervention. Via this catheter, contractility was sequentially increased by the administration of dobutamine, it was decreased by the administration of the beta-blocker esmolol and preload was significantly increased with a plasma expander. A software exclusively developed by the Institute of Experimental Physics was used for data acquisition as well as data presentation and analysis (Fig. 3). During the examination we began to realize that we were generating loop diagrams and could calculate elastance.

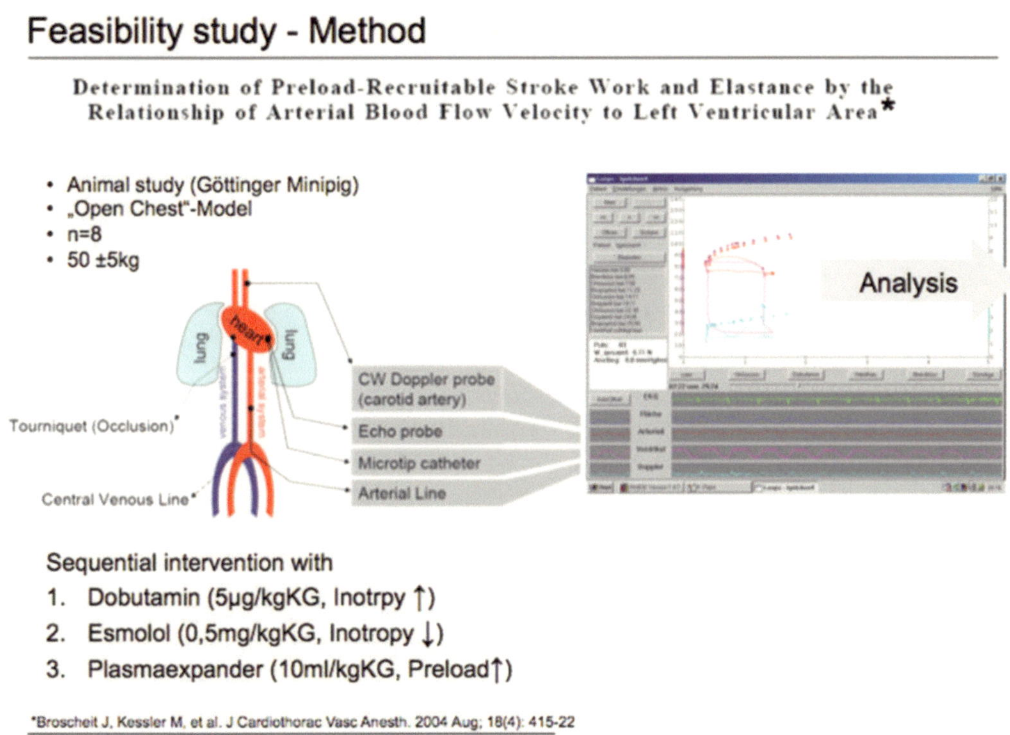

Fig. 3. Diagram for the experiment set-up of the study "Determination of Preload Recruitable Stroke Work and Elastance by the Relation of Arterial Blood Flow Velocity to Left Ventricular Area".

The data in table 2 (3b) show that the change in contractility was reliably detected through the change of slope of the individual elastance curves. A change of preload through the plasma expander did not influence the slope of the elastance curves.

To sum up, this study showed that contractility can be estimated with parameters which are deduced from flow-area relationships.

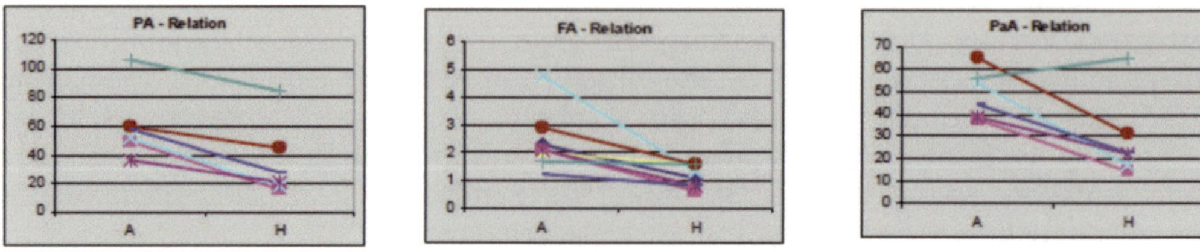

Abbreviations: PA – LVpressure vs. LVarea relation [mmHg/cm^2]
FA – blood flow velocity vs. LVarea relation [cm/s/cm^2]
PaA- art. rad vs. LVarea relation [mmHg/cm^2]

	PA - Relation			**FA - Relation**			**PaA- Relation**		
	B	**E**	**Δ**	**B**	**E**	**Δ**	**B**	**E**	**Δ**
Mean	**60.0**	**34.5**	**45.4***	**2.4**	**1.2**	**45.3***	**49.2**	**29.9**	**42.6 ***
± SD	**± 24.0**	**± 22.7**	**± 20.0**	**± 1.1**	**± 10.8**	**± 24.2**	**± 15.9**	**± 0.4**	**± 30.2**

B = baseline, E = Esmolol 0.5 mg/kgBW,
Δ = increase of the slope in %, * =signtest p < 0,05

→ Inotropic changes can be detected by the flow-area relation

Fig. 3b. Feasibility study - Results

5. Time-varying elastance concept applied to the relation of carotid arterial flow velocity and left ventricular area

In the previous study, changes in inotropy could in fact be detected with the help of the flow-area relationship and the following study was to answer the question as to how this procedure corresponds to the standard procedure.

In an animal experiment, 25 Göttinger minipigs were studied in a closed chest preparation. After a puncture of the femoral artery, the conductance catheter was placed in the left ventricle under fluoroscopy. The cross-sectional LV area was determined in this study using a transthoracic probe and the arteria carotis communis was studied as before. A pulmonalis catheter was used for the calibration of the conductance catheter and a Forgarty catheter, which was advanced into the inferior vena cava, was used for preload reduction. The central venous catheter served as a line for the pharmacological interventions. Like in the previous study, contractility was sequentially increased by the administration of dobutamine, it was decreased by the administration of the beta-blocker esmolol and preload was significantly increased with a plasma expander. Additionally, afterload reduction was induced through akrinor.

For the collection and processing of data, software developed by Paul Steendijk from the experimental cardiology of the University Leiden was used in this study. Pressure volumes and flow-area relationships could be described using this software. The elastance of the LV pressure-volume relationship is referred to as E_{es} in literature and we called the elastance of the flow-area relationship E'_{es}.

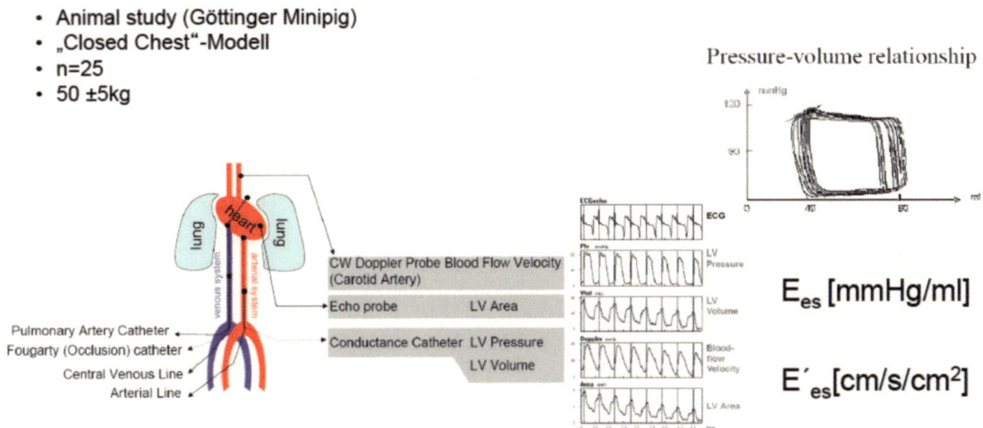

Fig. 4. Diagram for the experiment set-up of the study "Time-Varying Elastance Concept Applied to the Relation of Carotid Arterial Flow Velocity and Left Ventricular Area"

n = 25	Baseline	Dobutamine	Esmolol	Akrinor	Volume
HR (bpm)	64 ± 11	94 ± 32*	56 ± 7	64 ± 23	60 ± 19
E_{es} (mmHg/mL)	5.8 ± 3.04	10.1 ± 4.19*	3.7 ± 2.4*	8.31 ± 3.58	6.1 ± 2.8
E'_{es} (cm³/min)	0.68 ± 0.288	1.24 ± 0.458*	0.44 ± 0.15*	0.98 ± 0.379	0.69 ± 0.283

NOTE. All interventions were performed after complete reversal of hemodynamic changes to baseline. HR, heart rate; Ees, time-varying elastance; E´es, time-varying elastance of velocity; LV, area relation; *$p < 0.05$ versus baseline.

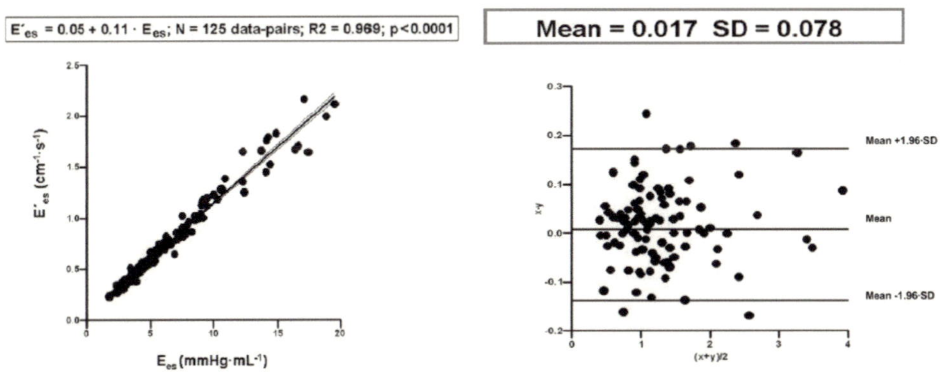

→ acceptable agreement of both methods

Broscheit J, Steendijk P, et al. J Cardiothorac Vasc Anesth. 2006 Jun;20(3):340-6.

Fig. 4b. Validational study (Conductance-Catheter) - Results

In relation to the initial values, the values obtained from both procedures displayed changes in inotropy. A regression analysis was carried out using the pooled data. A significant linear correlation between the two measuring methods became evident. The Blant-Altman analysis showed that both methods correspond to each other acceptably.

6. The relationship between carotid blood-flow velocity and left ventricular area during acute regional ischemia

This study was to answer the question as to how the two measuring methods would correspond to each other in the case of a myocardial wall motion abnormality.

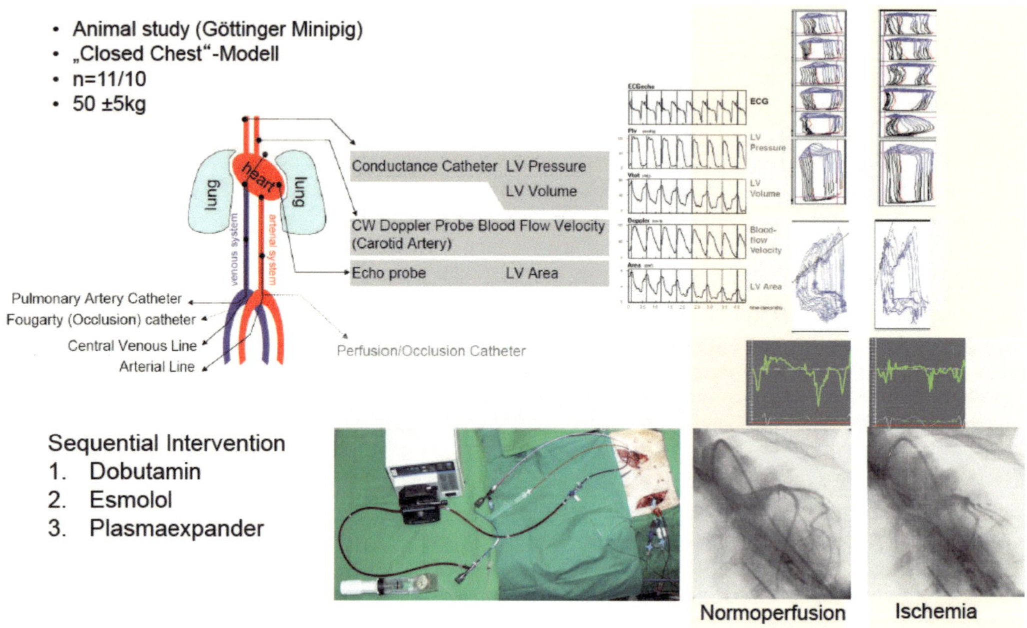

Fig. 5. Diagram for the experimental set-up of the study "The Relationship between Carotid Blood-flow Velocity and Left Ventricular Area during Acute Regional Ischemia".

In an animal experiment, 11 Göttinger minipigs were studied in a closed chest preparation. We advanced a coronary occlusion-perfusion catheter into the ramus circumflexus of the left coronary artery from the arteria femoralis. This catheter makes it possible to occlude a coronary artery while at the same time perfusing it with arterial blood using an adjustable roller pump. Standardized reduction of myocardial wall motion in the circulation area of the coronary artery was monitored by determining the systolic, radial strain rate. The strain rate is the rate of myocardial deformation and thus a unit of measurement for myocardial function. As the arteria femoralis was being used by the catheter, we advanced the conductance catheter through the right arteria carotis communis. Apart from that, preparation was the same as in the previous study.

Fig. 4 shows the loop diagram under normal perfusion and under ischemic conditions. The segmental loops of the conductance catheter deform under ischemia in the corresponding areas. This deformation was used for the calculation of an internal flow fraction, which arises when myocardial contraction cannot be completely transformed into an arterial flow.

	Baseline	Dobutamine	Esmolol	Ringer's Lactate	Perfusion State
E_{es} (mmHg/mL)	6.9 ± 2.7	12.8 ± 5.4*	4.4 ± 1.[illegible]*	6.4 ± 2.3	Normal
E_{es} (mmHg/ mL)	7.7 ± 4.2	11.8 ± 5.9*	4.9 ± 2.[illegible]*	5.0 ± 1.5	Ischemic
E'_{es} (mL/s/cm²)	0.54 ± 0.18	1.15 ± 0.42*	0.38 ± 0.14*	0.56 ± 0.13	Normal
E'_{es} (mL/s/cm²)	0.59 ± 0.12	0.88 ± 0.32*	0.37 ± 0.15*	0.41 ± 0.11*†	Ischemic
IFF_{sys} (%)	10 ± 17.7	12 ± 14	11 ± 8.9	21 ± 12.9	Normal
IFF_{sys} (%)	37 ± 24.7†	27 ± 24.5	35 ± 20.7†	21 ± 12.9*	Ischemic

NOTE. Normal perfused myocardium n=11; ischemic conditions, n=10. Abbreviations: Ees, end-systolic elastance calculated from the pressure-volume relation; E=es, end-systolic elastance calculated from the flow-area relation; IFFsys, systolic internal flow fraction. *Significance versus corresponding baseline value ($p<0.05$), †Significance versus corresponding nonischemic value ($p<0.05$).

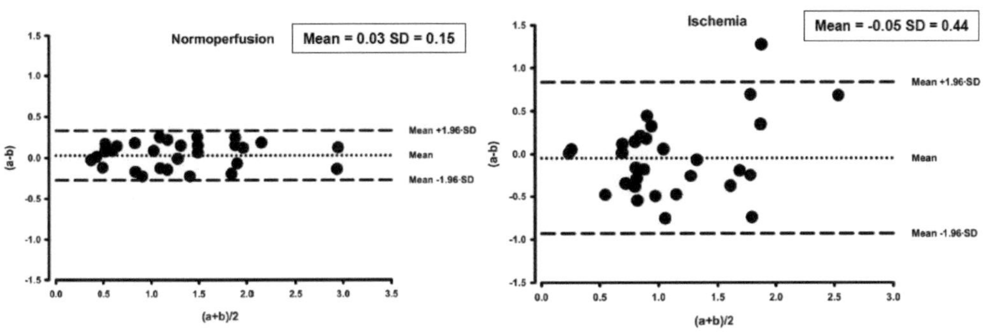

→ Decreasing agreement of both methods

Broscheit J, Weidemann F, Strotmann J, et al. J Cardiothorac Vasc Anesth. 2008 Dec;22(6):823-31.

Fig. 5b. Validational study during regional ischemia - Results

As the graph is directly taken from another journal, please get the copyright. I do realize that the author for this chapter is also the author for that article. However, the copyright need to be obtained as a formality from the journal. Table 1 (III 5b) shows that both procedures, independent of myocardial perfusion, could detect changes in inotropy. What stands out, however, is that the application of a plasma expander under myocardial ischemia leads to significant changes of the slope of the flow-area relationship compared to the initial values. The internal flow fraction also changed significantly under these conditions. Regression analysis in Fig. 5 (do you mean 5b? 5 is not a statistical analysis under ischemic conditions showed a decrease in the regression coefficient, linear correlation remained significant, however. The Bland-Alman analysis in Fig. 6 showed that the correspondence of the two parameters decreases.

The results of the study carried out showed that a valid assessment of myocardial contractility is possible with the flow-area relationship. Myocardial wall motion abnormalities constitute a limitation of the procedure.

7. Dobutamine induces ineffective work in regional ischaemic myocardium: An experimental strain rate imaging study

This study is to answer the question as to whether the results of the previous study can also be reflected by parameters of regional contractility.

In an animal experiment, 11 Göttinger minipigs were studied in a closed chest preparation. We advanced a coronary occlusion-perfusion catheter into the ramus circumflexus of the left coronary artery from the arteria femoralis. This catheter makes it possible to occlude a coronary artery while at the same time perfusing it with arterial blood using an adjustable roller pump. Standardized reduction of myocardial wall motion in the circulation area of the coronary artery was monitored by determining the strain rate. Apart from that, radial strain of the myocardium during systole was also determined. Strain is a unit of measurement for myocardial deformation. As the arteria femoralis was occupied by the catheter, we advanced the conductance catheter through the right arteria carotis communis.

The results show that a decrease of radial strain in the ischemic region can be documented under regional ischemia. Parallel to this, regional ischemia led to an increase in radial strain in the non ischemic myocardium. The stimulation of contractility with dobutamine intensifies the effect.

The present results confirm those of the previous study, i.e. that regional ischemia of the myocardium of 30% does not lead to a decrease of global contractility because contractility of the myocardium of the non-ischemic region is increased in a compensatory way. The increase of internal flow fraction is based on this effect, as has been shown in the previous study.

8. The relationship between carotid arterial flow and the left ventricular area is valid to indicate contractility in states of cerebral autoregulation and decreased arterial pressure

The present study is based on the question as to whether both measuring methods correspond under the condition of an arterial hypotension. Hypotension can activate mechanisms which, independent of systemic blood pressure, ensure constant blood flow in important organs such as the heart. To determine the flow-area relationship, we measure flow velocity in large vessels which supply the brain with blood; for this reason these mechanisms could have an effect on the flow-area relationship.

In an animal experiment, we studied 9 merino sheep and measured cortical microperfusion (flux) with the laser Doppler and we also determined tissue oxygen partial pressure ($p_{(ti)}O_2$) and tissue metabolism through microdialysis. We proceeded as in a validation study, the difference being that we fixed the TEE probe onto the myocardium with a minithoracotomy.

Arterial blood pressure was, on the one hand, decreased by esmolol and on the other hand by the pure vasodilator sodium nitroprusside. Both pharmaceuticals were dosed in such a way that a mean arterial pressure of 50mmHg could be maintained for 20 minutes.

The table shows that the hypotension triggered by sodium nitroprusside did not lead to any other changes of the circulatory system and of the cortical and myocardial parameters. The hypotension triggered by esmolol, however, led to a decrease in cardiac output and to an increase in LV end-diastolic pressure. This was associated with a decrease in cortical microcirculation as well as with a decrease in tissue oxygen partial pressure. During the decrease in tissue oxygen partial pressure, the metabolites of the anaerobic metabolism increased. Furthermore an increase in internal flow fraction (IFF_{sys}) could be observed, indicating myocardial wall motion abnormalities. The hypotension triggered by esmolol led to a critical decrease of oxygen being supplied to the cortex and to the myocardium.

As in the previous studies, a linear correlation between flow-area relationship and LV pressure could be detected under the influence of sodium nitroprusside. The correlation between the two relationships was acceptable as the Bland-Altman analysis shows. The decrease of contractility induced by esmolol was also detected through the flow-area relationship. But the degree of correlation and the degree of correspondence of both parameters decreased significantly. This decrease probably results from an increase of the internal flow fraction as an indication of myocardial wall motion abnormalities. This correlation could already be detected in the previous studies. It remains unclear, however, which hemodynamic constellation led to the wall motion abnormalities - the increase in end-diastolic volume and/ or the decrease of cardiac output. Both parameters determine myocardial perfusion.

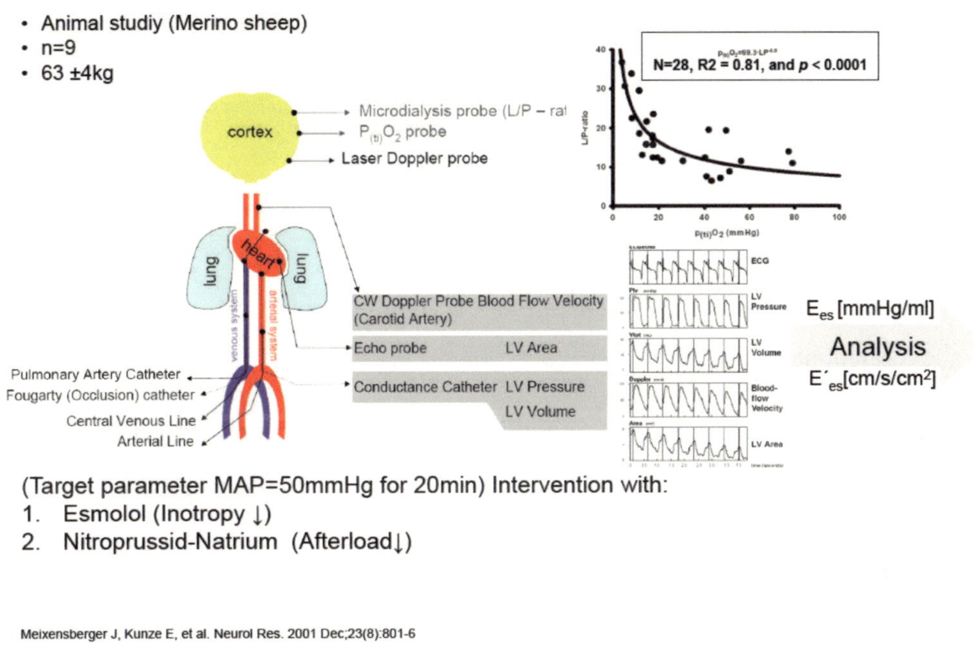

Fig. 6. Diagram for the experiment set-up of the study "The Relationship between Carotid Arterial Flow and the Left Ventricular Area is valid to indicate contractility in states of cerebral autoregulation and decreased arterial pressure

An increase in end-diastolic volume is connected with an increase in left ventricular radius. According to the law of Laplace, the increase in radius is tantamount to an increase in myocardial wall tension in diastole. During diastole the myocardium is perfused an increase in wall tension can lead to a decrease of coronary blood flow which means that oxygen supply is higher than oxygen demand. In this context, myocardial wall motion abnormalities can occur as an indication of hypoperfusion. A decrease in cardiac output is directly connected to a decrease of oxygen supply to all organs, i.e. also to the myocardium, which can result in insufficient oxygen supply.

The results of the study carried out showed that a valid assessment of myocardial contractility is possible with the flow-area relationship.

	Baseline	SNP	Esmolol
MAP [mmHg]	90 ±16	50 ±1#	48 ±6#
E_{es} [mmHg·cm^{-3}]	3.0 ±0.9	3.0 ±0.7	1.0 ±0.2#,+
E'_{es} [cm^{-3}]	0.89 ±0.24	0.76 ±0.27	0.36 ±0.21#,+
Flux [mm·s^{-1}]	1	0.84 ±0.20	0.63 ±0.30#
$p_{(ti)}O_2$ [mmHg]	33 ±23	34 ±7	14 ±13#,+
L/P-ratio [-]	12 ±3	19 ±8	28 ±15#,+

NOTE: Mean ± standard deviation; n = 9

Abbreviations: Ees, endsystolic elastance; E´es end-systolic elastance of the flow velocity-area relationship; Flux – cortical microcirculation; L/P-ratio, ratio of cortical lactate and pyruvate values; MAP, mean arterial pressure; p(ti)O2, cortical partial oxygen pressure in the tissue; SNP, sodium nitroprusside. # $p < 0.05$ compared with baseline. + $p < 0.05$ compared with SNP.

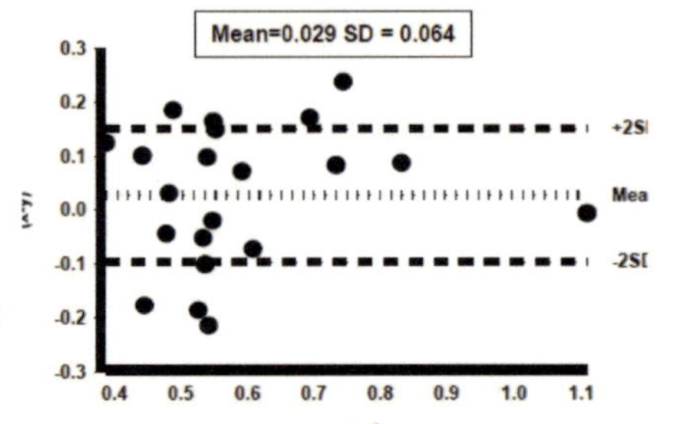

Bland-Altman analysis showing the limits of agreement and bias comparing conductance catheter derived Ees and ultrasonic based E`es. The limits of agreement (1.96 SD) were 0.13

→ acceptable agreement of both methods

Broscheit J, Kunze E, et al. I J Anesthesiology. 2008 Jan;18 (1):1-16

Fig. 6b. Validational study during arterial hypotension - Results

9. Association of increased myocardial contractility and elevated end-diastolic wall tension with short-term myocardial ischemia: A pressure-volume analysis

The present study is to answer the question whether myocardial hypoperfusion can be triggered by an LV hypervolemia, even if arterial pressure as well as cardiac output are in an "adequate" range - as literature usually calls it.

To answer this question, 15 Göttinger minipigs were studied in an open chest preparation. A catheter was placed in the arteria femoralis to measure pressure and a probe ,similar to those used for transoesophageal echocardiography, was fixed on the myocardium. A microtip catheter was inserted from the apex of the left ventricle for continuous pressure measurement. A catheter for microdialysis was implanted into the myocardium in the flow area of the left coronary artery. Finally, the arteria carotis communis was dissected to fix a U-shaped 8-MHz CW Doppler probe on it. A catheter in the femoral vein was used for pharmacological interventions.

Myocardial contractility was increased permanently through continuous application of dobutamine. A steady state was assumed after 20 minutes. Esmolol was administered in such a way that the heart rate - in relation to frequency - was lowered by at least 25% for 20 minutes under continuous infusion of dobutamin. Subsequently esmolol application was stopped so that dobutamin could again unfold its contractility-increasing effect. For comparison, only Esmolol was subsequently administered to another group - to the same amount as dobutamine and esmolol had been administered in the dobutamin-esmolol group. As expected, the table shows that when dobutamine and esmolol are administered at the same time, the heart rate decreases and contractility decreases later as well. Through the decrease in heart rate, LV volume increases in this phase and thus - according to the law of Laplace - diastolic myocardial wall tension increases as well. Dobutamine initially stimulates contractility but despite sufficient arterial pressure and cardiac output, oxygen supply is still lower than oxygen demand. Oxygen demand is then lowered by the decrease in contractility and the indications of hypoperfusion recede under identical wall tension. When the effect of esmolol starts to wear off, the contractility-stimulating effect of dobutamin comes back first and later the heart rate increases again. During this phase, increased wall tension leads to myocardial hypoperfusion again. Esmolol alone induces increased wall tension but no myocardial hypoperfusion.

The results of the present study show that an increase in myocardial wall tension alone is not necessarily associated with myocardial hypoperfusion. If, however, oxygen demand increases in this situation, or, as in the previous study, cardiac output and arterial pressure are reduced, the oxygen supply to the myocardium can sink below its oxygen demand. In this context, myocardial wall motion disorders can form as an indication of such an imbalance which in turn can lower the correlation of the two relations.

10. Conclusion and outlook

The results of the examination carried out allow the conclusion that a valid estimation of myocardial contractility is possible. Myocardial wall motion abnormalities limit the measuring accuracy of this new procedure. These myocardial wall motion abnormalities can occur if increased LV end-diastolic volume is associated with low cardiac output or an increased myocardial oxygen requirement.

In further investigations we would like to try to answer the question as to whether the acute afterload reduction necessary for the determination of elastance can also be induced through a Valsalva maneuver.

By using a 3-dimensional transoesophageal echocardiography, we would like to answer the question if measuring accuracy can possibly be significantly improved. On the one hand, using 3-dimensional echocardiography, similar to what is possible with a conductance catheter, could make it possible to determine internal flow fraction and consequently to develop a corrective factor for measurement. On the other hand, using 3-dimensional echocardiography makes it possible to estimate intraventricular volumes much more precisely than with the cross-sectional LV area.

Finally the use of this procedure should be verified in clinical studies.

11. References

[1] Suga H, Sagawa K, Shoukas AA. Load independence of the instantaneous pressure-volume ratio of the canine left ventricle and effects of epinephrine and heart rate on the ratio. Circ Res 1973;32:314-22.

[2] Gorcsan J, III, Morita S, Mandarino WA, et al. Two-dimensional echocardiographic automated border detection accurately reflects changes in left ventricular volume. J Am Soc Echocardiogr 1993;6:482-9.
[3] Deneault LG, Kancel MJ, Denault A, et al. A system for the on-line acquisition, visualization, and analysis of pressure-area loops. Comput Biomed Res 1994;27:61-7.
[4] Danielsen M, Ottesen JT. Describing the pumping heart as a pressure source. Journal of Theoretical Biology 2001;212:71-81.
[5] Ottesen JT, Danielsen M. Modeling ventricular contraction with heart rate changes. Journal of Theoretical Biology 2003;222:337-46.
[6] Paladino, J, Mulier, J, and Noordergraaf, A. Defining Ventricular Elastance. 1-11-0098.
[7] Strobeck JE, Sonnenblick EH. Myocardial and ventricular function. Part II: Intact heart. Herz 1981;6:275-87.
[8] Strobeck JE, Sonnenblick EH. Myocardial and ventricular function. Part I: Isolated muscle. Herz 1981;6:261-74.
[9] Frank O. Zur Dynamik des Herzmuskels. Z Biol 1895;32:370-447.
[10] Starling EH. The Linacre Lecture of the Law of the Heart. London: Longman, Greens and Co, Ltd, 1918.
[11] Seelen, P. J. A human circulatory analog computer. VIII Considerations leading to a preliminary analog of the left ventricle of the heart. 1961. Physics Lab, Univ. Utrecht. Ref Type: Internet Communication
[12] Beneken, J. E. W. A mathematical approach to cardio-vascular function. 1965. Univ. Utrecht. Ref Type: Thesis/Dissertation
[13] Liljestrand GLENG. The immediate effect of muscular work on the stroke and heart volume in man. Skand Arch Physiol 1938;80:265-82.
[14] Hill AV. The maximum work and mechanical efficiency of human muscles, and their most economical speed. J Physiol (London) 1922;56:19-41.
[15] Olufsen MS, Nadim A, Lipsitz LA. Dynamics of cerebral blood flow regulation explained using a lumped parameter model. Am J Physiol Regul Integr Comp Physiol 2002;282:R611-R622.
[16] Baan J, Jong TT, Kerkhof PL, et al. Continuous stroke volume and cardiac output from intra-ventricular dimensions obtained with impedance catheter. Cardiovasc Res 1981;15:328-34.
[17] Suga H, Sagawa K. Instantaneous pressure-volume relationships and their ratio in the excised, supported canine left ventricle. Circ Res 1974;35:117-26.
[18] Broscheit JA, Greim CA, Kessler M, Weidemann F, Roewer N: J Cardiothorac Vasc Anesth. 18(4): 415-22.
[19] Broscheit J, Greim CA, Weidemann F, Strotmann J, Steendijk P, Karle H, Roewer N: J Cardiothorac Vasc Anesth. 2006 Jun; 20(3): 340-346.
[20] Broscheit J, Weidemann F, Strotmann J, Steendijk P, Eberbach N, Karle H, Schuster F, Roewer N, Greim CA: J Cardiothorac Vasc Anesth Epub 2008 Jun 22.
[21] Weidemann F, Broscheit J, Eberbach N, Steendijk P, Voelker W, Greim C, Ertl G, Roewer N, Strotmann JM: Clin Sci (Lond). 2004 Feb; 106(2): 173-81.
[22] Broscheit JA, Weidemann F, Grein B, Lange M, Muellenbach R, Schuster F, Lindner C, Kunze E, Steendijk P, Roewer N, Greim CA: I Anesthesiology. 2009;18(1):1-16
[23] Broscheit JA, Rinck A, Anetseder M, Kessler M, Roewer N, Greim CA: J Cardiothorac Vasc Anesth. 2007 Feb;21(1):8-17

5

Electrical Heart Instability Evaluation in Conditions of Diastolic Heart Failure Suffered by Coronary Heart Disease Patients

E.P. Tatarchenko, N.V. Pozdnyakova, O.E. Morozova and E.A. Petrushin
Penza Extension Course Institute for Medical Practitioners
Russia

1. Introduction

In 1965 WHO experts singed out coronary heart disease (CHD) in a separate group. It was dictated by the growing epidemic incidence rate and high mortality from disease complications. Besides, it was urgent to take measures to treat the disease. However, the end of the XX century and the beginning of the XXI century have not brought any significant changes. The heart and vessel diseases complicated by atherosclerosis are still one of the main problems in most countries. The main reasons are high incidence of disease, stabile director disability and mortality among employable population. Each year, cardiovascular diseases cause 4.3 million deaths in Europe in general, and over 2 million in the EU, accounting for 48 and 42% of the total number of deaths respectively. Mortality from coronary heart disease among of men in the age of 65 is 3 times higher than among women. In older age mortality rate is equalized, and after 80 years of age it is 2 times higher among women.

In its essence, all the pathophysiological manifestations of coronary heart disease are caused by an imbalance between myocardial oxygen demand and oxygen delivery.

CHD may start abruptly with myocardial infarction (MI) or sudden cardiac death (SCD), but almost 50% of patients suffer immediately a chronic form of coronary heart disease. It is called exertional angina [2, 3]. In absolute figures it means approximately 30,000 - 40,000 patients with angina per 1 million population [4]. According to some reports men suffering angina live on average eight years less than those who do not have this pathology [5].

According to epidemiological studies, CHD patients suffer blood circulation blocking in most cases; it leads to approximately 90% sudden deaths. About half of patients with diagnosticated CHD die suddenly without a preceding pain syndrome.

Meanwhile, M.R.Cowie and others [2002] argue, the main risk factor for sudden death is left ventricular dysfunction. The prognosis of chronic heart failure (CHF) is still extremely serious, regardless of its etiology, but you should agree with J.N. Cohn and others [1999] who wrote that "...coronary disease may be an independent predictor of poor prognosis for patients suffering heart failure". Traditionally, CHF was considered to have connection with systolic dysfunction, however, in recent years the main subject of research of clinicians and physiologists is mechanisms of myocardium diastolic dysfunction (DD) development and its role in the onset of heart failure. Nowadays heart failure is considered as a syndrome which develops from various pathological heart changes, neuroendocrinal regulation disorders and represents a complex of circulatory reactions because of systolic or diastolic cardiac dysfunction.

About 50% of patients with chronic heart failure die within 5 years after the onset of clinical symptoms despite the use of combination therapy. According to the Framingham study, 75% of men with CHF and 62% of women die within 5 years after establishing diagnosis. Only half of patients with CHF die from heart failure which is refractory to therapy. The second half of patients with heart failure dies suddenly because of ventricular tachyarrhythmia. Oxymortia is the main death mechanism (in 30-80% of cases) among patients with CHF of II-III of functional class [8]. These facts allowed us to formulate an assumption that heart failure is the most the arrhythmogenic factor in cardiology and the most important sign of sudden death risk [9, 10].

Thus, the prediction and solution of sudden cardiac death (SCD) problem is only possible with the full study of the structural abnormalities and functional diseases which cause life-threatening arrhythmias acoording to modern model. Pathological changes of myocardium go with various dysfunctions of electrical heart activity. They are prognostically unfavorable in terms of the occurrence of fatally dangerous rhythm disturbances. The validity of the assumption is based on the fact that electrophysiological alternation of cells and cell membranes boosts the development of electrical heart instability (EHI) after the cases of transient coronary heart disease and myocardial infarction having developed in areas of myocardial dysfunction.

Though this problem is intensively investigated, the search of pathogenic mechanisms causing electrophysiological properties disorder and associated with pathological electrocardiographic and electrophysiological phenomena going with structural remodeling of myocardium in CHD is still important.

The research objective was to study the indicators characterizing electrical instability of myocardium suffered by CHD patients who have diastolic heart failure.

According to protocol adopted by local Ethical Committee a number of patients who had suffered myocardial infarction more than a year ago took part in the research. They had a stabile clinical course of coronary heart disease and clinical implications of chronic cardiac failure syndrome with left ventricle ejection fraction of 45% during the previous month. Each patient signed an agreement to take part in our research as a volunteer. We observed the group of 128 patients (36 women and 92 men). The average age of patients was 57.3±5.6 years.

The elimination criteria were coronary revascularization or cerebral stroke during the last 6 months, symptoms of VI class cardiac failure according to NYHA classification, clinically significant cardiac defects and lung diseases, dysfunctions of liver and nephros, atrial fibrillation.

Besides standard clinical research, we did the whole complex of work including electrocardiography in 12 derivations, echocardiography, Holter monitoring, registration of average signaling electrocardiography with identification of ventricular late potential, analysis of variability of cardiac rhythm, evaluation of ventricle repolarization-interval dispersion Q-T (QT_d), resolved interval Q-T (QT_C).

We evaluated left ventricular geometry and left atrium (end-diastolic size - EDD, size - ESD; end-systolic volume - EDV, end-systolic volume - ESV; left ventricular mass index – LVMI, relative thickness of the left ventricular wall; left atrium volume change index); left ventricular systolic function (ejection fraction - EF, %; stroke index – SI, ml/m^2; systolic shortening`s fraction of the front-back size aortic ventricle - ΔS,%); myocardium regional contractility (diacrisis of zone with regional contractility dysfunction). We used ultrasound cordis investigation with Doppler spectral echocardiography mode and color Doppler mapping.

Analyzing left ventricular diastolic function we studied indeces of transmitral diastolic flow in incipient and delayed diastole (E, A, m/s), their ratio (E/A), time of flow delay(DT, ms) and flow acceleration during the phase of rapid inflow(AT, ms), is ovolumic relaxation time (IVRT, ms) and duration of diastole (ET, ms) - Figure 1.

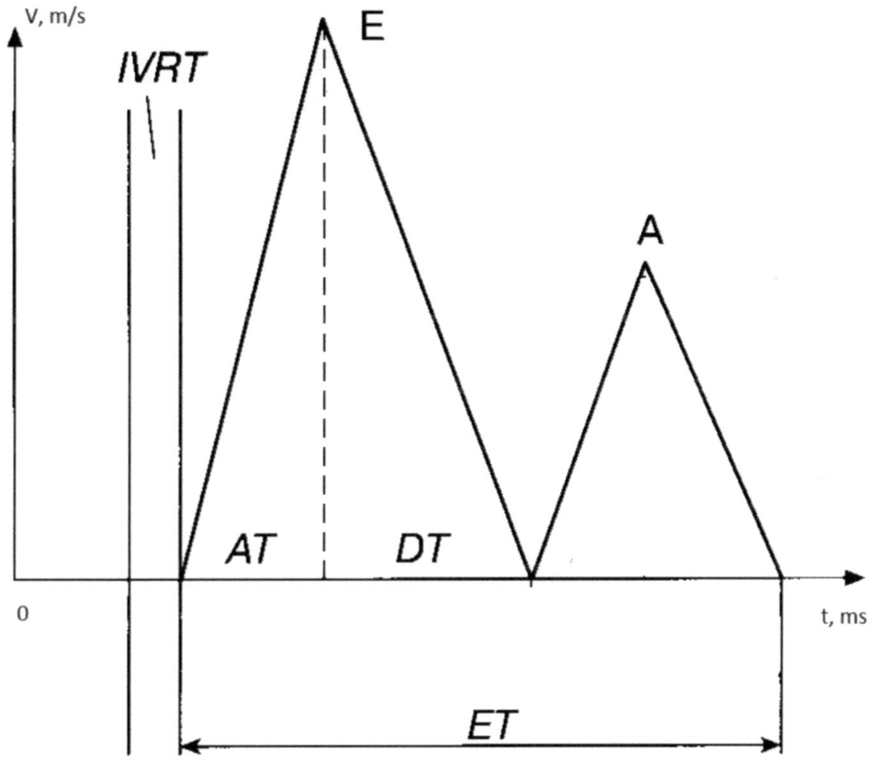

Fig. 1. Estimation of trancmitral diastolic flow

We also evaluated blood flow at the mouth of the pulmonary veins (D, cm / s; Ar, cm / s; Adur / Ar) – Figure 2.

We used tissue Doppler sonography to detect signs of inflow disorder, loss of elasticity, the increase of the left ventricular rigidity. We defined the maximum speed of mitral annulus: peak systolic speed - S '(cm / s) peak speed of incipient diastolic relaxation - E' (cm / s) peak speed in atrial systole phase - A '(cm / s), the ratio of maximum speed of incipient LV inflow (E) to the maximum speed of the fibrous ring kinesis in incipient diastole (E') - Figure 3.

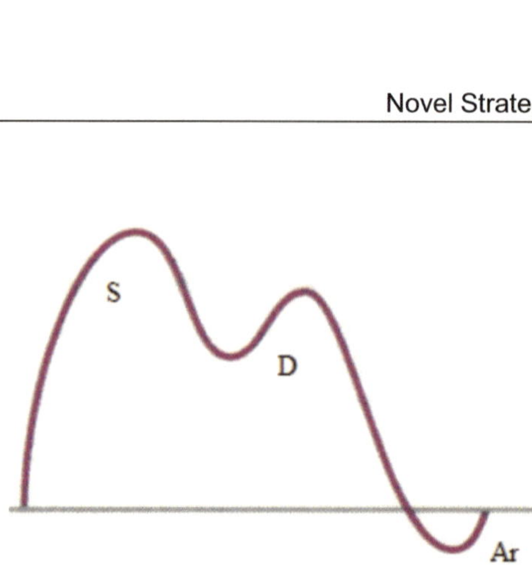

Fig. 2. Estimation of bloodstream at the mouth of the pulmonary veins

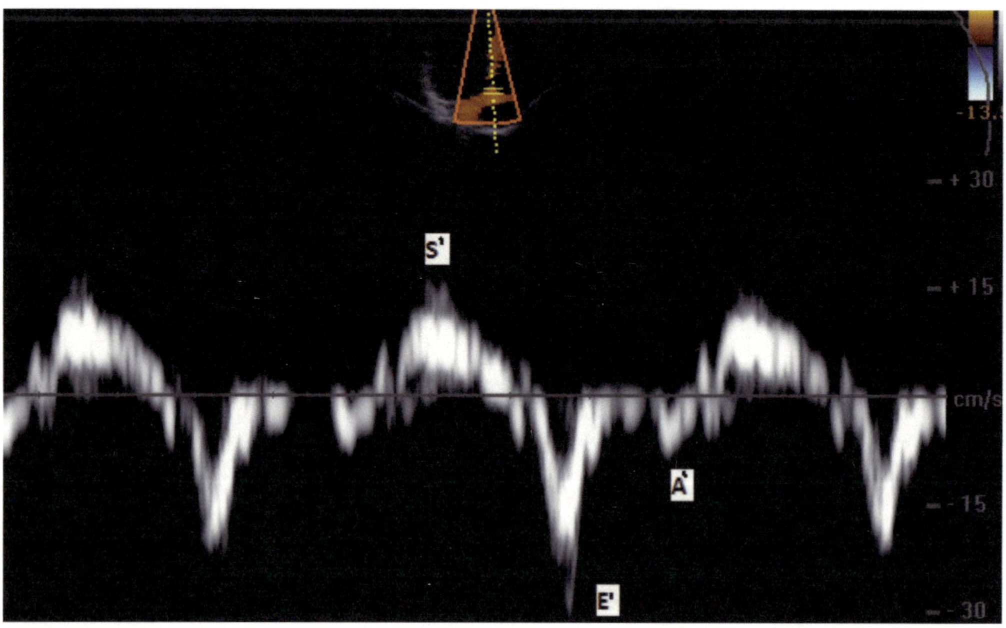

S' (cm/s) – peak diastolic speed; E' (cm/s) – peak speed of incipient diastolic relaxation; A' (cm/s) – peak speed in atrial systole phase.

Fig. 3. Fibrous ring`s movement of the mitral valve in pulse-wave mode histic doppler

Using Holter monitoring ECG we took into account the nature of rhythm disturbance and asequence, we estimated the quantity of pain assessed and painless ischemic episodes, the daily duration of ischemia, the maximum depth of segment ST depression.

Time-line analysis of ventricular late potential was performed by method of M. Simson [1981]. We calculated numerical quantitative values of three indicators: the duration of the filtered complex QRS (HF QRS-Dauer), the rms amplitude of the last 40 ms of the complex QRS (RMS 40), the duration of the low amplitude signals at the end of the filtered complex QRS (LAH Fd). We took HF QRS-Dauer which is more than 114 ms, RMS 40 which is less than 25 mV, LAH Fd which is more than 38 ms as pathological parameters of the signal averaged ECG - Figure 4.

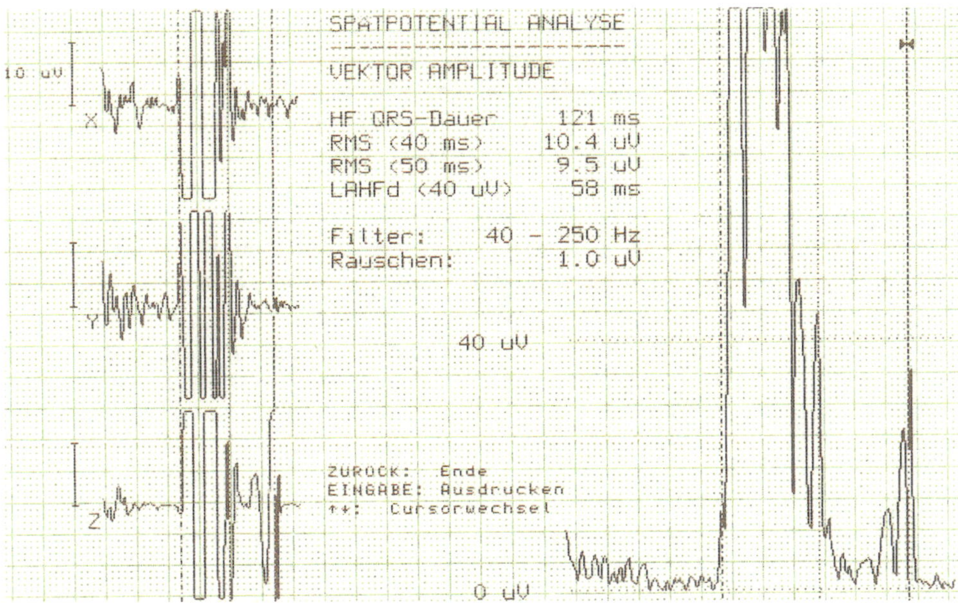

Fig. 4. Analysis of the signal-averaged ECG with elimination late potentials of the ventricles

Performing heart rate variability analysis we evaluated rMSSD (mean square difference between the duration of contiguous sinus intervals RR, BB 50 (proportion of contiguous sinus intervals RR which differ more than 50ms,%), SDNN (standard derivation of average duration of sinus intervals RR, ms).

Performing spectral analysis of heart rate variability analysis we estimated frequency ranges: high frequency (HF), low frequency (LF), the ratio of sympathetic and parasympathetic influences on heart rate variability (LF/HF).

We examined the following heart rate turbulence indicants:

- turbulence onset (TO,%). We estimated the value-of sinus rhythm acceleration after ventricular arrhythmia;
- turbulence slope (TS, ms / RR). We studied the intensity of the sinus rhythm deceleration, following its quickening.

In assessing ventricular repolarization we calculated corrected interval Q-T (QTs) using Bazeta. The dispersion of the interval Q-T (QTd) was defined as the difference between the maximal and minimal value of Q-T interval in different leads of standard ECG.

T-test of Student, entry criteria applied by static data handing. Gotten results have been presented in the form of an average arithmetical significance ± is standart devition. Differences considered reliable at $p < 0,05$.

In case of CHD left ventricle diastole indices and diastole functions undergo complex changes which are connected with both worsening of diastolic disorders and the development of hemodynamic adaptive responses acting through an increase in pressure in the left atrium and/or left ventricular end diastolic pressure and leading to the formation of various types of diastolic dysfunction.

We divided our patients into 3 groups according to the type of diastolic dysfunction of left ventricle: the first group (n=36) included patients with abnormal relaxation of left ventricle, the second group (n=28) consisted of patients with pseudonormal type of diastolic dysfunction and the third group (n=22) was formed from the patients who suffered restrictive type of diastolic dysfunction of left ventricle.

The average duration of disease was 6.9±3.9 years (3 to 12 years). Medical history and electrocardiographic criteria indicated macrofocal myocardial infarction (with Q tooth) suffered by 68 patients (53.1%).9 out of 68 patients had a chronic aneurysm of the anterior wall according to electrocardiographic and echocardiographic features. Fine-focal MI (without Q tooth) is marked in 60 cases according to medical documentation (hospital records, discharge summary). 82 patients (64%) had coronary heart disease accompanied by arterial hypertension (AH). 92 patients (72%) had burdened familial history. Lipid exchange violations were indicated in 112 cases (87.5%).

Figure 1 shows the gradation of patients with different variants of the left ventricle diastolic dysfunction according to functional classes of chronic heart failure (CHF). 42 patients had signs of I FC CHF, 51 patients had II FC and 35 patients had III FC.

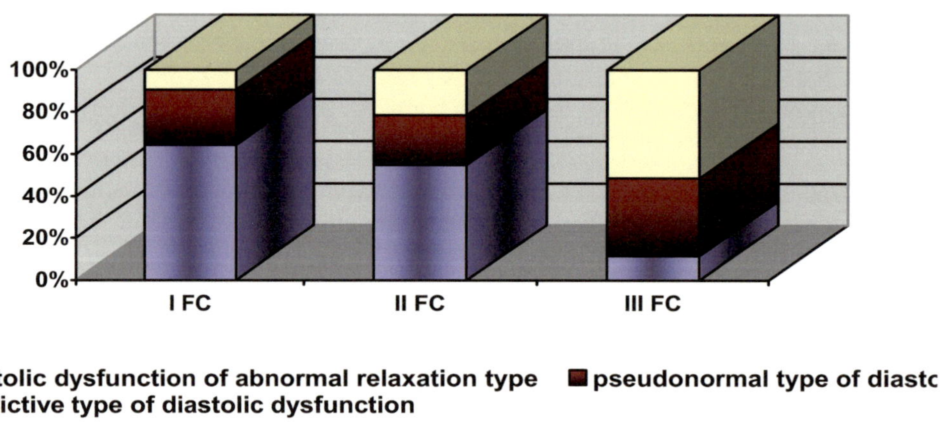

Fig. 5. The gradation of patients suffering coronary heart disease with left ventricle diastolic dysfunction according to functional classes of chronic heart failure (CHF).

In cases of heart failure clinical manifestations we have received the relation of r = 0,620 (p <0.01) of the frequency of CHF FC to the type of diastolic dysfunction. When FC increases the disturbances of LV DF become more pronounced: restrictive type of LV DD was detected in III FC (51% observations); in I FC it was observed on 11.4%; patients had the type of abnormal relaxation in 9.5% and 64.3% respectively, pseudonormal type was detected in 21.6% and 55% of cases.

The analysis of the structural and geometric parameters of left heart chambers (Table 1) showed that group III had an increase of the dilation of the cavities of the left ventricle and left atrium, increased left ventricle myocardial mass, reduction in contractile function (ejection fraction of III group was more than 45% but less than 50%, in group I it was 50%) in comparison with group I.

Indicators	I group	II group	III group
Number of patients, n	59	36	33
E, m/s	0.65±0.06*	0.81±0.03	1.07±0.05**
A, m/s	0.93±0.09*	0.65±0.02	0.36±0.03*
E/A,	0.82±0.05*	1.25±0.02	3.15±0.08**
AT, ms	99.47±2.1	94.1±3.2	97.3±3.3
DT, ms	267.6±11.4*	169.6±7.9	143.5±3.2**
IVRT, ms	116.8±7.4*	88.3±2.3	58.9±4.8**
Ar, cm/s	24.1±2.2°	36.6±1.3	55.3±1.6
SI, ml/m2	40.3±2.8	41.2±1.4	41.7±2.6
EDVI, ml/m2	82.1±5.3*	85.8±4.58	100.8±6.7
ESVI, ml/m2	37.85±2.1*	39.2±1.1	41.61±2.5
LVEF, %	55.93±2.7*	53.1±2.17	49.6±2.06
ESVILA, ml/m2	39.5±2.3*	44.37±3.2	50.43±3.61
ICVLA,%	37.65±1.5 *	34.1±2.1	24.9±2.7
LVMI, g/m2	126.35±9.7*	132.1±6.3	148.2±11.1
left ventricular RT, cm	0.44±0.06*	0.45±0.05	0.50±0.02

SI – stroke index, EDVI - end-diastolic volume index, ESVI - end systolic volume index, LVEF - left ventricular ejection fraction, ESVILA - end systolic volume index of left atrium, the ICVLA - an indicator of changes in the volume of the left atrium, LVMI - left ventricular mass index, left ventricular RT is the relative thickness of the left ventricular wall, *-p <0.05 - reliability of differences between patients with DD of abnormal relaxation type and patients with pseudonormal type of DD, ** p <0.05 - reliability of differences between the group of patients with restrictive type of DD and the groups with pseudonormal type of DD and abnormal relaxation, ° - p <0.05 - reliability of the indicator difference between group with DD of abnormal relaxation type and groups with DD of pseudonormal and restrictive type.

Table 1. Echocardiographic indicators of patients with coronary heart disease

We believe that one of the determinants of heart failure is diastolic dysfunction of the heart, which can be viewed both as the initial stage and as a pathophysiological link in the "vicious circle" of circulatory inefficiency, which affects negatively on the prognosis of patients with coronary heart disease [11].

The violation of left ventricular diastolic properties is essential, along with other structural and functional changes (dilation and hypertrophy), which form the concept of "remodeling". Patients had eccentric hypertrophy (43.75% of cases) and concentric hypertrophy of LV (37.5% of cases) as predominant types of LV remodeling after MI.

We established the correlation between the severity of LV DD and exponent change in the volume of the left atrium - r = -0.43 (p = 0.032), with left ventricular ejection fraction - r = -0.48 (p <0.04), with an index of end diastolic volume - r = 0,51 (p = 0.02), with left ventricular mass index - r = 0.45 (p = 0.034).

We associate the appearance and progression of LV DD with violation of diastolic relaxation on the back of acute or long-lasting ischemia with increased stiffness of the myocardium, including the location of postinfarction scar. We spotted the following law: a degree of LV DF disorder was growing in patients having macrofocal myocardial infarction versus patients having fine-focal myocardial infarction, respectively, it was 30.5% with abnormal relaxation type and 69.5% (p = 0.047), 58.3% and 41.7% (p = 0.05) with pseudonormal, 87.9% and 12.1% (p = 0.0476) with restrictive type. We believe that patients with previous Q-infarction had long-lasting deterioration of LV function during myocardial hibernating, which is characterized by a chronic reduction in cardiomyocyte contractility, while their viability is maintained. In these conditions viable myocardium which is far from infarction zona undergoes diastolic myocardial stress.

We detected the dependence of manifestation degree of diastolic dysfunction with an index of contractility WMSI - r = 0.91 (p = 0.01) among patients with a history of MI. We pointed the positive correlation of restrictive type of LV DD with Q- myocardial infarction r = 0.638 (p <0.001). In group III (restrictive type) Q-infarction occurred in 87.9% of cases, which is significantly lower in comparison with group I – 30.5%, p <0.01.

In conditions of limited blood flow the possibility of injury and death of cardiomyocytes because of their necrotization and apoptosis [12] is the main unfavorable result of myocardial hypoxia in case of coronary heart disease. However, death of cardiomyocytes is accompanied by compensatory hypertrophy of survived myocardial cell and the development of connective tissue [13]. There is an opinion that left ventricle hypertrophy may lead to myocardial dysfunction. It is an individual risk factor for high cardiovascular case rate, including ischemia myocardial infarction, heart failure, ventricular arrhythmias and sudden death.

We tend to assume that the process of cardiac remodeling affects all myocardium components. Changes occur at the level of cardiac myocytes and in the extracellular matrix. Typically, ischemic myocardial injuries develop leading to the coagulation and apoptosis. In this case, as approved by the J.Soto, G.Beller [2001], responsive genes are activated immediately, especially c-fos, and the program of "programmed death", apoptosis, starts to run. In the peripheral areas ischemic injury usually results in colliquative necrosis with cell edema and myocytolysis. It is especially true for reperfusion injury. The formation of connective tissue (fibrosis) may have redundant diffuse or interstitial nature in addition to substitution (focal), with interstitial spread perivascular.

Different biomechanical properties of myocardium in chronic ischemic zone and so-called intact myocardium generate special effects according to the type of stress concentration on their border. The type of stress concentration is connected with further progression of degenerative and sclerotic changes, significant changes in the shape and size of remodeled heart chambers. Further LV remodeling with the expansion of the cavity in postinfarction period is caused by involving of myocardium in the "transition zone" in the process of remodeling. The data obtained from pathophysiological studies suggest that patients suffering coronary heart disease have clinical picture determined by not only the heterogeneity of causes, but also the diversity of adaptive and disadaptive changes in metabolism and contractile condition of cardiomyocytes [16]. The most significant adaptive myocardium reactions in response to myocardial ischemia include the "new ischemic syndromes": hibernate, stupor.

The defining condition for the occurrence of lethal arrhythmias is considered to be structural disease of heart, which becomes electrically unstable under the influence of various functional factors. Ischemia and necrosis, hypertrophy and dilatation of the ventricles, the inflammation and swelling of the myocardial tissue can act as the structural changes that determine the development of ventricular tachycardia. According to the results of many studies [17, 18, 19] these changes constitute anatomical substrate for appearance of malignant arrhythmias with the participation of the various triggering and modulating factors.

Ventricular late potential with a stable disease course was recorded among 35 patients (27.3%) with a history of MI (Table 2). We believe that structural cardiomyocyte changes, programmed apoptosis and secondary hypertrophy, increased diastolic stiffness and active myocardium relaxation violation, reactive changes of connective tissue skeleton of the myocardium, decrease in diastolic filling and remodeling with segmental structure violation, i.e. all these processes, lead to the formation of electrical myocardium heterogeneity and cause greater frequency of recording of late potentials among CHD patients in conditions of progression of LV DD: with abnormal relaxation (18.6%), with pseudonormal type (27.8%), and restrictive type of LV DD (42.4%, $p < 0.05$).

Indicator	Variations of diastolic dysfunction		
	Type I	Type II	Type III
The number of patients, n	59	36	33
The number of patients with ventricle late potential, n	11	10	14
The number of patients with ventricular arrhythmia, n	50	35	33
analysis of ventricular extrasystole			
I gradation, n/%	29/49.1%	10/27.8%	2/6.1%
IIgradation, n/%	7/11.9%	7/19.4%	5/15.1%
IIIgradation, n/%	10/16.9%	13/36.1%	12/36.4%
IV-V gradations, n/%	4/6.8%	5/13.9%	14/42.4%
analysis of Q-T interval			
RRNN, ms	810 ± 64	798 ± 98	753 ± 132
QT_c, ms	405.5 ± 5.2*	422.3 ± 2.6**	450.2 ± 5.4
QT_d, ms	39.7 ± 2.7*	49.6 ± 3.3**	64.2 ± 3.1

I type- LV DD of abnormal relaxation type, II type - LV DD of pseudonormal type; III type - LV DD of restrictive type, VLP ventricular late potential, VA- ventricular arrhythmia, RRNN - the duration of sinus RR intervals; n / % - the absolute number of patients with given symptom/percentage of the number of patients of this group.

Table 2. The comparative analysis of ventricular arrhythmias, cardiac late potentials, QT intervals among patients with coronary heart disease

Ventricular arrhythmias are considered to be one of the factors determining the poor prognosis and high mortality among CHD patients. Ventricular arrhythmias may be the cause of death among patients with heart failure symptoms even in conditions of adequate control of decompensation symptoms.

Cardiac arrhythmias were detected among 99.2% of patients (Table 2), while supraventricular arrhythmias (SA) were detected among 7% of patients, ventricular arrhythmias were detected among 56.2% of patients, a combination of ventricular arrhythmias (VA) with various forms of supraventricular arrhythmias (SA) were indicated among 36% of patients. Complex forms of VA (ventricular extrasystole of grades IV-V) were found in 23 cases (18%). Polymorphic ventricular extrasystole was detected among 35 CHD patients with left ventricular diastolic dysfunction (27.3%). In 41 cases (32%) the revealed ventricular extrasystole was assigned to I gradation when the frequency of episodes did not exceed 220 per day.

Having analyzed ventricular arrhythmias we noted the following law: early, paired, volley ventricular extrasystoles were detected among patients with slow fragmented activity more frequently in comparison with patients without ventricular late potential, respectively, 19 (54.3%) and 4 (4.3%) with $\chi 2 = 7.4$, $p < 0.001$.

Ventricular late potential and ventricular arrhythmias were recorded more often with an increase in the degree of diastolic dysfunction and end-diastolic volume of left ventricle. When DD had a restrictive type, ventricular extrasystole was found in 100% of cases and ventricular extrasystole of IV-V grades was detected among 14 patients (42.4%), 13 of them had a diagnosed slow fragmented activity at the end of the ventricular complex. In group I (with abnormal left ventricular relaxation) ventricular extrasystole was observed among 84.7% of patients and complex forms of ventricular extrasystole were detected among 4 patients with abnormal rates of Holter ECG (6.8%).

The most common mechanism for tachyarrhythmias of high grades is the mechanism of re-entry momentum. It means the presence of unilateral and delayed passage of the depolarization wave front because of the violation of inter-cell contacts in parallel-oriented fibers [20], proliferation heterogeneity and fragmentation of the depolarization wavefront, which is a marked by ventricular late potential. That's what we explain the significant prevalence of complex forms of ventricular extrasystole among patients with slow fragmented ventricular activity (54.3%).

To study the effect of reversible ischemia on myocardial electrophysiological properties we analyzed daily myocardial ischemia and indicators of Holter ECG among patients with coronary heart disease having left ventricular DD. Correlation analysis revealed the dependence of the daily duration of ischemia on the duration of filtered set of HF QRS Dauer ($r = 0.53$, $p = 0.01$), with duration of low-amplitude signals at the end of filter-centered complex QRS LAH Fd ($r = 0.49$ $p = 0.03$), duration of painless myocardial ischemia with HF QRS Dauer ($r = 0.57$, $p = 0.01$). A positive correlation was obtained by estimating the depth of segment depression in HF QRS-Dauer ($r = 0.45$, $p = 0.03$), with LAH Fd ($r = 0.41$, $p = 0.05$); number of painless ischemic episodes per day with HF QRS-Dauer ($r = 0.51$, $p = 0.04$).

The results confirm that the presence of slow fragmented activity focus, marked by ventricular late potential is connected with heterogeneous areas of myocardium in CHD patients: profound disturbances in the processes of relaxation and recovery of cardiomyocytes occur in both acute and chronic ischemia because of degenerative changes and apoptosis. But it should be noted that studying the complex mechanisms of late potentials formation and the functions and metabolism of cardiac muscle, we traditionally pay much attention to cardiomyocytes. However, we tend to assume that extracellular matrix plays a insignificant role in the genesis of fragmented ventricular activity. Fibrosis is an essential component of cardiac muscle remodeling; the development of reparative (replacement) fibrosis may not only violate cardiomyocytes supply but also impede the electrical contact between them [21] in case of ischemia and myocardial necrosis.

The results of our studies have shown that myocardial dysfunction in ischemic area leads to the inhomogeneity of repolarization processes in conditions of limited coronary blood flow. However, the increase of QT dispersion in patients with coronary heart disease is associated with the duration of daily myocardial ischemia (DMI). We received a positive relationship of DMI with QT_d ($r = 0.485$, $p = 0.05$). When the DMI was more than 60 minutes the duration of QTc and QT_d interval was 449.2±4.1 ms and 67.2±2.7ms, p <0.05,when the DMI was 30 to 60 min analogous figures corresponded to the values of 412.5±3,2ms and 46.8± 2,4 ms.

While studying QTd we observed higher values in patients with ventricular arrhythmia of III-V grades (67.5±4.2 ms) in comparison with patients without ventricular arrhythmia (44.3±2.5ms), p <0,05. The analysis revealed a dependence of the variance of QT interval with gradation of ventricular extrasystole ($r = 0.6432$, $p < 0.01$), with exponents of Holter ECG: LAH Fd ($r = 0.4831$, $p < 0.05$) HF QRS-Dauer ($r = 0.5744$, $p < 0.05$).

The proportion of patients with restrictive type of LV DD with QTc interval which was over 440 ms (69%), and QTd which was more than 50 ms (72%) was significantly higher in comparison with those values in group II, it was 30.6% and 33% ($p<0.05$) respectively, and in Group I it was 19% and 17% ($p<0.03$) respectively.

The performance analysis of electrical and structural remodeling among patients havingcoronary heart disease with different variants of left ventricular DD allowed us to establish a clear pattern (Figure 6): ventricular late potential and ventricular arrhythmias of higher grades were detected more often with increasing degree of diastolic function disturbance. Inhomogeneity of repolarization processes was heightened with an increase in QT interval dispersion. In our view, the resulting dependence reflects inhomogeneity of repolarization processes and depolarization of the ventricles in chronic ischemia, the conditions for malignant arrhythmias in CHD patients having left ventricular DD were created. We assume that the electrical stability of myocardium and its global-sustaining capacity are integral characteristics that determine the functioning of the heart as a self-regulating system. The violation of bioelectrical activity of the myocardium inevitably leads to its mechanical failure.

The discussion of the pathogenesis of coronary heart disease was always connected with neurogenic component. The theory of "punctuated antagonism" of the interaction of two divisions of the autonomic nervous system (ANS) and their impact on the regulation of the pacemaker in the sinus node (SN) is complicated by the activity of all the structures of the peripheral segmental heart ANS. In conditions of limited coronary blood flow morpho-functional component is considered to be slowly-varied, and pathologically altered regulation of heart rate variability is one of the earliest and most obligate manifestations of ischemic process [22, 23]. Sympathetic distress is a critical drop in power of neurohumoral regulation with a shift in the sympathovagal balances to the sympathetic component. It is regarded as a predictor of sudden death which is independent from left ventricular ejection fraction [22].

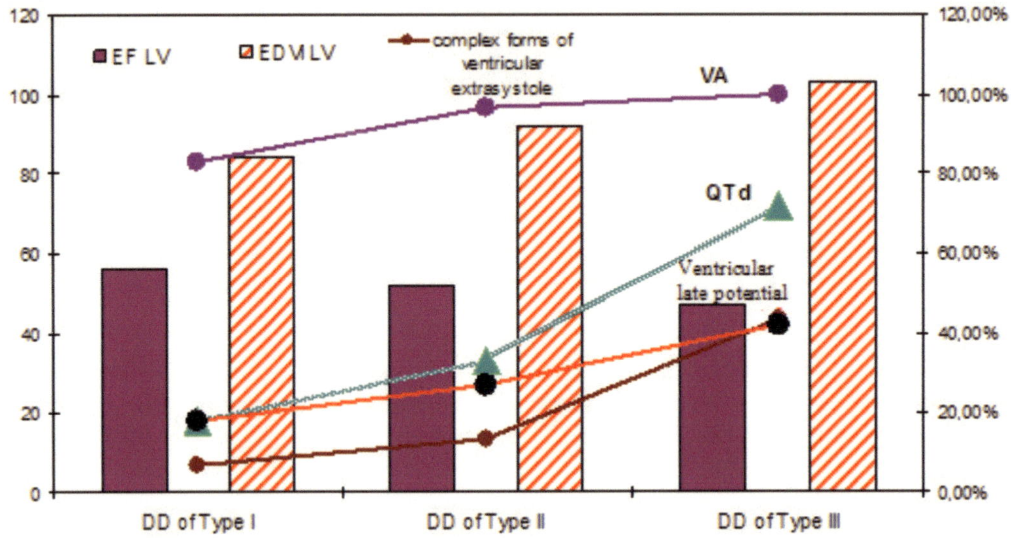

DD of Type I - diastolic dysfunction according to the type of abnormal relaxation, DD of Type II- diastolic dysfunction of pseudonormal type, DD of Type III - diastolic dysfunction of restrictive type; EDVI LV - end-diastolic volume index of left ventricle, EF LV - ejection fraction left ventricular, QTd - the dispersion of Q-T interval.

Fig. 6. The performance analysis of structural and geometrical and eletrical remodeling in CHD patients with left ventricle diastolic dysfunction.

Assessing the neurohumoral regulation of heart rate, we conducted the analysis of quantitative indicators of HRV and HRT (Table 3).

HRV indices in the group with impaired relaxation did not differ significantly from those in the group with pseudonormal type, once-reliable differences were obtained in comparison with III group of diastolic heart failure.

Rates BB50, SDNN index, rMSSD are drastically reduced in patients of group III. These values indicate a disorder of vagal protective effect on the value of "threshold of heart fibrillation". Disorders of neurohumoral regulation were diagnosed in conditions of the restrictive version of the DD LV, they pointed the increased sympathetic activity (SDNN - 24.7±3,2ms, LF/HF - 5.46±0,61 conventional units, BB50 - 0%).

During our study we pointed out the following pattern: autonomic imbalance with increased sympathetic activity grew with an increase in the degree of LV DD. The excess of the balance of ANS of sympathetic type LF / HF was observed in 39% of patients in group I who had abnormal left ventricular relaxation, it was detected in 58.3% of patients in group II with pseudonormal type of DD LV and it was indicated in 94% cases in group III with restrictive type, p <0.05.

And, if the HRV is a proven non-invasive method of quantitative analysis of the functioning of ANS in patients with coronary heart disease with preserved sinus rhythm, HRT is a fairly new noninvasive method of estimation the modulating autonomic influences on the sinus node in patients with ventricular arrhythmias, which resulted from the progressive fading of the carotid baroreflex [24]. Schematically, the formation of HRT can be represented by the following sequence: compensatory pause occurs after ventricular extrasystole, and, as a result, heart rate and blood pressure increase are caused by baroreflex, then blood pressure increase leads to the subsequent decrease in heart rate through baroreflex.

Indicators	Group I	Group II	Group III
The number of patients, n	59	36	33
RRNN, ms	810±64	798 ± 98	753 ± 132
analysis of heart rate variability			
SDNN, ms	41.4± 2.7	36.6± 2.3	24.7± 3.2*
SDNN index, ms	22.6 ±1.9	19.3 ±1.3	8.7±1.6*
rMSSD, ms	23.1±2.1	21.1±1.4	16 ±1.3*
BB50, beats per minute	10.3±3.2	8.8±1.4	3.4±1.2*
LF/HF, conv.	2.93±0.54	3.51±0.68	5.16 ±0.61*
analysis of heart rate turbulence			
TO more 0% , n/%	10/17	9/25	17/51.5
TS less 2,5мс/RR, n/%	9/15.2	9/25	16/48.5

RRNN - the average duration of sinus RR intervals between contractions, SDNN-standard deviation from the mean duration of RR intervals between sinus contractions, BB50 - the number of adjacent sinus RR intervals, which differ by more than 50 ms, SDNN index-average standard deviations, rMSSD - square root of the sum of squared differences of successive sinus RR intervals, LF/HF - index of the balance of sympathetic and parasympathetic nervous systems; TO is more than 0%; TS is less than 2.5 ms / RR * - p <0, 05 – the difference is reliable when indicators of group III are compared with indicators of I and II groups.

Table 3. Quantitative indices of HRV in patients with coronary heart disease

HRT indicators reflect early acceleration of sinus rhythm (TO) and the subsequent decrease in heart rate (TS) after ventricular arrhythmia. Studies in recent years characterized HRT as effective method of predicting the outcomes of patients with coronary pathology, which is comparable with HRV, and in some cases it is superior to HRV in its diagnostic capabilities [25, 26].

During our study we reported the value of TO> 0% in 36 patients (28%) from the group of 128 patients with previous MI history, we detected TS <2.5 ms / RR in 34 cases (26.6%), and we observed the combination of pathological values of TO and TS in 19 cases (14.8%). The frequency of registration TO> 0% and TS <2.5 ms / RR significantly dominated in the group with restrictive type of LV DD in comparison with group I (DD type of abnormal relaxation) and group II (DD of pseudonormal type), $p < 0.05$.

We have established a connection of HRT violation with left atrium volume change indicator- $r = -0.43$ ($p = 0.032$), with left ventricular ejection fraction- $r = -0.49$ ($p = 0.03$), with end-diastolic volume index - $r = 0.51$ ($p = 0.02$), with left ventricular mass index - $r = 0.45$ ($p = 0.04$). We marked the correlation of TS with HRV indicators: SDNN ($r = 0.41$, $p = 0.02$) and LH/HF ($r = 0.332$, $p = 0.02$). The absolute values of TO significantly correlated with QTd ($r = 0.349$, $p = 0.04$).

Pathophysiologic ground for coronary heart disease is a discrepancy between myocardial oxygen demand and opportunities in meeting the needs in oxygen because of a limitation of acute or chronic coronary blood flow. Admittedly, the provision of myocardial blood through the coronary arteries occurs in the phase of diastole. That is why we suggest to consider diastolic dysfunction not only as an initial stage, but also as a pathological link in the "vicious circle" of the development of cardiac events in CHD patients.

Rates of diastole and its function undergo complex changes caused by the violation of diastolic relaxation in the background of acute or chronic ischemia, with increased stiffness of the myocardium at the site of postinfarction scar during the coronary heart disease. Necrosis of cardiomyocytes and activation of the cascade of biochemical reactions which occur in the postinfarction period, cause a significant change in mechanical properties of tissues. However, we should take into account different biomechanical properties of myocardium in the areas of chronic ischemia and so-called intact (healthy) myocardium. The specific effects are generated on their borders according to the type of stress concentration. They cause the further progression of degenerative and sclerotic changes, the formation of connective tissue in conditions of limited blood flow. In conditions of chronic ischemia, the changes occur not only in cardiomyocytes but also in cells of connective tissue skeleton. Increased rigidity of myocardium, change in the myocardium viscoelastic properties are the consequences of disorganization and reorganization of connective tissue skeleton of ischemic nature. Progressive hypertrophy and dilation of the heart are accompanied by a further violation of the diastolic left ventricular function, then it is accompanied by systolic dysfunction, they cause an increase in myocardial oxygen demand and a change in subendocardial blood flow, impaired myocardial bioenergetics.

The evaluation of the changes of myocardium electrophysiological properties seems for us to be an important aspect in the search for new diagnostic tests of severity of ischemic myocardial damage in patients with coronary heart disease. The validity of these approaches is based on the notion that electrophysiological alternation of cells and their membranes is associated with remodeling after an episode of ischemia or myocardial infarction and is involved in genesis of arrhythmia That is why we examined the relationship of electrical and structural myocardium remodeling with left ventricular diastolic function in CHD patients who had myocardial infarction history.

The analysis of ventricular late potentials and dispersion of QT interval allows to assess arrhythmogenic substrate in patients having CHD with left ventricular diastolic dysfunction. Persistent deterioration of left ventricular diastolic function during myocardium hibernating among CHD patients increases the manifestation of inhomogeneity of depolarization and repolarization processes.

The increase of the sympathetic influence has an effect on myocardium active relaxation and diastolic phase structure during the subsequent abuse of metabolic pathways accompanied by destabilization of connective tissue skeleton and secondary changes of contractile myocardium. Neurohumoral regulation violations caused by diastolic dysfunction in CHD patients are the same as when they are generated by heart failure. They are evident in increase of sympathetic activity, reduced parasympathetic and pressosensitive activity.

Even single ventricular extrasystole can be a trigger factor of fatally dangerous arrhythmias in conditions of chronic myocardial ischemia with arrhythmogenic substrate, which is the marked by ventricular late potential and QTd, when autonomic nervous system is activated according to the sympathetic type.

Complex analysis of parameters reflecting the functional conditions of myocardium and the interrelation of electrical and structure-geometrical myocardium remodeling is necessary to improve the diagnostics and the prognostication of risk degree among CHD patients in conditions of increasing of left ventricle diastolic dysfunction, given the multifactorial genesis of the problem of myocardial electrical instability

The use of integrated risk markers may contribute to the development of an integrated approach to risk stratification of SCD and arrhythmic complications prevention in CHD patients.

2. Abbreviations

ANS - autonomic nervous system

CHD - coronary heart disease

CHF - chronic heart failure

DD - diastolic dysfunction

DF - diastolic function

EDD - end-diastolic size

EDV - end-diastolic volume

ESD - end- systolic size

EHI - electrical heart instability

ESV - end- systolic volume

EF - ejection fraction

HRT - heart rate turbulence

HRV - heart rate variability

IVRT – isovolumic relaxation time

LV - left ventricle

LVMI - left ventricular mass index

MI - myocardial infarction

SA - supraventricular arrhythmias

SCD - sudden cardiac death

SI – stroke index

ΔS - systolic shortening's fraction of the front-back size aortic ventricle

VA - ventricular arrhythmia

VLP - ventricular late potential

3. References

[1] Allender S., Scarborough P., Peto V., Rayner M., Leal J., Luengo-Fernandez R., Gray A. . European cardiovascular disease statistics 2008 // Eur. Heart Network. -2008.- Vol. 4. – P. 76–78.

[2] Kannel W.B., Feinleib M. Natural history of angina pectoris in the Framingham study. Prognosis and survival // American Journal of Cardiology. – 1972.- Vol. 29.- P. 154-163.

[3] Pepine C.J., Abrams J., Marks R.G. et al. Characteristics of a contemporary population with angina pectoris: TIDES Investigators // Am. J. Cardiol. – 1994.- Vol. 74.- P. 226-231.

[4] Williams S.V., Fihn S.D., Gibbons R.J. Guidelines for the management of patients with chronic stable angina: diagnosis and risk stratification// Ann. Intern. Med. – 2001.- Vol. 135.- P. 530-547.

[5] Oganov R.G., Maslennikova. G.Y. Demographic situation and cardiovascular diseases in Russia: ways to solve problems// Cardiovascular therapies and prevention. .- 2007.- №6. – P.7-14.

[6] Cowie M.R., Fox K.F., Wood D.A. et al. Hospitalization of patients with heart failure: a population–based study. //Eur Heart J. - 2002.- Vol. 23.- P. 877–85.

[7] Cohn, J.N., Johnson G. Veterans Administration Cooperative Study Group. Heart failure with normal ejection fraction: V-HEFT Study // Circulation. - 1990.- Vol. 81.- P. 48-53.

[8] O'Callaghan P.A., Camm A.J. Treatment of arrhythmias in heart failure // Europ. J. Heart Failure.- 1999.- Vol.1 (2).- P. 133-137.

[9] Mareev V.Y. Heart failure and ventricular arrhythmias: the problem of treatment.// Cardiology.-1996.- № 12.- P.4–12.
[10] Cowie M.R., Mosterd A., Wood D.A. et al. The epidemiology of heart failure // Eur Heart J. – 1997. - Vol. 18.- P. 208-255.
[11] Devereux R.B. Left ventricular diastolic dysfunction: early diastolic relaxation and late diastolic compliance. J. Am. Coll. Cardiol 1989; 13: 337-339.
[12] Kapelko V.E. The evolution of concepts and metabolic basis of ischemic myocardial dysfunction.// Cardiology. - 2005. - № 9. – P. 55–61.
[13] Wainwirght C.L. Matrix metalloproteinases? Oxidative stress and the acute response to acute myocardial ischemia-reperfusion // Curr Opin Pharmacol. - 2004.- Vol. 4.- P. 132 – 138.
[14] Molkentin J.D., Lu J-R, Antos C.L. et al. A calcineurin-dependent transcriptional pathway for cardiac hypertrophy // Cell.- 1998. – Vol. 93.- P. 215 - 228.
[15] Soto J., Beller G. Clinical Benefit of Noninvasive Viability Studies of Patients with Severe Ischemic Left Ventricular Dysfunction // Clin. Cardiol. – 2001. - Vol. 24. - P. 428-434.
[16] Opie L.H. Newly identified ischemic syndromes and myocardial endogenous cytoprotection and their role in clinical cardiology in the past and future. // Medicography. - 1999. - № 21(2). - P. 65–73.
[17] Hohnloser S.H., Franck P., Klingenheben T. et al. Open infarct artery, late potentials, and other prognostic factors in patients after acute myocardial infarction in the thrombolytic era: a prospective trial // Circulation. – 1994.- Vol. 90.- P. 1747-1756.
[18] Goldstein S., Brooks M. M., Ledingham R. et al. Association between ease of suppression of ventricular arrhythmia and survival// Circulation. – 1995.- Vol. 91.- P. 7979 – 7983.
[19] Petersen S., Peto V., Rayner M. et al. European cardiovascular disease statistics // Eur. Heart J. – 2005. - Vol. 21. - P. 1261-1272.
[20] Kramer J.B., Saffitz J.E., Witkowsky F.V., Corr P.B. Intramural reentry as a mechanism of ventriculartachycardia during evolving canine myocardial infarction.// Circ. Res.- 1985 - Vol. 56 - P. 736-754.
[21] Tatarchenko E.P., Pozdnyakova N.V., Morozova O.E. Late potentials of the heart: clinical and electrophysiological evaluation. Penza: Elma.- 2000. – P. 144 .
[22] Maisch B. Ventricular remodeling // Cardiology.- 1996.- Vol. 8(7).- P. 2-10.
[23] Bigger J., Fleiss J.L., Steiman R.C. Correlation among time and freguency domain measures of heart period variability two week after acute myocardial infarction. Am. J. Cardiol 1992; 69: 891 - 898.
[24] Tatarchenko E.P., Pozdnyakova N.V., Morozova O.E., Shevyryov V.A. Prognosis of patients with coronary heart disease (clinical and instrumental aspects). Penza: Elma.- 2002. – P. 206.
[25] Schmidt G., Malik M., Barthel P. et al. Heart-rate turbulence after ventricular premature beats as a predictor of mortality after acute myocardial infarction // Lancet.- 1999.- Vol.353.- P.1390-1396.

[26] Ghuran A., Reid F., La Rovere M.T. et al. Heart rate turbulence-based predictors of fatal and nonfatal cardiac arrest (The Autonomic Tone and Reflexes After Myocardial Infarction substudy) // Am. J. Cardiol.- 2002.- Vol.89.- P.184-190

[27] Bauer A., Barthel P., Schneider R., Schmidt G. Dynamics of heart rate turbulence // Circulation.- 2001.- Vol.104, Supplement II-339.- P.1622.

Part 3

Pharmacotherapy of Ischemic Heart Disease

6

Prehospital Thrombolysis: It's All About Time

Raveen Naidoo and Nicholas Castle
Durban University of Technology
South Africa

1. Introduction

Prehospital emergency care personnel can play a crucial role in the identification and management of patients presenting with ST Elevation Myocardial Infarction (STEMI). Specifically, prehospital thrombolysis by emergency medical personnel such as paramedics/nurses/prehospital doctors has been identified as being a successful and safe approach for the provision of accelerating reperfusion strategies for acute STEMI. Moreover, prehospital thrombolysis has no added specific risks (arguably, it is safer as delayed thrombolysis increases the risk of myocardial rupture) as compared to inhospital thrombolysis; nor is it an obstacle for later percutaneous coronary intervention (PCI). This chapter will focus on the general management of STEMI, the potential benefits related to prehospital thrombolysis and alternative, adjunctive therapies and provide some useful hints to drug administration.

Prehospital thrombolysis is an established emergency treatment and has been classified as a Class IIa recommendation therapy for acute STEMI by the leading international cardiology societies like European Society of Cardiology (2008). Prehospital thrombolysis research is ongoing with a large multi-center trial currently recruiting patients in 112 locations worldwide - STREAM - Strategic Reperfusion Early After Myocardial Infarction. STREAM aims to evaluate, in a proof of concept approach, the outcome of prehospital patients presenting with acute STEMI within 3 hours of symptom onset. Following randomization, a treatment strategy of early (prehospital) tenecteplase and additional antiplatelet and antithrombin therapy followed by catheterization within 6-24 hours with timely coronary intervention as appropriate (or by rescue coronary intervention if required) compared to primary angioplasty. This intention to treat study will therefore place patients into two groups; Group A will receive primary PCI performed according to local standards and Group B will receive prehospital thrombolysis supported by optimal supportive adjunctive therapy (http://clinical trials.gov.show/NCT00623623).

2. Development of prehospital thrombolysis

The first published study of prehospital thrombolysis involved the intravenous administration of 750,000 units of streptokinase by physicians was undertaken in 1985. This study demonstrated that patients treated less than 1.5 hours after the onset of pain had a significantly higher ejection fraction (56±15 vs. 47±14 %; $P<0.05$), improved infarct-related regional ejection fraction (51±19 vs. 34±20 %; $P<0.01$) and a lower QRS score (5.6±4.9 vs.

8.6±5.5; P<0.01) than patients receiving treatment between 1.5 and 4 hours from the onset of pain. Patients in the prehospital arm of the study also had better-preserved left ventricular function than patients treated in the hospital. The study concluded that thrombolytic therapy with streptokinase is most effective when administered within 1.5 hours from onset of symptoms of acute myocardial infarction. Although this study produced positive results it lacked statistical power (due to small sample size) but it served to highlight the importance of timely thrombolysis (Koren et al., 1985).

Arguably, the Grampian Region Early Anistreplase Trial (GREAT) was the most influential prehospital thrombolysis based study. The aim of GREAT was to determine the time saved by thrombolysis when initiated at home by trained general practitioners (GPs) / family physicians as compared to thrombolysis inhospital. The GPs randomly assigned thrombolytic therapy to 311 patients with suspected acute myocardial infarction into two groups; prehospital thrombolysis and thrombolysis after arrival at the hospital. GPs selected patients on the basis of a history of chest pain from 20 minutes to 4 hours with treatment initiated within 6 hours from onset of pain. Patients in the prehospital treatment group received thrombolysis up to 130 minutes earlier than patients at hospital (101 vs 240 minutes from the onset of symptoms) with a 50% reduction in mortality in the prehospital group; 17 (10.4%) vs 32 (21.6%). The greatest saving of time was seen in the rural environment as well as in areas where there were significant inhospital treatment delays (Rawles, 1994). Importantly, during the GREAT study, prehospital thrombolysis was undertaken using a single bolus thrombolytic agent.

Patients enrolled in the GREAT study were followed up at five years where investigators noted 25% of the prehospital treatment group had died compared to 36% in the inhospital treatment group (Rawles, 1997). The GREAT study reconfirmed the negative impact of time delays by demonstrating that delaying thrombolysis by one hour increased the hazard ratio of death by 20%, with the equivalent loss of 43 lives per 1000 patients treated at five years. In a subset analysis of GREAT patients who met current ECG criteria for thrombolysis undertaken after 10 years, a 16% difference in mortality was maintained between the two groups (Rawles, 2003). The benefits seen in GREAT were significantly higher than those seen in any other thrombolysis study. The long-term mortality patterns has not been replicated in other long-term (inhospital) follow up studies, like ISIS-2 (1988) or GUSTO-1 (1993).

Treatment delays and the potential time savings of prehospital thrombolysis are key factors in the decision-making process around reperfusion with a meta-analysis by Morrison et al. (2000) of six randomized controlled trials clearly demonstrating the impact of the time savings to be achieved with prehospital treatment over inhospital treatment. Morrison et al. reported on all-cause hospital mortality as well as symptom to treatment time and adverse events. Although individual trials failed to demonstrate a statistically significant difference in all cause inhospital mortality; the meta-analysis involving 6434 patients showed a pooled benefit with prehospital thrombolysis. Morrison et al. demonstrated that prehospital thrombolysis saved approximately 60 minutes ($p = 0.07$) per patient compared to inhospital thrombolysis (104 versus 162 minutes) thereby reducing all-cause hospital mortality by 17%. If we consider the data from the five year follow up of the GREAT study, such time-savings can be extrapolated into significant numbers of lives saved.

Bjorklund et al. (2006) evaluated treatment delays and outcome in a large cohort of acute STEMI patients transported by ambulance who were either thrombolysed by paramedics in the prehospital environment or thrombolysed inhospital. Importantly, Björklund et al. utilized data from the Swedish / Register of Cardiac Intensive Care drawing data from 75 hospitals. Although register based data lacks the scientific controls seen within clinical trials, it is arguably more reflective of 'real life' clinical care. Following this study, Bjorklund et al. were able to conclude that prehospital thrombolysis by paramedics in ambulances was associated with reduced time to thrombolysis by almost 1 hour and reduced adjusted 1-year mortality by 30%.

Minimizing treatment delays in the administration of thrombolysis is key to optimizing patient outcomes. Although the LATE study (Becker, 1995) demonstrated clinical benefits of thrombolysis up to 12 hours, the greatest benefits were seen within 6 hours with the highest mortality reduction seen in those patients treated within the first 3 hours from onset of symptoms. The most commonly perceived post thrombolysis risks of stroke or major haemorrhage remain static regardless of when within the 12 hour period thrombolytic therapy is administered. However, the typically lethal complication of myocardial rupture exponentially increases after six hours. As demonstrated in the GREAT, WEST (Armstrong, 2006) and CAPTIM (Bonnefoy et al., 2009) studies prehospital thrombolysis is more likely to recruit patients within the first 6 hours of symptom onset; typically within the first 3 hours were the clinical benefit of treatment is at its highest.

These trails and others help to confirm the feasibility and safety of prehospital thrombolysis in a wide variety of circumstances and settings ranging from traditional ambulance services through to use by ship-based medical teams (cruise ships) and deployed military medicine. However, the choice between reperfusion strategies to manage acute STEMI remains a topic of interest. While it is agreed that primary PCI is the best strategy for acute STEMI it is still time sensitive and therefore needs to be performed in a timely manner and by experienced centres. This is not always achievable in developing countries, in rural health care settings or in remote medical facilities such as cruise ships.

3. Prehospital thrombolysis supported by early intervention

A number of mixed strategies for reperfusion have been studied; to include prehospital thrombolysis (full dose thrombolytic therapy) supported by rescue PCI for failed thrombolytic reperfusion (a hybrid reperfusion strategy) plus pre-discharge or symptom/ischaemia driven PCI, reduced dose thrombolysis supported by immediate PCI (facilitated PCI) and primary PCI. The ASSENT-4 PCI (2006) study demonstrated that facilitated thrombolysis, that is, thrombolysis immediately followed by PCI has been proven to be an unsuccessful intervention and will not be discussed further.

A hybrid reperfusion service involves implementing the best combination of reperfusion options to meet the unique requirements of the patient and typically involves early prehospital thrombolysis for those patients with the greatest benefit e.g. anterior STEMI presenting within 2-3 hours supported by rescue PCI and pre-discharge angioplasty with a system of primary PCI for the remaining patients. It must be re-iterated that primary PCI does still offer a superior treatment option when it is available in a timely manner.

The WEST trial investigated the use of a number of different reperfusion strategies, immediate prehospital thrombolysis plus usual inhospital care (excluding routine PCI), prehospital thrombolysis with compulsory rescue PCI for failed thrombolysis against primary PCI strategy. A key finding of the WEST study was a lower incidence of cardiogenic shock in patients who received thrombolysis early (within 3 hours) and the importance of prehospital triage/decisions for reperfusion with delays to definitive treatment being shorter when a decision was made in the prehospital setting. The WEST study also highlighted that thrombolysis used timeously remains an important treatment modality in the early management of acute STEMI.

The larger CAPTIM study used a similar design to the WEST study utilizing prehospital triage/decision to prehospital thrombolysis (this time supported by compulsory rescue PCI) with pre-discharge coronary intervention compared to primary PCI. The long term 5 year follow up of the CAPTIM study confirmed a significant reduction in mortality when thrombolysis was administered within 2 hours in the prehospital group when compared with primary angioplasty. The relationship between reperfusion strategy and the time from symptom onset on 1 year mortality was examined in a pooled analysis of patients from the CAPTIM and WEST studies. Mortality benefit was observed time (< 2 hours) (2.8% vs 6.9%, p = 0.021, hazard ratio 0.43, 95% CI 0.20-0.91) emphasizing that time from symptom onset was a key determinant when selecting the reperfusion strategy for acute STEMI (Westerhout et al., 2011). The optimal design of a hybrid reperfusion service is yet to be determined but the data from WEST and CAPTIM would support prehospital thrombolysis within the first 3 hours as along as all patients were delivered to a receiving hospital with interventional cardiology capability.

Prehospital thrombolysis can clearly be initiated earlier that inhospital thrombolysis or primary PCI and it can be performed with limited equipment. In fact, the same minimum equipment is required to perform prehospital thrombolysis as is required to identify prehospital patients requiring direct admission for primary PCI. Data from WEST (paramedic decision-makers), CAPTIM (doctor decision-makers) and projected findings from STREAM (paramedic/nurse/doctor decision-makers) are intended to inform the debate as to whether a hybrid reperfusion system is appropriate within developed countries. Regardless of the reperfusion strategy put into place, empowering the prehospital clinician is pivotal to success.

4. Education, training & equipment

The efficacy and safety of pre-hospital thrombolysis is dependent on several pre-requisites (Birkhead, 2004; Björklund et al., 2006; Mehta et al., 2002; Weaver, 1997; Welsh et al., 2006):

1. Prehospital personnel being trained to recognize symptoms and management of STEMI and its early complications (pain, ventricular fibrillation/ventricular tachycardia and bradycardic arrhythmias).
2. Diagnoses of STEMI using a 12 lead ECG with or without computer assistance for diagnosis and/or data transmission.
3. Intravenous access to be established and the administration of reperfusion therapy to be initiated within a treatment protocol / clinical guideline and supported by a thrombolysis checklist.

4. During transportation rhythm monitoring, availability of a defibrillator and advanced cardiac life support are mandatory
5. Pre-alerting receiving hospital of impending arrival of the patient supported by (if available) electronic transmission of the 12 lead ECG
6. Consultation for on-line support can support decision-making
7. On-going quality assurance

4.1 Education and training

The foundation for the practice of thrombolysis requires an understanding of anatomy and physiology of cardiovascular system and the pathophysiology of acute coronary syndromes. The complications of acute coronary syndromes / acute myocardial infarction must be covered as this will prepare the paramedic/nurse/prehospital doctor for complications that may arise during clinical practice. The ability to analyze a 12 lead ECG with a particular focus on recognition of AMI is required along with an understanding of thrombolytic therapy. An evidence based thrombolysis protocol which is subject to regular review is required taking into consideration the operational requirements for the practical implementation of the protocol. Classroom practice through the use of simulated clinical patient scenarios for stable angina, unstable angina, infarctions of the various territories including right ventricular infarction and scenarios where thrombolysis is contra-indicated will prepare and improve clinical practice. This theoretical and practical classroom education and training will need to be supported by clinical exposure within coronary care units and cardiac catheterization facilities.

4.2 Diagnosing acute STEMI

Van't Hof et al. (2006) demonstrated that prehospital diagnoses, triage and treatment in the ambulance is feasible in 95% of acute STEMI patients when undertaken by highly trained paramedics using a validated computerized ECG software. Prehospital decision-making can also be improved with the electronic transmission of an ECG although systems that support autonomous prehospital thrombolysis are well established and electronic data transmission can be problematic as they tend to rely on mobile telephone technology. The availability of prehospital 12 lead ECG capabilities serves to improve cardiac care in general and increased use of recording and subsequent interpretation of the 12 lead ECGs by prehospital clinicians improves overall confidence in using the prehospital ECG as a diagnostic tool. A particularly important aspect of the prehospital 12 lead ECG is that it is often obtained in the early phase of the patient's illness and becomes a useful ECG to compare against ECGs obtained later on in the patient's care.

The availability of diagnostic software and more importantly data transmission introduces an interesting concept for remote medical management of STEMI as the formal diagnosis of STEMI can be made by a distant clinician with the attending clinician acting primarily as a technician. This would involve the practical skills of cannulation, obtaining a 12 lead ECG and resuscitation skills (e.g. defibrillation) being undertaken by a junior clinician, but the decision to treat being made by a supervising clinician. This concept would expand the provision of prehospital thrombolysis whilst minimizing the education burden of the attending clinician and would be suitable for use in remote medical sites such as off shore oil platforms or small remote communities (e.g. Scottish Islands). Such a system is not dissimilar to the early use of defibrillation by paramedics where external supervision was required before defibrillation was performed.

5. Protocols, checklists & consent

5.1 Protocols

The use of clinicians empowered to make individual thrombolysis decisions removes the requirement for fixed protocols, however at the very least an evidence-based clinical guidelines for thrombolysis will be required. The availability of a clinical guideline or protocol will depend on the level of training provided to the prehospital clinician as guidelines support lateral thinking, whereas protocols tend to be more prescriptive.

The development of the thrombolysis protocol / guidelines needs to incorporate adjunctive therapy such as anti-thrombotic agents (e.g. heparin) and anti-platelets agents. This is an important aspect of patient care as to date none of the completed prehospital or inhospital thrombolysis studies have incorporated optimal anti-platelet and anti-thrombotic therapy. However, STREAM is currently utilizing the most up-to-date thrombolysis strategy.

5.2 Checklist

A thrombolysis checklist (Table 1), as part of a protocol / guideline, can support rapid decision-making whilst acting as a prompt to steps in the patient's management. However, care must be taken to ensure that the checklist is not overly restrictive as this can lead to under treatment of appropriate patients and careful consideration of the checklist layout can rapidly identify those patients where prehospital thrombolysis is deemed inappropriate e.g. advanced age (Castle et al., 2007a).

All contra-indications to thrombolysis need to be carefully considered and weighted. Often the type and number of contra-indications selected will reflect the risk adverse nature of the service delivering prehospital thrombolysis and, therefore, the list of contra-indications may change as the prehospital service becomes more established. It is now agreed that previous contra-indications such as prior cardiac compressions (Castle et al., 2007b; Cross et al., 1991) are no longer barriers to thrombolysis (in fact post cardiac arrest survivors with STEMI require urgent reperfusion with either PCI or hrombolysis); nor is diabetic retinopathy. (Mahaffey et al., 1997). Furthermore, complete heart block (CHB) is an indicator for rapid reperfusion therapy with thrombolysis being an accepted form of treatment as prompt reperfusion of the AV node (inferior STEMI with CHB) or intra-ventricular septum/Bundle of His (anterior STEMI with CHB) will resolve the arrhythmia thereby removing the need for a temporary pacing wire (Castle et al., 2007b) - the very reason typically quoted for with-holding thrombolytic therapy. All contra-indications to thrombolysis, with the exception of myocardial rupture as shown by the LATE Study (1993), are static/not affected by time whereas the benefit of thrombolysis is time dependent. Therefore, denying prehospital thrombolysis in a patient with STEMI based on one contra-indication only for the patient to be transferred to hospital for thrombolytic therapy to be administered will be counter-productive.

	Primary assessment: Can you confirm the following?	**Yes**	**No**
1	The patient is conscious and coherent, and able to understand that clot dissolving drugs will be used?		
2	The patient has symptoms that are characteristic of a heart attack (severe, continuous pain in a typical distribution of 15 minutes duration or more without remission)?		
3	The symptoms started less than 12 hours ago? NOTE: Consider "stuttering start" MI – many infarcts start this way.		
4	The pain built up over seconds and minutes rather than starting totally abruptly?		
5	Breathing does not influence the severity of the pain?		
6	The systolic blood pressure is more than 80mmHg and less than 180mmHg and that the diastolic is below 110mmHg despite treatment? i.e. Analgesia & GTN for blood pressure and fluid challenge / atropine for hypotension).		
7	The electrocardiogram ECG shows abnormal ST elevation of 2mm or more in at least 2 standard leads or in at least 2 adjacent precordial leads, not including V1? NOTE: ST elevation can sometimes be normal in V1 and V2.		
8	The QRS width is 0.16 seconds (4 small squares) or less, and that left bundle branch block is absent from the tracing? NOTE: RBBB is permitted only with qualifying ST elevation. LBBB = QRS 140 ms or greater; small narrow R wave in V1 & V2 with big S wave; tall upright monophasic R in standard Lead 1 and V6.		
	Secondary assessment (contra-indications): Can you confirm the following?	**Yes**	**No**
9	The patient is **not** likely to be pregnant, nor has delivered within the last 2 weeks?		
10	The patient has **not** had an active peptic ulcer within the last 6 months?		
11	The patient has **not** had a stroke of any sort within the last 12 months and does not have any permanent disability from a previous stroke?		
12	The patient has **no** diagnosed bleeding tendency, has had no recent blood loss (except normal menstruation) and is not taking warfarin (anticoagulant) therapy?		
13	The patient has **not** had any surgical operation, tooth extractions, significant trauma, or head injury within the last 4 weeks?		
14	The patient has **not** been recently treated for any other serious head or brain condition?		
15	The patient is **not** being treated for liver failure, renal failure, or any other severe systemic illness?		

Table 1. An example of a thrombolysis checklist

5.3 Consent

It is standard practice to obtain consent from the patient for thrombolytic therapy. The complications from thrombolysis are well documented. The patient will need to be appraised of the risks in undergoing thrombolysis. A standard statement that is simple, clear and concise is used in most established prehospital settings. An example of such a statement is as follows (Table 2):

However, it remains arguable whether a patient in pain or post opiate administration is in a position to give informed consent. It, therefore, falls to the attending clinician to ensure that they are working in the patient's best interest.

Initial Consent

"It is likely that you are having a heart attack and the best treatment available to you is a clot dissolving drug called (***specify agent***). The quicker you receive this drug, the lower the risks of a heart attack-which is why Doctors recommend that the treatment is started as soon as possible. These drugs can cause serious side effects in a small minority of patients which I can explain to you in more detail if you so wish, but the risks attached to this treatment are very much less than the likely benefit. Would you like me to give you the injection or would you prefer to have more details?'

I hereby consent to the treatment:

________________	_____/_____	____________________
Name of patient	Date / Time	Signature / Thumbprint

In the unlikely event that the patients do want more information they should be given the following information:

Further information

"Treatment at this stage saves the lives of about 1 in every 25 treated. But it can sometimes cause serious bleeding. The biggest risk is stroke which affects about 1 patient in every 200 treated. Some patients also have allergic and other effects that do not usually cause any major problems. Would you like me to give you the injection?"

Table 2. An example of consent

6. Drugs

6.1 Thrombolytic agents

There are a number of thrombolytic agents available, however Tenecteplase (TNK) is the only single-use bolus agent available making it the most suitable for prehospital use. Despite this, the ideal thrombolytic agent currently does not exist.

The characteristics of an "ideal thrombolytic agent" are as follows:

- Rapid reperfusion (15 - 30 minute)
- 100% efficacy at achieving 100% TIMI 3 in 30 minutes
- Administered as a single intravenous bolus
- Lower incidences of intracranial haemorrhage
- Lower incidences of systemic bleeding and other complications.
- Specific for recent thrombi
- Lower incidences for re-occlusion
- Long-term sustained patency
- No antigenicity
- No negative interaction with adjunctive therapy
- Affordable

The GUSTO trial (1993) demonstrated the superiority of the accelerated regimen of tissue plasminogen activator (tPA, Alteplase) over Streptokinase (STK), however, this came at a price of slightly greater risk of intracranial haemorrhage especially in female patients over the age of 75 years. However, stroke after thrombolysis is a known risk and in the GUSTO trial the stroke rate with STK was 1.19% compared to 1.55% with tPA (Gore et al., 1995). The issue of stroke is an important consideration as denying thrombolysis does not decrease the stroke rate as STEMI is an independent risk factor for stroke - unrelated to thrombolysis primarily due to the higher incidence of atrial fibrillation (AF) and poor left ventricular (LV) function caused by STEMI. Therefore, early treatment of STEMI with reperfusion that reduces the incidence of AF and LV dysfunction is an important aspect of stroke and morbidity reduction.

Single bolus TNK is now the most widely used thrombolytic agent in the developed world partly due to its improved efficacy but also because of ease of administration and variable dosing. TNK and Alteplase are equivalent in regard to 30 day mortality, but non-cerebral bleeding and blood transfusions are less with TNK.

The dose of TNK is weight adjusted and administered in a single bolus over 5 seconds as compared to 90 minutes of variable rate infusion with tPA or a 30 - 60 minute infusion of STK. Although a 30 minute regime for STK exists, it is associated with an increased risk of hypotension but by slowing the infusion rate of STK, the incidence of hypotension tends to decrease. Reteplase is a more fibrin specific agent administered as a 10 unit twin bolus given 30 minutes apart. However, the time sensitive nature of the twin bolus administration of Reteplase can be problematic. Reteplase is equivalent with reduction in mortality and hemorrhage rates achieved with Alteplase.

The major benefit of the bolus agents lies in the ease of administration and in the simplified dosing regimen that reduces the risk of dosing errors. However, the cost of TNK and its manufacturer's recommendation for use up to 6 hours makes the cheaper STK a more practical drug of choice for use in the developing world as for each patient treated with TNK five patients could be treated with STK (Table 3) (BNF, 2011). Its use as a prehospital thrombolytic is worth consideration, particularly in static remote health care settings, although its requirement for an infusion plus the incidence of hypotension makes it more labour intensive.

	Streptokinase (STK)	Alteplase (tPA)	Reteplase (rtPA)	Tenecteplase (TNK)
Fibrin selective	No	Yes	Yes	Yes
Plasminogen binding	Indirect	Direct	Direct	Direct
Duration of infusion (minutes)	60	90	10 + 10	5-10 seconds
Half life (minutes)	23	<5	13-16	20
Fibrinogen breakdown	4+	1-2+	Not known	>tPA
Early heparin	Yes	Yes	Yes	Yes
Hypotension	Yes	No	No	No
Allergic reactions	Yes	No	No	No
Approximate cost/dose	£83.44/1.5 MU	£600/100 mg	£627.27/20 unit kit	£502.25/50 mg
TIMI reflow grade 3 at 90 min	32	45-54	60	>tPA
Recommended use	Up to 12 hours	Up to 12 hours	Up to 12 hours	Up to 6 hours (typically used up to 12 hours)

Table 3. Characteristics of commonly used thrombolytic agents. Adapted from Opie (2009).

There are two key considerations for the use of STK in the prehospital environment. The first is duration of infusion and second the requirement for an expensive infusion pump. Although an infusion pump offers better control of drug delivery, this is less of an issue with STK as the delivery of STK is less time sensitive when compared to tPA. In static medical care environments (e.g. remote medical center) the infusion can be completed before hospital transfer as STK can be safely delivered without an infusion pump using either a small intravenous bag (100/250ml 0.9% saline) or a pediatric burette supported by close clinician supervision. The use of a pediatric burette or a 100/250ml bag of saline is not an option for administration during ambulance transfer as the low ceilings in ambulances lack the height to ensure fluid flow and this is further aggravated by ambulance movement. Novel techniques involving the use of low cost drip counters (that restrict flow through an administration set) supported by a pressure infusion bag to maintain a constant pressure through the drip counter is feasible but as yet, is unproven.

The second consideration is the much higher incidence of hypotension and bradycardia. This is due to the release of bradykinin and not as commonly thought as an allergic reaction (although anaphylaxis is more common with STK, it remains rare). Therefore, the treatment of hypotension consists of slowing or stopping the infusion and the administration of a 250-500ml crystalloid bolus. The routine use of intravenous steroids and anti-histamines offers no clinical benefit and in the case of intravenous steroids, it may adversely affect patient outcome by affecting myocardial scar tissue formation, thereby potentially increasing the risk of myocardial rupture.

Streptokinase	Tenecteplase
1.5 mega units over 30-60 minutes (requires an infusion pump)	Single weight adjusted bolus
Aspirin 300mg	Aspirin 300mg
Clopidogrel age adjusted (75-300mg)	Clopidogrel age adjusted (75-300mg)
No heparin (local policy my vary)	Weight adjusted heparin bolus followed by infusion or weight adjusted subcutaneous injection of heparin: 4000 unfractionated heparin bolus followed by infusion (an infusion pump is mandatory) Age adjusted enoxaparin.
Bradycardia (common) reversed by atropine	Bradycardia (less common than STK) reversed by atropine
High risk of drug induced hypotension responsive to fluid challenge stopping/slowing infusion	No specific drug induced hypotension
Labour intensive	Not labour intensive
Affordable (if no infusion pump used)	Expensive

Table 4. Comparison of a STK and TNK treatment regime

6.2 Adjunctive drug treatment

6.2.1 Oxygen

Oxygen is commonly administered during the management of patients during thrombolysis. Its routine use in patient with pulse oximetry above 95% has been questioned primarily due to the possibility of vasoconstriction and limited evidence of benefit (O'Driscoll, 2008). Oxygen remains an important adjunctive therapy in the presence of left ventricular failure although it is better provided as part of continuous positive airway pressure. Oxygen should routinely be administered in the presence of arrhythmias (e.g. ventricular tachycardia) (Neumar, 2010), hypotension/hypo-perfusion and any post cardiac arrest.

6.2.2 Analgesia

Analgesia is a priority therapy in the management of STEMI and intravenous opiates (morphine, diamorphine or fentanyl) offer the most effective analgesia although the legal framework for administration of these drugs can be problematic resulting in drugs such as Tramadol or Nubain being used if legal barriers to opiates do exist. The use of inhaled nitrous oxide (Entonox™) remains a useful supplementary analgesic (or primary analgesic if prehospital opiates are not available) providing both supplementary oxygen and analgesia and the use of Pentrane (common in Australia) is also a useful inhaled analgesic allowing higher percentage of inhaled oxygen if required. Thrombolysis also represents effective analgesia as the restoration of myocardial blood flow results in pain relief reflecting successful reperfusion.

Non-pharmacological interventions (re-assurance, calm professional mannerism of the care provider) are important aspects of pain relief. The use of rapid road transfer with lights and sirens may induce greater patient anxiety (as well as the risk of road traffic collision). If prehospital thrombolysis has been administered (with appropriate adjunctive therapy) there is little to be gain from rapid transfer to hospital.

6.2.3 Nitrates

Although there is no survival benefit to be gained from nitroglycerin it remains a common early therapy primarily providing analgesia. Nitroglycerin (0.4mg) is typically administered sublingually although intravenous nitrates are also used to manage on-going ischaemic chest discomfort, control of hypertension and for the management of pulmonary oedema (nitrates are a Class I recommendation for left ventricular failure). Nitrates should not be administered to patients who have received phosphodiesterase inhibitor within 24 to 48 hours and should be administered with care in patients with suspected right ventricular infarction as they may induce marked hypotension. Despite this, nitrates are very safe drugs for use by prehospital clinicians and it must be remembered that known cardiac patients may have already treated themselves with varying doses of nitrates prior to the arrival of the prehospital clinician.

6.2.4 Antiplatelet agents

Antiplatelets are vital in the management of all acute coronary syndromes (unstable angina, non-STEMI and STEMI). Within the context of STEMI management anti-platelet therapy is as important as thrombolytic therapy. This is because the intra-coronary thrombus responsible for re-infarction tends to be platelet rich and thrombolysis may raise the possibility of thrombolytic-induced platelet aggregation (Keeley et al., 2006).

6.2.4.1 Aspirin

All patients with suspected acute coronary syndrome (unstable angina, non-STEMI and acute STEMI), should be considered for prehospital aspirin treatment as there are relatively few contra-indications to a single dose of aspirin (Class I recommendation). Despite this, aspirin is often withheld either due to concerns over allergy, adverse drug interactions (e.g. Warfarin), confusion due to chronic ongoing use of aspirin or uncertainty of diagnosis. Typically unless a patient has a known documented allergic reaction (not just gastric irritation) to aspirin or is actively bleeding from a gastrointestinal tract ulcer, aspirin at the 300mg dose should be given. The choice of 300mg is typically the dose of a single aspirin with the administration being initiated as early as possible with consideration being given to emergency call takers being empowered to recommend aspirin before the arrival of emergency personnel (Class IIb recommendation).

The benefit of aspirin was established in the ISIS 2 trial (1988) where 162.5 mg aspirin resulted in 25 lives saved per 1000 patients primarily by reducing the incidence of re-infarctions (10 non-fatal re-infarctions per 1000) as well as preventing 3 non-fatal strokes per 1000 patients. The results from ISIS 2 highlighted that the effectiveness of aspirin alone was nearly as effective as STK without aspirin (23% v 25% odds reduction of death) and that by combining aspirin with STK, the magnitude of benefit was highly significant (42% odds reduction of death). It is noteworthy that aspirin administration during the ISIS 2 trial was anytime within the first 24 hours but a meta-analysis by Freimark et al. (2002) demonstrated that early aspirin administration (before thrombolysis) was an independent factor in patient survival at 1 year (5% vs 11% survived with early aspirin; odds ratio 0.41; 95% CI 0.21-0.74).

The benefits of aspirin for acute STEMI are attributed to its inhibition cyclo-oxygenase dependent platelet activation. The administration of an initial dose of 160-300mg aspirin ideally non-enteric coated formulation chewed is a Class I recommendation for acute STEMI. Intravenous or rectal aspirin are also acceptable routes of administration.

Although over-treatment of patients or the administration of an unnecessary treatment cannot be endorsed, the benefits of early use of aspirin in any patient with symptoms suspected of a STEMI (or other acute coronary syndrome) is such that the potential of over-treatment of patients is arguably worth the risk, especially when comparing the maximum acute anti-platelet dose of aspirin (300mg) to the analgesic dose of aspirin of 600-900mg.

6.2.4.2 Clopidogrel

Clopidogrel is a potent platelet inhibitor and the anti-platelet benefits of clopidogrel in combination with aspirin is to reduce ischaemic events in non ST-elevation acute coronary syndromes (Yusuf et al., 2001) and in patients undergoing percutaneous coronary intervention - PCI CLARITY (2005). The COMMIT-CCS 2 (2005) trial involving more than 45 000 patients (many post thrombolysis) demonstrated that administration of Clopidogrel (75mg daily) with aspirin and standard treatment safely reduced mortality and major vascular events. In the CLARITY-TIMI 28 Trial (2006), patients 75 years and younger with acute STEMI received thrombolysis supported by a loading dose of 00mg Clopidogrel followed by 75mg once daily and either low molecular weight heparin (LMWH) or unfractionated heparin (UFH). The combination of dual anti-platelet therapy (aspirin/clopidogrel) with thrombolytic treatment demonstrated more favorable angiographic patency of the infarct related artery and a reduction in mortality. A major contributor to mortality reduction was the reduction in the re-infarction rate in those patients receiving dual anti-platelet therapy. This was without an associated increase in the rate of bleeding.

The importance of improved patency and lower incidence of re-infarction was confirmed in the ECG CLARITY-TIMI 28 Study (2006) where the use of clopidogrel was shown to improve late coronary patency and clinical outcomes in those patients who achieve ST-segment resolution by preventing re-occlusion of open arteries rather than by facilitating early reperfusion. The administration of 300mg loading dose of clopidogrel in association with thrombolysis to patients less than 75 years of age is a Class IIa recommendation and it is common practice to adjust the dose in the over 75 year old patients to 75mg based on the COMMIT data.

Newer oral antiplatelets such Prasugrel and Ticagrelor are now available with potentially improved antiplatelet as Ticagrelor produces a more profound and consistent antiplatelet effect than clopidogrel (Wallentin et al., 2003), but as yet to be studied in conjunction with thrombolytic therapy.

6.2.5 Anticoagulants

Heparin is considered to be effective and is routinely given as an adjunct for PCI and thrombolytic therapy although it is commonly withheld in the first 24 hours in those patients receiving STK. The role of heparin is primarily to reduce re-infarction but the combination of dual anti-platelet therapy, thrombolysis and heparin may increase the risk of bleeding. The American Heart Association guidelines call for careful weight based dosing of heparin with thrombolytic therapy in STEMI (Antman et al., 2008).

The timing of heparin therapy when using fibrin specific thrombolytic agents (tPA, reteplase and TNK) is an important aspect of patient management. In an observational study of the United Kingdom (UK) national registry the frequency of re-infarction during hospital admission after thrombolytic treatment of 35, 356 STEMI patients during 2005–2006 was analyzed. Re-infarction rates with inhospital treatment were similar for reteplase (6.5%) and TNK (6.4%) but were higher for those patients treated by paramedics in the community. When the interval from prehospital treatment to hospital arrival was greater than 30 minutes re-infarction rates were 12.5% for reteplase, and 11.4% for TNK. For intervals shorter than 30 minutes the re-infarction rates were significantly greater for TNK (9.3% than reteplase (4.2%). Overall, re-infarction rates were higher after prehospital treatment with TNK than reteplase (9.6% vs 6.6%, p=0.005).

The differences in re-infarction rates were considered to be primarily due to the different uses of adjunctive anti-thrombotic therapy as UK paramedic thrombolysis protocols only allowed a single bolus dose of heparin prior to thrombolysis but did not allow for ongoing heparinization until arrival inhospital as compared to inhospital practice which resulted in either an infusion of UFH (800-1000 IU per hour adjusted to aPTT) or weight adjusted LMWH. It was also noted that on arrival at hospital there was often a delay in the commencement of heparin therapy, either due to confusion about the prehospital protocol or other time related pressures. In addition, clopidogrel was commonly administered early in association with inhospital thrombolysis but only after arrival at hospital for those patients receiving prehospital thrombolysis (Horne et al., 2009). This may also have been a confounding factor as Keeley (2006) noted that thrombolysis induced platelet aggregation was a possible cause of re-infarction following thrombolysis.

UFH has long been regarded as the anti-thrombotic agent of choice in the adjunctive treatment of patients with STEMI until the introduction of enoxaparin. The ASSENT-3 PLUS Trial (2003) evaluated the feasibility, efficacy and safety of prehospital enoxaparin or UFH with tenecteplase. There was a reduction in the composite of 30 day mortality, inhospital re-infarction or inhospital refractory ischemia in the enoxaparin group (14.2% vs 17.4%., p = 0.08). However, there was a tendency towards higher rates of intracranial haemorrhage (ICH) and major bleeding in the enoxaparin group. The risk for ICH and major bleeding was mainly confined to patients > patients over 75 years. It must be noted that in ASSENT-3 PLUS, the dose of enoxaparin was not weight adjusted. The safety concern of enoxaparin among elderly patients was addressed by the ExTRACT-TIMI-25 Trial (2005) that randomized more than 20 000 thrombolysed patients to receive either enoxaparin or UFH. The ExTRACT-TIMI 25 study was significantly changed from the ASSENT 3 study with patients > to greater than 75 years of age not receiving the IV bolus of enoxaparin as well as receiving a reduced dose of subcutaneous enoxaparin (75%) with a maximum ceiling dose of subcutaneous enoxaparin for the patients under 75 being set at 100mg and 75mg for the over 75 age group. The primary endpoint of this study was all cause mortality or non-fatal reinfarction at 30 days. Treatment with enoxaparin was found to be superior to UFH but was associated with an increase with major bleeding episodes. A telephone follow up at 1 year showed a sustained reduction in mortality or re-infarction when using the enoxaparin strategy (Morrow et al., 2010). Data from a meta-analysis from 12 earlier trials involving more than 49 000 patients support these results (Murphy et al., 2007). Enoxaparin is administered as an initial dose of 30mg intravenous bolus, followed by 1mg/kg subcutaneously within 15 minutes and is a Class I recommendation.

The likely reason for both the reduction in re-infarctions but also the increased risk of bleeding associated with enoxaparin is that enoxaparin (in fact all LMWHs) provide more predictable anticoagulation. Whereas UFH is both dose and person sensitive typically requiring frequent dose changes as dictated by aPTT and commonly results in either under or over anti-coagulation.

Enoxaparin offers a number of operational benefits for use with prehospital thrombolysis; primarily the absence of an infusion pump that is required when administering an infusion of UFH. Two single 100mg dose syringes of enoxaparin is adequate to support prehospital thrombolysis with one syringe being used for the 30mg IV dose followed by subsequent subcutaneous dose (the maximum subcutaneous dose of enoxaparin remains 100mg). The intravenous dose of enoxaparin can be simply administered by decanting all of a 100mg dose of enoxaparin into a 10ml syringe and then diluting with water for injection to a total volume of 10mls thereby providing 10mg enoxaparin per ml. A multiple use vial of enoxaparin for IV administration is also available.

6.2.6 Steroids and antihistamines

The routine administration of steroids and antihistamines to prevent hypotension/bradycardia especially in association with Streptokinase complicates the administration process and is unlikely to prevent hypotension as the cause of Streptokinase induced hypotension is primarily due to speed of administration (Lew et al., 1985; Tatu-Chiţoiu et al., 2004) and the action of bradykinin activated by Streptokinase (Hoffmeister et al., 1998).

Tatu-Chiţoiu et al (2004) noted that the incidences of hypotension occurred in nearly half of all patients treated with Streptokinase but it did not adversely affect patient outcome whereas the prophylactic use if steroids is linked with an increased risk of myocardial rupture (Mannisi et al., 1987) and is not recommended by the leading international cardiology societies (Van de Werf et al., 2008).

7. Support systems

Studies have clearly demonstrated that thrombolytic therapy can be safely administered in the prehospital environment by doctors, paramedics and nurses. The most effective system will depend on population demographics, geographical factors, the structure and financial resources of the emergency medical services. Regardless of who undertakes thrombolysis, the personnel need to be capable of rapid diagnosis, early risk stratification, minimal treatment delay and rapid administration of a thrombolytic agent. EMS systems vary throughout the world. In 75% of Europe thrombolysis is undertaken by emergency physicians while in many other settings like United Kingdom, Australia and United States of America, it is undertaken by paramedics. In most countries, the use of non-doctors in the prehospital environment seems to be the most practical and cost effective option.

The practice of paramedic thrombolysis may be undertaken independently or under direct supervision depending on the local emergency medical system. A system of consultation and 12-lead ECG transmission with CCU nurses/a senior paramedic/specialist clinician experienced in STEMI management is highly recommended at the initial implementation of thrombolysis and for on-going clinical support in difficult cases (Liem et al., 2007; McLean et al., 2008). Furthermore, paramedics can also fast track acute STEMI patients to CCU by by-passing the emergency department as well as by-passing local hospitals to deliver the patient to a hospital with an on-site catheter laboratory for either rescue angioplasty or pre-discharge angioplasty. These strategies have demonstrated reductions in door-to-balloon time and mortality (Afolabi et al., 2007; Bång et al., 2008; Le May et al., 2006).

The transmission of 12-lead ECG may be challenging and is dependent of the use of cellular technology which may result in the inability to transmit the ECG due to poor coverage or drop zones. The transmission of the ECG may involve the pairing of cellular phones and ECG machines therefore will need to be tested and practiced to prevent user error.

8. Quality assurance

An on-going continuous professional development programme which incorporates quality improvement measures obtained by on-going monitoring of prehospital thrombolysis via clinical audit and feedback should be mandatory for continued safe prehospital thrombolysis and staff development. A clinical review team incorporating all role players would need to meet regularly to appraise all cases of prehospital thrombolysis. In settings where the frequency of the performance of thrombolysis is low, an on-going programme of refresher training is essential to maintain skill competence. External surveillance registries like MINAP and the Swiss registries provide valuable information on trends in management of acute STEMI and should be used to guide treatment timeframes and clinical outcomes.

9. Other uses for prehospital thrombolysis

Prehospital thrombolysis is primarily aimed at the treatment of patients with symptoms and ECG diagnosis of STEMI. Although this will remain the mainstay of the use of thrombolytic therapy, thrombolysis is also used in the treatment of other clinical emergencies.

9.1 Stroke

Although stroke thrombolysis is not suitable for initiation in the community due to the need for a CT scan and in a small subset of patients an MRI, the early identification of patients with a possible stroke is vital. This has required a change in emphasis within emergency departments and ambulance services where an acute stroke has now been identified as a time-sensitive clinical emergency. The UK has just completed a mass TV awareness campaign for the recognition of stroke, building on the brain attack model developed in

America. Prehospital clinicians are, therefore, pivotal in the early identification of suspected stroke patients typically using the **F**ast, **A**rm, **S**peech, **T**est (FAST) supported by pre-arrival alerts to hospitals equipped to deliver stroke thrombolysis (with 3-4 hours of onset of symptoms).

9.2 Cardiopulmonary resuscitation (CPR)

The use of thrombolysis during resuscitation is also a potential treatment option but the routine administration of thrombolysis during cardiac arrest management is not endorsed (Class III recommendation). However, its use to treat a confirmed or suspected massive pulmonary embolism or STEMI should be considered on a case-per-case bases (Class IIa recommendation) (Neumar, 2010). Confirmation of diagnosis remains challenging but is primarily based on clinical history supported by clinical suspicion although the use of bedside ECHO for the diagnosis of massive pulmonary embolism is worth consideration (typically to look at the right ventricle) but the expertise for this is limited in the prehospital environment.

Following the administration of thrombolytic therapy, during CPR, the period of resuscitation should be extended to a minimum of 60 minutes (Neumar, 2010) and this protracted period of resuscitation is an important consideration when initiating thrombolytic therapy. The administration of thrombolysis during resuscitation does not replace the need for effective compressions and supportive ventilation but represents a targeted treatment for a small subset of patients.

10. Conclusion

Prehospital thrombolysis offers two unique clinical pathways for the patient presenting with STEMI. Prehospital thrombolysis can be the preferred reperfusion strategy in developing countries or countries without rapid access to primary angioplasty facilities or can provide ultra-early reperfusion as part of a hybrid reperfusion service. Key to the success of any prehospital service is the recruitment and training of appropriately qualified personnel although in remote areas the use of telemedicine and electronic data transmission can support the administration of thrombolysis by junior clinicians. Although thrombolysis offers significant patient benefits, it needs to be appropriately delivered and supported by adjunctive therapy which should include dual anti-platelet therapy for all patients supported by heparin (ideally LMWH) as appropriate.

11. References

Afolabi, B. A., G. M. Novaro, S. L. Pinski, K. R. Fromkin and H. S. Bush (2007). Use of the prehospital ECG improves door-to-balloon times in ST segment elevation myocardial infarction irrespective of time of day or day of week. *Emergency Medicine Journal*, Vol. 24,No. (8), pp. 588-591.

Antman, E. M., M. Hand, P. W. Armstrong, E. R. Bates, L. A. Green, L. K. Halasyamani, J. S. Hochman, H. M. Krumholz, G. A. Lamas, C. J. Mullany, D. L. Pearle, M. A. Sloan and S. C. Smith, Jr. (2008). 2007 Focused Update of the ACC/AHA2004 Guidelines for the Management of Patients With ST-Elevation Myocardial Infarction: A Report of the American College of Cardiology/American Heart Association Task Force on

Practice Guidelines Developed in Collaboration With the Canadian Cardiovascular Society Endorsed by the American Academy of Family Physicians. *Journal of American College of Cardiology*, Vol. 51,No. (2), pp. 210-247.

Antman, E. M., D. A. Morrow, C. H. McCabe, F. Jiang, H. D. White, K. A. A. Fox, D. Sharma, P. Chew and E. Braunwald (2005). Enoxaparin versus unfractionated heparin as antithrombin therapy in patients receiving fibrinolysis for ST-elevation myocardial infarction: Design and rationale for the Enoxaparin and Thrombolysis Reperfusion for Acute Myocardial Infarction Treatment-Thrombolysis In Myocardial Infarction study 25 (ExTRACT-TIMI 25). *American Heart Journal*, Vol. 149,No. (2), pp. 217-226.

Armstrong, P. W. (2006). A comparison of pharmacologic therapy with/without timely coronary intervention vs. primary percutaneous intervention early after ST-elevation myocardial infarction: the WEST (Which Early ST-elevation myocardial infarction Therapy) study. *European Heart Journal*, Vol. 27,No. (13), pp. 1530-1538.

Bång, A., L. Grip, J. Herlitz, S. Kihlgren, T. Karlsson, K. Caidahl and M. Hartford (2008). Lower mortality after prehospital recognition and treatment followed by fast tracking to coronary care compared with admittance via emergency department in patients with ST-elevation myocardial infarction. *International Journal of Cardiology*, Vol. 129,No. (3), pp. 325.

Becker, R. C., Charlesworth, A., Wilcox, R.G., Hamptom, J., Skene, A., Gore, J.M., Topol, E.J. (1995). Cardiac Rupture Associated with Thrombolytic Therapy: Impact of time to Treatrment in the Late Assessment of Thrombolytic Efficacy (LATE) Study. *Journal of American College of Cardiology* Vol. 25, pp. 1063-1068.

Björklund, E., U. Stenestrand, J. Lindbäck, L. Svensson, L. Wallentin and B. Lindahl (2006). Pre-hospital thrombolysis delivered by paramedics is associated with reduced time delay and mortality in ambulance-transported real-life patients with ST-elevation myocardial infarction. *European Heart Journal*, Vol. 27,No. (10), pp. 1146-1152.

BNF (2011). *British National Formulary*, BMJ Group. London

Bonnefoy, E., P. G. Steg, F. Boutitie, P.-Y. Dubien, F. Lapostolle, J. Roncalli, F. Dissait, G. Vanzetto, A. Leizorowicz, G. Kirkorian and for the CAPTIM investigators (2009). Comparison of primary angioplasty and pre-hospital fibrinolysis in acute myocardial infarction (CAPTIM) trial: a 5-year follow-up. *European Heart Journal*, pp. ehp156.

European Society of Cardiology, (2008). Management of acute myocardial infarction in patients presenting with persistent ST-segment elevation: The Task Force on the management of ST-segment elevation acute myocardial infarction of the European Society of Cardiology. *Europen Heart Journal*, Vol. 29,No. (23), pp. 2909-2945.

Castle, N., C. Porter and B. Thompson (2007b). Acute myocardial infarction complicated by ventricular standstill terminated by thrombolysis and transcutaneous pacing. *Resuscitation*, Vol. 74,No. (3), pp. 559-562.

Castle, N. R., R. C. Owen and M. Hann (2007a). Is there still a place for emergency department thrombolysis following the introduction of the amended Joint Royal Colleges Ambulance Liaison Committee criteria for thrombolysis? *Emergency Medicine Journal*, Vol. 24,No. (12), pp. 843-845.

Chen, M., L. X. Jiang, Y. P. Chen, J. X. Xie, H. C. Pan, R. Peto, R. Collins and L. L.S (2005). Addition of clopidogrel to aspirin in 45 852 patients with acute myocardial infarction: randomised placebo-controlled trial. *The Lancet*, Vol. 366,No. (9497), pp. 1607-1621.

Cross, S. J., H. S. Lee, J. M. Rawles and K. Jennings (1991). Safety of thrombolysis in association with cardiopulmonary resuscitation. *British Medical Journal*, Vol. 303, pp. 1242.

Freimark D, M. S., Leor J, Boyto V et al. 2002; . (2002). Timing of aspirin administration as a determinant of survival of patients with acute myocardial infarction treated with thrombolysis. *American Journal of Cardiology*, Vol. 89, pp. 381-385.

Gore, J. M., C. B. Granger, M. L. Simoons, M. A. Sloan, W. D. Weaver, H. D. White, G. I. Barbash, F. Van de Werf, P. E. Aylward, E. J. Topol and R. M. Califf (1995). Stroke After Thrombolysis : Mortality and Functional Outcomes in the GUSTO-I Trial. *Circulation*, Vol. 92,No. (10), pp. 2811-2818.

EMIP Group. (1993). Prehospital thrombolytic therapy in patients with suspected acute myocardial infarction. *N Engl J Med* Vol. 329, pp. 383-390.

GUSTO (1993). An International Randomized Trial Comparing Four Thrombolytic Strategies for Acute Myocardial Infarction. *New England Journal of Medicine*, Vol. 329,No. (10), pp. 673-682.

Hoffmeister, H. M., M. Ruf, H. P. Wendel, W. Heller and L. Seipel (1998). Streptokinase-Induced Activation of the Kallikrein-Kinin System and of the Contact Phase in Patients with Acute Myocardial Infarction. *Journal of Cardiovascular Pharmacology*, Vol. 31,No. (5), pp. 764-772.

Horne, S., C. Weston, T. Quinn, A. Hicks, L. Walker, R. Chen and J. Birkhead (2009). The impact of pre-hospital thrombolytic treatment on re-infarction rates: analysis of the Myocardial Infarction National Audit Project (MINAP). *Heart*, Vol. 95,No. (7), pp. 559-563.

ISIS-2 (1988). Randomised Trial Of Intravenous Streptokinase, Oral Aspirin, Both, Or Neither Among 17 187 Cases Of Suspected Acute Myocardial Infarction: ISIS-2. *Lancet* Vol. 332,No. (8607), pp. 349.

Keeley, E. C., J. A. Boura and C. L. Grines (2006). Comparison of primary and facilitated percutaneous coronary interventions for ST-elevation myocardial infarction: quantitative review of randomised trials. *The Lancet*, Vol. 367,No. (9510), pp. 579-588.

Koren, G., A. T. Weiss, Y. Hasin, D. Appelbaum, S. Welber, Y. Rozenman, C. Lotan, M. Mosseri, D. Sapoznikov, M. H. Luria and M. S. Gotsman (1985). Prevention of Myocardial Damage in Acute Myocardial Ischemia by Early Treatment with Intravenous Streptokinase. *New England Journal of Medicine*, Vol. 313,No. (22), pp. 1384-1389.

Le May, M. R., R. F. Davies, R. Dionne, J. Maloney, J. Trickett, D. So, A. Ha, H. Sherrard, C. Glover, J.-F. Marquis, E. R. O'Brien, I. G. Stiell, P. Poirier and M. Labinaz (2006). Comparison of Early Mortality of Paramedic-Diagnosed ST-Segment Elevation Myocardial Infarction With Immediate Transport to a Designated Primary Percutaneous Coronary Intervention Center to That of Similar Patients Transported to the Nearest Hospital. *The American Journal of Cardiology*, Vol. 98,No. (10), pp. 1329-1333.

Lew, A., P. Laramee, B. Cercek, L. Rodriguez, P. Shah and W. Ganz (1985). The effects of the rate of intravenous infusion of streptokinase and the duration of symptoms on the time interval to reperfusion in patients with acute myocardial infarction. *Circulation*, Vol. 72,No. (5), pp. 1053-1058.

Liem, S.-S., B. L. van der Hoeven, P. V. Oemrawsingh, J. J. Bax, J. G. van der Bom, J. Bosch, E. P. Viergever, C. van Rees, I. Padmos, M. I. Sedney, H. J. van Exel, H. F. Verwey, D. E. Atsma, E. T. van der Velde, J. W. Jukema, E. E. van der Wall and M. J. Schalij (2007). MISSION!: Optimization of acute and chronic care for patients with acute myocardial infarction. *American Heart Journal*, Vol. 153,No. (1), pp. 14.e11-14.e11.

Mahaffey, K., C. Granger, C. Toth, H. White, A. Stebbins, G. Barbash, A. Vahanian, E. Topol and R. Califf (1997). Diabetic retinopathy should not be a contraindication to thrombolytic therapy for acute myocardial infarction: review of ocular hemorrhage incidence and location in the GUSTO-I trial. Global Utilization of Streptokinase and t-PA for Occluded Coronary Arteries. *J Am Coll Cardiol*, Vol. 30,No. (7), pp. 1606-1610.

Mannisi, J. A., H. F. Weisman, D. E. Bush, P. Dudeck and B. Healy (1987). Steroid administration after myocardial infarction promotes early infarct expansion. A study in the rat. *The Journal of Clinical Investigation*, Vol. 79,No. (5), pp. 1431-1439.

McLean, S., G. Egan, P. Connor and A. D. Flapan (2008). Collaborative decision-making between paramedics and CCU nurses based on 12-lead ECG telemetry expedites the delivery of thrombolysis in ST elevation myocardial infarction. *Emerg Med J*, Vol. 25,No. (6), pp. 370-374.

Mehta, R. H., C. K. Montoye, M. Gallogly, P. Baker, A. Blount, J. Faul, C. Roychoudhury, S. Borzak, S. Fox, M. Franklin, M. Freundl, E. Kline-Rogers, T. LaLonde, M. Orza, R. Parrish, M. Satwicz, M. J. Smith, P. Sobotka, S. Winston, A. A. Riba, K. A. Eagle and G. A. P. S. C. o. t. A. C. o. C. for the (2002). Improving Quality of Care for Acute Myocardial Infarction: The Guidelines Applied in Practice (GAP) Initiative. *JAMA*, Vol. 287,No. (10), pp. 1269-1276.

Morrison, L. J., P. R. Verbeek, A. C. McDonald, B. V. Sawadsky and D. J. Cook (2000). Mortality and Prehospital Thrombolysis for Acute Myocardial Infarction. *JAMA: The Journal of the American Medical Association*, Vol. 283,No. (20), pp. 2686-2692.

Morrow, D. A., E. M. Antman, K. A. A. Fox, H. D. White, R. Giugliano, S. A. Murphy, C. H. McCabe and E. Braunwald (2010). One-year outcomes after a strategy using enoxaparin vs. unfractionated heparin in patients undergoing fibrinolysis for ST-segment elevation myocardial infarction: 1-year results of the ExTRACT-TIMI 25 Trial. *European Heart Journal*, Vol. 31,No. (17), pp. 2097-2102.

Murphy, S. A., C. M. Gibson, D. A. Morrow, F. Van de Werf, I. B. Menown, S. G. Goodman, K. W. Mahaffey, M. Cohen, C. H. McCabe, E. M. Antman and E. Braunwald (2007). Efficacy and safety of the low-molecular weight heparin enoxaparin compared with unfractionated heparin across the acute coronary syndrome spectrum: a meta-analysis. *European Heart Journal*, Vol. 28,No. (17), pp. 2077-2086.

Neumar, R. W., Otto, C. W., Link, M. S., Kronick, S. L., Shuster, M., Callaway, C. W., Kudenchok, P. J., Ornato, J. P., McNally, B., Silvers, S. M., Passman, R. S., White, R. D., Hess, E. P., Tang, W., Davies, D., Sinz, E. & Morrison, L. J. (2010). Part 8: Adult Cardiovascular Life Support: 2010 American Heart Association Guidelines for Cardiopulmonary Resuscitation and Emergency Care. *Circulation*, Vol. Vol 122,No. (Supplement), pp. S729-S767.

O'Driscoll, B. R., Howard, L.S. & Davison, A.G. (2008). Guidelines for emergency oxygen use in adults: On behalf of the British Thoracic Society Emergency Oxygeng Guidelines Development Group. *Thorax*, Vol. 63,No. (Supplement VI), pp. VI 1-VI 73.

Opie, L. H. G., B. J. (2009). *Drugs for the heart.*, Saunders Elsevier. 978-4160-6158-8, Philadelphia

Rawles, J. (1994). Halving of mortality by domiciliary thrombolysis in the Grampian Reagion Early Anstreplase Trial (GREAT). *Journal of the American College of Cardiology*, Vol. 23, pp. 1-5.

Rawles, J. (2003). GREAT: 10 year survival of patients with suspected acute myocardial infarction in a randomised comparison of prehospital and hospital thrombolysis. *Heart*, Vol. 89,No. (5), pp. 563-564.

Rawles, J. M. (1997). Quantification of the Benefit of Earlier Thrombolytic Therapy: Five-Year Results of the Grampian Region Early Anistreplase Trial (GREAT). *Journal of the American College of Cardiology*, Vol. 30,No. (5), pp. 1181-1186.

Sabatine, M. S., C. P. Cannon, C. M. Gibson, J. L. López-Sendón, G. Montalescot, P. Theroux, B. S. Lewis, S. A. Murphy, C. H. McCabe and E. Braunwald (2005). Effect of Clopidogrel Pretreatment Before Percutaneous Coronary Intervention in Patients With ST-Elevation Myocardial Infarction Treated With Fibrinolytics. *JAMA: The Journal of the American Medical Association*, Vol. 294,No. (10), pp. 1224-1232.

Scirica, B. M., M. S. Sabatine, D. A. Morrow, C. M. Gibson, S. A. Murphy, S. D. Wiviott, R. P. Giugliano, C. H. McCabe, C. P. Cannon and E. Braunwald (2006). The Role of Clopidogrel in Early and Sustained Arterial Patency After Fibrinolysis for ST-Segment Elevation Myocardial Infarction: The ECG CLARITY-TIMI 28 Study. *Journal of American College of Cardiology*, Vol. 48,No. (1), pp. 37-42.

Tatu-Chiţoiu, G., C. Teodorescu, M. Dan, M. Guran, P. Căpraru, O. Istrăţescu, A. Tatu-Chiţoiu, A. Bumbu, V. Chioncel, S. Arvanitopol and M. Dorobanţu (2004). Streptokinase-induced hypotension has no detrimental effect on patients with thrombolytic treatment for acute myocardial infarction. A substudy of the Romanian Study for Accelerated Streptokinase in Acute Myocardial Infarction (ASK-ROMANIA). *Romanian Journal of Internal Medicine*, Vol. 42,No. (3), pp. 557-573.

van 't Hof, A. W. J., S. Rasoul, H. van de Wetering, N. Ernst, H. Suryapranata, J. C. A. Hoorntje, J.-H. E. Dambrink, M. Gosselink, F. Zijlstra, J. P. Ottervanger and M.-J. de Boer (2006). Feasibility and benefit of prehospital diagnosis, triage, and therapy by paramedics only in patients who are candidates for primary angioplasty for acute myocardial infarction. *American Heart Journal*, Vol. 151,No. (6), pp. 1255.e1251-1255.e1255.

Van de Werf, F., J. Bax, A. Betriu, C. Blomstrom-Lundqvist, F. Crea, V. Falk, G. Filippatos, K. Fox, K. Huber, A. Kastrati, A. Rosengren, P. G. Steg, M. Tubaro, F. Verheugt, F. Weidinger, M. Weis, E. C. f. P. Guidelines, A. Vahanian, J. Camm, R. De Caterina, V. Dean, K. Dickstein, C. Funck-Brentano, I. Hellemans, S. D. Kristensen, K. McGregor, U. Sechtem, S. Silber, M. Tendera, P. Widimsky, J. L. Zamorano, D. Reviewers, F. V. Aguirre, N. Al-Attar, E. Alegria, F. Andreotti, W. Benzer, O. Breithardt, N. Danchin, C. D. Mario, D. Dudek, D. Gulba, S. Halvorsen, P. Kaufmann, R. Kornowski, G. Y. H. Lip and F. Rutten (2008). Management of acute myocardial infarction in patients presenting with persistent ST-segment elevation. *European Heart Journal*, Vol. 29,No. (23), pp. 2909-2945.

Van de Werf, P., A. Ross, P. Armstrong and C. Granger (2006). Primary versus tenecteplase-facilitated percutaneous coronary intervention in patients with ST-segment elevation acute myocardial infarction (ASSENT-4 PCI): randomised trial. *The Lancet*, Vol. 367,No. (9510), pp. 569-578.

Wallentin, L., P. Goldstein, P. W. Armstrong, C. B. Granger, A. A. J. Adgey, H. R. Arntz, K. Bogaerts, T. Danays, B. Lindahl, M. Mäkijärvi, F. Verheugt and F. Van de Werf (2003). Efficacy and Safety of Tenecteplase in Combination With the Low-Molecular-Weight Heparin Enoxaparin or Unfractionated Heparin in the Prehospital Setting. *Circulation*, Vol. 108,No. (2), pp. 135-142.

Weaver, W. D., Simes R.J., Betriu, A., Grines, C.L., Zijistra, F., Garcia, E., Grinfield, L., Gibbons, E.E., DeWood, M.A., Ribichini, F. (1997). Comparison of primary coronary angioplasty and intravenous thrombolytic therapy for acute myocardial infarction: a quantitative review. *Journal of American Medical Association* Vol. 278,No. (23), pp. 2093-2098.

Welsh, R. C., A. Travers, M. Senaratne, R. Williams and P. W. Armstrong (2006). Feasibility and applicability of paramedic-based prehospital fibrinolysis in a large North American center. *American Heart Journal*, Vol. 152,No. (6), pp. 1007.

Westerhout, C. M., E. Bonnefoy, R. C. Welsh, P. G. Steg, F. Boutitie and P. W. Armstrong (2011). The influence of time from symptom onset and reperfusion strategy on 1-year survival in ST-elevation myocardial infarction: A pooled analysis of an early fibrinolytic strategy versus primary percutaneous coronary intervention from CAPTIM and WEST. *American Heart Journal*, Vol. 161,No. (2), pp. 283-290.

Yusuf, S., F. Zhao, S. R. Mehta, S. Chrolavicius, G. Tognoni and K. K. Fox (2001). Effects of Clopidogrel in Addition to Aspirin in Patients with Acute Coronary Syndromes without ST-Segment Elevation. *New England Journal of Medicine*, Vol. 345,No. (7), pp. 494-502.

7

Thrombolysis in Myocardial Infarction

Ajay Suri[1], Sophia Tincey[2],
Syed Ahsan[1] and Pascal Meier[1]
[1]*The Heart Hospital, University College Hospital, London*
[2]*North Middlesex Hospital, London*
UK

1. Introduction

Worldwide around 7 million people suffer myocardial infarctions per year according to White et al. (2008). Around one third of these patients having acute myocardial infarction die within the first hour of having symptoms usually due to fatal arrhythmia. Characteristic ST segment elevation in the 12 lead electrocardiogram (ECG) accompanied by clinical symptoms of chest pain provide the most rapid way to diagnose those patients who should receive thrombolysis to help dissolve thrombus and restore blood flow. In fact, since the early 1980s, thombolysis has been the cornerstone of treatment for patients having ST segment elevation myocardial infarctions (STEMI) by improving outcomes and preserving left ventricular function. There are in fact many large randomised clinical trials which support early thrombolysis and these can be found in the Fibrinolytic Therapy Trialists' (FTT) Collaborative Group publication from 1994. This document reinforces the importance of early reperfusion with 30 lives per 10000 being saved by thrombolysis given within 6 hours of presentation and 20 lives per 1000 saved if initiation is between 6 and 12 hours.

2. Pathophysiology of myocardial infarction

Acute myocardial infarction which is commonly known as a heart attack is the interruption of blood supply and therefore oxygen to heart muscle thereby potentially causing cell death or necrosis. This is usually due to the occlusion of the coronary artery lumen by clot called thrombus. This thrombus is formed by the rupture of unstable arteriosclerotic plaque which consists of white blood cells (mainly macrophages) which engulf lipids to form foam cells covered with a fibrous cap in the arterial wall. The plaque can rupture as a result of many factors including the mechanical shear stress from blood flow and flexion and tension of the fibrous causing it to be injured and thinned. Rupture exposes adhesion molecules in the sub-endothelium which form thrombus when exposed to flowing blood. This allows primary haemostasis to occur, resulting in platelet adhesion, platelet activation and aggregation forming thrombus. Thrombolytic drugs break down this thrombus thereby restoring blood flow and preventing further damage to myocardium. It is therefore obvious to see that the sooner myocardial infarction is diagnosed and the earlier thrombolysis can be given the greater the myocardial salvage.

3. Clinical indications

The indications for thrombolysis in myocardial infarction rely on eliciting a history of typical clinical symptoms (mainly but not exclusively chest pain) and diagnosing characteristic changes in the 12-lead electrocardiogram (ECG) which is a non-invasive means of recording the electrical activity of the heart over seconds using transthoracic electrodes. The prompt recognition of the characteristic symptoms and ECG changes are required to institute rapid reperfusion therapy through thrombolysis.

The main clinical symptom of acute myocardial infarction is central or left-sided chest pain which can be described as dull, squeezing or tightness. This is called angina pectoris. The pain most commonly radiates to the left arm but can radiate to the neck, jaw, epigastrium, back and the right side of the chest. The management of myocardial infarction also requires prompt relief of the ischaemic pain with oxygen, opiates and sublingual or intravenous nitrates which act through vasodilatation. Other symptoms are shortness of breath from left ventricular dysfunction and resultant pulmonary oedema due to myocardial ischaemia. The remaining symptoms are due to surges of catecholamines from sympathetic overdrive such as palpitations, nausea, vomiting, light-headedness, weakness, anxiety and excessive sweating termed diaphoresis. Loss of consciousness may also occur and is usually due to arrhythmia as a consequence of ischaemia or cerebral hypoperfusion due to poor left ventricular output and cardiogenic shock. Notably women tend to report more atypical symptoms and so when making a diagnosis clinicians should bare this in mind. To complicate matters further around one quarter of patients suffering an acute myocardial infarction do not have any symptoms at all. These 'silent' myocardial infarctions most commonly occur in the elderly and diabetic patients. This can cause problems when selecting out patients that are suitable for thrombolysis as the clinician would have to rely on the ECG criterion and any other relevant history that is available at that time.

Other scenarios where a history may be difficult to obtain are patients that are acutely breathless from pulmonary oedema or those that have been successfully resuscitated or are being resuscitated from cardiac arrest. In these situations if the ECG shows characteristic changes and the bleeding risk from chest compressions is felt to be low then an experienced clinician can make the decision to proceed with thrombolysis. In cardiac arrests with refractory ventricular fibrillation and a prior history of chest pain or ischaemic heart disease then also in these cases a decision may be taken to give thrombolysis.

4. Electrocardiogram criterion

The ECG criterion for thrombolysis are well validated and need to be met before initiation of therapy. As mentioned earlier the ECG is a recording of electrical activity as it spreads through the heart muscle. The ECG can be daunting in its interpretation and in itself a massive topic but here we focus specifically on the parts of the ECG that are relevant for diagnosing acute myocardial infarction suitable for thrombolysis.

Ventricular depolarisation and contraction are represented on the ECG by a waveform termed the QRS complex which is later followed by a smaller deflection termed the T wave which constitutes ventricular repolarisation and relaxation. In fact, repolarisation begins with the ST segment which connects the QRS complex to the T wave. The beginning of the ST segment is termed the J point.

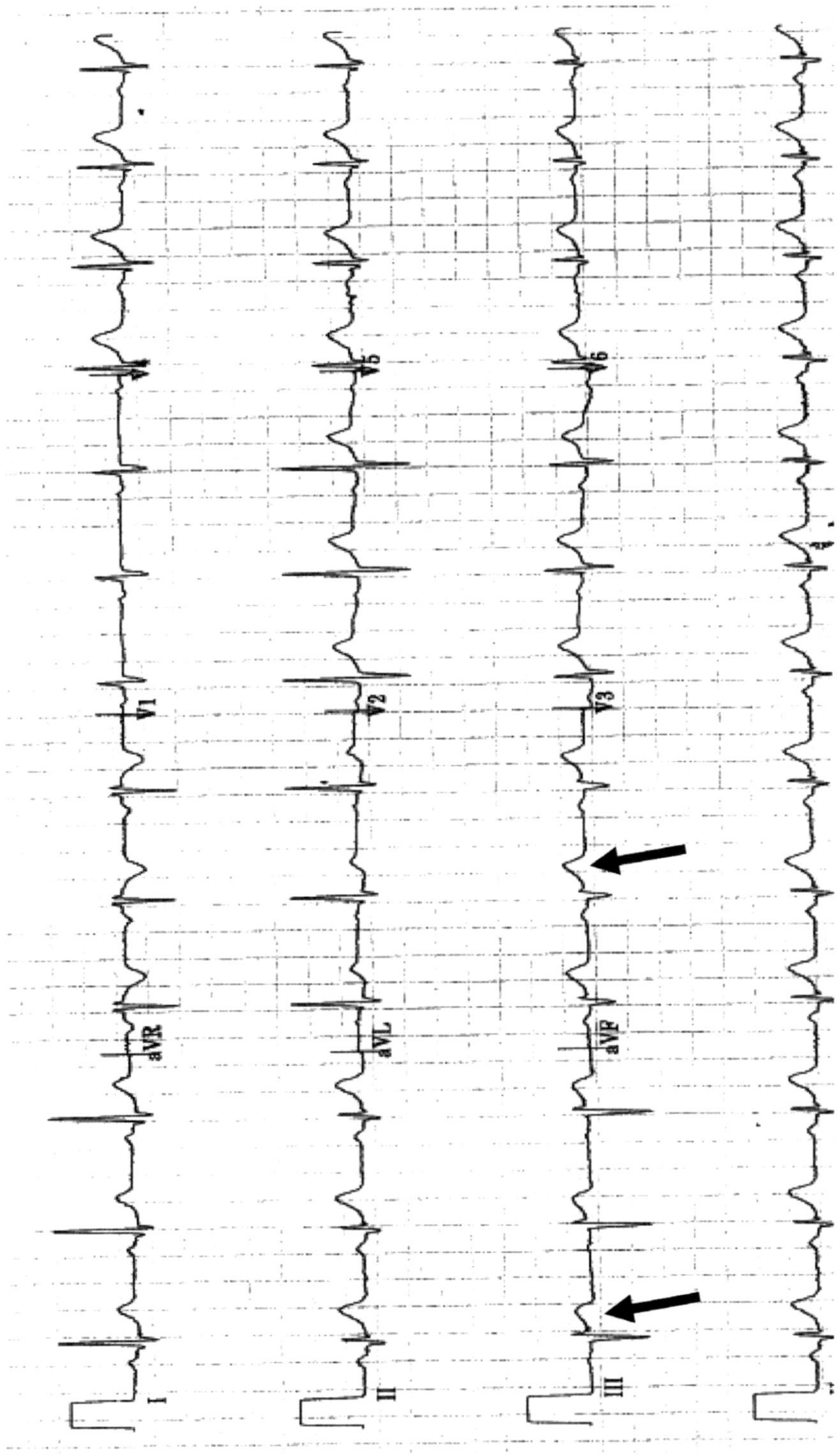

Fig. 1. An electrocardiogram showing ST elevation in leads III and AVF.

The criterion for thrombolysis refer to the QRS complex and ST segments and are as follows:

1. 1mm of ST segment elevation from the J point in at least 2 contiguous limb leads (I, II,III, AVF and AVL)
2. 2mm of ST segment elevation from the J point in at least 2 contiguous chest leads (any two of V1 to V6)

New onset left bundle branch block. This is recognised as characteristic deflections of the QRS complex and an increased width of greater than 120 milliseconds which is 3 small squares on the ECG when the recording speed is set to the usual 25mm/second.

The various limb leads and chest leads pick up electrical signals by literally overlying and 'pointing' towards various parts of the heart. Therefore ECG changes in certain leads represent ischaemia affecting certain territories or areas of heart muscle. ECG changes in leads I and AVR represent ischaemia in the anterior wall of the left ventricle while II, III, and aVF represent the inferior aspect of the heart. The V leads or chest leads show if the anterior-septal area is affected (V1-V4) and the late V leads signify infarction of the lateral wall of the ventricle. Leads I and AVL also represent the lateral territory of the heart. The criterion requires that these changes are in at least two contiguous leads because this is more likely to represent a significant area or 'territory' of myocardium. ST segment changes in a single lead are more likely to be due to other causes the most likely being normal variant due to an earlier repolarisation of the myocardium. Clinicians also need to bear in mind alternative diagnoses which could present with ST elevation by ECG. Acute pericarditis, which is a usually benign condition of pericardial inflammation, can present with ST elevation but typically the ST segment has a saddle-shaped appearance. The clinical symptoms may also mimic myocardial infarction but the classical description is of pain is different in that it is sharp and stabbing which varies with respiration and is also positional. Clinically the patient may also have an audible rub on auscultation using a stethoscope. This is a scratchy noise caused by the inflamed layers of pericardium rubbing against each other. The other condition in which ST elevation may be present is when the patient has an outpouching of the left ventricle termed an aneurysm. Again the ECG can have a more characteristic Clinicians should keep the possibility of these alternative diagnoses at the forefront of their minds to avoid misdiagnosis and therefore inappropriate administration of thrombolysis.

Other ECG changes that accompany ST elevation may also be present and aid the diagnosis of acute ST elevation myocardial infarction. The T waves may become hyperacute and lose their normal concavity. There may also be the presence of a pathological Q wave at the start of the QRS complex which is represented by a negative deflection of at least 1 small square on the ECG (40 milliseconds). This is said to represent infarcted non-viable myocardium. The other common abnormality which can accompany ST elevation is ST depression in reciprocal leads. Essentially, this means that leads looking at the opposite aspect of the heart show a mirror image of the leads showing ST elevation.

5. Contraindications for thrombolysis

Contraindications to thrombolysis in myocardial infarction can be separated into absolute and relative ones. Absolute contraindications are suspected dissecting aortic aneurysm, ischaemic stroke within 3 months (except if acute and within 3 hours of symptom onset when it is a treatment), intracranial neoplasm or arterio-venous malformation, active bleeding diathesis, uncontrolled hypertension (systolic>180mmHg or diastolic >100mmHg), significant closed-head trauma or facial trauma within 3 months.

Rigorous cardiopulmonary resuscitation or compressions of greater than 10 minutes duration is a relative contraindication to thrombolysis. Other scenarios which require precaution include active peptic ulceration, therapeutic anticoagulation with warfarin therapy, active menstruation, pregnancy, recent streptococcal infection of less than five days, controlled severe hypertension, haemorrhagic or diabetic retinopathy and invasive or surgical procedure in the preceding three weeks.

6. Evidence base for thrombolysis and alternative strategies

Initially, streptokinase infusion produced conflicting results until the (GISSI) trial in 1986, which validated streptokinase as an effective therapy and established a fixed regime for its use in acute myocardial infarction. As mentioned earlier the evidence supporting thrombolysis as opposed to not giving thrombolysis is outlined in the Fibrinolytic Therapy Trialists' (FTT) Collaborative Group publication from 1994. This combined the data from 9 trials and included a total of 58,600 patients. Here, the obvious survival advantage of thrombolysis in ST segment elevation in myocardial infarction and left bundle branch block was established. However, excess deaths were noted in the elderly and those thrombolysed after 12 hours of symptom onset. Most notably, it was clearly seen that the earlier thrombolysis was given the greater the benefit. The reason being that the earlier reperfusion is achieved the smaller the infarct size and the greater the myocardial salvage, which in turn has a significant impact on morbidity and mortality. This has led to targets for thrombolysis to be initiated within 20 to 30 minutes of arrival at hospital ("door to needle" time) and within 60 minutes of calling for help ("call to needle" time) across the UK and in Europe.

Primary percutaneous coronary intervention (PPCI) has evolved as an alternative emergency treatment for patients with STEMI. This is an invasive keyhole procedure which involves the passing of thin catheters from the femoral or radial arteries in to the aorta and then in to the openings of the coronary arteries to act as a conduit for various specialized equipment that can be used to treat the acute thrombus. The equipment used for this purpose are primarily clot extraction catheters termed extraction catheters, inflatable balloons and metal stents which act as a scaffold for keeping the arteries open. Although the number of patients receiving this treatment is steadily increasing because of the potential benefits, not all hospitals have the facilities to provide this therapy and so most patients in Europe still receive thrombolysis as initial management.

Once thrombolysis was established as a mode of treatment it was initially given in hospital by clinicians but with the extensive data that early thrombolysis yielded better outcomes there was a move towards pre-hospital thrombolysis (PHT). This involved emergency services giving thrombolysis at the scene on arrival to the patient.

Meta-analyses of RCTs show that PHT is superior to in-hospital thrombolysis (IHT) as it saves on average 30 minutes to 1 hour from the time between calling for medical help and initiation of thrombolysis. The time benefit is even more apparent where ambulance transport times are long. For this reason IHT is only reserved for those places that that do not offer PHT or PPCI. When PPCI is not available or offered around the clock then PHT becomes the treatment modality of choice to ensure the maximal myocardial salvage.

Comparison of Angioplasty and Prehospital Thrombolysis in Acute Myocardial Infarction (CAPTIM) compared PHT directly against PPCI. This showed that if thrombolysis was administered within 2 hours of symptom onset mortality data at 30 days strongly favoured this treatment over PPCI. However, after 2 hours the trend of outcomes reversed and PPCI became the treatment of choice. This was mirrored in the PRAGUE-2 trial which showed the benefits of IHT up to 3 hours.

In contrast to this the Primary Coronary Angioplasty vs. Thrombolysis (PCAT)-2 Trialists Collaborative Group meta-analysis looked at IHT versus an invasive strategy and showed that PPCI was superior to thrombolysis with lower mortality rates and risk of re-infarction. In the USA, guidelines favour the data on PHT over PPCI but also focus on the time factor with regards to reperfusion. They recommend that PHT should be given within 30 minutes after the arrival of emergency services at the scene and if this is not available and the patient is transferred to a hospital without PPCI facility then IHT should be given within 30 minutes of arrival at the centre (this is termed to door-to-needle time). If PPCI is offered in the hospital then actual disruption of the acute thrombus in the coronary artery should take place within 90 minutes (termed door-to-balloon time). European guidelines differ in that they prefer PPCI as the primary mode for reperfusion but with the several caveats. They stipulate that the procedure should be performed by a skilled operator in a high volume centre (operator performing more than 75 PCIs a year and the centre performing more than 200 PCIs) within 120 minutes of the first medical contact or within 90 minutes in patients receiving medical help within 2 hours from the onset of symptoms. If PPCI is not available then thrombolysis should be given within 3 hours of symptom onset with preference given to PHT over IHT.

7. Rescue PCI, routine PCI and facilitated PCI

When thrombolysis fails then rescue PCI should be considered. In the REACT trial patients that had not been successfully treated by thrombolysis after 90 minutes from initiating therapy (signified by less than 50% resolution of ST segment resolution by ECG) were randomized between conservative management, repeat thrombolysis and rescue PCI. This trial showed a clear benefit of the latter in all outcome data including 6 month mortality. Rescue PCI should therefore be offered to all patients within 12 hours of symptom onset. This may therefore involve patient transfer to a centre that offers a PCI service if not available at the hospital where the patient was thrombolysed or where they were taken after PHT. The exact definition of failed thrombolysis is controversial but the absence of chest pain is considered as misleading as opiates, analgesics and vasodilators may contribute to this. Generally accepted markers are taken as ST segment resolution of less than 50-70% and the time taken to assess whether thrombolysis has taken effect is between 45 and 90 minutes.

All patients should receive PCI subsequent to this, ideally within a period of 24 hours, but a benefit is even seen up to 30 days as evidenced by the CAPTIM trial. GRACIA-1, CARESS-in-AMI and the WEST trials all looked at PCI within a quicker time frame after thrombolysis and the overall results showed that this was comparable to PPCI outcomes when the post-thrombolysis PCI was performed within 24 hours. The very recent TRANSFER-AMI trial reinforced the benefits of a pharmaco-invasive strategy which compared PCI at 6 hours after thrombolysis with 'standard treatment' which involved thrombolysis with delayed angiography and PCI (after 24 hours). There was a statistically significant reduction in the primary endpoint of combined incidence of death, reinfarction, recurrent ischemia, new or worsening heart failure, or cardiogenic shock at 30 days for the pharmaco-invasive strategy (11% in the pharmaco-invasive arm vs. 17.2% in the standard treatment arm). There was also less recurrent ischaemia (0.2% vs. 2.1%) and reinfarction (3.4% vs. 5.7%) in the pharmaco-invasive strategy and fewer congestive heart failure (3.0% vs. 5.6%). On the other hand, there were more deaths and more patients experiencing cardiogenic shock in the pharmaco-invasive arm but these differences were not statistically significant. There were significantly more minor bleeding episodes in the combined strategy arm when compared to standard treatment but there was no difference in major bleeding. It is important to note that this pharmaco-invasive strategy is very different to thrombolysis followed by *immediate* PCI. This is called facilitated PCI and in fact has failed to shows clinical benefit and may in fact be harmful. The reason for this being that if PCI is performed too early then the thrombolytic administered is still active causing increased bleeding risk as well as resulting in more acute stent thrombosis (the potentially catastrophic blocking of a stent by thrombus within 24 hours of it being deployed) which is caused by the increased platelet activation and aggregation which accompanies thrombolytics.

The ideal setting for PHT in the USA involves an experienced physician being available to interpret the ECG by either being part of the Emergency Medical service team on the ambulance or being available to review a copy of a transmitted ECG. This has proved harder to achieve in Europe where more frequently, trained paramedics decide on whether the ECG meets criterion. Some UK studies have shown that this is safe and sometimes even better than the physician-assisted model due technological issues when transmitting the ECG or failure of mobile phones when trying to communicate to doctors from remote areas. However, in contrast a study in Finland has shown that having physicians on site for PHT is superior to paramedics alone. A checklist of contraindications should also be gone through prior to administration to ensure that the patient is not placed at increased risk of catastrophic bleeding. Therefore, this can also be used as a means of identifying those patients that are more suitable for PPCI.

8. Adjunctive therapies for thrombolysis

Aspirin is well established as an adjunctive therapy to thrombolysis and it is recommended that 150 to 325mg of chewable aspirin be given to the patient with thrombolysis. Clopidogrel is an oral, thienopyridine class antiplatelet agent which when given at a dose of 300 mg also provides prognostic benefit. The COMMIT-CCS-2 and CLARITY-TIMI 28 trials provided this evidence for adding clopidogrel to aspirin in patients undergoing fibrinolytic therapy.

It is recommended that unfractionated heparin, an intravenous anticoagulant is given intravenously with all of the thrombolytics to enhance clot dissolution and decrease the risk of re-occlusion. In vitro studies and animal models show discordant results regarding concomitant administration of heparin with thrombolysis suggesting that it may enhance, inhibit or have no effect. Hsia J et al.(1990) have shown that thrombolysis achieves faster lysis with greater vessel patency in combination with heparin (between 7 and 24 hours a patent vessel was found in 88% of those receiveing thrombolysis with heparin and aspirin vs. 52% in those treated with thrombolysis and aspirin alone). Unfortunately this does not translate into clinical outcome with a meta-analysis of the six trials by Muhaffey KW et al.

(1996) showing that there were similar rates of mortality and re-infarction before discharge. Despite this the general consensus from expert opinion is that heparin is beneficial in preventing re-occlusion and that it should be given as a bolus with all thrombolytics other than Streptokinase and then be given as a continuous IV infusion. With the advent of low molecular weight heparins (LMWHs) which only need once or twice daily subcutaneous administration without regular blood monitoring the continuous IV infusion of unfractionated heparin has been superseded by these newer anticoagulants. In fact there is evidence that the LMWH, Enoxaparin, appears superior to UFH in the EXTRACT-TIMI 25 trial when given during thrombolysis. In fact, patients under the age of 75 years can be given a 30 mg intravenous bolus followed by the subcutaneous dose every 12 hours. In practice this intravenous preparation LMWH is less widely available and UFH is more commonly given.

9. Thrombolytics used in clinical practice

9.1 Streptokinase

This was the first thrombolytic used in the treatment of STEMI and remains the cheapest and most commonly used. Two large trials were pivotal in demonstrating the efficacy of Streptokinase as a thrombolytic in myocardial infarction which reduces mortality when compared against placebo. The first of these was the GISSI trial mentioned earlier, published in 1986 and included 11,712 patients. This trial showed that at 21 days the mortality for patients treated with Streptokinase was 10.7% vs 13% for the placebo group which represented a statistically significant absolute reduction of 2.3% (risk ratio 0.81; 95% confidence ratio [CI] 0.72 to 0.9). The second trial, ISIS-2 trial included 17,187 patients and was published 2 years after GISSI in 1988. In this study, vascular mortality at 5 weeks was 9.2% in the streptokinase group and 12% in those treated with placebo which represented a statistically significant absolute reduction of 2.8%. Streptokinase is administered as an IV infusion over 1 hour. Streptokinase has a few side-effects which are namely low blood pressure termed hypotension, infrequent allergic reactions and sometimes although not commonly, anaphylaxis. Patients treated with streptokinase develop anti-streptococcal antibodies, which is why patients should only ever receive this drug once in a lifetime.

9.2 Alteplase

A meta-analysis of eight trials which compared alteplase with streptokinase found that there was no significant difference between the two drugs in terms of mortality up to 35 days. However, re-infarction rates were found to be in favour of alteplase but this was offset by a doubling in the risk of haemorrhagic stroke (odds ratio 2.13; 95% CI 1.04 to 4.36). In contrast to this, streptokinase was associated with a statistically significant higher risk of major bleeds than alteplase. However, the definitions of major bleeding varied between the trials and so it is difficult to judge the clinical significance of these findings.

9.3 Alteplase

Alteplase which is also known as recombinant human tissue plasminogen activator or rtPA can be delivered in a standard or accelerated regimen. The accelerated regimen, which is much more commonly used especially in PHT because of its ease of administration as it is delivered by an initial IV bolus injection. This is followed by only two IV infusions at 30 minutes and 60 minutes. The GUSTO-I trial was the only study in the meta-analysis mentioned above which looked at the more commonly used accelerated regimen rather than the standard regimen. This trial which included over 40000 patients was also the only trial to demonstrate superiority over different thrombolytics with an absolute reduction in mortality at 30 days of 1.0% (6.3% versus 7.3%; 95% CI 0.4% to 1.6%) in favour of accelerated alteplase when compared to streptokinase. However, this benefit was balanced by a statistically significantly higher incidence of haemorrhagic stroke (odds ratio 1.42; 95% CI 1.05 to 1.91). Using a combined outcome measure of mortality and disabling stroke, there was in fact a statistically significant absolute advantage of streptokinase over alteplase of 0.9%;p = 0.006). Interestingly, statistically significant rates of moderate bleeding or worse were lower in the alteplase group. Alteplase also fared better with regards to the common side effects experienced by streptokinase namely causing less allergic reactions, anaphylaxis, and sustained hypotension and these were also statistically significantly lower. Despite this a further meta-analysis of nine trials comparing standard alteplase with streptokinase, including the findings of GUSTO-I (i.e. accelerated alteplase), found no significant difference between the two drugs in terms of mortality up to 35 days (odds ratio 0.94; 95% CI 0.85 to 1.04).

9.4 Reteplase

This is the third most commonly used thrombolytic and one of the easiest to administer as it only involves two IV boluses administered 30 minutes apart. The INJECT study involving nearly 6000 patients compared reteplase to streptokinase. This study found an absolute difference in 35 day mortality of 0.5% (95% CI –1.98% to 0.96%) in favour of reteplase but this was not deemed as statistically significant. Similarly to alteplase, when a combined outcome measure using overall effects on mortality and disabling stroke is applied to the trial data then reteplase may in fact be inferior to streptokinase, as the trial also found a statistically significantly lower risk of haemorrhagic stroke in the streptokinase group (odds ratio 2.1; 95% CI 1.02 to 4.31). However, the trial also found that the in the reteplase group the rates of heart failure (23.6% vs 26.3%, $p<0.05$) and allergic reactions (1.1% vs 1.8%, $p<0.05$) were significantly lower. In one small study of 324 patients (RAPID-2), reteplase was compared to alteplase and this found that better vessel patency was achieved when coronary angiography was the endpoint. Subsequent to this the large GUSTO-III trial involving 15,059 was designed to test the clinical superiority of reteplase over accelerated alteplase. However, GUSTO-III found no statistically significant difference between the two drugs, in terms of survival or adverse effects but at 30 days mortality was 7.5% in the reteplase group and 7.2% in the accelerated alteplase group giving an absolute risk reduction of 0.23% in favour of accelerated alteplase (95% CI–1.10% to 0.66%). Therefore, reteplase cannot be considered as equivalent to accelerated alteplase.

9.5 Tenectaplase

This is the easiest of the thrombolytics to administer and only involves a single bolus. ASSENT-2 enrolled over 16,000 patients to compare tenecteplase and accelerated alteplase and found that 30-day mortality was the same in the tenecteplase group and the accelerated alteplase at 6.2% each, thereby showing equivalence in outcomes. In fact there was an absolute difference of 0.03% in favour of accelerated alteplase but this was not statistically significant (95% CI -0.55% to 0.61%). However, there was a small but statistically significant reduction in the incidence of bleeding with tenecteplase of 26.4% compared with 28.9% in the accelerated alteplase group. This resulted in fewer blood transfusions in the tenecteplase group (4.3% of patients compared with 5.5% in the accelerated alteplase group.

In summary, with regards to clinical effectiveness and mortality, standard alteplase and reteplase are as effective as streptokinase, and tenecteplase is as effective as accelerated alteplase. According to GUSTO-I, accelerated alteplase is believed to be superior to streptokinase and if this is the case then indirectly tenecteplase would also be considered to be superior to streptokinase (as tenectaplase was superior to accelerated alteplase in ASSENT-2). In practice, cost and availability is a significant issue with regards to what is ultimately used and also use may also go unchanged for long periods purely because of a specific thrombolytic having historical use in a certain area.

9.6 Other considerations

In the elderly, evidence suggests that thrombolysis provides a mortality benefit but that there is increased risk of adverse events and poor outcomes in those with advancing age. The main risk in the older age group is of intracerebral haemorrhage and this is why a clear benefit is seen for PPCI in patients above the age of 75 and in fact the benefit is maintained even when there are longer door-to-balloon times. Low body weight has also been found to be independently associated with increased mortality and morbidity. With regards to sex, it is accepted that there is no difference with regards to efficacy but studies have shown that for unknown reasons women are less likely to receive any type of reperfusion (thrombolysis or PPCI) than men. Anterior infarcts also seem to show an increased benefit with thrombolysis over other territories but this may simply reflect the increased baseline risk in this group. Overall, when clinicians are deciding who would benefit from thrombolysis it appears that patient selection is key and benefits should be balanced against any potential risks.

10. References

A comparison of reteplase with alteplase for acute myocardial infarction. The Global Use of Strategies to Open Occluded Coronary Arteries (GUSTO III) Investigators.. N Engl J Med 1997 Oct 16;337:1118-23

Armstrong P, WEST Steering Committee. A comparison of pharmacologic therapy with/without timely coronary intervention vs. primary percutaneous intervention early after ST-elevation myocardial infarction: the WEST (Which Early ST-elevation myocardial infarction Therapy) study. Eur Heart J 2006;27: 1530–1538.

Bode C, Smalling RW, Berg G, Burnett C, Lorch G, Kalbfleisch JM, Chernoff R, Christie LG, Feldman RL, Seals AA, Weaver WD. Randomized comparison of coronary thrombolysis achieved with double-bolus reteplase (recombinant plasminogen activator) and front-loaded, accelerated alteplase (recombinant tissue plasminogen activator) in patients with acute myocardial infarction. The RAPID II Investigators.. Circulation 1996;94:891-8

Cantor WJ, Fitchett D, Borgundvaag B, Heffernan M, Cohen EA, Morrison LJ, Ducas J, Langer A, Mehta S, Lazzam C, Schwartz B, Dzavik V, Goodman SG. Rationale and design of the Trial of Routine ANgioplasty and Stenting After Fibrinolysis to Enhance Reperfusion in Acute Myocardial Infarction (TRANSFER-AMI).. Am Heart J 2008;155:19-25

COMMIT collaborative group. Addition of Clopidrogel to aspirin in 45,852 patients with acute myocardial infarction: randomised placebo-controlled trial. *Lancet.* Nov 2005;366(9497):1607-21

Di Mario C, Dudek D, Piscione F, Savonitto S, Murena E, Dimopoulos K, Manari A, Gaspardone A, Ochala A, Zmudka K, Bolognese L, Steg PG, Flather M, on behalf of the CARESS-in-AMI investigatorsImmediate angioplasty versus standard therapy with rescue angioplasty after thrombolysis in the Combined Abciximab REteplase Stent Study in Acute Myocardial Infarction (CARESS-in-AMI): an open, prospective, randomised, multicentre trial. Lancet 2008;371:559–568.

"Effectiveness of intravenous thrombolytic treatment in acute myocardial infarction. Gruppo Italiano per lo Studio della Streptochinasi nell'Infarto Miocardico (GISSI)". Lancet 1 (8478): 397–402. 1986

Elliott M. Antman, M.D., David A. Morrow, M.D., M.P.H., Carolyn H. McCabe, B.S., Sabina A. Murphy, M.P.H., Mikhail Ruda, M.D., Zygmunt Sadowski, M.D., Andrzej Budaj, M.D., Jose L. López-Sendón, M.D., Sema Guneri, M.D., Frank Jiang, M.D., Ph.D., Harvey D. White, D.Sc., Keith A.A. Fox, M.B., Ch.B., and Eugene Braunwald, M.D. for the Enoxaparin versus Unfractionated Heparin with Fibrinolysis for ST-Elevation Myocardial Infarction (ExTRACT-TIMI 25) Investigators N Engl J Med 2006; 354:1477-1488April 6, 2006

Fernandez-Avile´s F, Alonso JJ, Castro-Beiras A, Vazquez N, Blanco J, Alonso-Briales J, Lopez-Mesa J, Fernandez-Vazquez F, Calvo I, Martinez-Elbal L, San Roman JA, Ramos B. Routine invasive strategy within 24 hours of thrombolysis versus ischaemia-guided conservative approach for acute myocardial infarction with ST-segment elevation (GRACIA-1): a randomised controlled trial. Lancet 2004;364:1045–1053.

Gershlick AH, Stephens-Lloyd A, Hughes S, Abrams KR, Stevens SE, Uren NG, de Belder A, Davis J, Pitt M, Banning A, Baumbach A, Shiu MF, Schofield P, Dawkins KD, Henderson RA, Oldroyd KG, Wilcox R; REACT Trial Investigators. Rescue angioplasty after failed thrombolytic therapy for acute myocardial infarction. N Engl J Med. 2005 Dec 29;353(26):2758-68.

Hsia J, Hamilton WP, Kleiman N, Roberts R, Chaitman BR, Ross AM. A comparison between heparin and low-dose aspirin as adjunctive therapy with tissue plasminogen activator for acute myocardial infarction. Heparin-Aspirin Reperfusion Trial (HART) Investigators. N Engl J Med. 1990; 323:1433-7.)

Muhaffey KW, Granger CG, Collins R, O'Connor CM, Ohman EM, Bleich SD, Col JJ, Califf RM. Overview of randomized trials of intravenous heparin in patients treated with thrombolytic therapy. Am J Cardiol 1996;77: 351-6.

Randomised, double-blind comparison of reteplase double-bolus administration with streptokinase in acute myocardial infarction (INJECT): trial to investigate equivalence. International Joint Efficacy Comparison of Thrombolytics. Lancet 1995;346:329-36

Sabatine MS, Cannon CP, Gibson CM, et al. Addition of clopidogrel to aspirin and fibrinolytic therapy for myocardial infarction with ST-segment elevation. *N Engl J Med*. Mar 2005;352(12):1179-89.

The GUSTO Investigators. An international randomized trial comparing four thrombolytic strategies for acute myocardial infarction. *N Engl J Med.* 1993;329:673-682.

Van De Werf F, Adgey J, Ardissino D, Armstrong PW, Aylward P, Barbash G, Betriu A, Binbrek AS, Califf R, Diaz R, Fanebust R, Fox K, Granger C, Heikkilä J, Husted S, Jansky P, Langer A, Lupi E, Maseri A, Meyer J, Mlczoch J, Mocceti D, Myburgh D, Oto A, Pao. Single-bolus tenecteplase compared with front-loaded alteplase in acute myocardial infarction: the ASSENT-2 double-blind randomised trial.. Lancet 1999 Aug 28;354:716-22

8

Platelet Activation in Ischemic Heart Disease: Role of Modulators and New Therapies

Mahdi Garelnabi[1], Javier E. Horta[1] and Emir Veledar[2]
[1]*Department of Clinical Laboratory and Nutritional Sciences University of Massachusetts Lowell, Lowell, MA*
[2]*Emory University School of Medicine Atlanta, GA*
USA

1. Introduction

Ischemic heart disease (IHD) remains the major cause of morbidity and mortality in developed countries, and has joined infectious diseases in developing countries as a leading cause of death (WHO 2008). Decades of research have shown conclusively that a number of determinants operating from early childhood onwards, most of them associated with lifestyle, are responsible for IHD.

IHD results when the oxygen demand of the myocardium cannot be met due to an inadequate blood supply. The most common cause of myocardial ischemia is atherosclerosis of epicardial coronary arteries. The major risk factors for atherosclerosis, and therefore IHD, are dyslipidemia (i.e., elevated low-density lipoprotein (LDL) and/or low high-density lipoprotein (HDL)), diabetes mellitus, hypertension, cigarette smoking, poor dietary habits, and lack of physical activity. These risk factors, particularly when more than one co-exists, can progressively damage the vascular endothelium, causing dysregulation of its anti-inflammatory and anti-thrombotic functions. The associated proliferation of underlying fibroblasts and vascular myocytes, together with the accumulation of extracellular matrix and lipids, result in the formation of what are known as atherosclerotic plaques that lead to a reduction in the luminal diameter. Some of the risk factors for atherosclerosis facilitate the development of atherosclerotic plaques, while others sustain or accelerate their formation, producing the clinical manifestations of IHD (Parthasarathy 2008, Garelnabi 2010).

By reducing the lumen of blood vessels, atherosclerosis causes an absolute decrease in myocardial perfusion in the basal state and hinders the required increase in perfusion when the demand for flow is augmented. As this process progressively worsens, the shear stress associated with blood flow through the reduced arterial lumen can cause plaques to erode or rupture, exposing the intimal layer to the luminal contents and thereby promoting frank thrombosis. Platelet activation, mobilization, and recruitment are central to this process. Luminal thrombi can trap red blood cells and acutely reduce coronary blood flow, producing a sudden myocardial ischemic event referred to as an acute coronary syndrome (ACS) that becomes manifest as either unstable angina or myocardial infarction (MI) if there is complete occlusion without prompt reperfusion. MI may also occur with embolization of platelet aggregates and/or atherosclerotic debris from a ruptured plaque.

Coronary blood flow can also be limited by vascular spasm, as well as by congenital abnormalities, such as anomalous origin of the left anterior descending coronary artery from the pulmonary artery, which may cause myocardial ischemia and infarction in infancy, but is very rare in adults.

Patients with IHD can be grouped into two broad categories: those having chronic coronary artery disease (CAD), who most commonly present with stable angina, and those who present with ACSs (i.e., unstable angina and MI). Chronic CAD is most commonly caused by slowly progressive coronary artery atherosclerosis, whereby a narrowing of the lumen of the coronary arteries limits their ability to adequately increase perfusion in response to an increase in demand for oxygen (e.g., during exertion). As the disease progresses in severity, perfusion of the myocardium can become compromised even at rest. ACSs, on the other hand, are the result of acute vasoocclusive events secondary to thrombosis at sites of erosion or rupture of atherosclerotic lesions.

2. Role of platelets in the etiology and pathophysiology of IHD

2.1 Structure of platelets

Blood platelets play an essential role in hemostasis, thrombosis, and coagulation of blood. They are engaged in a complex repertoire of biochemical and molecular activities designed to prevent hemorrhage.

On Wright-Giemsa-stained blood smears, platelets appear as small, anucleate, ovoid or round cells with a pale grayish blue cytoplasm that contains homogeneously distributed purple-red granules. After platelet spreading or aggregation, these dispersed granules become concentrated in the middle of the cell.

When platelet morphology is considered under functional subdivisions rather than purely anatomic terms, there are three major structural zones of the platelet, each related to specific aspect of platelet function. The peripheral zone is involved primarily in adhesion, the solgel zone in contraction, and the organelle zone in secretion.

The volumes of circulating platelets from a single individual are heterogeneous and exhibit a log normal size distribution. Circulating platelets have a volume of 7.06 ± 4.85 μm^3 (femtoliters), a diameter of 3.6 ± 0.7 µm (Mean ± SD), and a thickness of 0.9 ± 0.3 µm (Paulus et al. 1979, Frojmovic et al. 1976). Platelet size varies from one individual to another, although abnormally small or large platelets are present only in certain disease states. By scanning electron microscopy, circulating blood platelets appear as flat discs, with smooth contours and rare spiny filopodia, with random openings of a channel system, which invaginates throughout the platelet and is the conduit by which granule contents exocytose after stimulation. Although the platelet is anucleate, transmission electron microscopy reveals a cytoplasm packed with a number of different organelles essential to maintenance of normal hemostasis. Platelets contain four distinct populations of granules: α-granules, dense bodies, lysosomes, and microperoxisomes. α-granules and dense bodies are distinguished morphologically from one another by their electron density as revealed by electron microscopy.

Phospholipids constitute 80% of the total lipid content of platelets, although smaller amounts of neutral lipids and glycolipids are also present. Evidence suggests that these phospholipids move to the outer membrane leaflet after platelet activation, thereby functioning to promote clot formation. Platelet membrane glycoproteins mediate a wide number of adhesive cellular interactions. These glycoproteins function as receptors that can receive signals from outside the platelet, facilitating cell-cell interactions; binding of specific ligands to these receptors results in distinct platelet responses to the external environment. Several other proteins are unique to the platelet, including platelet factor 4 (PF4), low-affinity PF4, β-thromboglobulin (β-TG), and the calcium-binding proteins thrombospondin, calmodulin, and platelet-derived growth factor (PDGF) (Stenberg et al. 1984).

2.2 Function and biochemistry of platelets

In terms of dry weight, platelets are composed of approximately 60% protein, 15% lipid, and 8% carbohydrate. Platelet minerals include magnesium, calcium, potassium, and zinc. Platelets contain substantial amounts of vitamin B_{12}, folic acid, and ascorbic acid (Weiss et al. 1968). The concentration of sodium and potassium within the platelet are 39 and 138 mEq, respectively, a gradient against plasma that is maintained by active ion pumping, which derives energy from membrane adenosine triphosphatase of the Ouabain-sensitive, Na^+/K^+-dependent type. Potassium apparently is distributed in two discrete metabolic compartments (Cooley and Cohen 1967).

Non-stimulated platelets maintain a low cytoplasmic Ca^{2+} concentration, by limiting Ca^{2+} transport from plasma and promoting active efflux of this ion from the cell. Two pools of calcium are present in platelets: a rapidly-turning over cytosolic pool that is regulated by sodium-calcium antiporter in the plasma membrane, and a more slowly-exchanging pool that is regulated by a calcium-magnesium-ATPase and is sequestered in a dense tubular system. Platelets are therefore able to transport calcium from the cytosol by moving it against a gradient into the extracellular space or by sequestration in the dense tubular system (Brass 1984, Enouf et al. 1987).

There are several similarities between the energy metabolism of platelets and that of skeletal muscle. Both involve active glycolysis and the synthesis and use of large amounts of glycogen, and in both, the major mediator of intracellular energy use is ATP. Platelets, like muscle cells, are metabolically adapted to expend large amounts of energy rapidly during aggregation, the release reaction, and clot retraction (Karpatkin et al. 1970).

The presence of platelets in the hemostatic plugs that form to prevent bleeding suggests that platelets have a physiological role in hemostasis. Their presence in thrombi and emboli, however, suggests that they may have a pathological role as well. Platelets display certain properties that may be relevant to hemostasis and thrombosis. They have the capacity to adhere to foreign surfaces, they can be induced to aggregate, and they can synthesize or release a number of substances.

Platelet adhesion

The only structures with which platelets normally interact are red cells, white cells, and the endothelial lining of blood vessel walls. All other surfaces are thus foreign to them, but platelets have the ability to adhere to such surfaces. Platelets adhere to subendothelial structures that are exposed when the normal endothelial lining of the blood vessel wall is injured, which causes the deposition of a monolayer of platelets on the surface of the injured vessel. This is followed by the release of pro-coagulation substances, leading to platelet aggregation and formation of a fibrin clot over the adhered layer that results in thrombus formation (Heptinstall and Hanley 1985).

Platelet aggregation

Platelets circulate as disc-shaped cells, but when they come in contact with exposed subendothelium, agonists that activate platelets are exposed, generated, or released. These agonists include collagen, which is present in subendothelium; thrombin, which is generated on the surface of activated platelets and elsewhere; ADP, which is released from damaged red blood cells and secreted from activated platelet-dense granules; circulating epinephrine; and arachidonic acid, which is released from lipid stores in platelets and metabolized to the potent agonist thromboxane A_2 (TXA_2). These agonists generally cause platelets to change shape such that they form long pseudopodia, followed by platelet aggregation. Aggregation requires activation of platelet integrin adhesion receptor GP IIb/IIIa so that it can bind fibrinogen or von Willebrand factor (vWF) and link adjacent platelets together in an aggregate. Platelet agonists induce signal transduction events in platelets that cause the above events, although the signal transduction pathways are not completely understood (Leslie et al. 1999).

Platelet release reaction

Platelets store ATP, ADP, Ca^{2+}, and serotonin in dense granules as well as adhesive proteins such as platelet factor 4, β-thromboglobulin, platelet-derived growth factor (PDGF), fibrinogen, fibronectin, thrombospondin, and vWF in α-granules (Siess 1989). Upon activation by agonists, platelets undergo a release reaction, thereby secreting their granular contents. The release reaction is associated with the production of TXA_2, and the extent of the secretion depends on the strength of the agonist. Weak agonists (e.g., ADP and epinephrine) require both cyclooxygenase activity and primary aggregation to induce secretion that is observed at low Ca^{2+} concentrations (Smith et al. 1973, Banga et al. 1986). Agonists of intermediate strength (e.g., platelet activating factor, PAF) can induce secretion in the absence of formation of arachidonic acid metabolism and without primary aggregation. Interestingly, when collagen is added at low concentrations to platelet suspensions, secretion of ATP occurs before the onset of shape change. This secretion is not inhibited by cyclooxygenase blockers, but is sensitive to the extracellular Ca^{2+} concentration and is a direct consequence of platelet binding to collagen (Siess et al. 1983, Malmgren 1986).

Platelet activation

Some signaling pathways involved in various platelet activation events are reasonably well understood, whereas others are not. Many, but not all platelet agonists activate platelets by occupying seven transmembrane-spanning, G protein-coupled receptors. Activation of these receptors generally results in activation of phospholipase Cβ (PLC). PLC hydrolyzes phosphatidyl-inositol-4,5-bisphosphate (PIP_2), generating inositol-1,4,5-triphosphate (IP_3) and diacylglycerol (DAG). Both IP_3 and DAG appear to play important roles in pathways leading to various aspects of platelet activation. IP_3 is believed to interact with specific receptors to induce intracellular Ca^{2+} release from the dense tubular system, an intracellular

Ca^{2+} storage organelle analogous to the sarcoplasmic reticulum in skeletal muscle. However, the exact mechanism by which this response contributes to platelet aggregation is not entirely clear because IP_3-induced platelet aggregation is also dependent on thromboxane A_2 (TXA_2) production and ADP release (Knezevic et al. 1992). DAG interacts directly with protein kinase C (PKC) and appears to play a crucial role in the pathways of some agonists, leading to the activation of GP IIb/IIIa and fibrinogen binding. Specific inhibitors of PKC block fibrinogen binding and platelet aggregation induced by some agonists. Drivers for platelet activation include the signaling events that occur downstream of receptors for collagen (GP VI and GP Ibα), thrombin (PAR1 and PAR4), adenosine diphosphate (ADP; P2Y1 and P2Y12), and thromboxane A2 (TXA_2; TP) (Brass 2010).

Platelets are activated and stimulated to synthesize or release a number of substances, namely thrombin, arachidonic acid, PAF, and epinephrine which are of functional importance. When platelet ADP is released from platelet-dense granules during platelet activation by numerous agonists, secreted ADP potentiates the activating effects of other agonists (Hourani and Cusack 1991). ADP causes shape change, granular secretion, and aggregation. However, unlike strong agonists such as thrombin and collagen, ADP induces secretion usually only in conjunction with platelet aggregation. Strong agonists generally stimulate phosphoinositide hydrolysis, increase cytosolic free Ca^{2+}, and induce TXA_2 formation.

Platelet receptors and MicroRNA signaling

Platelet receptors are known to interact with external stimuli in the main blood stream leading to the regulation of platelet activation. Platelet adhesion receptors are the key initiators of platelet activation at sites of vascular injury, where platelets become exposed to adhesive proteins in the matrix, or on endothelial cells. Despite significant differences in their functions and signaling pathways, several major platelet adhesion receptors share many similarities in their signal transduction mechanisms (Li et al. 2010). The most studied platelet receptor is platelet integrin GP IIb/IIIa, which is reported to play an essential role in thrombus formation through interactions with adhesive ligands and has emerged as a primary target for the development of anti-thrombotic agents (Hagemeyer and Peter 2010). Successful blockade of this ligand binding has validated GP IIb/IIIa as a therapeutic target in cardiovascular medicine.

MicroRNAs (MiRs) molecules are a novel class of endogenous, small, noncoding RNAs that regulate gene expression via degradation, translational inhibition, or translational activation of their target messenger RNAs (Pan et al. 2010, O'Sullivan et al., 2011). Bioinformatics analysis predicts that each MiR can regulate hundreds of targets, suggesting that they play an essential role in almost every physiological and pathological pathway. Functionally, an individual MiR is important as a transcription factor because it is able to regulate the expression of its multiple target genes. MiRs are short (~20 nucleotides long), single-stranded RNAs initially transcribed by either RNA polymerase II or RNA polymerase III, as a long primary MiR transcript (pre-MiR). It is then cleaved in the nucleus by the microprocessor complex, Drosha-DGCR8, resulting in a precursor hairpin (pre-miRNA) ranging in length from 60 to 110 nucleotides. The pre-MiRNA is exported from the nucleus to the cytoplasm by exportin 5-Ran-GTP. In the cytoplasm, Dicer, a member of the RNase III family, in complex with TRBP, cleaves the pre-MiR hairpin to a 22 base pair MiR duplex.

The mature MiR is incorporated with argonaute (Ago2) proteins into the RNA-induced silencing complex (RISC), where MiR guides the complex to partial complementary binding sites located in the 3′ untranslated region (UTR) of target mRNAs to suppress gene expression. MiRs are able to directly regulate at least 30% of genes in a cell. In addition, other genes may also be regulated indirectly by MiRs. Therefore, MiRs are pivotal regulators in normal development, physiology, and pathology. Recent studies have identified a number of MiRs highly expressed in the vasculature and their expression is dysregulated in diseased vessels (Jamaluddin et al. 2011, Haver et al. 2010, Bonauer et al. 2010, Wierda et al. 2010, Urbich et al. 2008, Fang et al. 2010, Leeper et al. 2011). MiRs are also found to be critical modulators of cell differentiation, contraction, migration, proliferation, and apoptosis. Accordingly, MiRs have emerged as therapeutic targets in disease.

Platelets are also reported to have microRNA population that may regulate its activity. It is well known that platelets have mRNA and mRNA splicing machinery, and translate mRNA into proteins relevant to hemostasis and inflammation (Edelstein and Bray 2011). In silicon analysis work from Edelstein and Bray indicates that each platelet MiR targets an average of 307 distinct mRNAs, concluding in their review that platelet MiRs have ample opportunity to regulate platelet function.

2.3 Role of inflammation and oxidative stress in platelet activation

Involvement of inflammation in cardiovascular disease is well defined. Circulating platelets are affected by this metabolic disruption and by inflammatory mediators synthesized and/or released on contact with inflammatory signals. Platelets are known to play a major role in this process and have been identified as targets and players in inflammation-induced cardiovascular disease (Weksler 1983, Nurden 2011). It has been explicitly established that free radicals can cause metabolic disturbances and cell injury in a variety of ways, including lipid peroxidation, hydroxyl radical-induced modification of proteins and nucleic acids, changes in enzyme activity, and carbohydrate damage. Oxidative modification of lipids can be induced in vitro by a wide array of pro-oxidant agents and occurs in vivo during atherosclerosis and several other disease conditions (Parthasarathy et al. 2008). Alterations in the superoxide and glutathione oxidation-reduction system may lead to depleted antioxidant capacity and may result in oxidative stress. Previous studies have suggested that platelets and vascular endothelial cells could be the central target as well as the origin of oxygen free radicals or its metabolites (Dousset et al. 1983). Measuring the end products of lipid peroxidation is one of the most widely accepted assays for oxidative damage. These aldehydic secondary products of lipid peroxidation are generally accepted markers of oxidative stress.

Several studies suggest that the basal release of NO by the endothelium contributes to regulation of the vascular tone (Antoniades et al. 2008), blood flow, and blood pressure. NO inhibits platelet aggregation and adhesion to vascular endothelium. In addition, NO inhibits leukocyte adhesion to endothelium (Petidis et al. 2008). Alteration of cellular calcium homeostasis is also a critical event in ischemic heart injury. NO released by endothelium or synthesized by platelets participates in the regulation of Ca^{2+} signaling. Elevation of cGMP as a result of the activation of guanylate cyclase by NO stimulates a number of mechanisms that actively decrease calcium levels within the cell (Joseph et al. 1996). Although the NO-cGMP signaling system has been immensely investigated, sparse data is available pertaining to the role of platelet NO activity in coronary artery (CAD). We and others have studied the NO-cGMP system in patients with CAD, particularly the role of oxidative stress and NO-mediated platelet response in IHD (Garelnabi et al. 2010, Ikeda et al. 2000, Garelnabi et al. 2011). These studies have clearly indicated that lipid peroxidation is augmented in patients with ischemic heart disease. The increased oxidative stress seen in these patients was accompanied by platelet activation and impaired antioxidant enzymes activity. On the other hand, platelet aggregation, NO, cGMP, NO synthase activity, plasma NO, and ionized Ca^{2+} was profoundly increased in CAD. The increases in NO-cGMP components may have resulted as a compensatory response to ameliorate platelet activity and increased Ca^{2+} levels in CAD patients. Another interesting modulator of platelet activity is the recent description of platelet-derived microparticles (PMP) which are known as a heterogeneous population of vesicles (<1 mm) generated from the plasma membrane upon platelet activation by various stimuli. These PMPs have been shown to not only stimulate the response of platelets, but have also been reported to mediate the intercellular transfer of bioactive molecules such as lipids, surface receptors, and even enzymes (Siljander 2010).

3. Classes and mechanism of action of antiplatelet drugs

The main goals of pharmacological intervention in patients with IHD are to reduce the occurrence of anginal attacks by minimizing the rise in blood pressure and heart rate associated with physical activity so that patients can go about their daily activities without ischemic episodes. Given the prominent role that thrombosis plays in IHD, antiplatelet therapy is one of the most important modalities used in its treatment.

Antithrombotic drugs used for prevention and treatment of thrombosis include: (1) antiplatelet drugs, (2) anticoagulants, and (3) fibrinolytic agents. Given the predominance of platelets in arterial thrombi, which are the major source of IHD, the treatment and inhibition of arterial thrombosis focus mainly on antiplatelet agents, although anticoagulants and fibrinolytic drugs are often included in the acute setting.

Under normal conditions, the actions of vascular endothelial cells maintain platelets in the bloodstream in an inactive state, largely by their production of nitric oxide (NO) and prostacyclin, but also by their surface expression of adenosine diphosphatase (ADPase), which breaks down ADP released via degranulation of activated platelets. With the occurrence of injury to the vascular endothelium, production of these substances is compromised and certain components of the subendothelial matrix are exposed (e.g., collagen, von Willebrand factor (vWF), and fibronectin) to which platelets adhere via receptors constitutively expressed on their surface (e.g., GP IIb/IIIa). As discussed above, adhered platelets undergo a morphological change and then release the contents of their dense granules (e.g., ADP) and synthesize and release thromboxane A_2 (TXA_2), both of which serve to recruit and activate surrounding circulating platelets to the site of vascular injury.

Disruption of the vascular wall also exposes underlying cells and matrix that express pro-thrombotic factors to the circulation, which triggers the coagulation cascade. Activated platelets enhance coagulation by binding clotting factors and supporting the assembly of activation complexes that increase thrombin generation, which in addition to converting fibrinogen to fibrin, also acts as a potent platelet agonist and recruits more platelets to the site of vascular injury.

The most abundant receptor on the surface of platelets is GP IIb/IIIa, which undergoes a conformational change upon platelet activation that allows it to bind fibrinogen. Divalent fibrinogen molecules link adjacent platelets together to form aggregates, which are meshed together via fibrin strands generated via the action of thrombin to form a lattice composed of platelets plus fibrin. Antiplatelet drugs target various steps in this process. The most commonly used drugs include cyclooxygenase inhibitors, among which aspirin is the most common, thienopyridines and functionally related drugs, phosphodiesterase inhibitors, adenosine reuptake inhibitors, and GP IIb/IIIa antagonists, all of which are discussed below.

3.1 Cyclooxygenase inhibitors

The cyclooxygenases (COXs) are a family of isoenzymes responsible for the biosynthesis of various important and potent pro-inflammatory and pro-thrombotic mediators called eicosanoids, which include prostaglandins, leukotrienes, and thromboxanes. Non-steroidal anti-inflammatory drugs (NSAIDs), like aspirin and ibuprofen, exert their effects through inhibition of COX, and as such they relieve the symptoms of inflammation (e.g., pain, swelling).

COX converts arachidonic acid (AA, an ω-6 polyunsaturated fatty acid (PUFA)) to prostaglandin H_2 (PGH_2), the parent of the eicosanoids, which can then be converted to the other compounds via further enzymatic action that involves radical chemistry and the consumption of molecular oxygen. To date, three distinct COX isoenzymes have been identified: COX-1, COX-2, and COX-3. COX-1 and COX-3 are products of alternative splicing of the same gene, so COX-3 is referred to by some as COX-1b or COX-1 variant (COX-1v). Different tissues express varying levels of the different COXs, and although the isoenzymes basically catalyze the same transformations, selective inhibition can produce a different side-effect profile. COX-1 is nearly ubiquitous among mammalian cells, but COX-2 is undetectable in most normal tissues and is inducible in macrophages upon their activation, as well in endothelial cells at sites of inflammation, where it serves to produce prostacyclin, a potent vasodilator and inhibitor of platelet aggregation. COX-2 is also upregulated in various types of cancers, so it is believed to play a role in oncogenesis.

Both COX-1 and -2 also oxygenate two other essential fatty acids – dihomo-γ-linolenic acid (DGLA, ω-6) and eicosapentaenoic acid (EPA, ω-3) – to give eicosanoids with less potent pro-inflammatory properties than those derived from AA. Both DGLA and EPA competitively inhibit oxidation of AA by the COXs, which is believed to be the major mechanism by which dietary sources of DGLA and EPA (e.g., fish oil) can reduce inflammation.

The traditional COX inhibitors are not selective for any particular COX, resulting in widespread inhibition of eicosanoid synthesis that ultimately reduces inflammation, as well as providing antipyretic, antithrombotic, and analgesic effects. However, inhibition of the synthesis of gastroprotective prostaglandins can cause gastric irritation and increases the risk of development of peptic ulcer disease.

The development of selective COX-2 inhibitors was originally aimed at blocking the production of pro-inflammatory prostaglandins while minimizing any effects on platelet and gastric function. Selective inhibition of COX-2 has been accomplished with the "coxibs", which differ in their selectivity for COX-2 relative to COX-1 by selectively binding to a hydrophobic side-pocket on the COX-2 enzyme where a valine takes the place of what is an isoleucine on COX-1, allowing access to an otherwise sterically hindered site that causes inhibition of the enzyme's function. Since COX-2 is largely expressed selectively in inflamed tissue, there is much less gastric irritation and risk of peptic ulceration associated with COX-2 inhibitors. However, the selectivity of COX-2 causes an imbalance between thromboxane and prostacyclin, resulting in an increased risk of thrombosis, MI, and stroke. Thus, by blocking prostacyclin synthesis without concomitant inhibition of thromboxane A_2 (TXA_2) production, highly selective inhibitors of COX-2 increase the risk of cardiovascular events. These effects seemed most notable with rofecoxib (Vioxx®) and valdecoxib (Bextra®), which were removed from the market in 2004 and 2005, respectively. Other COX-2 selective NSAIDs, such as celecoxib (Celebrex®), and etoricoxib (Arcoxia®), are still on the market as they continue to be investigated for these adverse effects. Even with short-term use, COX-2 inhibitors have been found to increase the risk of atherothrombosis, most notably manifested as a 2-to-5-fold increased risk of myocardial infarction. Furthermore, high-dose regimens of some traditional NSAIDs such as diclofenac and ibuprofen are associated with a similar increase in risk of vascular events. Thus, although NSAIDs, particularly COX-2 inhibitors, have demonstrated benefits, the risks associated with their use should be seriously considered when prescribing them to a patient having risk factors and/or a personal or family history of IHD.

3.1.1 Aspirin

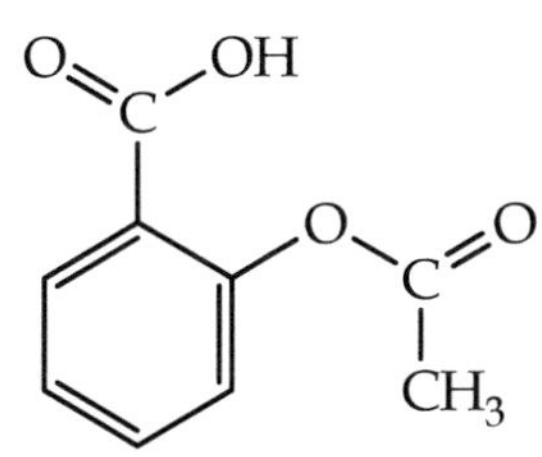

Aspirin (acetylsalicylic acid, ASA), is the oldest and most widely used antiplatelet drug due to its low cost, wide availability, and proven effectiveness. It is a salicylate drug whose mechanism of action serves as the model of most antiplatelet therapeutic strategies.

Mechanism of action

Aspirin, a non-selective COX inhibitor, is one of the most commonly used drugs in IHD that can reduce the development of thrombosis associated with the rupture of atheromatous plaques. Aspirin interferes with the activation of platelets by irreversibly inhibiting COX, thereby interfering with the biosynthetic pathway of thromboxanes. Unlike other NSAIDs, whose antiplatelet action is transient (i.e., in the order of hours), aspirin irreversibly acetylates COX-1 in platelets, thereby inhibiting the biosynthesis of thromboxane A_2 (TXA_2) and in that manner producing a long-lived antithrombotic effect (i.e., days, until new platelets are produced by the bone marrow). At higher doses (e.g., 1 g/d), however, aspirin also inhibits COX-2, which can ultimately produce a prothrombotic effect by inhibiting the synthesis of prostacyclin in endothelial cells.

Indications, dosage, and side effects

Aspirin is widely used for the primary prevention of ischemic events in patients at risk, as well as secondary prevention of cardiovascular events in patients with IHD and cerebrovascular and peripheral vascular disease. Aspirin is usually administered once a day at a dose between 75-325 mg, with 75-100 mg being recommended for most indications. When fast platelet inhibition is needed, a dose of at least 160 mg should be given orally. Higher doses of aspirin have not been shown to be more effective than lower doses, and in fact, reduced efficacy has been reported with higher doses. As discussed above, very high doses of aspirin (i.e., 1 g/d) can have a paradoxical prothrombotic effect due to the inhibition of COX-2.

Long-term daily oral enteric-coated aspirin has been demonstrated to reduce (1) the incidence of anginal episodes in patients with chronic stable angina, as well as in survivors of unstable angina and myocardial infarction (MI), and (2) the risk of recurrent infarction, stroke, or cardiovascular mortality by 25% following an MI compared with placebo. It has also been established that low doses of aspirin may be given immediately after an MI to reduce the risk of another MI or of the death of the myocardium.

Aspirin is equally effective in men and women, although in men it mainly reduces the risk of MI, while in women it lowers the risk of stroke. Although aspirin also raises the risk of hemorrhagic stroke and other major bleeds, these events are rare, and are by far outweighed by aspirin's positive effects.

The most common side effects of aspirin use are gastrointestinal, ranging from simple stomach upset, to erosive gastritis, to peptic ulcers with bleeding and perforation, all of which are dose-dependent. For these reasons, aspirin should never be administered to individuals with a history of gastrointestinal bleeding or severe stomach upset. Although the use of enteric-coated or buffered aspirin may relieve some of these symptoms, they do not eliminate the risk of gastrointestinal complications due to the inhibition of gastroprotective prostaglandins as part of the actions of aspirin. The overall risk of major bleeding with aspirin is low, however, estimated at 1-3% per year, but is increased when aspirin is given in conjunction with anticoagulants (e.g., warfarin). In these situations, a lower dose of aspirin should be given (e.g., 75-100 mg/d). In patients with a documented history of peptic ulcer disease caused by Helicobacter pylori infection, treatment of the infection and administration of a proton pump inhibitor (PPI) may reduce the risk of aspirin-induced gastrointestinal bleeding. Aspirin should also never be given to individuals with a history of allergic responses to salicylates, particularly those associated with bronchospasm.

3.2 Thienopyridines

A second class of antiplatelet drugs commonly used in IHD is the thienopyridines. These structurally related drugs have similar benefits as aspirin in patients with stable chronic IHD and may be used instead of aspirin when aspirin is contraindicated. The thienopyridines include clopidogrel (Plavix®), ticlopidine (Ticlid®), and prasugrel (Effient®). A structurally unrelated but functionally similar drug is ticagrelor (Brilinta®).

Mechanism of action

The thienopyridines are prodrugs that must first be metabolized by the hepatic cytochrome P450 enzyme system before they can exert any biological activity, so their onset of action can be delayed for several days. They interfere with the aggregation of platelets by competitively and irreversibly inhibiting the adenosine diphosphate (ADP) chemoreceptor P2Y12 on the surface of platelets, which is crucial for the conformational change that activates GP IIb/IIIa and ultimately leads to platelet aggregation and cross-linking by fibrin.

3.2.1 Clopidogrel (Plavix®)

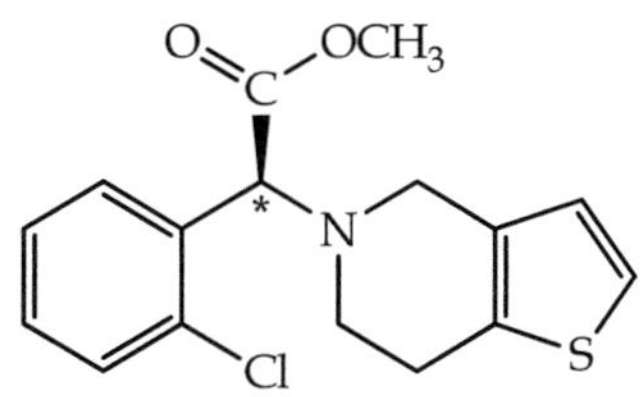

Clopidogrel is an oral thienopyridine marketed under the trade name Plavix by Bristol-Myers Squibb and Sanofi-Aventis as 75 mg oral tablets.

Indications, dosage, and side effects

Clopidogrel is indicated for the prevention of vascular ischemic events in patients with symptomatic atherosclerosis, acute coronary syndromes, and MI. When compared with aspirin in patients with recent ischemic stroke, MI, or peripheral arterial disease, clopidogrel further reduced the risk of cardiovascular death, MI, and stroke by nearly 10%. Thus, although clopidogrel is actually more effective than aspirin in reducing morbidity and mortality of IHD, it is also considerably more expensive and not as readily available. It is also used, together with aspirin, for the prevention of thrombotic events after placement of intracoronary stents, or as an alternative to aspirin in patients who have a contraindication for aspirin.

Combination therapy consisting of aspirin and clopidogrel has been shown to reduce morbidity and mortality in patients with angina and it also reduces the risk of thrombosis in patients who have undergone coronary artery stenting (the risk of gastrointestinal bleeding in these patients can be reduced by also prescribing a PPI while on this combination therapy). The combination therapy of clopidogrel and aspirin capitalizes on the capacity of these drugs to inhibit complementary pathways of platelet activation and is associated with a highly statistically significant 20% relative risk reduction when comparing each drug alone.

In patients with a history of acute coronary syndrome, it is standard medical practice to administer aspirin indefinitely, and it is recommended that combination therapy with clopidogrel be given for 1-3 months after the implantation of a bare metal stent. With the use of drug-eluting stents, which deliver antiproliferative drugs locally (e.g., rapamycin or paclitaxel), combination therapy should continue for at least one year because these drugs are associated with delayed endothelial healing that prolongs the window during which there is an increased risk for thrombosis around the area where the stent was placed. Although aspirin and clopidogrel may help prevent coronary thrombosis associated with stenting, there is no evidence that these drugs reduce the occurrence of re-stenosis. However, the use of drug-eluting stents can reduce re-stenosis to near zero within the stent itself and less than 10% at its edges.

There is little evidence of additional benefit of adding clopidogrel to the routine regimen of aspirin in patients with chronic stable IHD that have not undergone stenting. However, "aspirin resistance" has been noted in up to 10% of patients, more frequently in patients treated with lower doses of aspirin. In these cases, the use of higher doses of aspirin and/or combination therapy with clopidogrel should be considered. Although the routine management of patients with IHD is medical, many patients show greater improvement after undergoing interventional coronary revascularization. These invasive procedures should not take the place of the required ongoing modification of risk factors and medical therapy but rather should be performed in combination with them.

Combination therapy of aspirin and clopidogrel increases the risk of major bleeding to about 2% per year, a risk that will exist even if the daily dose of aspirin is reduced to 100 mg. Thus, the combination of clopidogrel and aspirin should only be used when there is a clear benefit. For example, combination therapy has not been shown to reduce the risk of acute ischemic stroke relative to clopidogrel alone or to reduce the risk of primary cardiovascular events when compared to aspirin alone.

As mentioned above, the onset of action of clopidogrel is slow, so even though platelet inhibition can be seen within a few hours after a single oral dose of the drug, a loading-dose between 300-600 mg is commonly given when prompt inhibition of the ADP receptors is desired, which is continued as a once daily oral dose of 75 mg for maintenance.

The documented adverse effects of clopidogrel include bleeding, severe neutropenia, and thrombotic thrombocytopenic purpura (TTP). Patients with a history of resolved aspirin-related peptic ulcers who received aspirin plus a PPI (e.g., esomeprazole) were shown to have a lower incidence of recurrence of peptic bleeding when compared to patients receiving clopidogrel instead. Another study suggested that prophylaxis with PPIs when undergoing treatment with clopidogrel following an acute coronary syndrome (ACS, i.e., unstable angina or MI) may increase the incidence of adverse cardiac events, perhaps as a result of the inhibition of the cytochrome P450 variant CYP2C19, which is required for the conversion of clopidogrel to its pharmacologically active form. However, even after some government health agencies issued a statement on a potential drug interaction between clopidogrel and PPIs, people within the cardiology community manifested concerns regarding the possible existence of flaws in the studies that served as the basis for these conclusions and subsequent warnings, putting into question the veracity of an adverse drug interaction between clopidogrel and PPIs.

Clopidogrel, was issued a black box warning from the FDA on March 12, 2010 because it is estimated that 2-14% of the US population have low levels of the CYP2C19 liver enzyme needed to activate clopidogrel and, therefore, may not get the full effect from the drug. However, there are tests available to predict if a patient will be susceptible to this reduced pharmacological effect.

3.2.2 Ticlopidine (Ticlid®)

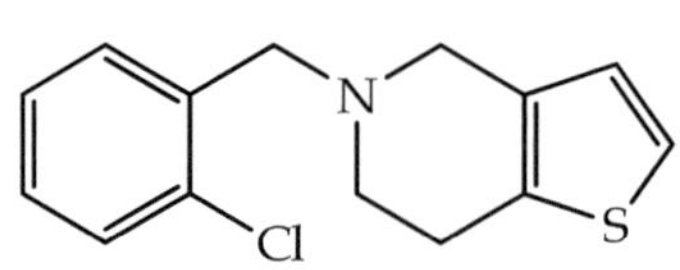

Ticlopidine is an oral thienopyridine marketed under the trade name Ticlid by Roche Pharmaceuticals as 250 mg oral tablets.

Indications, dosage, and side effects

Ticlopidine is typically administered as an oral twice-daily dose of 250 mg. Like aspirin, ticlopidine is more effective than placebo at reducing the risk of cardiovascular death, MI, and stroke in patients with atherosclerotic disease, but due to its delayed onset of action, ticlopidine is not recommended for patients with acute MI. Ticlopidine has been routinely used in addition to aspirin after coronary artery stenting, and as a substitute for aspirin in patients with a contraindication to aspirin. However, because ticlopidine is less potent than clopidogrel and is associated with greater risk of hematologic disorders (e.g., neutropenia, TTP, thrombocytopenia, aplastic anemia), it has largely been replaced by clopidogrel. Due to the known hematologic side effects, which usually become manifest within the first few months of beginning therapy, frequent blood counts must be carefully performed when taking ticlopidine. As with clopidogrel, it is contraindicated in patients having hypersensitivity reactions to thienopyridines, as well as bleeding disorders, active bleeding, and liver disease.

3.2.3 Prasugrel (Effient®)

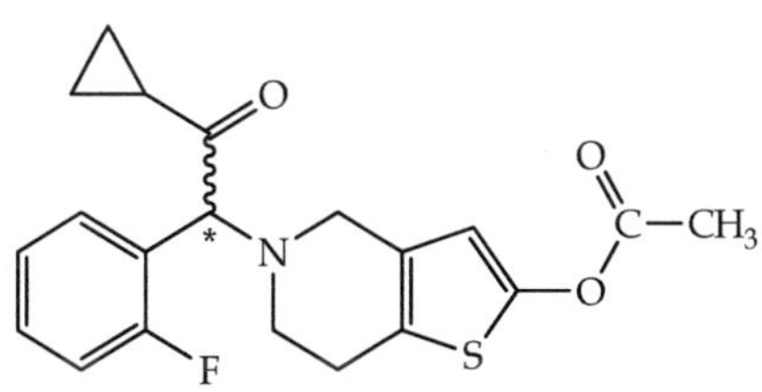

Prasugrel is an oral thienopyridine marketed under the trade names Effient, Efient, Apagrel, and Prasita. It was developed by Daiichi Sankyo Co. and is currently marketed in the United States in cooperation with Eli Lilly and Co. as 5 mg and 10 mg oral tablets.

Indications, dosage, and side effects

Prasugrel was approved for patients with acute coronary syndrome who will be undergoing a percutaneous coronary intervention (PCI) to reduce the occurrence of cardiovascular thrombotic events. Prasugrel is faster than clopidogrel at inhibiting ADP-induced platelet aggregation and does so to a greater extent than both normal and higher doses of clopidogrel in healthy individuals, as well as in patients with coronary artery disease, including those undergoing PCI. Unlike clopidogrel, prasugrel has not been shown to produce a lesser effect in patients who have a low level of hepatic CYP2C19 enzyme. Prasugrel should be administered as a single 60 mg oral loading dose and then continued at a dose of 10 mg orally once daily. Patients should also take aspirin (75-325 mg) per day.

A study published in the New England Journal of Medicine that compared prasugrel with clopidogrel in patients with acute coronary syndromes, both in combination with aspirin, found that prasugrel was a more potent anti-platelet agent, demonstrating a 1.2-fold reduction in the combined rate of cardiovascular mortality, nonfatal myocardial infarction, and nonfatal stroke. However, prasugrel was associated with a 1.6-fold rate of serious bleedings and 4-fold rate of fatal bleedings, even though overall mortality did not differ between the two patient groups.

3.2.4 Ticagrelor (Brilinta®)

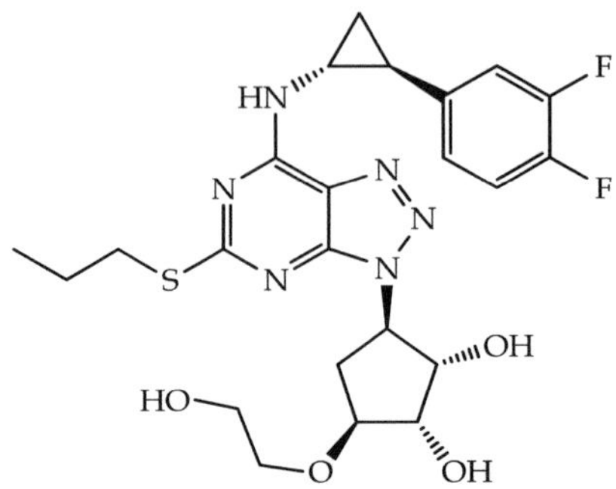

Ticagrelor is an oral cyclopentyltriazolopyrimidine (CPTP) agent marketed under the trade names Brilinta, Brilique, and Possia. The drug was approved for use in the European Union on December 3, 2010 and by the US Food and Drug Administration on July 20, 2011, being marketed in the United States by AstraZeneca as 90 mg oral tablets.

In contrast to the other antiplatelet drugs clopidogrel, ticlopidine, and prasugrel, ticagrelor is a reversible allosteric inhibitor that does not require hepatic activation, making it a better choice for patients with hepatic insufficiency or those carrying low levels or genetic variants of the CYP2C19. Due to its reversible mode of action, ticagrelor is both faster and shorter acting than clopirogrel, making it a easier to discontinue (e.g., surgery, hypersensitivity), but typically requiring more frequent dosing, which can present an issue with compliance.

In a study by AstraZeneca, ticagrelor was associated with ~2% lower mortality rate than clopidogrel in patients with ACS and it was found that taking ticagrelor displayed a lower mortality rate from vascular causes, heart attack, or stroke. However, patients taking ticagrelor was associated with 1.5% higher propensity of non-lethal bleeding.

Indications, dosage, and side effects

Treatment with ticagrelor should be initiated as an oral loading dose of 180 mg, and then continued at 90 mg orally twice daily. Patients should also take aspirin (75-100 mg) daily. Ticagrelor is indicated for the prevention of thrombotic events in patients with ACS or MI, in combination with aspirin unless the latter is contraindicated. Compared with clopidogrel, ticagrelor significantly reduces the mortality rate in patients with ACS. The drug is contraindicated in patients with hepatic insufficiency and a history of pathological bleeding. It also should not be given in combination with other drugs that affect the CYP3A4 liver enzyme, since the drug is metabolized by CYP3A4 and is mainly excreted via bile and feces.

The most common side effects of ticagrelor are dyspnea as well as bleeding (e.g., gastrointestinal, nasal, subcutaneous/dermal). To date, less than 1% of patients taking ticagrelor have reported allergic reactions.

Inhibitors of hepatic CYP3A4 enzyme (e.g., ketoconazole and (?) grapefruit juice), increase blood plasma levels of ticagrelor and can therefore cause bleeding and other adverse effects. Conversely, activators of hepatic CYP3A4 (e.g., rifampicin and (?) St. John's wort), can reduce the effectiveness of ticagrelor. Furthermore, drugs that are also metabolized by CYP3A4 (e.g., simvastatin), will display higher plasma levels, which can result in an increase of the side effects of these drugs when combined with ticagrelor.

3.2.5 Thienopyridine resistance

There is variability among different individuals in the ability of the thienopyridines to inhibit ADP-induced platelet aggregation. To a certain extent this variability reflects genetic polymorphisms in the CYP isoenzymes associated with the metabolic activation of these drugs. For example, individuals carrying the CYP2C19*2 allele have been shown to display a lower responsiveness to clopidogrel, in a similar fashion as those having a lower activity of hepatic CYP3A4. These observations have resulted in the proposal that genetic testing may lead to the identification of individuals that may experience resistance to the effects of thienopyridines.

3.3 Phosphodiesterase inhibitors and adenosine reuptake inhibitors

As the name implies, phosphodiesterase inhibitors interfere with the function of the enzyme phosphodiesterase, which breaks down the intracellular second messenger cyclic adenosine monophosphate (cAMP). This results in increased levels of cAMP, ultimately leading to the inhibition of platelet activation and vasodilation.

3.3.1 Cilostazol (Pletal®)

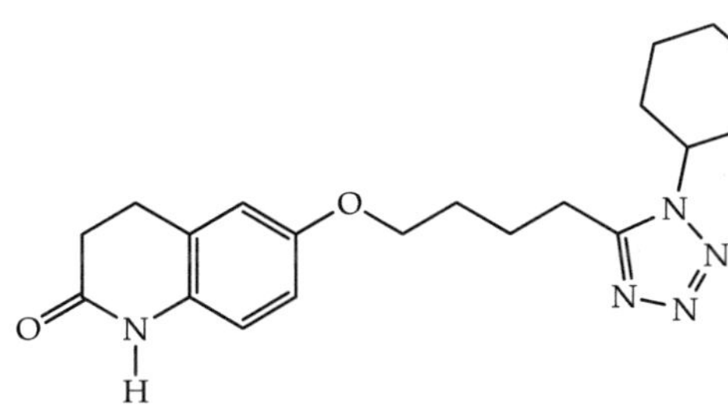

Cilostazol is an oral phosphodiesterase inhibitor marketed under the trade name Pletal. The drug is marketed in the United States by Otsuka Pharmaceutical Co. as 50 and 100 mg oral tablets. Cilostazol is not used in the treatment of ischemic heart disease but rather in the relief of intermittent claudication in patients with peripheral vascular disease.

3.3.2 Dipyridamole (Persantine® and Aggrenox® (in combination with aspirin))

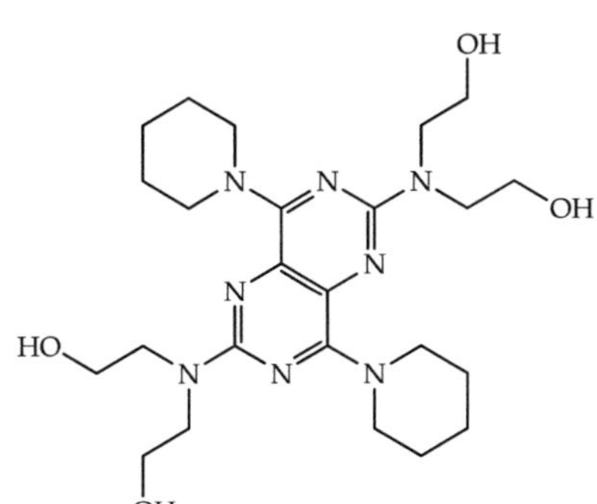

Dypyridamole is an oral phosphodiesterase inhibitor marketed as a single drug under the trade name Persantine, and as an extended-release combination with low-dose aspirin under the name Aggrenox. Persantine drug is marketed in the United States by Boehringer Ingelheim Pharmaceuticals, Inc. as 25, 50, and 75 mg oral tablets, while Aggrenox contains 200 mg of extended-release dipyridamole and 25 mg of aspirin.

Dypiridamole also inhibits the reuptake of adenosine by platelets, red blood cells, and vascular endothelial cells, as well as the enzyme adenosine deaminase, which metabolizes adenosine into inosine. Both of these effects increase the extracellular concentration of adenosine, which causes smooth muscle relaxation and is, at least in part, responsible for the vasodilatory effects of dipyridamole. Persantine causes vasodilation when given at high doses over a short time and it inhibits thrombosis when given long term by also acting as a thromboxane synthase inhibitor.

Indications, dosage, and side effects

The recommended dose of dipyridamole is 75-100 mg four times daily as an adjunct to warfarin therapy. Dipyridamole is a relatively weak antiplatelet agent on its own and thus is not used for the treatment of IHD. However, dipyridamole has been shown to increase myocardial perfusion and left ventricular function in patients with ischemic cardiomyopathy. In combination with low-dose aspirin (i.e., Aggrenox) it is used for prevention of stroke in patients with a history of transient ischemic attacks given as a twice-daily dose.

When given by intravenous infusion over 3-5 minutes, dipyridamole is associated with a rapid increase in the local concentration of adenosine in the coronary circulation, which has a vasodilatory effect. However, this vasodilation largely occurs in healthy coronary arteries, while those arteries that are stenosed remain so. This results in an imbalance of coronary perfusion that can become clinically manifest by symptoms of chest pain as well as electrocardiographic signs of ischemia.

Dipyridamole combined with aspirin reduces the risk of stroke by 22.1% compared with aspirin and by 24.4% compared with dipyridamole alone in patients with a history of cerebrovascular disease (i.e., TIA and/or stroke). With regard to secondary prevention in patients with a history of ischemic stroke, combination therapy resulted in 13% of patients having vascular death, stroke, or MI as opposed to 16% of those treated with aspirin alone. Based on all this data, Aggrenox is often used for stroke prevention. However, because it has vasodilatory effects, combination therapy of dipyridamole with aspirin (i.e., Aggrenox) should not be used for the prevention of stroke in patients with symptomatic coronary artery disease. A triple therapy of aspirin, clopidogrel, and dipyridamole has been investigated, but an increase in adverse bleeding events was observed with this combination.

The major side effects documented with the use of dipyridamole are gastrointestinal, headache, facial flushing, dizziness, and hypotension, which often disappear with continued use of the drug.

3.4 GP IIb/IIIa receptor antagonists

As a member of the integrin family of adhesion receptors, GP IIb/IIIa is found on the surface of platelets and megakaryocytes. With about 80,000 copies, GP IIb/IIIa is the most abundant receptor on platelets. GP IIb/IIIa consists of a non-covalently linked heterodimer that is inactive on resting platelets. When platelets are activated, a signal transduction pathway triggers a conformational change on the receptor that leads to its activation. Activated GP IIb/IIIa can bind other adhesion molecules (e.g., fibrinogen, vWF) under conditions of high shear stress. Binding is mediated by an Arg-Gly-Asp (RGD) sequence found on both fibrinogen and vWF, and by a Lys-Gly-Asp (KGD) sequence located within a unique dodecapeptide domain on fibrinogen. Once GP IIb/IIIa is bound to fibrinogen and/or vWF, adjacent platelets can be bridged together and lead to platelet aggregation.

Abciximab, eptifibatide, and tirofiban all target the GP IIb/IIIa receptor, but as described below, they are structurally and pharmacologically distinct. Abciximab has a long half-life and can be detected on the surface of platelets for a couple of weeks, while eptifibatide and tirofiban have shorter half-lives.

All of the GP IIb/IIIa antagonists are administered by intravenous (IV) infusion following an IV bolus. The dosage of eptifibatide and tirofiban must be reduced in patients with renal insufficiency since they are cleared by the kidneys.

The most serious complications of GP IIb/IIIa inhibitors are bleeding and thrombocytopenia, which is immunoglobulin-mediated as a result of antibodies directed against neoantigens on GP IIb/IIIa that form upon binding of the drug.

3.4.1 Abciximab (ReoPro®)

Abciximab is manufactured by Centocor and distributed by Eli Lilly. As with all of the GP IIb/IIIa antagonists, it is administered by intravenous (IV) infusion. It is a humanized murine monoclonal immunoblogulin Fab fragment directed against the activated form of GP IIb/IIIa that binds to the activated receptor with high affinity and blocks the binding of adhesion molecules.

Indications, dosage, and side effects

Abciximab is used in the setting of percutaneous coronary interventions (e.g., angioplasty, with or without stenting) to prevent platelet aggregation and thrombosis. It is administered as an IV bolus at 0.25 mg/kg, 10 to 60 min before PCI followed by continuous infusion of 0.125 μg/kg/min (to a max of 10 μg/min) for 12 h. Its use is associated with a reduction in both the incidence of ischemic complications, as well as the necessity for repeated interventional procedures within the first thirty days. Patients with diabetes and chronic renal insufficiency can be given abciximab, but its use is contraindicated in patients who shall be undergoing an emergent surgical procedure (e.g., coronary artery bypass grafting), since bleeding time may remain elevated for up to 12 hours.

Abciximab has a relatively short half-life (i.e., ~10-30 min), but its pharmacological effects on platelet function persist for up to 48 hours after cessation of IV infusion, followed by a low degree of GP IIb/IIIa receptor blockade that can continue for up to two weeks.

Many of the side effects of abciximab are due to its anti-platelet effects, including an increased risk of bleeding (e.g., gastrointestinal hemorrhage). Thrombocytopenia is a rare but known serious risk that occurs in up to 5% of individuals receiving the drug, which can be severe in ~1% of these patients. Abciximab-induced thrombocytopenia can typically be treated with transfusion of platelets. Abciximab induced thrombocytopenia can last for seven days after initial drug administration. Transfusing platelets is the only known treatment and may have limited effectiveness as the drug may also bind to the new platelets. Platelet counts, which should average 250,000-400,000, can effectively drop to zero.

In addition to targeting the GP IIb/IIIa receptor, abciximab also inhibits the closely related v3 receptor, which binds vitronectin, and M2, a leukocyte integrin. In contrast, eptifibatide and tirofiban are specific for GP IIb/IIIa. Inhibition of v3 and M2 may impart abciximab with anti-inflammatory and/or antiproliferative properties that extend beyond the inhibition of platelets.

3.4.2 Tirofiban (Aggrastat®)

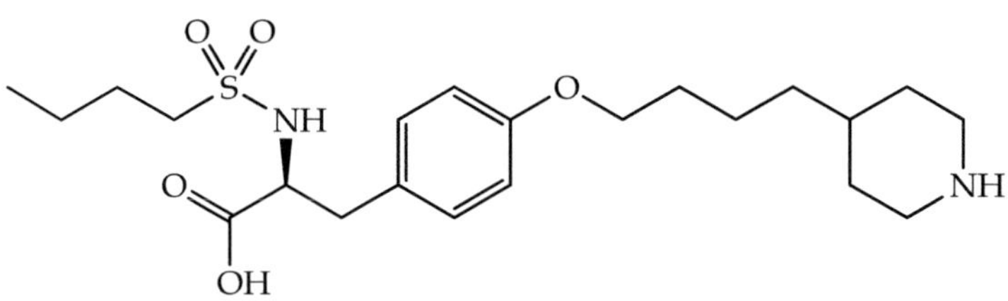

Tirofiban is marketed the United States by Medicure Pharma and the rest of the world by Irokocardio International SARL under the brand name Aggrastat as a parenteral solution for intravenous administration in dosages of forms 5 mg and 12.5 mg. Tirofiban is a non-peptidic tyrosine derivative that mimics the RGD motif found on the ligands of GP IIb/IIIa.

Indications, dosage, and side effects

Tirofiban is administered intravenously with an initial dose of 0.4 μg/kg/min for the first 30 minutes, followed by a maintenance dose of 0.1 μg /kg/min as a constant IV infusion for 12-24 hours following PCI. Tirofiban, in combination with aspirin and heparin, is indicated in the treatment of patients with acute coronary syndromes (i.e., unstable angina or acute MI), including those who may be undergo subsequent percutaneous coronary intervention, to reduce the occurrence of further ischemic damage, new myocardial infarction, and mortality.

Tirofiban has a fast onset and short duration of action, with coagulation parameters returning to normal within 4-8 hours after intravenous infusion is stopped.

The major side effect of tirofiban seen in clinical trials was bleeding, both locally and systemically, with major bleeding occurring in 1.4% of patients and minor bleeding in 10.5%. About 4.0% of patients needed a transfusion to stop intractable bleeding and to improve anemia secondary to it. Thrombocytopenia was seen in patients given tirofiban and heparin at a rate of about 1.5%, compared to only 0.8% in those receiving heparin alone. This side effect was usually reversible within a few days. Positive fecal and urine hemoglobin tests were also seen. After the drug entered the market, there have been reports of intracranial and retroperitoneal bleeding, pulmonary hemorrhage, spinal-epidural hematoma, and hypersensitivity reactions including acute anaphylaxis. Fatal bleedings have been rarely reported.

3.4.3 Eptifibatide (Integrilin®)

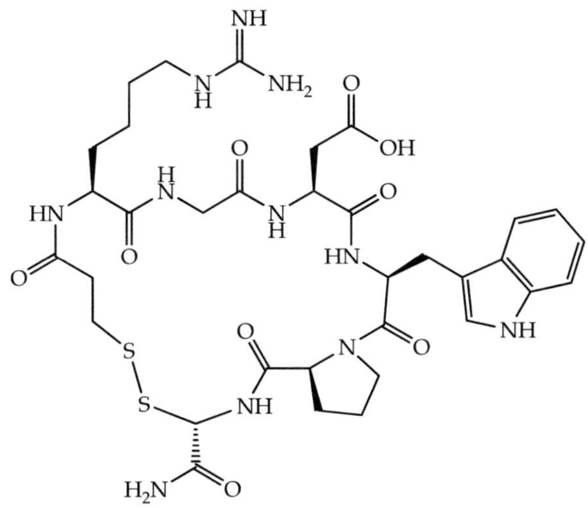

Eptifibatide is a cyclic heptapeptide that binds GP IIb/IIIa because it contains the KGD motif. It is manufactured by Millennium Pharmaceuticals and co-promoted by Schering-Plough/Essex. Eptifibatide is supplied as a sterile solution in 10-mL vials containing 20 mg of the drug, and 100-mL vials containing either 75 mg or 200 mg of eptifibatide.

Indications, Dosage, and Side Effects

The recommended adult dosage of eptifibatide in patients with acute coronary syndrome that have normal renal function is an intravenous bolus of 180 μg/kg as soon as possible following diagnosis, followed by a continuous infusion of 2.0 μg/kg/min for up to 72 hours until hospital discharge or initiation of coronary artery bypass graft (CABG) surgery. For patients who are to undergo a percutaneous coronary intervention (PCI) while receiving eptifibatide, the infusion should be continued up to hospital discharge, or for up to 18 to 24 hours after the procedure, whichever comes first, allowing for up to 96 hours of therapy.

Eptifibatide is used to reduce the risk of acute cardiac ischemic events (i.e., death and/or myocardial infarction) in patients with unstable angina or non-ST-segment elevation (i.e., non-Q-wave) myocardial infarction (i.e., non-ST-segment elevation acute coronary syndromes) both in patients who are to receive non surgery (conservative) medical treatment and those undergoing percutaneous coronary intervention (PCI). The drug is always applied together with aspirin or clopidogrel and (low molecular weight or unfractionated) heparin.

The side effects of eptifibatide are very similar to those of abciximab.

4. Ongoing trials of antiplatelet therapy

According to the International Committee of Medical Journal Editors (ICMJE):

"Any research study that prospectively assigns human participants or groups of humans to one or more health-related interventions to evaluate the effects on health outcomes."

Over the past ten years, government agencies and the IMCJE have issued laws and directives on the subject of trial registration. All parties have consistently agreed that the purpose of trial registration is to promote the public good by ensuring that the existence and design of clinically directive trials are publicly available. The registration effort began with the development of a publicly available website, ClinicalTrials.gov, which is a service of the NIH, developed by the National Library of Congress.

In 1997, the FDA/NIH began requiring registration for only a limited number of trials. In September, 2007, the Food and Drug Amendments Act (Title VIII. Sec. 801) significantly expanded the scope of clinical trials that must be registered. Penalties for failing to register "applicable trials" may include civil monetary penalties.

In 2004, the International Committee of Medical Journal Editors (ICMJE) defined trials that must be registered in order to be considered for publication in journals that adhere to ICMJE standards. In 2007 the ICMJE expanded the definition of trials that must be registered. Scores of journals (not limited to medical journals) have adopted the registration policy.

The best way to obtain information about clinical trials in platelet activation in ischemic heart disease is by accessing two renowned sources:

http://clinicaltrials.gov

http://www.clinicaltrialresults.org/

Clinicaltrials.gov is a site organized by US government and their webpage states:

"ClinicalTrials.gov offers up-to-date information for locating federally and privately supported clinical trials for a wide range of diseases and conditions. A clinical trial (also clinical research) is a research study in human volunteers to answer specific health questions."

ClinicalTrials.gov currently contains 112,970 trials sponsored by the National Institutes of Health, other federal agencies, and private industry. Studies listed in the database are conducted in all 50 States and in 175 countries. ClinicalTrials.gov receives over 50 million page views per month and 65,000 visitors daily.

The U.S. National Institutes of Health (NIH), through its National Library of Medicine (NLM), has developed this site in collaboration with the Food and Drug Administration (FDA), as a result of the FDA Modernization Act, which was passed into law in November 1997. See the FDA document - Guidance for Industry: Information Program on Clinical Trials for Serious or Life-Threatening Diseases and Conditions (March 2002).

This site allows for selection of all important characteristics of clinical trial to be displayed. We can choose any combination of next characteristics: condition, intervention, sponsor, gender, age group, phase, number enrolled, funded by, study type, study design, NCT ID, other IDs, first received date, start date, completion date, last updated date, last verified date, acronym, primary completion date, and outcome measure.

The second site, http://www.clinicaltrialresults.org/, can be used as excellent source of slides, movies, reports, and other useful information about clinical trials. The 'cardiology' section contains divisions into subspecialty news, with listing about: acute coronary syndromes, angina, anticoagulants, antiplatelet agents, antithrombins, congestive heart failure, electrophysiology, imaging, interventional cardiology, prevention, and patient resources. Since access to these sources is in the public domain, we decided not to cite individual trials by other sources although we went deeper and extracted information from from individual trials. We advise our readers to visit these two sites frequently.

A reasonably informative overview of ongoing trials of antiplatelet therapy is supposed to list name and registry number for trial, to describe study population, specify primary end point, and define study arms. This data is presented in table 4.1

Clinical Trial (Registry No.)	Study Population	Primary End Point	Study Arms
ACCOAST (NCT01015287)	4,100 patients with NSTEMI planned to undergo PCI	CV death, MI, stroke, urgent revascularization, or GP IIb/IIIa inhibitor bailout at 7 days	Randomized to pre-treatment with prasugrel (30 mg at time of diagnosis with additional 30 mg atPCI) vs. prasugrel (60 mg) at PCI. Maintenance therapy in both arms will be 10 mg daily with dose reduction to 5 mg in patients >75 yrs and body weight <60 kg
ARCTIC (NCT00827411)	2,500 patients undergoing elective PCI with DES	Death, MI, stroke, urgent coronary revascularization, or stent thrombosis assessed at 1 yr; death, MI, stroke, urgent coronary revascularization, or stent thrombosis at 6–18 months after second randomization	Initial randomization to tailored antiplatelet therapy with VerifyNow P2Y12 vs. standard dual antiplatelet therapy. Subsequent randomization after 12 months of patients who remain eventfree to discontinuation of antiplatelet therapy or continuation of therapy
DANTE Trial (NCT00774475)	442 patients with NSTE-ACS undergoing PCI with stent implantation found to have high residual platelet reactivity with the VerifyNow P2Y12	CV death, MI, or target vessel revascularization at 6 months and 1 yr	Randomized to 75 mg of clopidogrel or 150 mg of clopidogrel
DAPT (NCT00977938)	20,645 subjects undergoing PCI	CV death, MI, and stroke at 33 months; stent thrombosis at 33 months	Subjects in the overall cohort who are free from death, MI, stroke, repeat revascularization, stent thrombosis, or major bleeding at 12 months will be randomized to 18 additional months of dual antiplatelet therapy or aspirin and placebo

Clinical Trial (Registry No.)	Study Population	Primary End Point	Study Arms
GRAVITAS (NCT00645918)	2,783 subjects after DES placement for stable CAD or NSTE-ACS will have platelet function testing done with VerifyNow P2Y12	CV death, MI, and definite/ probable stent thrombosis at 6 months	Patients with high residual platelet reactivity will be randomized to receive standard-dose clopidogrel (75 mg daily) or high-dose clopidogrel (600 mg load, 150 mg daily). A random sample of patients without high residual platelet reactivity will also be enrolled and will receive 75 mg of clopidogrel daily
INNOVATE-PCI (NCT00751231)	Phase II trial in 800 patients undergoing elective PCI	No pre-specified primary end point	Randomized to clopidogrel (300/600 mg load, followed by 75 mg daily) or elinogrel (80 mg IV bolus administered before PCI, followed by twice daily dosing of oral 50 mg, 100 mg, or 150 mg)
LANCELOT 201 (NCT00312052)	Phase II trial of 600 patients with CAD	Safety and tolerability (6 months)	Randomized to E5555 (50 mg, 100 mg, or 200 mg daily) or placebo
LANCELOT 202 (NCT00548587)	Phase II trial of 600 patients with CAD	Safety and tolerability (12 weeks)	Randomized to E5555 (50 mg, 100 mg, or 200 mg daily) or placebo
TRA-CER (NCT00527943)	12,500 subjects with ACS	CV death, MI, stroke, recurrent ischemia with repeat hospital stay, and urgent coronary revascularization at end of study	Randomized to SCH 530348 (40 mg loading dose, 2.5 mg daily) vs. placebo
TRA-2P-TIMI 50 (NCT00526474)	26,450 patients with history of CAD, CVA, or PAD	CV death, MI, stroke, and urgent coronary revascularization at end of study	Randomized to SCH 530348 (2.5 mg daily) vs. placebo
TOPAS-1 (NCT00914368)	Phase II trial of 450 patients who have either had or not had stent thrombosis or MI within 6 months of PCI while on dual antiplatelet therapy	Establish VerifyNow P2Y12 (PRU) and VASP (PRI, %) cutoff level of platelet inhibition in patients with and without clinical events.	All subjects will undergo platelet function testing with both VerifyNow P2Y12 and VASP assays

Clinical Trial (Registry No.)	Study Population	Primary End Point	Study Arms
TRIGGER-PCI (NCT00910299)	2,150 subjects with high residual platelet reactivity with the VerifyNow P2Y12 after elective PCI with DES	CV death or MI at 6 months	Randomized to prasugrel (60 mg load, 10 mg daily) vs. clopidogrel (75 mg daily)
TRILOGY-ACS (NCT00699998)	10,300 patients with NSTE-ACS being initially medically managed	CV death, MI, or stroke at end of study	Randomized to prasugrel (30 mg load ifadministered, followed by 5 mg or 10 mg maintenance) or clopidogrel (300 mg load if administered, followed by 75 mg daily)

Table 4.1

5. Abbreviations

ACCOAST: Comparison of Prasugrel at PCI or Time of Diagnosis of Non-ST Elevation Myocardial Infarction Trial

ACS: acute coronary syndrome

ARCTIC: Double Randomization of a Monitoring Adjusted Antiplatelet Treatment Versus a Common Antiplatelet Treatment for DES Implantation, and Interruption Versus Continuation of Double Antiplatelet Therapy Trial

ARMYDA: Antiplatelet Therapy for Reduction of Myocardial Damage During Angioplasty

CIPAMI: Clopidogrel Administered Prehospital to Improve Primary PCI in Patients with Acute Myocardial Infarction

CAD: coronary artery disease

CLARITY-TIMI: Clopidogrel as Adjunctive Reperfusion Therapy-Thrombolysis in Myocardial Infarction

CREDO: Clopidogrel for the Reduction of Events During Observation

CURE: Clopidogrel in Unstable Angina to Prevent Recurrent Events

CURRENT/OASIS: Clopidogrel Optimal Loading Dose Usage to Reduce Recurrent Events/Optimal Antiplatelet Strategy for Interventions

CV: cardiovascular

CVA: cerebrovascular accident

DANTE: Dual Antiplatelet Therapy Tailored on the Extent of Platelet Inhibition

DAPT: Dual Antiplatelet Therapy

DES: drug-eluting stents

GP IIb/IIIa: glycoprotein IIb/IIa

GRAVITAS: Gauging Responsiveness With A VerifyNow Assay—Impact On Thrombosis And Safety

INNOVATE-PCI: A Phase 2 Safety and Efficacy Study of PRT060128, a Novel Intravenous and Oral P2Y12 Inhibitor, in Non-Urgent PCI

LANCELOT 201: Safety and Tolerability of E5555 and Its Effects on Markers of Intravascular Inflammation in Subjects With Coronary Artery Disease

LANCELOT 202: Safety and Tolerability of E5555 and Its Effects on Markers of Intravascular Inflammation in Subjects With Acute Coronary Syndrome

MI: myocardial infarction

NSTE-ACS: non–ST-segment elevation acute coronary syndrome

NSTEMI: non–ST-segment elevation myocardial infarction

PAD: peripheral artery disease

PCI: percutaneous coronary intervention

PRI: platelet reactivity index

PRINCIPLE: Prasugrel in Comparison to Clopidogrel for Inhibition of Platelet Activation and Aggregation

PRU: platelet reactivity unit

STEMI: ST-segment elevation myocardial infarction

TIMI: Thrombolysis In Myocardial Infarction

TOPAS-1: Tailoring Of Platelet Inhibition to Avoid Stent Thrombosis

TRA-CER: Trial to Assess the Effects of SCH 530348 in Preventing Heart Attack and Stroke in Patients With Acute Coronary Syndrome

TRA-2P-TIMI 50: Trial to Assess the Effects of SCH 530348 in Preventing Heart Attack and Stroke in Patients With Atherosclerosis

TRIGGER-PCI: Testing Platelet Reactivity In Patients Undergoing Elective Stent Placement on Clopidogrel to Guide Alternative Therapy With Prasugrel

TRILOGY-ACS: Comparison of Prasugrel and Clopidogrel in Acute Coronary Syndrome Subjects

TRITON: Trial to Assess Improvement in Therapeutic Outcomes by Optimizing Platelet Inhibition with Prasugrel

VASP: Vasodilator-stimulated phosphorprotein

6. References

Antman, E. M. & Loscalzo, J. (2012). Chapter 245. ST-Segment Elevation Myocardial Infarction, In: *Harrison's Principles of Internal Medicine, 18e*, Fauci, A. S., Braunwald E., Kasper D. L., Hauser S. L., Longo D. L., Jameson J. L., & Loscalzo J., McGraw-Hill, Retrieved from http://www.accessmedicine.com/content.aspx?aID=9104591.

Antman, E. M., Selwyn, A. P., & Loscalzo, J. (2012). Chapter 243. Ischemic Heart Disease, In: *Harrison's Principles of Internal Medicine, 18e*, Fauci, A. S., Braunwald E., Kasper D. L., Hauser S. L., Longo D. L., Jameson J. L., & Loscalzo J., McGraw-Hill, Retrieved from http://www.accessmedicine.com/content.aspx?aID=9104321

Antoniades, C., Shirodaria, C., Van Assche, T., Cunnington, C., Tegeder, I., Lötsch, J., Guzik, T. J., Leeson, P., Diesch, J., Tousoulis, D., Stefanadis, C., Costigan, M., Woolf, C. J., Alp, N. J., & Channon, K. M. (2008). GCH1 haplotype determines vascular and plasma biopterin availability in coronary artery disease effects on vascular superoxide production and endothelial function. *J. Am. Coll. Cardiol.*, Vol. 52, pp. 158-165.

AstraZeneca (22 August 2011). BRILINTA™ (ticagrelor) tablets now available in U.S. pharmacies for patients with acute coronary syndrome, In: *http://www.astrazeneca-us.com/*, Available from: http://www.astrazeneca-us.com/search/?itemId=12475851

AstraZeneca (August 2011). Brilinta, In: *http://www.astrazeneca-us.com/our-medicines/*, Available from: http://www1.astrazeneca-us.com/pi/brilinta.pdf

Banga, H. S., Simons, F. R., Brass, L. F., & Rittenhouse, S. E. (1986). Activation of phospholipases A and C in human platelets exposed to epinephrine: role of glycoproteins IIb/IIIa and dual role of epinephrine. *Proc. Natl. Acad. Sci.*, Vol. 83, pp. 9197-9201.

Bassenge, E. (1996). Endothelial function in different organs. *Progress in Cardiovascular Diseases*, Vol. XXXIX, No. 3, pp. 209-228.

Beckman, J. S. & Koppenol, W. H. (1996). Nitric oxide, superoxide, and peroxynitrite: the good, the bad, and ugly. *Am. J. Physiol.*, Vol. 271, pp. C1424-C1437.

Bonauer, A., Boon, R. A., & Dimmeler, S. (2010). Vascular microRNAs. *Curr. Drug Targets*, Vol. 11, No. 8, pp. 943-949.

Brass, L. F. (1984). The effect of Na^+ on Ca^{2+} homeostasis in unstimulated platelets. *J. Biol. Chem.*, Vol. 259, pp. 12571-12575

Brass, L. F. (2010). Understanding and Evaluating Platelet Function Hematology. *Am. Soc. Hematol. Educ. Program.*, pp. 387-396

Cannon, C. P. & Braunwald, E. (2012). Chapter 244. Unstable Angina and Non-ST-Segment Elevation Myocardial Infarction, In: *Harrison's Principles of Internal Medicine, 18e*, Fauci, A. S., Braunwald, E., Kasper, D. L., Hauser, S. L., Longo, D. L., Jameson, J. L., & Loscalzo, J., McGraw-Hill, Retrieved from http://www.accessmedicine.com/content.aspx?aID=9104518

clinicaltrials.gov: http://clinicaltrials.gov/ct2/results?flds=Xt&flds=a&flds=b&term=Antiplatelet+Therapy&show_flds=Y

Cooley, H. & Cohen, P. (1968). Potassium transport in human blood platelets. *J. Lab. Clin. Med.*, Vol. 70, pp. 69-79.

Dousset, J., Trouilh, M., & Fogliett, M. (1983). Plasma malonaldehyde levels during myocardial infarction. *Clinica. Chimica. Acta*, Vol. 129, pp. 319-322.

Edelstein, L. C. & Bray, P. F. (2011). MicroRNAs in platelet production and activation. *Blood*, Vol. 17, No. 20, pp. 5289-5296.

Enauf, J., Bredoux, R., Bourdeau, N., & Levy, S. (1987). Two different Ca^{2+} transport systems are associated with plasma and intracellular human platelet membranes. *J. Biol. Chem.*, Vol. 262, pp. 9293-9297.

Fang, Y., Shi, C., Manduchi, E., Civelek, M., & Davies, P. F. (2010). MicroRNA-10a regulation of proinflammatory phenotype in athero-susceptible endothelium in vivo and in vitro. *Proc. Natl. Acad. Sci. USA*, Vol. 107, No. 30, pp. 13450-13455.

Frojmovic, M. & Panjwani, R. (1976). Geometry of normal mammalian platelets by quantitative microscopic studies. *Biophys. J.*, Vol. 16, pp. 1071-1089.

Garelnabi, M. (2010). Emerging Evidences from the Contribution of the Traditional and New Risk Factors to the Atherosclerosis Pathogenesis. J. Med. Sci., Vol. 10, pp. 136-144.

Garelnabi, M., Gupta, V., Mallika, V., & hattacharjee, J. (2010). Platelets oxidative stress in Indian patients with ischemic heart disease. *J. Clin. Lab. Anal.*, Vol. 24, No. 1, pp. 49-54.

Garelnabi, M., Gupta, V., Mallika, V., & Bhattacharjee, J. (2011). Platelet Nitric Oxide Signaling System in Patients with Coronary Artery Disease. *Ann. Vasc. Dis.*, Vol. 4, No. 2, pp. 99–105.

Hagemeyer, C. E. & Peter, K. (2010). Targeting the platelet integrin GP IIb/IIIa. *Curr. Pharm. Des.*, Vol. 16, No. 37, pp. 4119-4133.

Haver, V. G., Slart, R. H., Zeebregts, C. J., Peppelenbosch, M. P., & Tio, R. A. (2010). Rupture of vulnerable atherosclerotic plaques: microRNAs conducting the orchestra? *Trends Cardiovasc. Med.*, Vol. 20, No. 2, pp. 65-71.

Heptinstall, S. & Hanley, S. (1985). Blood platelets and vessel walls, In: *Hemostasis and Thrombosis, 1st Ed.*, pp. 36-74, Butterworths, USA.

Hourani, M. & Lausck, J. (1991). Pharmacological Receptors on Blood Platelets. *Pharmacol. Rev.*, Vol. 43, pp. 243-298.

Ikeda, H., Takajo, Y., Murohara, T., Ichiki., K., Adachi, H., & Haramaki, N. (2000). Platelet-derived nitric oxide and coronary risk factors. *Hypertension*, Vol. 35, pp. 904–907.

Jamaluddin, M. S., Weakley, S. M., Zhang, L., Kougias, P., Lin, P. H., Yao, Q., & Chen, C. (2011). miRNAs: roles and clinical applications in vascular disease. *Expert Rev. Mol. Diagn.*, Vol. 11, No. 1, pp. 79-89.

Karpatkin, S., Charmatz, A., & Langer, M. (1970). Glycogenesis and glyconeogenesis in human platelets. Incorporation of glucose, pyruvate, and citrate into platelet glycogen, glycogene synthetase and fructose-1,6-diphosphate activity. *J. Clin. Invest.*, Vol. 49, pp. 140-149.

Knezevie, I., Dieter, P., & Le Breton, C. (1992). Mechanism of inositol 1,4,5-triphosphate-induced aggregation in saponin-permeabilized platelets. *J. Pharmacol. Exp. Ther.*, Vol. 260, pp. 947-955.

Leeper, N. J., Raiesdana, A., Kojima, Y., Chun, H. J., Azuma, J., Maegdefessel, L., Kundu, R. K., Quertermous, T., Tsao, P. S., & Spin, J. M. (2011). MicroRNA-26a is a novel regulator of vascular smooth muscle cell function. *J. Cell. Physiol.*, Vol. 226, No. 4, pp. 1035-1043.

Leslie, V., Christel, B., Patricia, J., & Ulhas, N. (1999). Platelets in Hemostasis and thrombosis, In: *Wintrobe's Clinical Hematology, 10th Edition,* Vol. 1, pp. 661-683, Williams & Wilkins, Maryland, USA.

Malmgren, R. (1986). ATP-Secretion occurs as an initial response in collagen induced platelet activation. *Thromb. Res.,* Vol. 43, pp. 445-453.

Nurden, A. T. (2011). Platelets, inflammation and tissue regeneration. *Thromb. Haemost.,* Vol. 105, Suppl. 1, pp. S13-S33.

O'Sullivan, J. F., Martin, K., & Caplice, N. M. (2011). Microribonucleic acids for prevention of plaque rupture and in-stent restenosis: "a finger in the dam". *J. Am. Coll. Cardiol.,* Vol. 57, No. 4, pp. 383-389.

Pan, Z. W., Lu, Y. J., & Yang, B. F. MicroRNAs: a novel class of potential therapeutic targets for cardiovascular diseases. *Acta Pharmacol. Sin.,*Vol. 31, No. 1, pp. 1-9

Parthasarathy, S. Litvinov, D. Selvarajan, K., Garelnabi, M. (2008). Lipid peroxidation and decomposition—conflicting roles in plaque vulnerability and stability, *Biochimica et Biophysica Acta,* Vol. 1781, pp. 221–231.

Paulus, M., Bur, J., & Grosdent, C. (1979). Control platelet territory development in megakaryocytes. *Blood Cells,* Vol. 5, pp. 59-88.

Petidis, K., Douma, S., Doumas, M., Basagiannis, I., Vogiatzis, K., & Zamboulis, C. (2008). The interaction of vasoactive substances during exercise modulates platelet aggregation in hypertension and coronary artery disease. *BMC Cardiovasc. Disord.,* Vol. 27, No. 8, pp. 11.

Selwyn, A. P., & Braunwald, E. (1994). Ischemic Heart disease. In: *Harrison's Principles of Internal Medicine, 13th Ed.,*Vol. 1, pp. 1077, McGraw-Hill, Inc. New York, USA.

Siess, W., Cautrecasas, P., & Lapetina, G. (1983). A role for cyclooxygenase products in the formation of phosphatidic acid in stimulated human platelets. Differential mechanism of action of thrombin and collagen. *J. Biol. Chem.,* Vol. 258, pp. 4683-4686.

Siess, W. (1989). Molecular mechanism of platelet activation. *Physiol. Rev.,* Vol. 69, pp. 58-177.

Siljander, P. R. M. Platelet-derived microparticles–an updated perspective. (2011). *Thrombosis Research,* Vol. 127, Suppl. 2, pp. S30–S33

Smith, B., Ingerman, C., Kocsis, J., & Silver, M. (1973). Formation of prostaglandins during aggregation of human blood platelets. *J. Clin. Invest.,* Vol. 52, pp. 965-969.

Stenberg, E., Shuman, A., Levine, P., & Bainton, F. (1984). Redistribution of alphagranules and their contents in thrombin-stimulated platelets. *J. Cell Biol.,* Vol. 98, pp. 748-760.

Urbich, C., Kuehbacher, A., & Dimmeler, S. (2008). Role of microRNAs in vascular diseases, inflammation, and angiogenesis. *Cardiovasc. Res.,* Vol. 79, No. 4, pp. 581-588.

Weiss, J., Kelly, A., & Herbert, V. (1968). Vitamin B_{12} and folate activity in normal human platelets. *Blood,* Vol. 31, pp. 258-262.

Weitz, J. I. (2012). Chapter 118. Antiplatelet, Anticoagulant, and Fibrinolytic Drugs, In: *Harrison's Principles of Internal Medicine, 18e,* Fauci, A. S., Braunwald, E., Kasper, D. L., Hauser, S. L., Longo, D. L., Jameson, J. L., Loscalzo J., McGraw-Hill, Retrieved from http://www.accessmedicine.com/content.aspx?aID=9101027

Weksler, B. B. (1983) Platelets and the inflammatory response. *Clin. Lab. Med.,* Vol. 3, No. 4, pp. 667-76.

WHO (2008). The World Health Report 2008: Primary Health Care Now More Than Ever. World Health Organization, Geneva, Switzerland, p. 119.

Wierda, R. J., Geutskens, S. B., Jukema, J. W., Quax, P. H., & van den Elsen, P.J. (2010). Epigenetics in atherosclerosis and inflammation. *J. Cell. Mol. Med.*, Vol. 14, No. 6A, pp. 1225-40.

Wikipedia (21 August 2011). Antiplatelet drug, In: *http://en.wikipedia.org/*, 5 September 2011, Available from: http://en.wikipedia.org/wiki/Antiplatelet_drug (including all links and references cited within).

Zehnder, J. L. (2009). Chapter 34. Drugs Used in Disorders of Coagulation, In: *Basic & Clinical Pharmacology, 11e*, Katzung, B. G., Masters, S. B., Trevor, A. J., pp. 598-600, McGraw-Hill, ISBN 978-0-07-160405-5, New York, NY, USA

Zhenyu, L., Delaney, M. K., O'Brien, K. A., & Du, X. (2010). Signaling During Platelet Adhesion and Activation. *Arterioscler. Thromb. Vasc. Biol.*, Vol. 30, pp. 2341-2349.

9

Myocardial Ischemia-Reperfusion/Injury

Nermine Saleh and Magda Youssef
Faculty of Medicine, Ain Shams University, Physiology Department
Egypt

1. Introduction

Refers to myocardial, vascular, or electrophysiological dysfunction that is induced by the restoration of blood flow to previously ischemic tissue. Tissue damage caused when blood supply returns to the tissue after a period of ischemia. The absence of oxygen and nutrients from blood during the ischemic period creates a condition in which the restoration of circulation results in inflammation and oxidative damage through the induction of oxidative stress rather than restoration of normal function.

Early reperfusion of ischemic myocardium is an accepted approach for the management of patients with acute coronary syndromes. In addition, surgical interventions requiring interruption of blood flow to the heart, out of necessity, must be followed by restoration of perfusion. Reperfusion, although essential for tissue and/or organ survival, is not without risk due to the extension of cell damage as a result of reperfusion itself.

Since rupture of the plasma membrane is a prominent feature of necrosis and ischemia-reperfusion injury and is a lethal event, it is worth considering what might lead to rupture of the plasma membrane. Rupture of the plasma membrane could be facilitated by calpain or some other protease cleavage of the cytoskeleton. Complete loss of ATP would also inhibit ion pumps, which would result in swelling perhaps rupturing the plasma membrane, particularly if the cytoskeleton has been weakened (Murphy & Steenbergen, 2008).

It is possible that a combination of protease activation with loss of ATP, ion dysregulation and cell swelling all conspire to rupture the plasma membrane. A rise in cytosolic free Ca^{2+} concentration $[Ca^{2+}]_i$ has been consistently observed in ischemia and early reperfusion. A rise in $[Ca^{2+}]_i$ will lead to activation of calpains, which could be involved in cleaving proteins leading to plasma membrane rupture. Calpain activates the proapoptotic BID, and also cleaves Atg5, shifting the balance from autophagy to apoptosis. An increase in $[Ca^{2+}]_i$ and ROS can lead to activation of an inner mitochondrial large-conductance channel known as the Mitochondrial permeability transition (MPT). Opening of this channel would lead to loss of ATP and mitochondrial function, which would quickly lead to mitochondrial swelling and release of cytochrome *c*, which could activate apoptosis. If a large number of mitochondria in a cell undergo opening of the MPT, the cell will lose the capacity to make ATP, and the cell will lose ion homeostasis, resulting in cell swelling, membrane rupture, and cell death (Murphy & Steenbergen, 2008).

Platelet-dependent thrombus formation is a key event in the pathogenesis of acute myocardial infarction (AMI). Platelets mediate both thrombotic occlusion of the entire epicardial coronary artery and also accumulate in the microcirculation resulting in impairment of microcirculation and provoking myocardial ischemia during reperfusion (Gawaz, 2004)..

Despite an improved understanding of the pathophysiology of this process and encouraging preclinical trials of multiple agents, most of the clinical trials to prevent reperfusion injury have been disappointing. Despite these problems, adjunctive therapies to limit reperfusion injury remain an active area of investigation. In these studies vitamin E has been tried to ameliorate lethal reperfusion injury.

2. Protective effects of vitamin E against myocardial ischemia/reperfusion injury in rats

Prevention of ischemia-reperfusion (I/R) injury is crucial for successful cardiac surgery. In cardiac surgery, it is reported that pharmacological agents can be administered prior to ischemia, enabling them to exert their protective effects on mitochondria prior to ischemia and reperfusion. The role of α-tocopherol (vitamin E) as a chain-breaking antioxidant is well characterized in vitro; it is considered the major lipophilic antioxidant in the human body, specifically by its reaction with peroxyl free radicals (Navarro et al., 2005). It has been demonstrated that vitamin E deficiency is responsible for increased myocardial injury caused by oxidative stress and that I/R of the heart is associated with a blunting in cardiac α-tocopherol levels (Altavilla et al., 2000). Vitamin E has been extensively assayed in experimental animal diseases, and in the protection and treatment of human diseases.

Research provided evidence that vitamin E intake much higher than the current recommended dietary allowance could contribute to or improve human health. It has been reported that dietary requirements to prevent deficiency and maintain apparent health is substantially less than optimal amounts necessary to provide protection against degenerative conditions and chronic diseases. Results of a number of studies suggested that increased vitamin E intake is associated with decreased risk of coronary heart disease, and certain types of cancer as well as enhancement of immune function (Ricciarelli et al., 2002 ; Dong et al., 2009). Literatures concerning safety, and tolerance of oral vitamin E demonstrated that vitamin E is relatively nontoxic (Dong et al., 2009; Hanson et al., 2007). In a 91-day study of rats receiving up to 316-443 mg vitamin E/animal/day, vitamin E had no adverse effects on weight gain, food intake, organ weights, hematology or serum chemistry values (Krasavage et al., 1977). In the heart and cardiovascular system, nitric oxide (NO) plays a significant role. The specific roles of NO in the heart in general and on cardiac mitochondria in particular remain controversial. It has been reported that both endogenous and exogenous sources of NO exert important modulatory effects on mitochondrial function (Davidson & Duchen, 2006). Nitric oxide donors have been shown to induce a powerful cardioprotection against I/R injury in mice (Wang et al., 2005). However, literature reporting varying results of NO therapy, with some investigators reporting cardioprotective effects, whereas others report cardiotoxic effects (Bell et al., 2003). Mitochondrial permeability transition (MPT) is a nonspecific pore in the inner mitochondrial membrane. It has been reported that the opening of the MPT converts the mitochondria from an organelle that provides adenosine triphosphate to sustain heart function into an instrument of cell death by apoptosis if the insult is mild, and to necrosis if the insult is profound (Halestrap et al., 2004). It is hypothesized that a major component of I/R injury is necrotic cell death, which is widely thought to be the consequence of opening the MPT as reported by previous literature (Costa et al., 2006). Functional recovery of the Langendorff-perfused heart from ischemia inversely correlates with the extent of the opening, and inhibition of the MPT provides protection against reperfusion injury (Halestrap et al., 2004). Previous literature (Kim et al., 2006) reported that radical oxygen species (ROS) generated during early reperfusion is the primary activator of the MPT, and cardiomyocyte death. Some recently developed, intracellularly targeted scavengers have been reported to provide some reduction in infarct size (Sheu et al., 2006). Antioxidants such as vitamins C, and E have also been suggested to scavenge ROS and reduce ischemic injury (Qin et al., 2006). A study, therefore, was performed with the following objectives, first, to determine whether a short course of oral administration of vitamin E in a megadose as compared to a NO donor nitroglycerin (GTN) can provide sufficient protection of the heart against reperfusion induced injury, and second, to determine whether a combined regimen of vitamin E and a NO donor confound superior protection to the hearts against this insult, and to investigate the effect of each of these pharmacological preconditioning agents on mitochondria and MPT.

2.1 Methods

This study was undertaken on female Wistar rats weighing 150-200 gm. Rats were allocated into 4 groups: a- Control group, non-treated , b- GTN-treated group, rats received GTN intraperitoneal 25 minutes before sacrifice, in a dose of 120 μg/kg bw (Zhou et al., 2002) ,c- Vit E-treated group, rat received vitamin E by oral tubal feeding 16-20 hours before sacrifice, in a dose of 250mg/rat d- Vit E and GTN-treated group, rats received vitamin E and GTN as in both GTN-treated group and vit E -treated group.

Experimental procedures; On the day of the experiments, rats were weighed and injected intraperitoneally with heparin sodium, 1000 IU. One hour later, the rats were anesthetized with thiopental sodium 40 mg/kg intraperitoneally.

In vitro studying of isolated hearts: Hearts were excised and perfused in a Langendorff preparation with the standard Krebs-Henselite Bicarbonate (KHB) buffer, pH 7.4 equilibrated with O2:CO2 (95%:5%) at 37 ° C (Ayobe &Tarazi, 1983). After 20 minutes stabilization period, baseline cardiac activities were recorded using isometric force transducer connected to a two-channel oscillograph.

Ischemia Reperfusion Technique:: After recording baseline cardiac activity, 30 minutes of ischemia was induced by stopping the perfusing fluid, and at 30-minute reperfusion, the cardiac activity was recorded again.

Cardiac activity was assessed by the following parameters: heart beating rate (BR), rate of tension development (dT/dt) and half relaxation time (1\2 RT). Myocardial flow rate (MFR) was measured at the same intervals by timed volumetric collection. Results were expressed as the percentage change of the measured parameters relative to baseline values to normalize individual differences between basal values among each group.

The cardiac chambers were weighed. The ventricles were used to isolate mitochondria. Mitochondria were isolated by conventional procedures of differential centrifugation. Hydrolysis of mitochondrial nicotinamide adenine dinucleotide (NAD^+) directly reflects MPT opening. The NAD^+ was measured after perchloric acid extraction (Di Lisa et al., 2001; Yamazaki et al., 2004). The malondialdehyde (MDA) was estimated in cardiac homogenates by the double heating method of Draper and Hadley (Draper & Hadley, 1990). Data for MDA and NAD^+ was calculated by non-parametric Mann -Witney test.

Electron microscopic study: Parts of the lower half of the left ventricle were fixed in 4% glutaraldehyde, dehydrated and embedded in resin. Sections of 60 nm thickness were cut on copper grids and stained with uranyl acetate followed by lead citrate for examination by the electron microscope (Hunter, 1984).

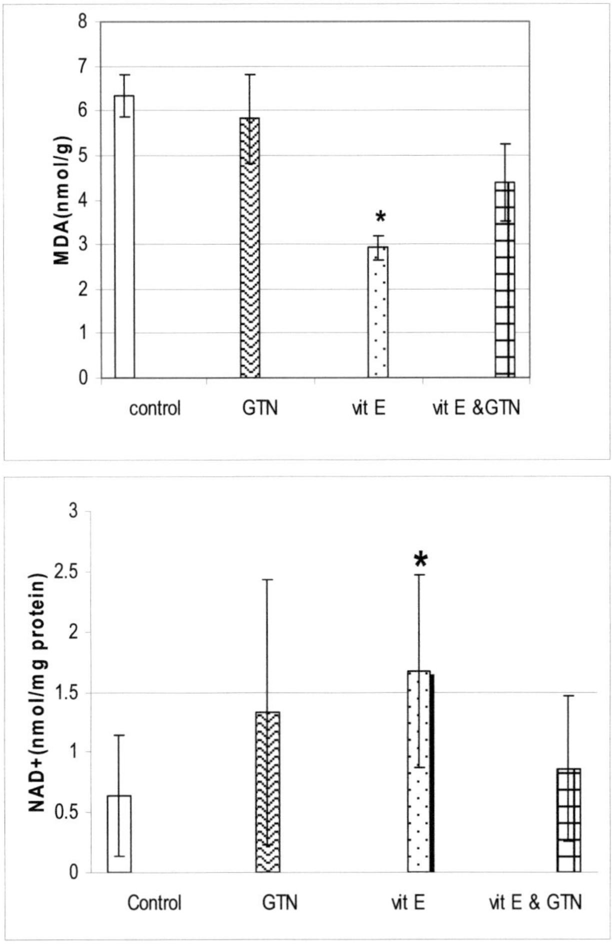

Fig. 1. The malondialdehyde (MDA) and mitochondrial nicotinamide adenine dinucleotide (NAD^+) levels after 30 minutes reperfusion in control rats, nitroglycerine-treated rats (GTN), vit E-treated rats and vit E & GTN-treated rats. Data are presented as means ± SD * P = 0.004 as compared to control rats.

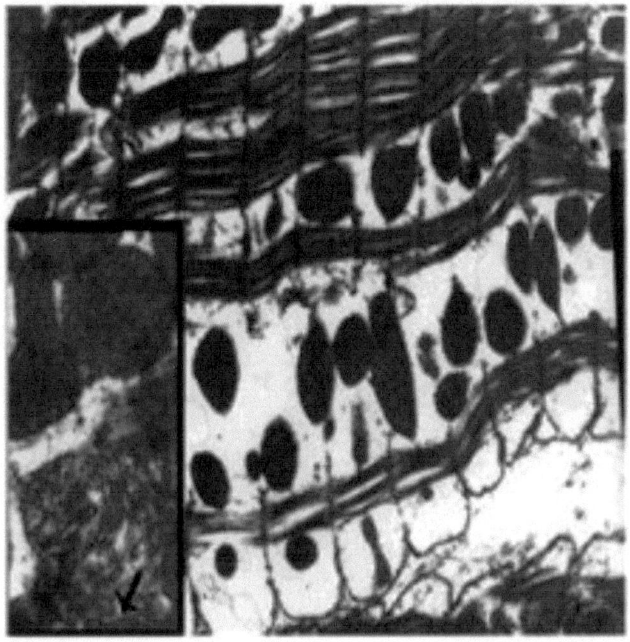

Fig. 2. Showing irregular, disorted myofilaments. They appear loose and discontinuous.Mitochondiae are pleomorphic and idely spaced (controll group x60000). Arrow shows disruption in the mitochondrial membrate (x15000).

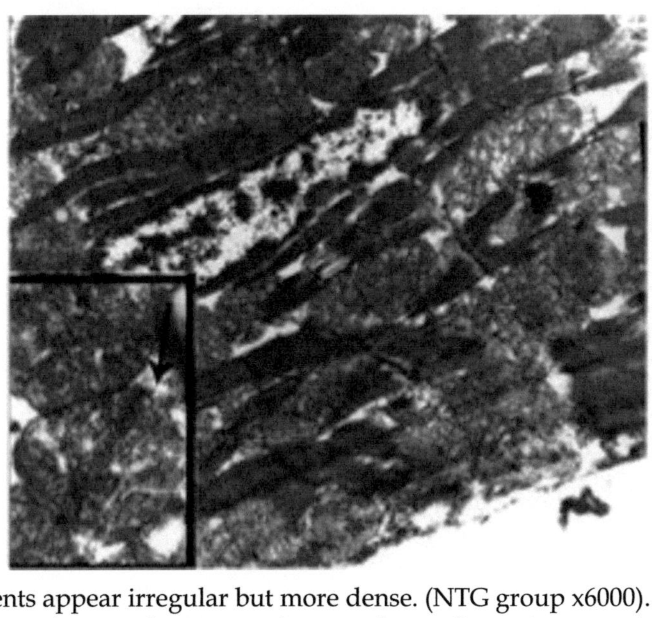

Fig. 3. Myofilaments appear irregular but more dense. (NTG group x6000). Inset - mitochondriae show disrupted cristae and arrow shows discontinuous mitochondrial membrane (x15000). GTN group - group received nitroglycerin

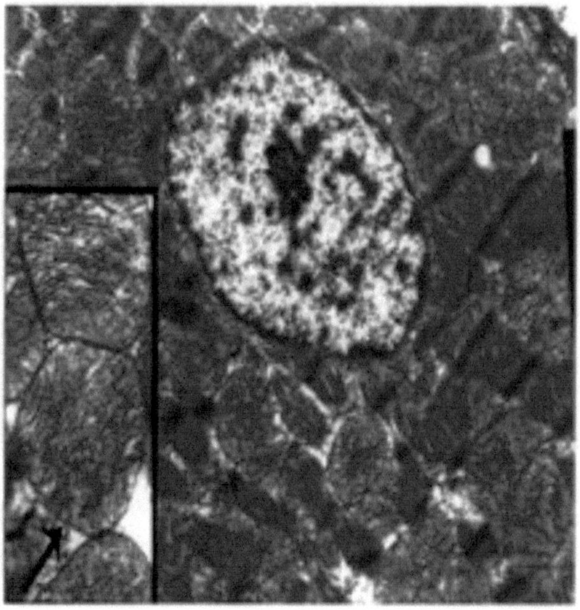

Fig. 4. Showing regular dense and continuous myofilaments. (Vit E group x6000). Inset - mitochondriae are regular in shape. They reveal transverse, parallel cristae.Arrow shows continuous mitochondrial membrane. (x15000). Vit E group - received vitamin E.

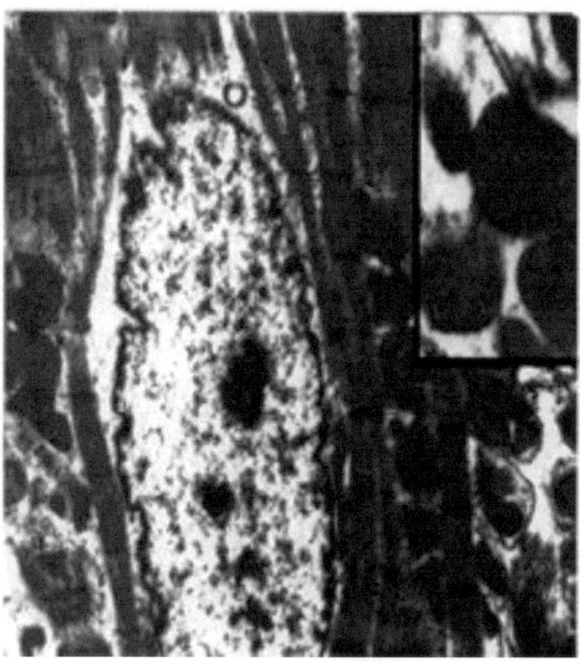

Fig. 5. Showing regular and dense myofilaments (GTN and Vit E group x6000.). Inset - mitochondriae are electron dense with unclear cristae. (x15000). GTN and Vit E group - received nitroglycerin and vitamin E.

Group (n=7)	%BR	%dT/dt	%½RT	%MFR
Control	-16.21±4.93	-23.75±6.88	22.85±9.84	-21.78±13.07
GTN-tr.	-21.16±11.04	22.94±20.64	46.43±19.57	-53.31±9.74
Vit E-tr.	15.37±26.21	39.66±24.43[a]	10.71±12.02	-17.57±17.68[b]
Vit E and GTN-tr.	-15.10±7.11	38.48±23.67[a]	14.29±5.04	-25.44±4.24

Data are presented as mean ± SEM. n: is the number of rats. a:Significance calculated by least significant difference (LSD) at P=0.03 from control group, b:Significance calculated by LSD at P=0.04 between vit E-tr., and GTN-tr groups. BR - beating rate, dT/dt - rate of tension development, ½ RT -half relaxation time, MFR - myocardial flow rate.

Table 1. Percentage changes from baseline values of cardiac activity at 30 minutes reperfusion after 30 minutes of ischemia (I/R) of perfused hearts isolated from; control rats, GTN-treated rats (GTN-tr.),vitamin E-treated rats (vitE-tr.), and vitamin E & nitroglycerin-treated rats (vit E and GTN-tr.).

2.2 Effects of vitamin E versus nitroglycerine on I/R injury

Our results demonstrated that a short course of vitamin E treatment induced preconditioning in the hearts. The vitamin E therapy, enhanced contractile, and vascular recovery, and attenuated oxidative stress in cardiac tissue, as demonstrated by the decrease of MDA in cardiac tissue. Moreover, this therapy protected the hearts against MPT opening as indicated by significant increase of NAD^+ in cardiac tissue. Histological examination showed less mitochondrial injury induced by reperfusion in the hearts of this group, with preservation of the myocytes structure. Moreover, the present study clearly demonstrated that preischemic treatment with GTN; a NO donor did not provide significant protection of hearts against I/R-induced contractile dysfunction and tissue injury. Peroxynitrite ($ONOO^-$), the reacting product of NO and O_2^-, is apotent cytotoxic agent. It is highly reactive with a wide variety of molecules, including deoxyribose, cellular lipids, and protein sulfhydryls, and results in oxidative tissue damage (Farshid et al., 2002). In this study, GTN treatment did not attenuate the reperfusion-mediated increase of MDA in cardiac tissues of GTN-treated rats. This finding suggested that $ONOO^-$ might be formed excessively in post-ischemic myocardial tissue. In the current study, supplementation of NO donor could have raised cardiac tissue NO concentration, with the coincident increase in free radical generation at reperfusion established the conditions of $ONOO^-$ formation. Therefore, we suggest that exogenous NO failed to provide cardioprotection, due to concomitant increase of $ONOO^-$. In this study, the non significant increase of NAD^+ content in isolated hearts from GTN-supplemented rats indicated failure of GTN to attenuate MPT opening. The opening of that channel lead to mitochondrial swelling, release of apoptotic molecules and eventually cell death. This suggestion was further confirmed by histological examination of isolated hearts from GTN-supplemented rats. Previous literature (Dhalla et al., 2000) reported a depletion of endogenous antioxidants in the ischemic hearts upon reperfusion. Various studies have reported the beneficial effects of antioxidants as these agents render resistance to the hearts against I/R injury. However, other investigators have failed to observe such results. The slow incorporation of vitamin E into tissues, due to its marked lipophilicity, is probably responsible for its failure as a cardioprotective compound as shown during the acute administration of α-tocopherol after

I/R injury induced in the pig (Altavilla et al., 2000). Several studies reinforce the importance of localization and timing in cardioprotection. Delivery of the antioxidants to the right compartment in the right time period is very difficult to achieve in controlled animal studies, and even more difficult in patients. As a result of the controversy in the animal studies, and the failed clinical trials, it is often concluded that inhibition of ROS will not influence infarct size. A more realistic assessment is that to have a significant benefit in reducing infarct size requires the correct delivery of mitochondrial targeted antioxidants perhaps in conjunction with other therapies. So in this study, we tried to give the animals vitamin E in a large dose, with a sufficient time to provide its effects. The demonstration that prior exposure to a low concentration of H_2O_2 protects against MPT opening may be of pathophysiological importance for cardioprotection (Costa et al., 2006). By the same reasoning, in preconditioning, we speculate the need for an antioxidant that attenuates the large burst of oxidative stress at the start of reperfusion without completely neutralizing free radicals.

We suggest that vitamin E as a physiological antioxidant acted to scavenge free radicals without completely neutralizing them, thereby affording a significant preconditioning effect. Reduction of free radical formation inhibits MPT opening, thereby affording preconditioning. This is clearly demonstrated in the current study, since there was a significant increase of NAD+ content of reperfused hearts in the vitamin E-treated groups. Histological examination confirmed this result, as it revealed marked protection of the normal structure of myocytes and mitochondria. Addition of GTN treatment to vitamin E attenuated its cardioprotective effect. In summary, the findings of the present study provide evidence that a short course of vitamin E treatment protected the heart against reperfusion-injury compared to a NO donor. The MPT is an important target of this protection.

3. Effects of vitamin E treatment on age-associated changes in cardiac responses to the injury of post I/R

Aging is one of the most important risk factors for the development of cardiovascular disease. Aging is characterized by loss of myocytes, remodeling and impaired contractile function in the heart. The rate of programmed cell death in the left ventricle increases with age (Kwak et al., 2006). Meanwhile the aged heart faces a high risk of free radical injury owing to slow generation of antioxidant enzymes by its cells, and a general decline in this system may be another reason for the development of myocardial dysfunction (Asha Devi et al., 2003 a).

It is well established that nitric oxide (NO), is constitutively generated within the heart, not only by the endothelium but also by the myocytes (Balligand et al., 1995). Numerous previous animal studies have reported that there is a loss of NO biological activity and /or biosynthesis during aging (Matz et al., 2000).

Oxygen free radicals increase in concentration upon reperfusion of ischemic cardiac tissue (Xia et al., 1996). It is well established that these reactive species can interact with and damage various cellular components (Berlett & Stadtman, 1997). Free radical production in the heart has also been reported to increase with age (Sohal et al., 1990). Thus, although restoration of blood flow is the sole method for salvaging ischemic tissue, oxidative damage may occur during reoxygenation and contribute to ischemia–reperfusion injury.

Regular exercise is a key component of cardiovascular risk prevention strategies. Physical activity is known to cause generation of free radicals. Exercise training in old animals failed to enhance antioxidant activity (Hatao et al., 2006). However swim training especially at low-intensity, was found to be beneficial as a major protective adaptation against oxidative stress particularly in the older myocardium (Kiran et al., 2004). The tocopherols (major vitamers of vitamin E) are believed to play a role in the prevention of human aging-related changes, and are of particular interest, mainly because of their antioxidative properties (Asha Devi et al., 2003 b).

From the aforementioned data, it seems possible that free radical - mediated injury is a major issue in the increase of aging related reperfusion-induced myocardial dysfunction. Exercise training program could not always protect the aging heart satisfactorily. We tried to test the hypothesis that using an antioxidant as vitamin E could lead to better protection of the aging hearts as compared with exercise training.

Therefore, a study was conducted to compare the effects of vitamin E treatment versus swim- exercise training on age- associated changes in cardiac responses to the injury of post I/R.

3.1 Methods

This work was undertaken on female Wistar rats aged 16-18 months. Rats were allocated into 3 groups: a) Control group of aged rats, b) Exercise -trained aged rats subjected to daily physical exercise by swimming in the water tank, for 2 hours daily, 6 days aweek for 2 weeks, and c) Vitamin E-treated aged rats subjected to daily injection of vitamin E (300 mg/kg) intraperitoneally, 6 days aweek for 2 weeks.

The swim-training program adopted was according to Refaat et al., (1989), in a swimming tank, filled with water and maintained at thermoneutral temperature of 30°c. A motor fan in the tank stirs strong water currents. This ensures uniformity of temperature and forces the rats to swim actively all the time.

3.1.1 Experimental procedures

They were done as previously described (Ayobe &Tarazi, 1983). Peak developed tension per left ventricular weight as well as coronary flow rate per left ventricular weight were calculated relative to left ventricular weight (PT/LV, g /100mg)& (CF/LV, ml /100mg/min).

Nitrate concentration in coronary effluents, as a stable product of nitric oxide (NO), was measured by an endpoint one-step enzymatic assay using nitrate reductase, as described by Bories and Bories, (1995), and modified in tissues by Kassim, (1997).

3.1.2 Effects of exercise on cardiac weights and post Ischemia-reperfusion (I/R) responses

In this study, exercise was found to exert a trophic effect on cardiac chambers manifested by significant increase of the absolute & relative weights of atria, right ventricle, and left ventricle. Swimming is well recognized for its effectiveness in inducing myocardial hypertrophy (Evangelista et al., 2003). Exercise can protect cardiac function of the aging heart by protection against; loss of cardiac myocytes, reduction in number of myonuclei, reactive hypertrophy of remaining myocytes, and increased connective tissue in left ventricle (LV) of the aging rat heart. This protection is achieved through attenuation of age-induced elevation in Bax/Bcl-2 ratio, thereby inhibits apoptosis (Asha Devi et al., 2003a), and exerts its trophic effect.

Although exercise-trained rats had significant increase in LV and LV/BW that indicates LV hypertrophy, they showed Peak developed tension similar to control which could be attributed to the increase of free radical in aged rats induced by exercise. Oxygen free radicals are known to have deleterious effects on contractile force of heart (Gao et al., 1996).

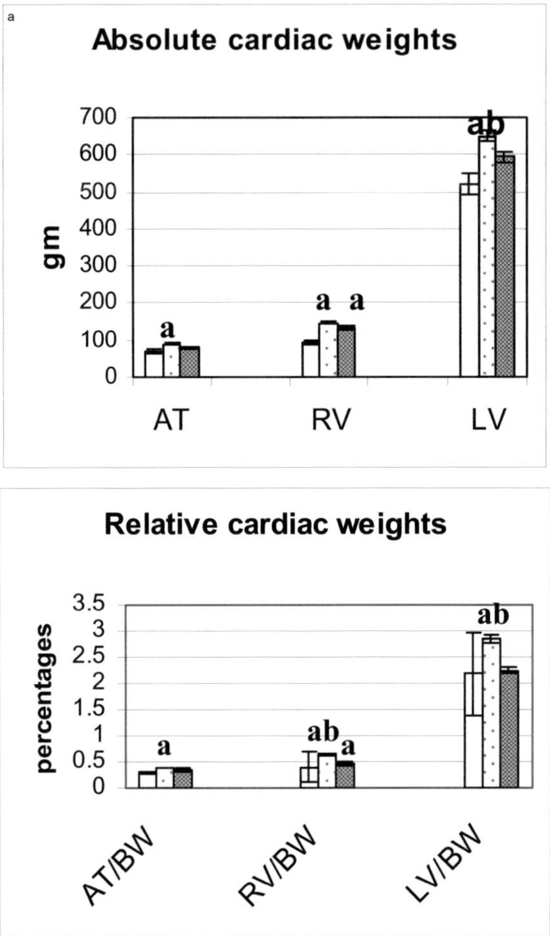

Fig. 6. Mean values± SEM of: absolute weights (mg) of atria (AT), right ventricle (RV), left ventricle (LV), and their relative weights (mg/g) (AT/BW), (RV/BW), (LV/BW) in control rats □ , exercise-trained rats □, and vit. E-treated rats ■.

a. Significance calculated by least significant difference (LSD) at $P < 0.05$ from control group.
b. Significance calculated by LSD at $P < 0.05$ between vit E-treated, and exercise-trained groups

The results of ischemia-reperfusion of isolated hearts from both control and exercise-trained aged rats have shown the lack of tolerance to ischemia-reperfusion injury as regard inotropic activities as well as myocardial flow rate. This could be explained in view of the increase in free radicals generation induced by exercise, even if small, was added to the increased free radicals generation induced by aging exceeding the antioxidant defense capacity of the heart leading to loss of beneficial cardio-protective effect of exercise on ischemia-reperfusion injury (Hatao et al., 2006).

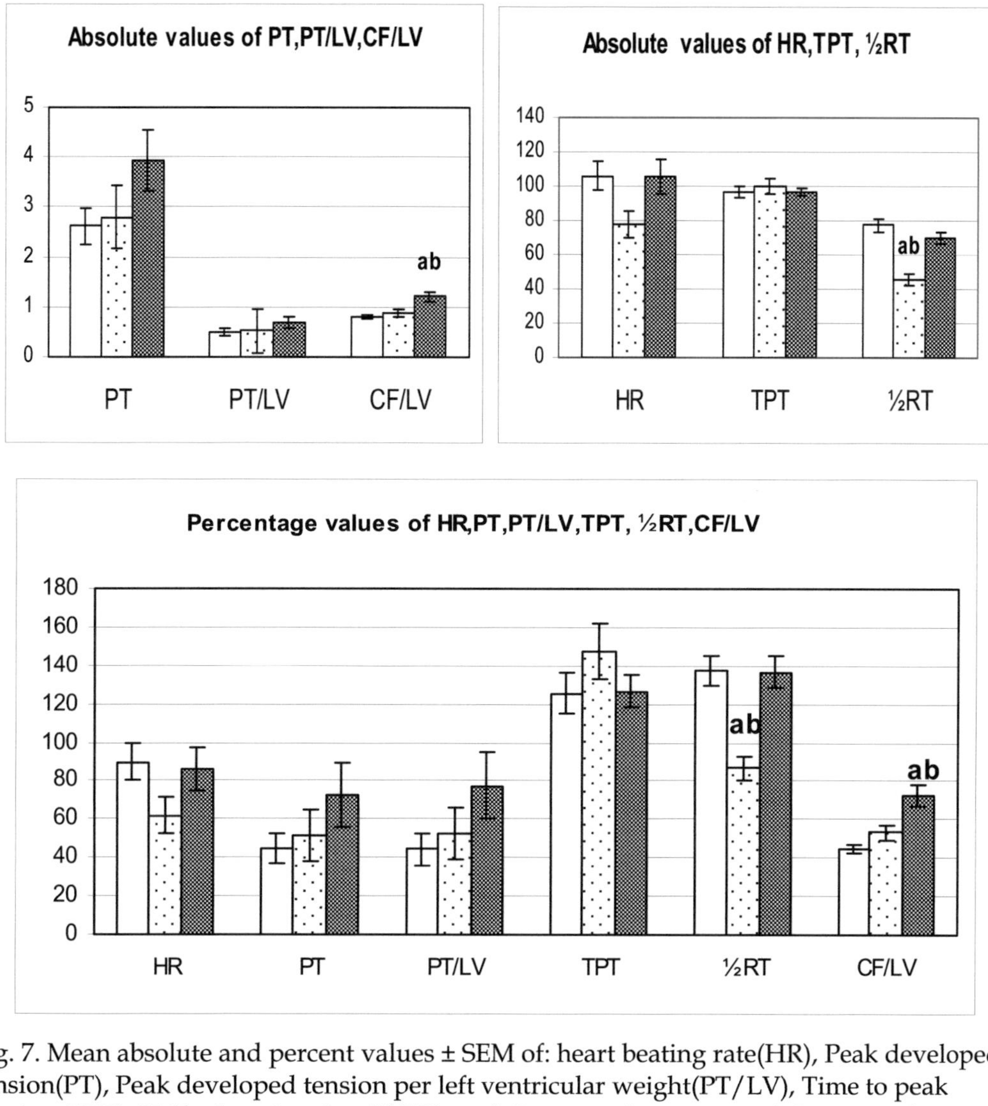

Fig. 7. Mean absolute and percent values ± SEM of: heart beating rate(HR), Peak developed tension(PT), Peak developed tension per left ventricular weight(PT/LV), Time to peak tension (TPT), Half relaxation time(½ RT), and Coronary flow rate per left ventricular weight (CF/LV), at 30 minutes reperfusion of hearts isolated from control rats ☐, exercise-trained rats ⬚, and vit. E- treated rats ▩.

a. Significance calculated by least significant difference (LSD) at $P < 0.05$ from control group.
b. Significance calculated by LSD at $P < 0.05$ between vit E-treated, and exercise-trained groups

The increased free radicals generation such as superoxide anion could react with NO to form peroxynitrate, decreasing NO biological activity. Peroxynitrate molecule by itself might play a significant role in oxidative tissue damage. This is supported in this study by the absence of increase of nitrates in the coronary effluent from exercise- trained aged rats at 30 min reperfusion.

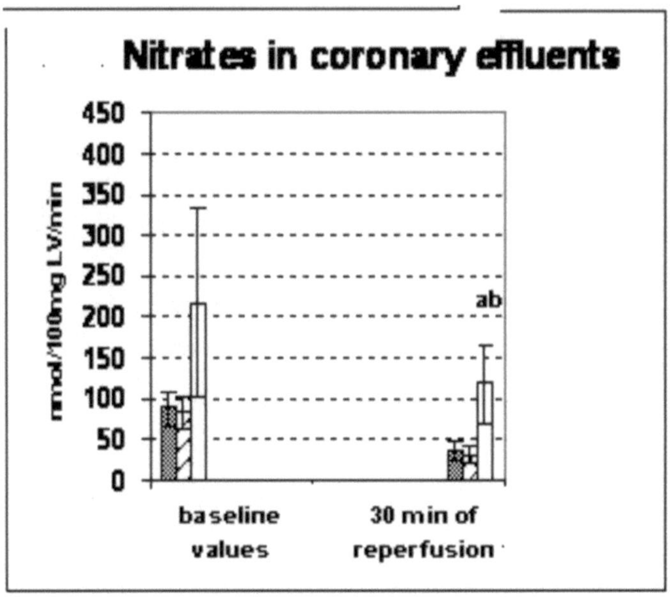

Fig. 8. Mean values ±SEM of nitrates in coronary effluents (nmol/100mg LV/min) at baseline values, and 30 minutes of reperfusion in control rats ▩, exercise-trained rats ⊠, and vit. E-treated rats □.

a. Significance calculated by least significant difference (LSD) at $P < 0.05$ from control group.
b. Significance calculated by LSD at $P < 0.05$ between vit E-treated, and exercise-trained groups

Also, the heart beating rate of the exercise-trained rats could not be preserved after 30 min of reperfusion. This could be attributed to the increased free oxygen radicals in these rats, since oxyradicals have been implicated as a possible cause of reperfusion arrhythmias (Tanguy et al., 1998). However, the rate of relaxation of hearts excised from exercise-trained rats showed better tolerance to I/R after initial intolerance, and such improvement is in accordance to a recent report by Libonati et al., (2005), who found that sprint training in rats improves post-ischemic left ventricular diastolic stiffness due to up-regulation of myocardial glycolysis, with ATP production that protects the heart from ischemia-reperfusion as it plays an important role in actin-myosin rigor bond dissociation, and regulating myocardial diastolic function.

Effects of vitamin E on cardiac weights and Post Ischemia-Reperfusion (I/R) responses:

Vitamin E has been reported to stimulate upregulation at the expression level of B cl-2 gene, B cl-2 molecule is involved in the inhibition of apoptosis (Azzi et al., 2004).

Therefore, vitamin E by preventing apoptosis of myocardial cells could be expected to induce hypertrophy of the heart (trophic effect). However in case of vitamin E-treated rats, results have shown that the effect of vitamin E on the rate of growth of right and left ventricles was not similar. While the rate of growth of right ventricle was increased by the anti-apoptosis effects of vitamin E. The increase in left ventricle & left ventricle/ body weight was insignificant. This could be attributed to the favorable effects of vitamin E on reduction of blood pressure and blood viscosity (Costa et al., 2005). These two factors have been claimed to induce growth of left ventricle during aging (Ghali et al., 1997). Thereby, by eliminating these two factors, the rate of growth of left ventricle was decreased under the influence of vitamin E supplementation counteracting its trophic effect in aged rats.

In contrast to aged control rats and exercise-trained aged rats, the isolated hearts from vitamin E-treated rats showed better tolerance as regard inotropic activity, especially force generation measured as peak developed tension as well as coronary flow rate. In accordance, Venditti et al., (1999) showed a protective action of vitamin E treatment against lipid peroxidation and cardiac dysfunction associated with ischemia- reperfusion in rats. Vitamin E decreases free radical deleterious effect on cell membrane, proteins, DNA, and decreases both ROS mediated direct ischemia-reperfusion mediated injury, as well as peroxynitrite-mediated injury and thereby preserving NO through preventing its inactivation by its transformation to peroxynitrite (Kamat, 2006). In support, this study showed significant increase of nitrates in coronary effluent from vitamin E- treated aged rats measured at 30 min of reperfusion.

In view of the aforementioned data, vitamin E proved to be a cardio-protective agent as it attenuated the injury of post ischemia-reperfusion on the aged myocardium. This beneficial effect of vitamin E could be partially attributable to preservation of NO biological activity by preventing its transformation to the toxic compound peroxynitrite.

On the other hand, the swim-training program adopted in this study, as regard tolerance to ischemia-reperfusion apart from improvement of half relaxation time, the swim-training program did not show other promising cardio-protective effects against cardiac changes associated with the aging process.

Therefore, vitamin E supplementation could be recommended to aged people especially patients suffering from ischemic heart disease. Vitamin E could be used either alone or in combination with exercise training taking into consideration the duration and intensity of exercise program.

Vitamin E and platelet function

Platelets play a critical role in the pathophysiology of reperfusion (Gawaz, 2004). Platelet function is not static during ischemia-reperfusion. Instead, during ischemia regional platelet aggregability is increased. Systemic and regional platelet aggregability also increases during myocardial reperfusion. The mechanism of these responses is unknown but may be related to regional endothelial dysfunction created by ischemia. The response observed could also be explained by the release of proaggregatory mediators in the coronary and/or systemic circulation during ischemia-reperfusion (Gurbel et al., 1995).

Reperfusion induces an important inflammatory response, characterized by a massive production of free radicals and by the activation of the complement and leucocyte neutrophils (Gourdin et al., 2009). Platelets and neutrophils act synergistically in provoking postreperfusion cardiac dysfunction (Lefer et al., 1998). Activated platelets play an important role in the process of myocardial ischemia-reperfusion injury, and platelet-derived P-selectin is a critical mediator (Xu et al., 2006), whereas platelet P-selectin promotes platelet interactions with leukocytes. Because platelets release potent proinflammatory chemokines and modulate leukocyte function, platelet accumulation in the postischemic microvasculature might significantly contribute to the manifestation of I/R injury (Massberg et al., 1998).

Reperfusion of the tissue, subsequent to ischemia, results in burst of oxygen consumption with consequent generation of oxygen derived free radicals; the oxidant-anti oxidant status of the tissue is thrown out of balance and multi dimensional free radical mediated damage ensues. Since vitamin E is a potent natural anti-oxidant, its administration is expected to restore the imbalance.

Effect of administration of 600 mg vitamin E each day, for six days, was observed on activity of some of the anti-oxidant enzymes and levels of malondialdehyde (as an index of free radical mediated damage) in the platelets of patients reperfused after myocardial infarction. It has been found that vitamin E administration significantly lowers the level of malondialdehyde in the patients. Vitamin E administration increases the activities of anti oxidant enzymes (superoxide dismutase, glutathione reductase and catalase) tested both in the patients and healthy controls. However, lowering of lipid peroxidation upon administration of vitamin E is specific for patients. These findings exhibit beneficial role of vitamin E administration in the management of the patients reperfused after myocardial infarction (Dwivedi et al., 2005).

The results of Chen et al, (2002) suggested that the reduction of myocardial I/R injury with vitamin E supplementation may be the result of the inhibition of polymorphonuclear neutrophil (PMN) CD11b expression.

Vitamin E supplementation in healthy subjects or patients with hypercholesterolemia was shown to diminish platelet function as assessed by ex vivo platelet aggregation of 11-dehydrothromboxane B_2, a marker of in vivo platelet activation (Calzada et al., 1997; Davi et al., 1997). Celestini et al., (2002) demonstrated that vitamin E can potentiate the antiplatelet activity of aspirin by inhibiting the early events of platelet activation pathway induced by collagen.

A study from our laboratory was to examine the possibility that vitamin E administration could exert an effect on blood elements and platelet aggregation.

Materials and Methods

Albino rats of both sexes weighing 180- 220 gm fed on a standard rat diet and fasted for 18-24 hours before sacrifice were used in this study.

In vivo study: A total of 30 rats were used in this study. They were divided in two groups. Group I: Saline control group; rats in this group were injected with saline instead of vitamin E, daily for 5 consecutive days. Group II: vitamin E treated group; rats were injected with vitamin E (300 mg/kg b.w.) intraperitoneally for five consecutive days. After 5 days all injections were stopped for 2 days. By the seventh day rats were anesthetized with pentobarbitone in a dose of 40 mg/kg b.w.

Collection of blood samples: blood samples were obtained by arterial puncture from the abdominal aorta. One ml samples were collected into tubes containing EDTA for examination of RBCs and platelet counts, hemoglobin content and hematocrite values.

Another blood samples were collected in chilled plastic tubes containing sodium citrate 3.8gm/100 ml (9 volumes of blood to 1 volume of sodium citrate) and gently shaken. These blood samples were used for study of platelet aggregation. The citrated blood was centrifuged at 1500 r.p.m. for 5 min. The supernatant platelet rich plasma (PRP) was pipetted into clean plastic tubes. The remaining blood sample was centrifuged at 10,000 r.p.m. for 10 min. to prepare platelet poor plasma (PPP). Standard PRP: the number of platelets in PRP was counted using coulter T-660 counter. The platelet number was adjusted to a standardized number of 3 x 10^5 platelet per µl by dilution with autologus platelet poor plasma.

Aggregation study: platelet aggregation was performed using Chrono-Log automatic aggregometer (model 540-VC, Chrono-Log Corp, Harvertown, USA) coupled with computer and printer. ADP as an aggregating agent was used at a final concentration of 10 uM. The maximum aggregation was recorded after 3 min.

In vitro of vitamin E on platelet aggregation

Collection of blood samples: blood was collected from normal rats, anaesthetized by pentobarbitone, by arterial puncture from abdominal aorta into chilled tubes containing sodium citrate 3.8 gm%. Preparation of standard PRP was carried out as described in the in vivo experiments.

The in vitro effect of vitamin E on ADP- induced platelet aggregation was studied by exposing PRP to rising concentrations of the vitamin 1,2,3,4 and 5 mg/ml. Equal volumes of saline were added to control samples.

Aggregation study: was carried as described above in vivo experiments.

Statistical analysis of the data was done using Student's "t" test for unpaired data according to Fisher and Yates (1957) $P < 0.05$ was considered significant.

Regression study: linear regression analysis was used to relate different parameters to a certain outcome (platelet aggregation) to find out the highest beta coefficient and the most important factor affecting this outcome. This analysis was performed on SPSS windows version eight.

Results

Table 1 portrays the results of in vivo effects of vitamin E on hematological parameters. RBCs count, Hb content and PCV showed slight and insignificant changes in vitamin E treated rats compared to their saline controls. The number of platelets was insignificantly decreased in vitamin E treated animals. However platelet aggregation induced by ADP showed a significant decrease ($P < 0.05$) in this group (table 2 and figure 9).

Regression analysis: as seen in fig. 10, multiple regression analysis of platelet aggregation against other parameters. Only a significant negative correlation between platelet number and platelet aggregation was seen in vitamin E treated group ($P < 0.03$).

In vitro effect of vitamin E on platelet aggregation: the platelet aggregation effect of ADP in presence of rising concentration of vitamin E showed significant inhibition ($P < 0.01$) only when vitamin E was added at a final concentration of 5 mg/ml. Addition of vitamin E in smaller concentrations of 2- 4 mg/ml final concentration produced insignificant inhibition of platelet aggregation. Almost no effect was seen when vitamin E was added at a final concentration of 1 mg/ml (table 3 and figure 11).

Parameters / Group treatment	RBCs $x 10^6$/ul	Hb gm/dl	PCV %	Platelet count $x 10^3$/ul	Platelet aggregation %
Saline control (15)	6.54±0.3	12.24±0.5	36.15±1.2	1146±71.12	68.1±1.9
Vitamin E treated rats (15)	6.33±0.2	11.93±0.3	35.3±0.9	1068±53.1	58.9±4
P	NS	NS	NS	NS	< 0.05

Data are mean± SEM In parenthesis is the number of observations NS: non significant

Table 2. Red blood cell count (RBCs), hemoglobin level (Hb), packed cell volume (PCV), platelet count and platelet aggregation in saline control and vitamin E treated rats.

Additions to normal PRP					
	Final concentration of vitamin E				
Saline control (12)	1mg/ml (8)	2mg/ml (9)	3mg/ml (11)	4mg/ml (11)	5mg/ml (13)
50.08±2.6	50.75±2	47.1±2.32	44.36±2.85	44.7±3.4	37.23±3
P	NS	NS	NS	NS	< 0.01

Data are mean± SEM In parenthesis is the number of observations NS: non significant

Table 3. In vitro effect of vitamin E on platelet aggregation of normal rat PRP in presence of different concentrations of vitamin E compared to saline control

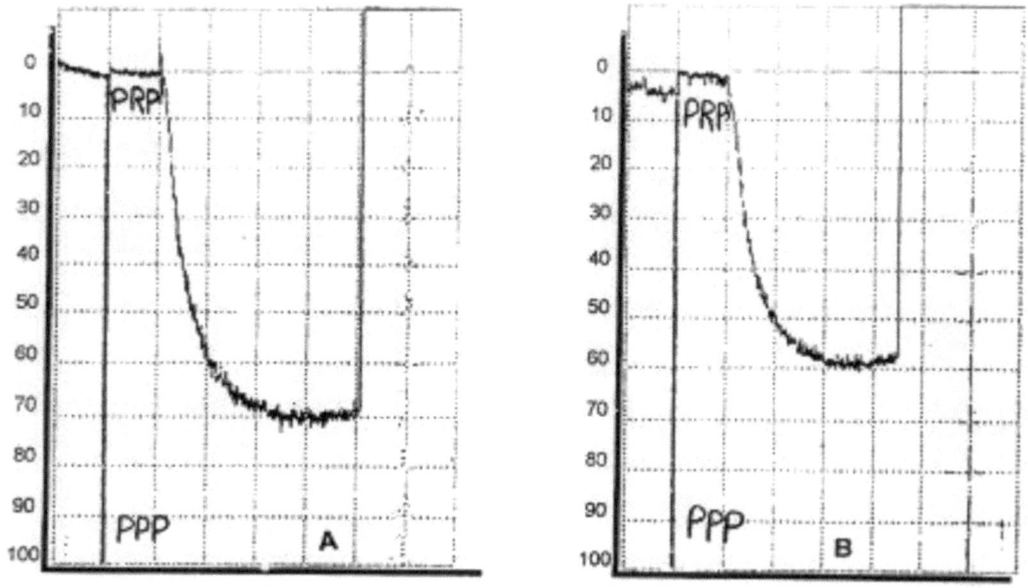

ADP-induced platelet aggregation%

Fig. 9. Tracing of ADP- induced platelet aggregation of Vitamin E-treated rats (B) compared to saline treated rats (A).

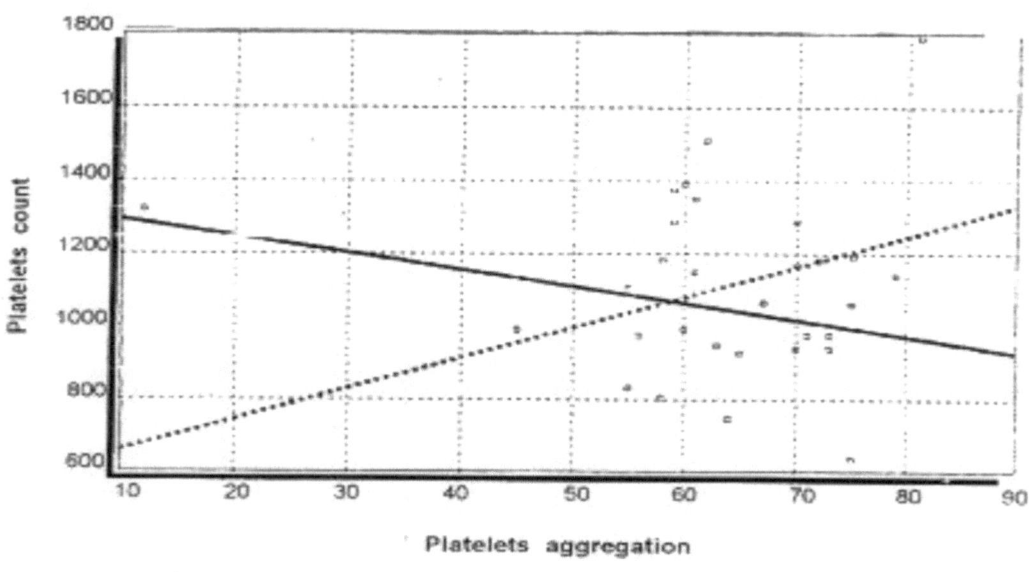

Vitamin E- treated rats ————

Saline- treated rats ....

Fig. 10. Correlation between platelet aggregation and platelet count among vitamin E-treated rats and saline treated rats (by multiple regression analysis)

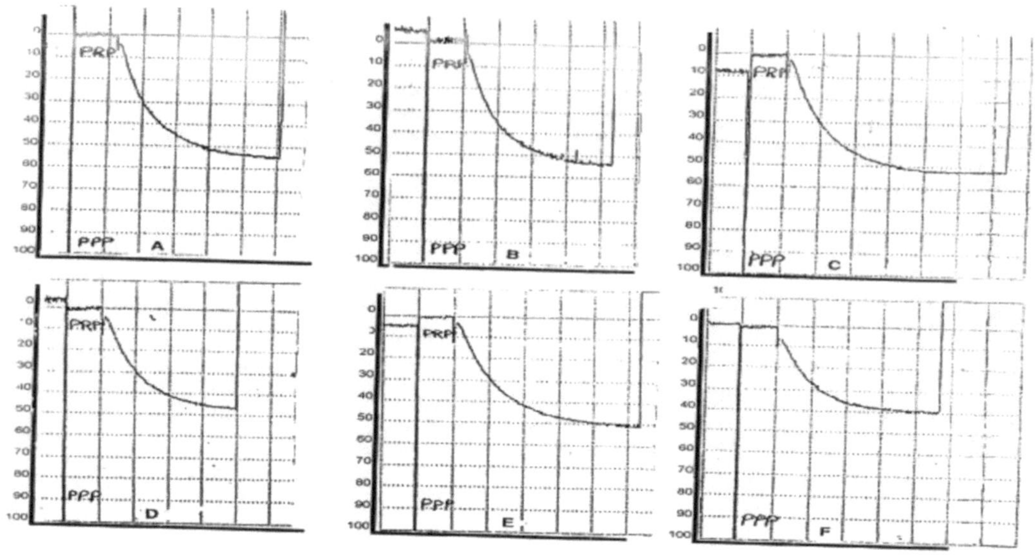

Fig. 11. Tracing of ADP- induced platelet aggregation of normal rats PRP in presence of vitamin E in concentrations of 1, 2, 3, 4 and 5 mg/ml respectively (B- F) compared to saline control (A)

The data reported here demonstrated that administration of megadose of vitamin E (300 mg/kg for one week) to rats, produced slight and nonsignificant changes in red blood cell counts, hemoglobin content, packed cell volume. Platelet counts showed an insignificant decrease. However, the platelet aggregation responses to ADP of PRP from treated rats were significantly inhibited. This finding shows the safety of vitamin E in this supra-physiological dose of 300 mg/kg on blood parameters tested.

On addition of vitamin E to normal PRP in vitro, the platelet aggregating effect of ADP showed significant inhibition only when vitamin E was added at a final concentration of 5 mg/ml. Addition of vitamin E in smaller concentrations of 2- 4 mg/ml produced insignificant inhibition of platelet aggregation. Almost no effect was seen when vitamin E was added at a final concentration of 1 mg/ml.

From these data, it can be concluded that this supra physiological dose of vitamin E is safe concerning the blood parameters tested.

The observation in the present study that vitamin E when added in vitro to normal rat PRP caused significant inhibition of platelet aggregation in response to ADP; illustrate that vitamin E by itself exerts a direct antiplatelet effect. Higashi & Kikuchi (1974) were the first to demonstrate that vitamin E inhibits the aggregation of platelets using hydrogen peroxide as the aggregating stimulus. Subsequent studies by Steiner & Anastasi, (1976) demonstrated that vitamin E also inhibited platelet aggregation response to epinephrine, collagen and ATP. Moreover, Freedman and Keaney, (2001) found that platelet incorporation of vitamin E both in vitro and in vivo leads to dose-dependent inhibition of platelet aggregation in response to agonists such as arachidonic acid and phorbol ester.

Although it is best known for its antioxidant activity the exact mechanism of the antiplatelet effect of vitamin E is not exactly known and one of the following mechanisms may operate. First, it can be attributed to altered metabolism of prostaglandins. The vascular generation of prostacyclin (PGI_2) is higher and the platelet thromboxane A_2 generation is lower than normal. This view is supported by the findings of Steiner and Anastasi (1976) and others (Karpen et al., 1981; Pritchard et al., 1982; Pignatelli et al., 1999) that vitamin E inhibits platelet thromboxane A_2 synthesis. On the other hand, PGI_2 synthesis is stimulated possibly by reduction of cellular peroxide level (Gilbert et al., 1983). Second, the inhibition of platelet aggregation can be explained by the ability of vitamin E to inhibit intracellular mobilization of sequestrated calcium from the dense tubular system of the cytoplasm (Srivastava, 1986). Third, by its membrane stabilizing action, vitamin E would impair platelet release reaction. This view is supported observations of Feki et al., (2001) that vitamin E by its antioxidant effect, protects molecules and tissue against the deleterious effect of free radicals and also contributes to the stabilization of biological membranes. Fourth, unrelated to its antioxidant action, vitamin E was shown to inhibit protein kinase C (PKC) in various cell types with consequent inhibition of platelet aggregation (Azzi et al., 2002; Freedman et al., 1996; Freedman and Keaney, 2001). Further, vitamin E includes inhibitory effects are the result of specific interactions with component of the cell e.g. proteins, enzymes and membranes (Ricciarelli et al., 2002).

Vitamin E attenuated P-selectin expression on activated human platelets and thus inhibited the P-selectin–dependent function, platelet–mononuclear cell (MNC) interaction. The mechanism probably was related to the inhibition of PKC activity in platelets. Since P-selectin is an important atherothrombogenic adhesion molecule, this finding will provide us new insights into the mechanism by which dietary vitamin E inhibits thrombosis and atherogenesis and thereby reduces the risk of coronary artery diseases (Murohara et al, 2004).

Although these studies from our laboratory have shown that vitamin E administered in megadose, could provide a protective effect against the cardiac responses to the injury of post I/R. Further studies should be conducted to test the possibility of using vitamin E in cardiac surgery.

4. References

Altavilla, D., Deodato, B., Campo, GM., Arlotta, M., Miano, M., Squadrito, G., Saitta, A., Cucinotta, D., Ceccarelli, S., Ferlito, M., Tringali, M., Minutoli, L., Caputi, AP. & Squadrito F. (2000). IRFI 042, a novel dual vitamin E-like antioxidant, inhibits activation of nuclear factor-kappaB and reduces the inflammatory response in myocardial ischemiareperfusion injury, *Cardiovasc Res* 47: 515-528.

Asha Devi, S., Prathima, S.& Subramanyam, MV. (2003 a). Dietary vitamin E and physical exercise: II, Antioxidant status and lipofuscin-like substances in aging rat heart, *Exp Gerontol*. 38: 291-297.

Asha Devi, S., Prathima, S.& Subramanyam, MV. (2003 b). Dietary vitamin E and physical exercise: I. Altered endurance capacity and plasma lipid profile in ageing rats, *Exp Gerontol*. 38: 285-290.

Ayobe, MH. & Tarazi, RC. (1983). beta-Receptors and contractile reserve in left ventricular hypertrophy, *Hypertension* 5: I192- I197.

Azzi, A., Gysin, R., Kempná, P., Munteanu, A., Negis, Y., Villacorta, L., Visarius, T.& Zingg, JM. (2004). Vitamin E mediates cell signaling and regulation of gene expression, *Ann N Y Acad Sci.* 1031:86-95.

Azzi, A., Ricciarelli, R. & Zingg, JM. (2002). Non-oxidant molecular functions of alpha-tocopherol (vitamin E), *FFBS Lett.* 22: 519.

Balligand, JL., Kobzik, L., Han, X., Kaye, DM., Belhassen, L., O'Hara, DS., Kelly, RA., Smith, TW.& Michel, T. (1995). Nitric oxide-dependent parasympathetic signaling is due to activation of constitutive endothelial (type III) nitric oxide synthase in cardiac myocytes, *J Biol Chem.* 270(24):14582-14586.

Bell, RM., Maddock, HL.& Yellon, DM. (2003). The cardioprotective and mitochondrial depolarising properties of exogenous nitric oxide in mouse heart, *Cardiovasc Res* 57: 405-415.

Berlett, B S. & Stadtman E R. (1997). Protein oxidation in aging, disease, and oxidative stress, *J Biol Chem.*;272:20313–20316.

Bories, PN. & Bories C.(1995). Nitrate determination in biological fluids by an enzymatic one-step assay with nitrate reductase, *Clin. Chem.* 41: 904-907.

Calzada, C., Bruckdorfer, KR. & Rice-Evans, C.A. (1997). The influence of antioxidant nutrients on platelet function in healthy volunteers, Atherosclerosis. 128: 97.

Celestini, A., Pulcinelli, FM., Pignatelli, P., Frati, G., Gazzaniga, PP. & Viol,i F. (2002). Vitamin E potentiates the antiplatelet activity of aspirin in collagen-stimulated platelets, *Haematologica.* 87(4):420.

Chen, Y. , Davis-Gorman, G. , Watson, RR. & McDonagh, PF. (2002). Vitamin E attenuates myocardial ischemia-reperfusion injury in murine AIDS, *Cardiovasc Toxicol.* 2 (2): 119- 27.

Costa, AD., Jakob, R., Costa, CL., Andrukhiv, K., West, IC.& Garlid, KD. (2006). The mechanism by which the mitochondrial ATP-sensitive K+ channel opening and H2O2 inhibit the mitochondrial permeability transition, *J Biol Chem* 281: 20801-20808.

Costa, VA., Vianna, LM., Aguila, MB.& Mandarim-de-Lacerda, CA. (2005). Alpha-tocopherol supplementation favorable effects on blood pressure, blood viscosity and cardiac remodeling of spontaneously hypertensive rats, *J Nutr Biochem* . 16: 251-256.

Davi, G., Alessandrini, P., Minotti, MG, Bucciarelli, T., Costantini, F., Cipollone F., Bittolo Bon, G., Ciabbattoni, G. & Patrono, C. (1997). In vivo formation of 8-epiprostaglandin F2a is increased in hypercholesterolemia, Arterioscler Thromb Vasc Biol. 17: 3230.

Davidson, SM. & Duchen, MR. (2006). Effects of NO on mitochondrial function in cardiomyocytes: Pathophysiological relevance, *Cardiovasc Res* 71: 10-21.

Dhalla, NS., Elmoselhi, AB., Hata, T.& Makino, N. (2000). Status of myocardial antioxidants in ischemia-reperfusion injury, *Cardiovasc Res* 47: 446-456.

Di Lisa, F., Menabò, R., Canton, M., Barile, M.& Bernardi, P. (2001). Opening of the mitochondrial permeability transition pore causes depletion of mitochondrial and cytosolic NAD+ and is a causative event in the death of myocytes in postischemic reperfusion of the heart, *J Biol Chem* 276: 2571-2575.

Dong, YH., Guo, YH. & Gu, XB. (2009). Anticancer mechanisms of vitamin E succinate, *Chin J Cancer* 28: 1114-1118.

Draper, HH.& Hadley, M. (1990). Malondialdehyde determination as index of lipid peroxidation, *Methods Enzymol* 186: 421-431.

Dwivedi, Vk. , Chandra, KM. , Misra, PC. & Misra, MK. (2005). Effect of vitamin E on platelet enzymatic anti-oxidants in the patients of myocardial infarction, *Indian Journal of Clinical Biochemistry*. 20 (1): 21- 25.

Evangelista, FS., Brum, PC.& Krieger JE. (2003). Duration-controlled swimming exercise training induces cardiac hypertrophy in mice, *Braz J Med Biol Res*.36:1751-1759.

Farshid, AA., Sadeghi-Hashjin, G.& Ferdowsi, HR. (2002). Histopathological studies on the effects of peroxynitrite on the lungs and trachea of rabbits, *Eur Respir J* 20: 1014-1016.

Feki, M., Souissi, M. & Mebazaa, A. (2001). Vitamin E: structure, metabolism, and functions, *Ann Med Interne (Paris)*. 152: 384.

Fisher, RA. & Yates, F. (1957). Statistical tables for biological structure and medical research, 5th edition:3.

Freedman, JE. & Keaney, JF. (2001). Vitamin E Inhibition of Platelet Aggregation Is Independent of Antioxidant Activity, *J Nutrition*. 131:374S-377S.

Freedman, JE., Loscalzo, J., Benoit, SE., Valeri, CR., Barnard, MR., and Michelson, AD. (1996). Decreased platelet inhibition by nitric oxide in two brothers with a history of arterial thrombosis, J. Clin. Invest. 97: 979–987.

Gao, WD., Liu, Y.& Marban, E. (1996). Selective effects of oxygen free radicals on excitation-contraction coupling in ventricular muscle. Implications for the mechanism of stunned myocardium, *Circulation* 15;94(10):2597-2604.

Gawaz, M. (2004). Role of platelets in coronary thrombosis and reperfusion of ischemic myocardium, Cardiovascular Research. 61: 498–511.

Ghali, JK. , Liao, Y.& Cooper, RS. (1997). Left Ventricular Hypertrophy in the Elderly, *Am J Geriatr Cardiol*. 6: 38-49.

Gilbert, VA., Zebrowski, EJ. & Chen, AC. (1983).Differential effects of megavitamin E on prostacyclin and thromboxane synthesis in streptozotocin-induced diabetic rats, *Horm Metab Res*. 15: 320.

Gourdin, MG.; Bree, B. & De Kock, M. (2009). The impact of ischaemia-reperfusion on the blood vessel, *Eu J Anaesthesiol*. 26(7):537- 47.

Gurbel, PA. , Serebruany, VL. , Komjathy, S F. , Collins, M E. , Sane, DC. ,Scott , H J., Schlossberg M L. & Herzog WR. (1995). Regional and systemic platelet function is altered by myocardial ischemia-reperfusion, *J Thromb Thrombolysis*. 1: 187-194.

Halestrap, AP., Clarke, SJ.& Javadov, SA. (2004). Mitochondrial permeability transition pore opening during myocardial reperfusion--a target for cardioprotection, *Cardiovasc Res* 61: 372-385.

Hanson, MG., Ozenci, V., Carlsten, MC., Glimelius, BL., Frödin, JE., Masucci, G., Malmberg, KJ.& Kiessling, RV.(2007).A short-term dietary supplementation with high doses of vitamin E increases NK cell cytolytic activity in advanced colorectal cancer patients, *Cancer Immunol Immunother* 56: 973-984.

Hatao, H., Oh-ishi, S., Itoh, M., Leeuwenburgh, C., Ohno, H., Ookawara, T., Kishi, K., Yagyu, H., Nakamura, H.& Matsuoka, T. (2006). Effects of acute exercise on lung antioxidant enzymes in young and old rats, *Mech Ageing Dev.* 127(4):384-390.

Higashi, O. & Kikuchi, Y. (1974). Effects of vitamin E on the aggregation and the lipid peroxidation of platelets exposed to hydrogen peroxide, *Tohoku J Exp Med.* 112: 271.

Hunter EE, editor. (1984) Practical electron microscopy. A beginner's illustrated guide. New York (NY): Praeger Publishers Inc.

Kamat, JP. (2006). Peroxynitrite: a potent oxidizing and nitrating agent, *Indian J Exp Biol.* 44: 436-447.

Karpen, CW., Merola, AJ., Trewyn, RW., Cornwell, DG. & Panganamala, RV. (1981). Modulation of platelet thromboxane A_2 and arterial prostacyclin by dietary vitamin E, *Prostaglandins.* 22: 651.

Kassim, SK.(1997). Determination of Cytosolic Nitrite and Nitrate as Indicators of Nitric Oxide Level in Ovarian Cancer Cells, *CMB*. 4: 1051-1059.

Kim, JS., Jin, Y. &, Lemasters, JJ. (2006). Reactive oxygen species, but not Ca2+ overloading, trigger pH- and mitochondrial permeability transition-dependent death of adult rat myocytes after ischemia-reperfusion, *Am J Physiol Heart Circ Physiol*;290: H2024-H2034.

Kiran, T., Subramanyam, MV. & Asha Devi S. (2004). Swim exercise training and adaptations in the antioxidant defense system of myocardium of old rats: relationship to swim intensity and duration, *Comp Biochem Physiol B Biochem Mol Biol.* 137: 187-196.

Krasavage, WJ. & Terhaar CJ.(1977). d-alpha-Tocopheryl poly(ethylene glycol) 1000 succinate, Acute toxicity, subchronic feeding, reproduction, and teratologic studies in the rat, *J Agric Food Chem* 25: 273-278.

Kwak, HB., Song, W.& Lawler JM. (2006). Exercise training attenuates age-induced elevation in Bax/Bcl-2 ratio, apoptosis, and remodeling in the rat heart, *FASEB J.* 20: 791-793.

Lefer, AM., Campbell, B., Scalia, R. & Lefer, DJ. (1998): Synergism between platelets and neutrophils in provoking cardiac dysfunction after ischemia and reperfusion: role of selectins, *Circulation.* 98: 1322– 8.

Libonati, J., Kendrick, Z.& Houser, R. (2005). Sprint training improves postischemic, left ventricular diastolic performance, *J Appl Physiol.* 99: 2121-2127.

Massberg, S.; Enders, G.; Leiderer, R.; Eisenmenger, S.; Vestweber, D.; Krombach, F. & Messmer, K. (1998). Platelet-Endothelial Cell Interactions During Ischemia/Reperfusion:The Role of P-Selectin, *Blood.* 92:507-515. Matz, RL., de Sotomayor, MA., Schott, C., Stoclet, JC.& Andriantsitohaina, R. (2000). Vascular bed heterogeneity in age-related endothelial dysfunction with respect to NO and eicosanoids, *Br J Pharmacol.* 131: 303-311.

Murohara, T., Ikeda, H., Otsuka, Y., Aoki, M., Haramaki, N., Katoh, A., Takajo ,Y. & Imaizumi, T. (2004). Inhibition of Platelet Adherence to Mononuclear Cells by α-

Tocopherol : Role of P-Selectin, *Circulation*.110:141-148. Murphy, E. & Steenbergen, C. (2008). Mechanisms Underlying Acute Protection From Cardiac Ischemia-Reperfusion Injury, *Physiol Rev* 88 (2): 581-609.

Navarro, A., Gómez, C., Sánchez-Pino, MJ., González, H., Bández, MJ., Boveris, AD.& Boveris, A. (2005).Vitamin E at high doses improves survival, neurological performance, and brain mitochondrial function in aging male mice, *Am J Physiol Regul Integr Comp Physiol* 289: R1392- R1399.

Pignatelli, P., Pulcinelli, FM., Lenti, L., Gazzaniga, PP. & Violi, F. (1999). Vitamin E inhibits collagen-induced platelet activation by plunting hydrogen peroxide, *Arterioscler Thromb Vasc Biol*. 19: 2542.

Pritchard, KA., Karpen, CW., Merola, AJ. & Panganamala, RV. (1982). Influence of dietary vitamin E on platelet thromboxane A_2 and vascular prostacyclin I_2 in rabbit, *Prostaglandins Leukot Med*. 9:373.

Qin, F., Yan, C., Patel, R., Liu, W., Dong, E. (2006).Vitamins C and E attenuate apoptosis, beta-adrenergic receptor desensitization, and sarcoplasmic reticular Ca2+ ATPase downregulation after myocardial infarction, *Free Radic Biol Med* 40: 1827-1842.

Refaat, MRA., El-Nasr, AS., Farrag, HF.& Ayobe, MH. (1989). Plasma libid changes following short term exercise program in rats, *Ain Shams Medical Journal*. 40:515-520.

Ricciarelli, R., Zingg, JM.& Azzi, A. (2002). The 80th anniversary of vitamin E: beyond its antioxidant properties, *Biol Chem* 383: 457-465.

Sheu, SS., Nauduri, D.& Anders, MW. (2006). Targeting antioxidants to mitochondria: a new therapeutic direction, *Biochim Biophys Acta* 1762: 256-265.

Sohal, R J., Arnold, L A.& Sohal, B H. (1990). Age-related changes in antioxidant enzymes and prooxidant generation in tissues of the rat with special reference to parameters in two insect species, *Free Radical Biol Med*. 10:495–500.

Srivastava, KC. (1986). Vitamin E exerts antiaggregatory effects without inhibiting the enzymes of the arachidonic acid cascade in platelets, *Prostaglandins Leukot Med*.21: 177.

Steiner, M. & Anastasi, J. (1976). Vitamin E. An inhibitor of the platelet release reaction, *J Clin Invest*. 57: 732. Tanguy, S., Boucher, F., Besse, S., Ducros, V., Favier, A.& de Leiris, J. (1998).Trace elements and cardioprotection: increasing endogenous glutathione peroxidase activity by oral selenium supplementation in rats limits reperfusion-induced arrhythmias, *J Trace Elem Med Biol*. 12(1):28-38.

Venditti, P., Masullo, P., Di Meo, S.& Agnisola C. (1999). Protection against ischemia-reperfusion induced oxidative stress by vitamin E treatment, *Arch Physiol Biochem*. 107: 27-34.

Wang, G., Liem, DA., Vondriska, TM., Honda, HM., Korge, P., Pantaleon, DM., Qiao, X., Wang, Y., Weiss, JN. &, Ping P. (2005). Nitric oxide donors protect murine myocardium against infarction via modulation of mitochondrial permeability transition, *Am J Physiol Heart Circ Physiol* 288: H1290-H1295.

Xia, Y., Khatchikian, G.& Zweier, J L. (1996). Adenosine Deaminase Inhibition Prevents Free Radical-mediated Injury in the Postischemic Heart, *J Biol Chem*. 271:10096–10102.

Xu, Y. , Huo, Y. ,Toufektsian , MC. , Ramos, SI. , Ma, Y. , Tejani, AD., French, BA. & Yang, Z. (2006). Activated platelets contribute importantly to myocardial reperfusion injury, *Am J Physiol Heart Circ Physiol.* 290: H692- 9.

Yamazaki, K., Miwa, S., Ueda, K., Tanaka, S., Toyokuni, S., Unimonh, O., et al. 2004 Prevention of myocardial reperfusion injury by poly(ADP-ribose) synthetase inhibitor, 3-aminobenzamide, in cardioplegic solution: in vitro study of isolated rat heart model, *Eur J Cardiothorac Surg* 26: 270-275.

Zhou, ZH., Peng, J., Ye, F., Li, NS., Deng, HW.& Li, YJ. (2002). Delayed cardioprotection induced by nitroglycerin is mediated by alphacalcitonin gene-related peptide, *Naunyn Schmiedebergs Arch Pharmacol* 365: 253-259.

Part 4

Novel Treatment Strategies

10

Connexin 43 Hemichannels and Pharmacotherapy of Myocardial Ischemia Injury

Ghayda Hawat and Ghayath Baroudi
Université de Montréal
Canada

1. Introduction

Connexin (Cx) is the basic unit in the composition of gap junction channels but also exist in non-junctional unapposed hemichannels (Hc). The gap junction channels are formed by apposition of two hexameric CxHc from adjacent cells and play an essential role in cardiac function by allowing conduction of electrical impulse and exchange of biologically important molecules between myocytes. While most CxHc are engaged in gap junction formation, some unapposed Hc are present in association with various organelles (mitochondria, ER, etc.) but also in sarcolemma where they connect the intracellular and extracellular spaces. Recent evidence indicates that unapposed Hc in the plasma membrane perform functions different from those achieved by gap junction channels, mainly by providing pathways between the cytosol and the extracellular space allowing movement of ions and other small metabolites (Bennett et al., 2003; Goodenough & Paul, 2003), release of ATP and NAD^+ (Bruzzone et al., 2001; Cotrina et al., 1998), regulation of cell volume (Quist et al., 2000), and the activation of survival pathways (Plotkin et al., 2002). These Hc are therefore believed to play a prominent role in cellular ion homoeostasis and signalling.

In normal myocardium, most of the Cx43 are phosphorylated (van Veen et al., 2001). However, under ischemic stress, the amount of non-phosphorylated Cx43 increases (Beardslee et al., 2000). Phosphorylation causes the unapposed Cx43Hc to close whereas, conversely, Cx43 dephosphorylation increases Hc conductance and permeability (Bao et al., 2007; Contreras et al., 2002; John et al., 1999b; Kondo et al., 2000; Li et al., 2001), an effect that can result in abnormal elevation of intracellular sodium and calcium loads (Li et al., 2001), release of ATP (Braet et al., 2003a; Braet et al., 2003b; Contreras et al., 2002), osmotic imbalance (John et al., 1999b; Li et al., 2001; Quist et al., 2000), swelling of myocytes (Jennings et al., 1986; Steenbergen et al., 1985; Tranum-Jensen et al., 1981) and lead to irreversible tissue injury (Shintani-Ishida et al., 2007) and cell death. Several kinases are involved in Cx43 phosphorylation (Cottrell et al., 2003; Duncan & Fletcher, 2002; Shi et al., 2001; TenBroek et al., 2001; Warn-Cramer et al., 1998), including protein kinase C (PKC) (Lampe et al., 2000). In humans and many other mammalian species, PKC is the protein kinase for which Cx43 contains the largest number of phosphorylation sites. For instance, rat Cx43 contains 14 putative sites for PKC whereas only 3 have been reported for PKA, 4 for PKG, and 3 for MAPK (van Veen et al., 2001). A major physiological importance of the PKC resides in the existence of multiple PKC isoforms that can selectively affect particular targets in different conditions. The apparent preferential activation in response to different conditions and stimuli suggests that various PKC isoforms have specific cellular and cardiovascular functions. For instance, data from several laboratories (Chen et al., 2001a; Dorn et al., 1999; Gray et al., 1997; Inagaki et al., 2003; Inagaki et al., 2005; Liu et al., 1999; Tanaka et al., 2004; Tanaka et al., 2005) shows that selective activation of εPKC isoform provides protection against ischemia damage, whereas activation of δPKC aggravates the injury. Indeed, PKC-selective modulator drugs are currently under development for the treatment of a variety of diseases involving PKC isoforms (Bar-Am et al., 2007; Casellini et al., 2007; Serova et al., 2006).

Until recently, unapposed CxHc were thought to remain closed and that their opening would induce metabolic stress and cell death. In fact, in the first study of Hc opening, which was conducted in Xenopus oocytes expressing Cx46, non-selective inward current, swelling, and cell death were observed (Paul et al., 1991). Subsequently, the opening of CxHc and consequent cell death following an ischemic insult were reported in different cell models including myocytes (Kondo et al., 2000; Li et al., 2001; Shintani-Ishida et al., 2007), astrocytes (Contreras et al., 2002; John et al., 1999a; John et al., 1999b), and renal tubule cells (Vergara et al., 2003). The involvement of Cx43Hc was also reported in cell lines, such HEK293 (John et al., 1999b) and HeLa (Contreras et al., 2002) cells, transfected with Cx43 that became more susceptible to death by simulated ischemia than non-transfected cells, a difference ascribable to Cx43Hc opening. Therefore, the delineation of PKC targets in the heart and the characterization of the functional role of the various PKC isoforms in the modulation of these targets will offer a mechanistic insight into the pathogenesis of ischemia/reperfusion injury and aid in the development of novel pharmacological interventions for cardioprotection.

The assessment of the functional role of PKC isoforms in the modulation of Cx43Hc and the role of Cx43Hc in cardiac protection against ischemia/reperfusion injury have largely been limited by the fact that selective modulators for PKC isoforms and selective inhibitors for Cx43Hc have not been available until recently. Therefore, two major objectives of the present study aimed respectively: 1) to determine the functional role of PKC isoforms - especially those involved in heart protection - in the regulation of Cx43Hc; and, 2) to reveal the importance of the inhibition of Cx43Hc in protection against ischemia/reperfusion injury. To this end, two unique sets of synthetic peptides were utilized in the course of the research: 1) a matrix of PKC isoform-selective activator and inhibitor peptides. In combination with the patch clamp technique, the peptides were individually delivered into the cytosol of the ion channels-deficient tsA201 cells exogenously expressing Cx43 to activate/inhibit each of the PKC isoforms and assess their specific roles in the modulation of Cx43Hc. 2) a pair of structural Cx43-mimetic peptides, Gap26 and Gap27. These peptides are presumed to have the ability to block Cx43Hc by binding to their extracellular loops and to have little or no immediate effects on gap junction channels (Evans et al., 2006; Leybaert et al., 2003; Martin et al., 2005; Pearson et al., 2005). The consequent effects of Cx43Hc inhibition following the administration of structural Cx43-mimetic peptides and their therapeutic potentials were assessed in isolated cardiomyocytes and in intact rat hearts under ischemic settings.

The use of Cx43-mimetic peptides to study unapposed CxHc encloses several benefits compared to other currently used techniques and represents an attractive pharmacological tool for *in vivo* studies. The specificity that Cx43-mimetic peptides have vis-à-vis Cx43Hc, and to a lesser extent gap junction channels, denotes a therapeutic advantage over PKC peptides and other compounds (e.g. heptanol) that are also involved in cardioprotection but concurrently affect a variety of other intracellular substrates. Furthermore, the accessibility to the binding sites on the extracellular loops of Cx43Hc eliminates the need to conjugate Cx peptides with cell penetrating carriers which may exert toxic effect on cells and delay the delivery process (Zorko & Langel, 2005). Finally, the use of transgenic or knockout animal models has been widely utilized to study the roles of multiple cell proteins and ion channels; however, using such techniques to identify the role of specific Cx during ischemia/reperfusion is challenged by the fact that sustained loss of Cx43 severely affects gap junctional communication and alters cardiac development. Therefore, we believe that if our hypothesis is confirmed, these peptides will represent a promising pharmacological tool with which to counteract cell death in the cardiac ischemia/reperfusion pathology.

2. Knowledge to date

2.1 Structure and expression of connexins in the heart

There is at least twenty-one known types of Cx identified in human (Goodenough & Paul, 2003; Saez et al., 2003; Willecke et al., 2002) usually named according to their molecular weight (Beyer et al., 1987). Each Cx is composed of four transmembrane segments, two extracellular and one intracellular loop as well as one amino-terminal and one carboxy-terminal regions located in the cytosol (Fig. 1). Connexins differ in the length of their cytosolic carboxy terminus, which is characterized by the presence of several phosphorylation sites. A connexin-formed Hc consists of an oligomeric assembly of six connexins that delineate an aqueous pore. Several connexins are expressed in cardiac myocytes in different amounts and combinations depending on regions of the heart (Zipes & Jalife , 2004). The ventricular muscle fibres express abundant amounts of Cx43 but only trace levels of Cx45 and no detectable Cx40. Most studies of connexins in the heart have focused on their role in gap junctions, but a few studies have also characterized Cx43Hc properties in isolated cardiac myocytes (John et al., 1999b; Kondo et al., 2000).

2.2 Unapposed Cx43Hc opening in ischemia/reperfusion injury

The conductance and permeability of Hc, as well as gap junction channels, are regulated by intracellular protons changes (Ek-Vitorin et al., 1996; Morley et al., 1997; Spray & Burt, 1990) and calcium concentrations (Spray et al., 1985; Spray & Burt, 1990) but also via phosphorylation of specific serine, threonine and tyrosine residues by several kinases (Lampe & Lau, 2000) especially PKC (Bowling et al., 2001; Doble et al., 2000; Lampe et al., 2000). As indicated above, the conductance and permeability of the unapposed Cx43Hc are increased once Cx43 becomes dephosphorylated (Burt & Spray, 1988; Lau et al., 1991; Saez et al., 1986), while being reduced with increased Cx43 phosphorylation (Kwak & Jongsma, 1996). The dephosphorylation of Cx43 has been proposed as a key mechanism to open Hc during metabolic inhibition in cortical astrocytes in culture (Fig. 2) (Contreras et al., 2002). While Cx43 is phosphorylated under physiological conditions (Schulz et al., 2003; van Veen et al., 2001) and remains so in the first few minutes of ischemia (Schulz et al., 2003), subsequent dephosphorylation of Cx43 occurs with increasing duration of myocardial ischemia (Beardslee et al., 2000; Jain et al., 2003; Jeyaraman et al., 2003; Miura et al., 2004; Schulz et al., 2003) a process that has been associated with the opening of unapposed Cx43Hc (John et al., 1999b; Li et al., 2001) which results in metabolic stress and cell death. Based on single Hc conductance measurements, it was suggested that opening of only 50 Hc is sufficient to drown the cell with Na^+ (John et al., 1999b). As a result, Na^+ overload induces the activation of reverse Na^+-Ca^{++} exchange and hence promotes intracellular Ca^{++} accumulation (Barry & Bridge, 1993; Silverman & Stern, 1994), irreversible cell injury and arrhythmogenic transient inward currents (Tani & Neely, 1989). Altogether, these data endorse the theory of the involvement of the unapposed Hc in ischemic-induced injury and support our hypothesis that inhibition of Hc during ischemia is an important determinant for cardioprotection against ischemia/reperfusion injury.

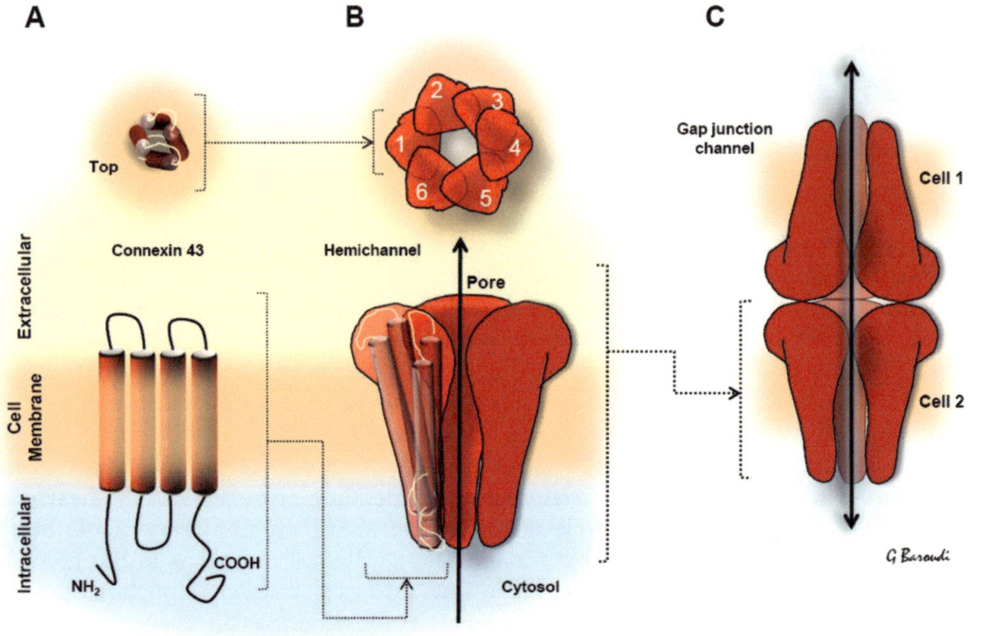

Fig. 1. Connexin 43 structures. A, secondary structure of Cx43 with insert showing a tridimensional view from the top; B, a single Hc is formed by the association of six connexins to form central permeable pore; C, a gap junction channel is formed when two Hc from adjacent cells appose and form a pathway between the cytosols of the neighbouring cells.

Ischemic preconditioning. The phosphorylation status of total Cx43 is affected by brief episodes of ischemia which reduce the adverse effects of subsequent myocardial ischemia (Cohen et al., 1991; Murry et al., 1986; Shiki & Hearse, 1987). In fact, ischemic preconditioned hearts from pigs (Schulz et al., 2003), rabbits (Miura et al., 2004), and rats (Jain et al., 2003) show preserved total Cx43 phosphorylation levels following prolonged ischemia. PKC is generally acknowledged as a key mediator of ischemic preconditioning (Schulz et al., 2003). One of the aims of this study is to establish that specific PKC isoforms are involved in the cascade of events leading to the preservation of the Cx43 phosphorylated state and cardioprotection. While cardioprotection is generally thought to involve phosphorylation of Cx43 gap-junction channels (Chen et al., 2005; Garcia-Dorado et al., 1997; Garcia-Dorado et al., 2004; Li et al., 2002; Rodriguez-Sinovas et al., 2006; Schwanke et al., 2002; Schwanke et al., 2003), experiments on isolated myocytes provided evidence that efficient ischemic preconditioning does not require the existence of gap junction channels (Li et al., 2004). Accordingly, we further hypothesize that unapposed Cx43 Hc (through their opening) are involved in ischemia-induced cell damage.

Other potential end-effectors of ischemic damage. Although this chapter focuses on the role of PKC isoform-dependent Cx43 HC phosphorylation in cardioprotection, one should be aware that several other mechanisms have been implicated in ischemia/reperfusion injury and cardioprotection. These include, but are not limited to, Na/H exchanger, mitochondrial permeability transition pore (MPTP) and K_{ATP} channels. While inhibition of Na/H exchanger has been shown to be beneficial for protection against ischemia (Xiao & Allen, 2000), PKC activation during ischemic preconditioning induces enhancement rather than inhibition of the Na/H exchanger (Kandasamy et al., 1995). The involvement of Na/H exchanger in heart conditioning is therefore uncertain (Avkiran, 1999). Another potential end-effector in ischemia-related protection is the MPTP (Hausenloy et al., 2002). While it has been proposed that MPTP inhibition in ischemia/reperfusion underlies the protection against injury in isolated rat hearts (Hausenloy et al., 2002), only a single study, thus far, has provided direct evidence for attenuated MPTP opening in preconditioned heart (Javadov et al., 2003). A significant number of studies support the involvement of the mitochondrial K_{ATP} channels in cardiac protection against ischemia (Gross & Fryer, 1999; Liu & O'Rourke, 2001; Sato & Marban, 2000). It has been suggested that opening of mitochondrial K_{ATP}

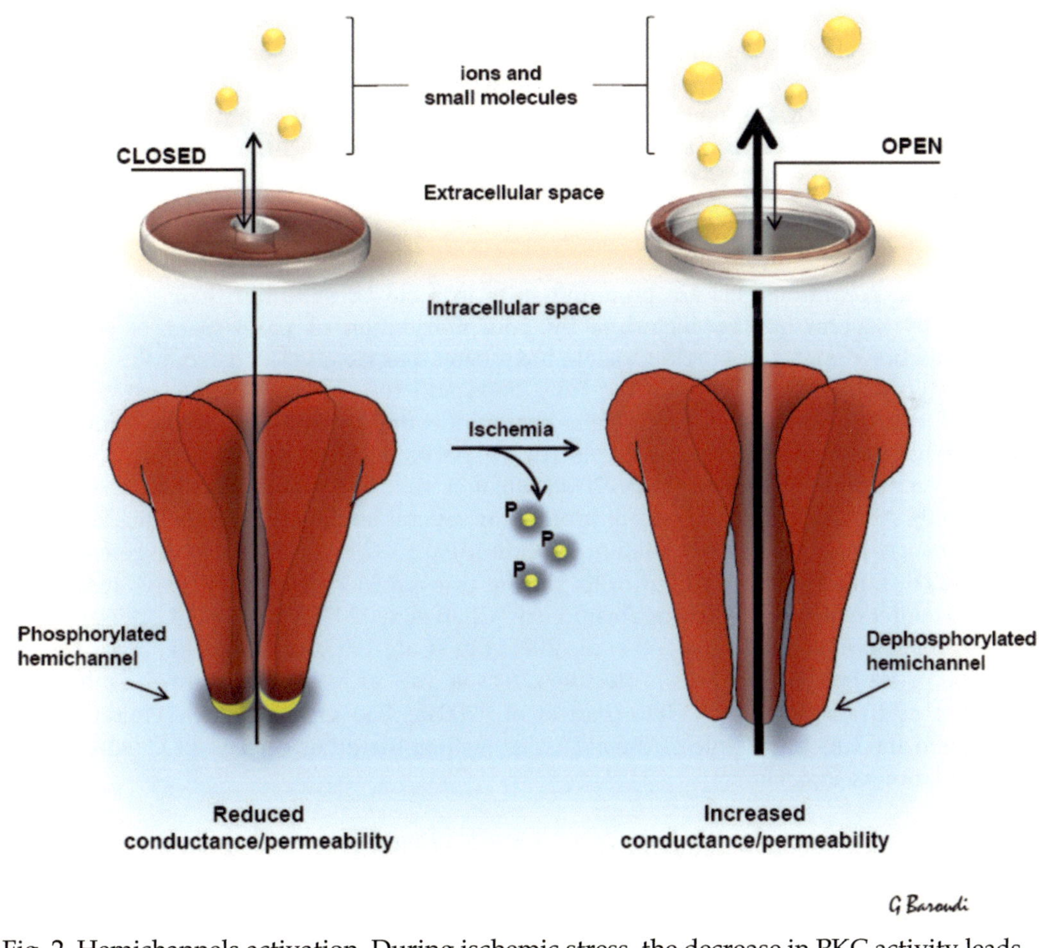

Fig. 2. Hemichannels activation. During ischemic stress, the decrease in PKC activity leads to increase in the dephosphorylated forms of Cx43, this causes the activation of Cx43Hc.

channels causes mitochondrial depolarisation, resulting in attenuated Ca overload during ischemia (Weiss et al., 2003). However, the protective effect of this reduction has never been experimentally demonstrated. Nevertheless, it should be noted here, that K_{ATP} channels are also modulated by PKC (Wang & Ashraf, 1999). Indeed, other end-effectors were also proposed to be directly involved in protection against ischemia/reperfusion injury. These include cGMP/PKG, calpains, cytoskeleton, and the tumor necrosis factor; the definitive evidence for their role on cardioprotection remains however obscure.

2.3 Function and regulation of CxHc

Currents from Hc have been successfully characterized in various native cell types (Hofer & Dermietzel, 1998; Kondo et al., 2000; Stout et al., 2002; Vergara et al., 2003) as well as in Xenopus oocytes (Ebihara & Steiner, 1993; Gomez-Hernandez et al., 2003; Gupta et al., 1994; Pfahnl et al., 1997; Pfahnl & Dahl, 1999; White et al., 1999; Zoidl et al., 2004) and in mammalian expression systems (Bukauskas et al., 2006; Contreras et al., 2003; Valiunas, 2002). Basically, they behave like large conductance ion channels that share properties with gap junction channels in terms of permeability and gating (DeVries & Schwartz, 1992; Li et al., 1996; Trexler et al., 1996). Nevertheless, opening of these channels is significantly facilitated by exposure to calcium-free extracellular solutions (DeVries & Schwartz, 1992; Li et al., 1996), membrane depolarization (Hofer & Dermietzel, 1998), or metabolic inhibition (Contreras et al., 2002; John et al., 1999b). Cx43Hc have been implicated in diverse functions including volume regulation (Quist et al., 2000), efflux of NAD^+ and ATP (Bruzzone et al., 2001; Cotrina et al., 1998; Stout et al., 2002), influx of Na^+ and Ca^{2+} ions (Contreras et al., 2002; John et al., 1999b; Kondo et al., 2000) and activation of survival pathways (Plotkin et al., 2002).

Under resting conditions, Hc are predominantly in a closed state but their gating can be regulated by several factors, including by phosphorylation of Cx43 (Saez et al., 2005). Several functional states of single Cx43Hc have been described; closed Hc, fully open Hc, and an intermediate state between the fully open and the closed states (Contreras et al., 2003). On western blot, Cx43 exhibits three bands reflecting the presence of three functional states of Cx43: a highly phosphorylated, a partially phosphorylated and a non-phosphorylated state (Hertzberg et al., 2000; Musil et al., 1990; Saez et al., 1997; VanSlyke & Musil, 2000). Although Cx43 is a target protein for several kinases (Lampe & Lau, 2000), we are particularly interested in modulation by individual PKC isoforms. Because activation of εPKC and/or inhibition of δPKC prior to, during or even following an ischemic insult was shown to confer cardioprotection against injury (Chen et al., 2001a; Dorn et al., 1999; Gray et al., 1997; Inagaki et al., 2003; Inagaki et al., 2005; Liu et al., 1999; Tanaka et al., 2004; Tanaka et al., 2005); we believe that this protective effect is due, at least in part, to the inhibitory effect that εPKC exerts on Cx43Hc (Bao et al., 2004a; Bao et al., 2004b). Therefore, we investigated the functional role of the εPKC, as well as the other cardiac PKC isoforms, in the modulation of Cx43Hc.

2.4 PKC Isoform-selective activator and inhibitor peptides

PKC consists of a family of at least twelve closely related isoforms (McDonald et al., 1994; Nishizuka, 1988; Osada et al., 1992) which regulate biochemical processes by phosphorylation of cellular proteins on serine or threonine residues. Molecular cloning has revealed that PKC family can be divided into three major groups (Fig. 3). The conventional PKCs or cPKC consist of α, βI, βII and γ and have activity strongly dependent on calcium (Ca), phospholipid, and diacylglycerol (DG) (Nishizuka, 1988). The second group (novel PKC or nPKC) comprises the ε, δ, η and θ isoforms and exhibits Ca-independent activity. And finally, members of the atypical PKC group or aPKC, ζ and λ/ι are insensitive to DG, phorbol esters and Ca. There is also a μPKC that does not fit into any of the above groups and is sensitive to phospholipids and phorbol esters but insensitive to Ca. Remarkable progress has been made in understanding how extracellular stimuli act as upstream triggers to induce activation of particular PKC isoforms in cardiomyocytes (endothelin, phenylephrine, etc.) (Clerk et al., 1994; Clerk & Sugden, 2001; Rybin et al., 1999). Moreover, there is much evidence supporting the concept that PKC functions in an isoform-dependent manner and that specific cardiac manifestations depend on the activation of individual isoforms, not the activity of the entire PKC family (Chen et al., 2001a; Clerk & Sugden, 2001; Hahn et al., 2002; Mochly-Rosen & Gordon, 1998). Indeed, the successful development of isoform-specific modulator peptides and their use in combination with patch clamp technology (Hu et al., 2000; Xiao et al., 2001; Xiao et al., 2003) have empowered the investigation of isoform-selective roles of PKC family in ion channels modulation. Briefly, activator peptides by binding to one particular PKC isoform cause a conformational change of the enzyme structure which exposes its catalytic site, and enables its anchoring to the target molecule. On the opposite side, inhibitor peptides mimic structurally the PKC isoform binding site on the target protein or the target protein binding site on PKC and therefore inhibit the function of that particular PKC isoform. The specificity and sequences of the activator and inhibitor peptides of PKC isoforms are listed in Table 1. These peptides can be obtained through commercial custom peptide synthesis.

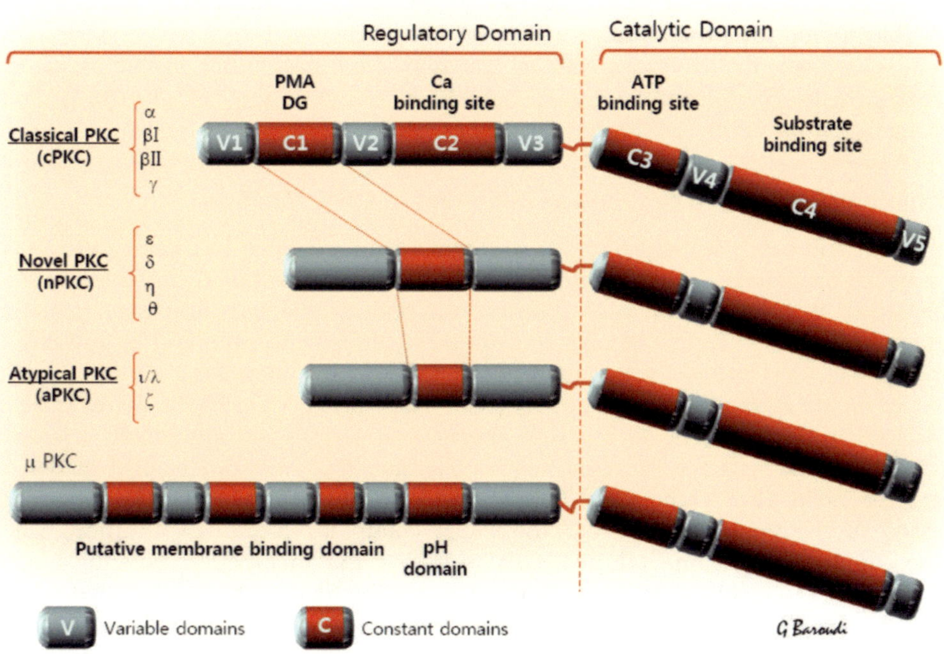

Fig. 3. Protein kinase C superfamily, classes of various PKC isoforms with corresponding structures.

Peptide	Specificity	Sequence
αC2-4	αPKC inhibitor	S-L-N-P-Q-W-N-E-T
βIV5-3	βIPKC inhibitor	K-L-F-I-M-N
βIIV5-3	βIIPKC inhibitor	Q-E-V-I-R-N
βC2-2	βPKC activator	S-V-E-I-W
δV1-1	δPKC inhibitor	S-F-N-S-Y-E-L-G-S-L
εV1-2	εPKC inhibitor	E-A-V-S-L-K-P-T
εV1-7	εPKC activator	H-D-A-P-I-G-Y-D
ηV1-2	ηPKC inhibitor	E-A-V-G-L-Q-P-T
Pentalysine	control	K-K-K-K-K

Table 1. PKC modulator peptides. List of the available PKC isoform-specific modulator peptides with their sequences and specificity.

2.5 Previous findings and implication for the current study

Previous data from several laboratories show that selective translocation/activation of the εPKC isoform provides protection against ischemic injury during ischemic/hypoxic preconditioning (Chan et al., 1995; Chou & Messing, 2005; Dorn et al., 1999; Gray et al., 1997; Liu et al., 1999; Ytrehus et al., 1994) and post-conditioning (Penna et al., 2006b; Philipp et al., 2006; Zatta et al., 2006) in different experimental paradigms. On the basis of the beneficial effects of εPKC translocation/activation and the fact that it can form a complex with Cx43 and phosphorylate the protein (Ping et al., 2001), we put forth that this particular isoform is critically involved in protection against ischemic injury. Therefore, the elucidation of the functional protective role of εPKC may allow for the identification of pharmacological agents that mimic the PKC isoform action on one particular target, i.e. Cx43Hc, without affecting other key molecules in cellular function. Certainly, other isozymes have been demonstrated to phosphorylate Cx43, notably αPKC (Bowling et al., 2001), but the functional implications in Cx43Hc regulation has not been assessed.

2.6 Structural Cx-mimetic peptides as inhibitors of CxHc function

Another experimental strategy using a different set of peptides has been utilized in the course of this study: the structural mimetics of Cx43. The conventional gap junction blockers (as heptanol) that are available to date act on both whole gap junction channels and unapposed Hc. Interestingly, Cx-mimetic peptides have recently emerged as powerful tools capable of blocking primarily the unapposed Cx43Hc by mimicking short amino acids sequences on the extracellular loops of Cx (references (Braet et al., 2003a; Evans et al., 2006; Leybaert et al., 2003; Martin et al., 2005; Pearson et al., 2005) testing ATP release from various non-cardiac cell types). Here, we investigated the consequent effect of two Cx43-mimetic peptides, Gap26 and Gap 27, on the electrophysiology of Cx43Hc exogenously expressed in the tsA201 cells using the patch clamp technique. In addition, we have designed multiple experimental protocols to assess the therapeutic potentials of these peptides against ischemia/perfusion injury in various settings including isolated cell model and intact hearts.

Initially, the Cx-mimetic peptides were designed with the intention of selectively blocking gap junction channels by intercepting the apposition of pairs of Hc from adjacent cells (Dahl et al., 1994; Warner et al., 1995), but have subsequently emerged as potent blockers for the unapposed CxHc with little or no immediate effect on gap junction (Braet et al., 2003a; Evans et al., 2006; Leybaert et al., 2003; Martin et al., 2005; Pearson et al., 2005).

Particularly, Gap26 and Gap27 peptides have recently emerged as powerful tools that block unapposed Cx43Hc (Braet et al., 2003a; Evans et al., 2006; Leybaert et al., 2003; Martin et al., 2005; Pearson et al., 2005) by mimicking short amino acids sequences on the first (VCYDKSFPISHVR) and second (SRPTEKTIFII) extracellular loops of Cx43, respectively (Fig. 4). Both sequences contain conserved motifs that are involved in connexin-connexin interaction in gap junction channels (Dahl et al., 1992; Warner et al., 1995). These motifs are not consistently found in other cell surface proteins suggesting that Gap26 and Gap 27 specifically interact with Cx43 without interfering with other Cx or surface proteins (Braet et al., 2003a; Isakson et al., 2006; Warner et al., 1995). In fact, the selective affinity of Gap26 and Gap27 toward Cx43Hc was first reported in 2003 by Braet and collaborators (Braet et al., 2003a; Braet et al., 2003b). In their studies, Gap26 and Gap27 were shown to selectively block the uptake of a reporter dye and the release of ATP in brain endothelial cells and Cx43-expressing HeLa cells without reducing gap junctional coupling. Subsequently, Cx-mimetic peptides were shown to consistently suppress the bi-directional permeability, i.e. dye uptake and ATP release, of the unapposed CxHc without affecting gap junctional coupling in several cell types including brain endothelium, retinal epithelium, and bladder cancer

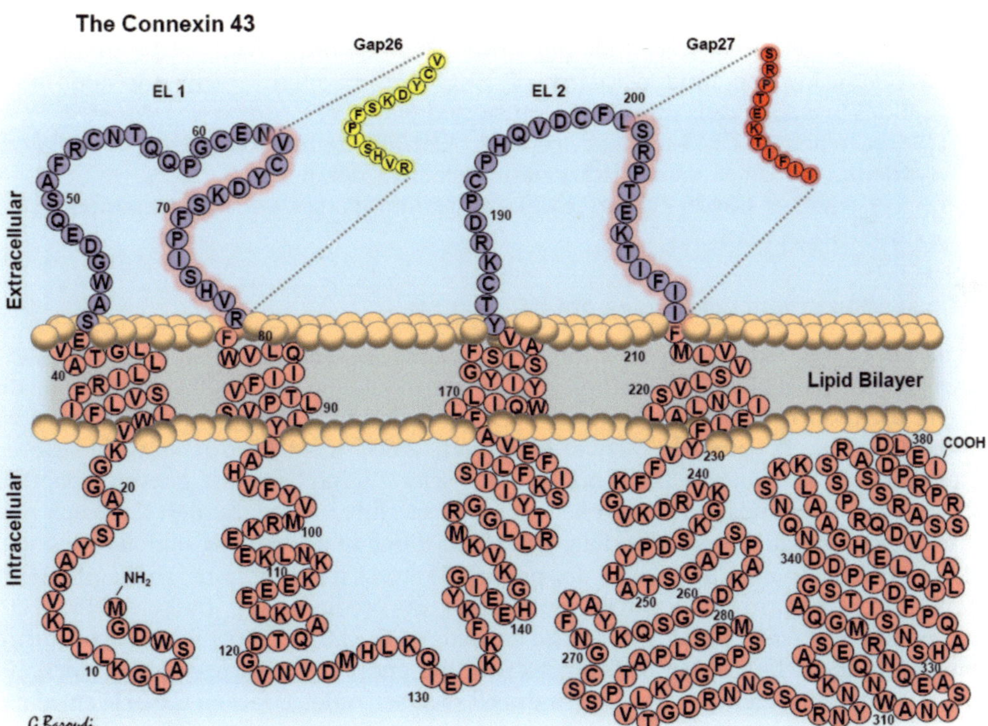

Fig. 4. Connexin 43 and its structural-mimetic peptides. Gap26 and Gap27 mimic the structure of first (EL 1) and second (EL 2) extracellular loops of Cx43, respectively.

epithelium cells, as well as transfected HEK293, HeLa, C6 glioma and ECV304 cell lines (De Vuyst et al., 2006; Leybaert et al., 2003; Pearson et al., 2005). Although, the mechanism that underlies the affinity of Cx-mimetic peptides toward Hc is currently not known, a possible explanation could be the accessibility of the extracellular loops of unapposed Hc compared to those of gap junction channels which are engaged in the Hc-Hc apposition and are therefore less accessible for interactions with exogenous peptides. On the other hand, it is still not clear how binding of these peptides to connexins causes a block of the Hc.

3. Experimental design and methods

In summary, this study was designed to test the hypothesis that the cardioprotective effect attributed to PKC activation is mediated, at least in part, through the closure of the unapposed Cx43Hc and their decreased conductance. Specifically, the study aims to assess the following:

1. Unapposed Cx43Hc function is selectively and differentially regulated by various isoforms of PKC. Particularly, phosphorylation of Cx43 by εPKC inhibits unapposed Cx43Hc.
2. Inhibition of the Cx43Hc, using the synthetic structural Cx43-mimetic peptides Gap26, confers sustained cardioprotection against ischemia/reperfusion injury by counteracting the ischemia-induced dephosphorylation effect on the unapposed Cx43Hc.

Therefore, our specific objectives are summarized as follows:

1. To dissect functional roles that individual PKC isoforms exert in the modulation of Cx43Hc using the unique matrix of PKC isoform-specific activator and inhibitor peptides in tsA201 cells transiently transfected with Cx43.
2. To test whether Cx43-mimetic peptide, Gap26, confers resistance to isolated rat ventricular myocytes against ischemia-induced cell death.
3. To test whether Gap26 confers cardioprotection against ischemia/reperfusion to the perfused intact heart.

3.1 Dissection of functional roles of PKC isoform

The matrix of PKC isoforms-specific modulator peptides (Table 1) was utilized to dissect and interrogate the individual PKC isoform roles in the modulation of Cx43Hc. Cx43Hc-mediated currents are recorded from transfected tsA201 cells using the patch clamp technique in whole cell configuration as described (Hawat & Baroudi, 2008). Cx43Hc currents were induced by incubating cells in a low-Ca bath solution. The selective inhibitor and activator peptides of PKC isoforms were individually applied to the intracellular space through the patch pipette. For each experiment, the cell was dialyzed with a different activator or inhibitor peptide (0.1 μM) for at least five minutes to allow for peptide to access the cytoplasm. The implication of a specific PKC isoform in Cx43Hc modulation is predicted by the capability of the corresponding activator peptide to reduce currents or the inhibitor peptide to abolish current inhibition induced by a general PKC activator, the phorbol myristate acetate (PMA, 10 nM applied in the bath solution). The PMA-induced PKC activation effect on Cx43Hc currents was assessed in the presence of each of the inhibitor peptides separately. To substantiate the specificity of PMA vis-à-vis PKC activation, the effect of PMA was compared with an inactive phorbol ester, the 4αPDD, that possesses all characteristics of PMA except for its capacity to activate PKC. Appropriate time was allowed for steady-state current levels to be reached before the application of PMA or 4αPDD. As negative controls, we used a scrambled version of active peptides to assess their effect on Cx43Hc-induced currents.

3.2 Study on isolated cardiomyocytes

To assess the functional effect of the Cx43-mimetic peptide Gap26 directly on Cx43Hc, currents were recorded using patch clamp from transfected tsA201 cells. Since peptides exert their effect by binding to the extracellular loops, these were added to the extracellular bath solution (0.5 μM). To determine the sensitivity of isolated myocytes to simulated ischemia/reperfusion, freshly isolated cardiac myocytes were incubated with saline, Gap26 or scrambled GAP26 (sGap26) 10 min before or 30 min after the initiation of ischemia as described (Hawat et al., 2010). Briefly, cells were pelleted by low speed centrifugation for 1 min and were washed twice with incubation buffer. Under these conditions, most of the non-myocyte cells remain in the supernatant, producing a pellet that contains >95% myocytes (Chen et al., 1999; Hawat et al., 2010). To simulate ischemic stress, cells were transferred to microcentrifuge tubes, washed twice with degassed glucose-free incubation buffer and pelleted as before. After centrifugation, 90% of supernatant was removed and microballoons were layered over the remaining buffer to create an air-tight environment. Tubes were incubated at 37°C for 180 min the damage to cardiac myocytes was assessed by trypan blue dye exclusion assay as previously described (Armstrong et al., 1994; Armstrong et al., 1997). The staining should correlate with myocytes rounding indicating cell death.

3.3 Study on intact heart

Using Langendorff technique, isolated Sprague-Dawley rat hearts were subjected to 20-min control stabilization followed by 40 min regional ischemia by ligation of the left anterior descending (LAD) coronary artery and then 180 min reperfusion by removing the ligation. The Cx43 structural mimetic peptide (0.5 μM) was administered either 10 min prior to the onset of ischemia or 30 min after (this is 10 min before reperfusion), as described (Hawat et al., 2010). For control, s Gap26 was utilized. Evans blue perfusion was used to determine the region at risk. The left ventricle was sectioned into 2-mm slices and incubated with triphenyltetrazolium chloride (TTC) to estimate the injured (infracting) myocardial zone. The results were confirmed by histology. Myocardial perfusate flow was also determined by measuring the volume of perfusate recovered from Langendorff-perfused heart during 1 min at 10 min after LAD occlusion or 10 min after reperfusion and compared to basal MPF (BMPF) as previously desrcibed (Hawat et al., 2010).

4. Results

4.1 PKC-mediated inhibition of Cx43Hc currents is primarily mediated through εPKC isoform

Application of the general PKC activator, PMA, in the bath solution consistently inhibited Cx43Hc currents (Fig. 5A, 5B, 5C). Averaged data show that PMA resulted in Cx43Hc current reduction by 74.0±4.3% (n=6, $P<0.05$). Superfusion of tsA201 cells with 4αPDD, an inactive phorbol ester analog that does not activate PKC, did not significantly affect Cx43Hc current amplitude (increase of 2.0±1.5%, n=5, P=NS; Fig. 5D), indicating that the PMA effect reported above is indeed mediated via PKC activation. To dissect the role of individual PKC isoforms in the regulation of Cx43Hc, we tested the ability of five PKC isoform-specific inhibitor peptides to antagonize the effect of PMA, i.e. αC2–4, βIV5–3, βIIV5–3, δV1–7, and εV1–2 targeting α-, βI-, βII-, δ-, and ε-PKC isoforms, respectively. Each of the tested peptides targets a corresponding native PKC isoform in tsA201 cells. Importantly, when cells were dialysed with the specific inhibitor peptide of the 'cardioprotective' εPKC, the PMA-induced current inhibition was completely abolished (118.5±15.8%, n=6, significantly different from the reference PMA effect; Fig. 5E) , this was in contrast with the other tested PKC isoforms inhibitors. In the presence of scrambled εV1–2, the inhibitory effect of PMA on Cx43Hc currents was not significantly different compared with the PMA effect alone (69.4±4.7%, n=3, *P*=NS). On the other hand, using an εPKC activator peptide εV1–7 (0.1 μM) alone was able to cause a 75.7±2.6% reduction in the basal Cx43Hc current (n=3, *P*<0.05; Fig. 5F), thus confirming the involvement of εPKC in Cx43Hc inhibition. Detailed results are reported (Hawat & Baroudi, 2008).

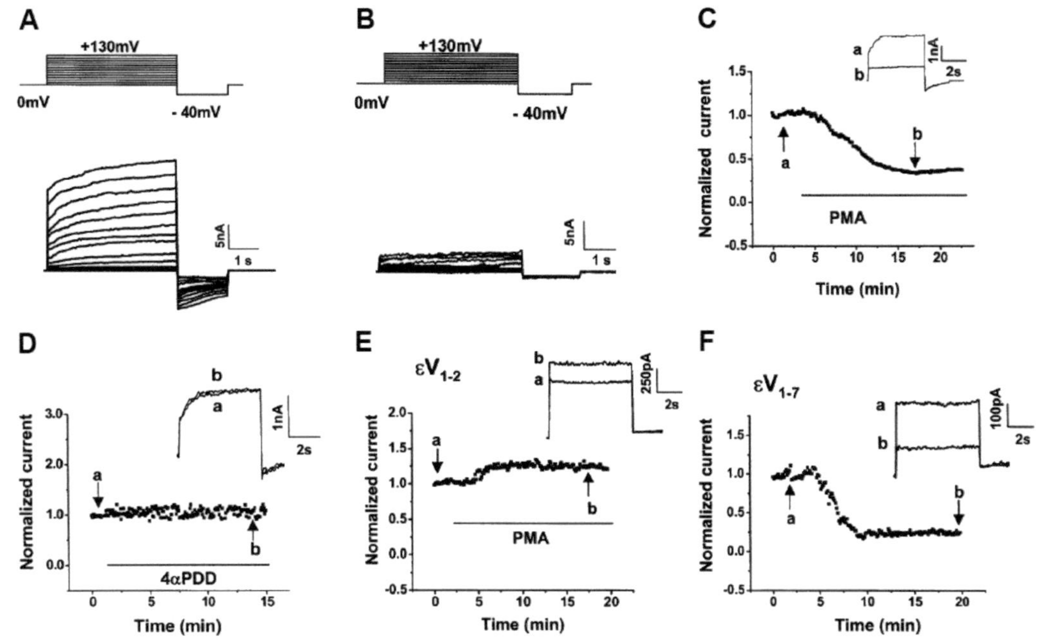

Fig. 5. Cx43Hc modulation by PMA and εPKC. A, whole-cell currents recorded from a typical tsA201 cell transfected with Cx43. B, traces from a non-transfected cell. Time course recording plotting Cx43Hc current amplitudes against time in the presence of C, PMA;. D, 4αPDD; E, PMA and the εPKC-specific inhibitor peptide; and F, εPKC activator peptide.

4.2 Gap26 inhibits Cx43Hc currents

Because we believed inhibition of Cx43Hc by εPKC may represent the basic key mechanism of cardioprotection during ischemic preconditioning, we next investigated the functional effect of the presumably specific inhibitor of Cx43Hc, the mimetic Gap26 peptide, on Cx43Hc mediated currents recorded from individual tsA201 cells transiently expressing Cx43. In Fig. 6A, a representative time course recording shows rapid Cx43Hc currents reduction when Gap26 was introduced in the bath solution. A steady-state inhibition was reached in all experiments. Averaged data indicate that Gap26 caused 60.1±4.6% (n=5, *P*<0.05) current reduction. In the presence of sGap26 peptide, the amplitude of Cx43Hc currents did not vary over a similar time frame (99.0±1.1%, n=5, $P>0.05$) (Fig. 6B). The histogram (Fig. 6C) summarizes the effects of both peptides on normalized Cx43Hc currents. Curves representing the current–voltage (I–V) relationship for Cx43Hc in the absence and in the presence of Gap26 are illustrated in Fig. 6D. I–V data were elicited by depolarizing cells with voltage steps ranging from +0 to +90 mV.

Because connexin 40 (Cx40) and connexin 45 (Cx45) may also form hemichannels in the heart, we examined whether Gap26 has effects on currents recorded from tsA201 cells transfected with either connexin isoforms. Importantly, the application of Gap26 did not cause a significant reduction in currents mediated by Cx40Hc (0.7±1.6%, n=4, $P>0.05$) or Cx45Hc (0.2±0.7%, n=4, $P>0.05$) over a time frame similar to that used in Cx43Hc experiments (Hawat et al., 2010).

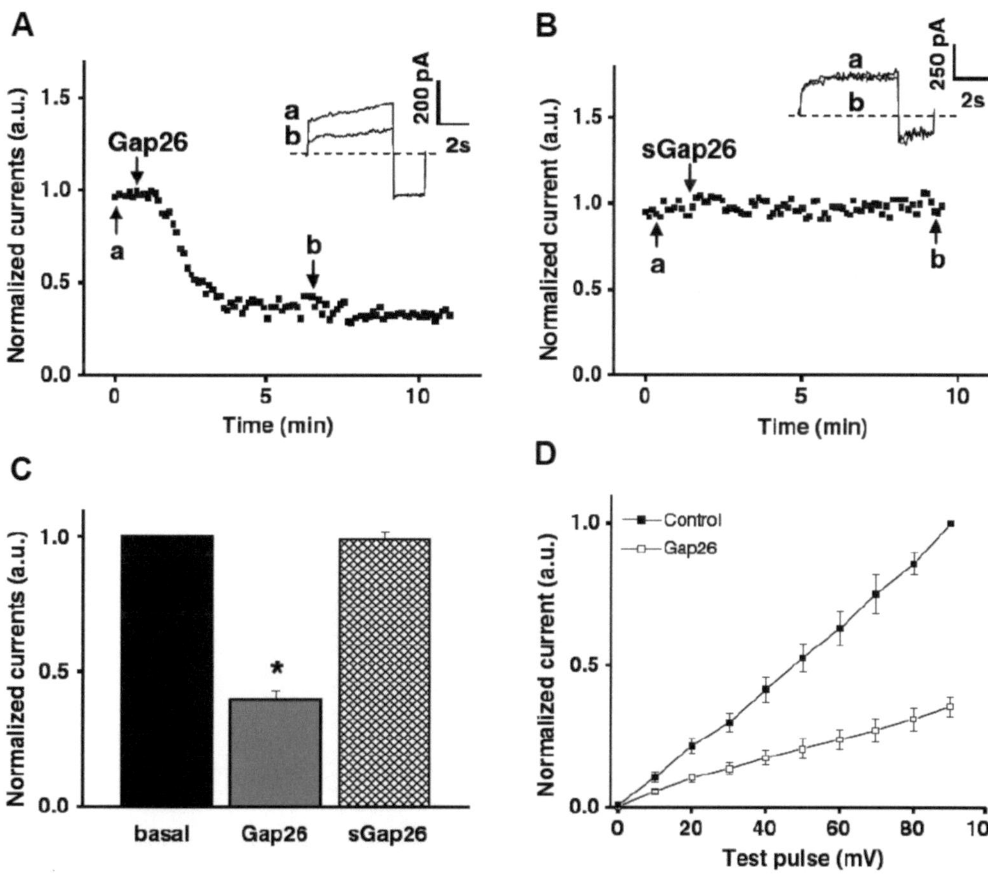

Fig. 6. Cx43Hc-mediated whole-cell current inhibition by Gap26 recorded from individual tsA201 cells. A, time course recording plotting current amplitudes in presence of Gap26 against time. B, a control time course recording in presence of sGap26. Insert in A and B show current traces recorded at time points indicated by arrows a and b. Current amplitudes are normalized against control and are represented in arbitrary units (a.u.). C, a histogram summarizing effects of Gap26 and sGap26 in comparison to basal current. D, current-voltage relationship obtained from tsA201 cells in absence and in presence of Gap26.

4.3 Connexin 43 mimetic peptide confers resistance to intact heart against ischemia injury

We next assessed the effect of Gap26 on intact ischemic heart. Administration of Gap26 before ischemia significantly decreased infarct size from 36.3±2.1 of area at risk in untreated hearts (n=7) to 18.8±1.9% (n=6, $P<0.05$) (Fig. 7A). In order to assess the peptide capability to counteract an existing ischemia, a separate group of hearts was studied in which Gap26 was introduced 30 min after the LAD coronary occlusion. Similarly, the infarct size was significantly reduced to 16.2±0.8% (n=7, $P<0.05$) of area at risk. These results correspond to infarct size reductions by 48.2% and 55.4% when Gap26 was introduced before or during ischemia, respectively. The size of area at risk to total ventricles did not change significantly in both experimental groups (41.3±4.5%, n=6, $P>0.05$ and 40.6±3.2%, n=7, $P>0.05$, respectively) compared to the group of untreated hearts (44.8±2.0%, n=7) (Fig. 7B). As negative control,

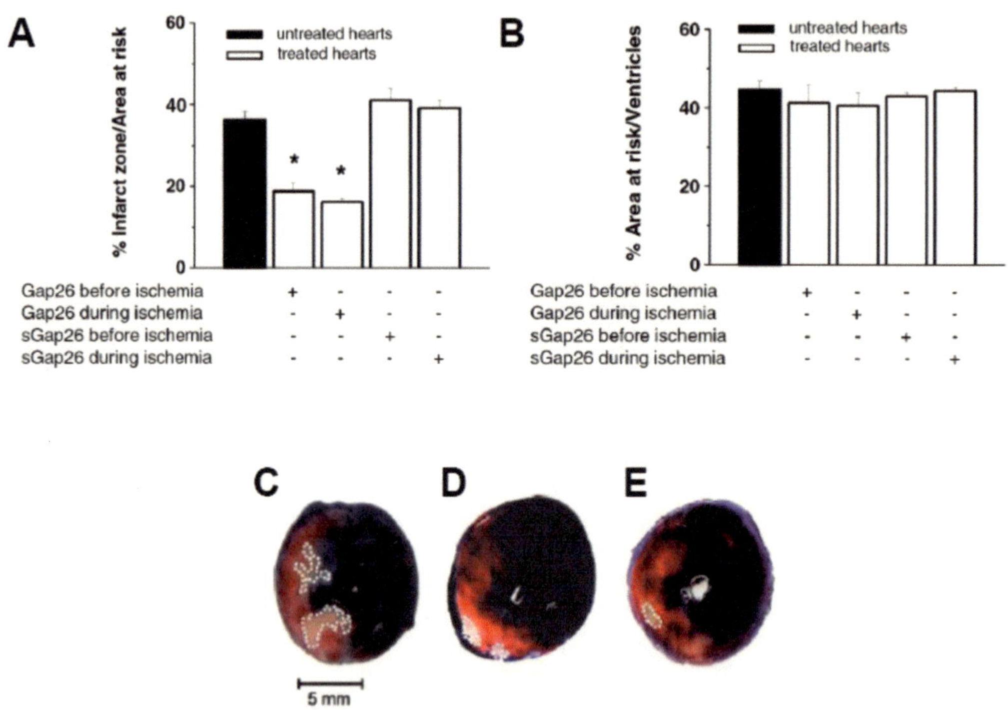

Fig. 7. Effect of synthetic peptides on intact hearts subjected to regional ischemia by LAD ligation. a Histogram representing the proportion of infarct zone to the area at risk, b histogram representing the proportion of area at risk to total ventricles. Values obtained from ischemic hearts in the presence of Gap26 or sGap26 added either 10 min before (n=6 and n=3, respectively) or 30 min after (n=7 and n=4, respectively) the occlusion of LAD are reported. *P<0.05 indicates statistically significant difference in comparison to untreated hearts (n=7). Photographs of TTC-stained heart sections after 40 min ischemia and 180 min reperfusion representing c untreated heart, d heart treated with Gap26 introduced 10 min before LAD occlusion, and e Gap26 introduced 30 min after LAD occlusion. c–e The infarct zone is the whitish area delimited with white dashed lines; the area at risk corresponds to the red region including the infarct zone; and the perfused area is in dark blue

sGap26 was also tested. Administration of sGap26 did not statistically affect the size of infarct area to area at risk when introduced before ischemia (41.1±3.0%, n=3, *P*>0.05) or during ischemia (39.2±2.0%, n=4, *P*>0.05) in comparison to untreated hearts (36.3±2.1%, n=7). The global size of total ventricles was comparable between groups of untreated hearts and hearts treated with Gap26 or sGap26 (data not shown). Percentage values for different heart areas obtained from various experimental groups are listed in Table 1. Transversal slices obtained from hearts representing the groups of untreated hearts, hearts treated with Gap26 before ischemia, and hearts treated with Gap26 during ischemia are shown in Fig. 7C, 7D, 7E.

In order to investigate the effect of Gap26 on the function of Langendorff-perfused hearts, we compared the MPF measured 10 min after LAD occlusion and 10 min after reperfusion to the BMPF. The BMPF is determined for each heart during normal conditions, i.e., before LAD occlusion in the absence of Gap26. Application of Gap26 to non-ischemic hearts during 1 h did not cause significant changes to MPF (data not shown). Importantly, addition of Gap26 in the perfusion solution increased MPF during reperfusion of ischemic hearts from 65.7±5.1% (n=7) of BMPF in untreated hearts to 89.8±4.9% (n=7, *P*<0.05) and 86.7±4.8% (n=4, *P*<0.05) in hearts treated with Gap26 before or during ischemia, respectively (Fig. 8). As negative control, sGap26 did not affect MPF when introduced before or during ischemia. Values for MPF variations in different experimental groups are listed in Table 2.

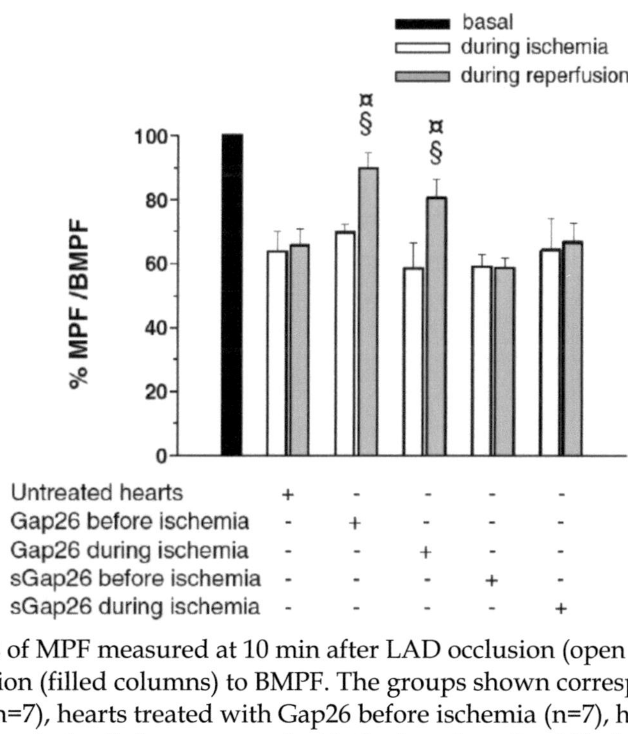

Fig. 8. Percentages of MPF measured at 10 min after LAD occlusion (open columns) or at 10 min after reperfusion (filled columns) to BMPF. The groups shown correspond to the untreated hearts (n=7), hearts treated with Gap26 before ischemia (n=7), hearts treated with Gap26 during ischemia (n=4), hearts treated with the inactive sGap26 before ischemia (n=3), and heart treated with sGap26 during ischemia (n=4). ¤*P*<0.05 indicates data significantly different from untreated hearts. §P<0.05 indicates data significantly different from MPF during ischemia.

Groups	IZ/AAR (%)	AAR/V (%)	N	MPFI/BMPF (%)	MPFR/BMPF (%)	N
Untreated hearts	36.3±2.1	44.8±2.0	7	63.8±6.2	65.7±5.1	7
Gap26 before ischemia	18.8±1.9	41.3±4.5	6	69.9±2.3	89.8±4.9	7
Gap26 during ischemia	16.2±0.8	40.6±3.2	7	58.5±7.4	86.7±4.8	4
sGap26 before ischemia	41.1±3.0	43.1±0.3	3	59.1±3.7	57.1±3.1	3
sGap26 during ischemia	39.2±2.0	44.4±1.0	4	64.2±9.9	66.7±5.9	4

IZ infarct zone, AAR area at risk, V ventricles, MPFI myocardial perfusate flow measured during ischemia, MPFR myocardial perfusate flow measured during reperfusion, BMPF basal myocardial flow

[a] Statistically different in comparison to untreated group

[b] Statistically different in comparison to MPF during ischemia

Table 2. Percentage values for heart areas and myocardial perfusate flows.

4.4 Effect of Gap26 on isolated cardiomyocytes

In order to elucidate the cellular basis for the Gap26-mediated cardioprotection observed in intact hearts, we investigated the effect of the peptide on isolated cardiomyocytes from adult rat hearts subjected to simulated ischemia-reperfusion. Application of Gap26 in the bath solution either 10 min before or 30 min after the initiation of simulated ischemia increased the number of surviving cardiomyocytes after 180 min reperfusion from 28.4±6.5% of total cells (n=8) to 53.1±6.8% (n=8, P<0.05) and 55.0±6.5% (n=8, *P*<0.05), respectively (Fig. 9A). The percentage of surviving cells did not differ statistically between groups treated with Gap26 before or during simulated ischemia. As negative control, the percentage of surviving cells following application of sGap26 before ischemia (22.9±6.9%, n=8) or during ischemia (26.0±6.6%, n=8) did not differ significantly in comparison to untreated cells (28.4±6.5%,

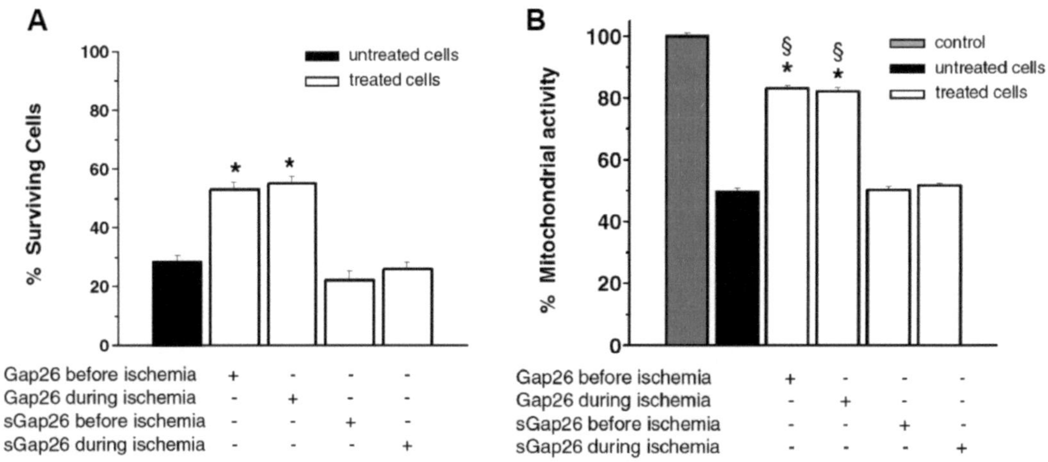

Fig. 9. Effect of Gap26 on viability of isolated adult rat cardiomyocytes during simulated ischemia-reperfusion. a The percentage of surviving cells to total cells after reperfusion was determined in the absence or presence of Gap26 or sGap26 added to the bath solution before or during ischemia (n=8 in each group). Data are expressed as mean ± SEM of eight experiments using myocytes from three different animals. b Mitochondrial dysfunction was determined with the MTT test (n=5 in each group, obtained from a single rat heart). *P<0.05 indicates significant difference in comparison to untreated cells. §P<0.05 indicates significant difference in comparison to control.

n=8, $P>0.05$). In order to substantiate these findings, we assessed mitochondrial activity in each experimental group of cardiomyocytes using the colorimetric MTT assay. To alleviate comparison, results are expressed as percentages of the mitochondrial activity measured in a control group of cardiomyocytes maintained at normoxic conditions during a similar time frame. Simulated ischemia-reperfusion reduced mitochondrial activity in untreated cardiomyocytes to 49.7±1.2%, n=5, $P<0.05$ in comparison to the control cardiomyocytes 100.0±1.2%, n=5. Treatment of cardiomyocytes with Gap26 prevented partially but significantly this mitochondrial dysfunction when introduced before or during ischemia (83.0±1.1%, n=5, $P<0.05$ and 82.1±1.1%, n=5, P<0.05, respectively). Application of sGap26 did not prevent the mitochondrial dysfunction when applied before ischemia (50.3±1.0%, n=5, P>0.05) or during ischemia (51.8±0.9%, n=5, $P>0.05$) in comparison to untreated cells. Results obtained from the different experimental groups are illustrated in the histogram (Fig. 9B).

5. Discussion

5.1 PKC isoform selective modulation of Cx43Hc

The first important observation here was the unraveling of selective and differential implication of PKC isoforms in the modulation of Cx43Hc conductance. The εPKC was found to be the isoform predominantly involved in the modulation of Cx43Hc conductance after PMA superfusion.

Cx43Hc dephosphorylation (Beardslee et al., 2000; Jain et al., 2003; Jeyaraman et al., 2003; Miura et al., 2004; Schulz et al., 2003) and opening (John et al., 1999b; Kondo et al., 2000; Shintani-Ishida et al., 2007) have been proposed as key mechanisms underlying cell injury in response to simulated ischemia in cardiomyocytes. Preservation of Cx43 phosphorylation by selective activation of the εPKC isoform occurs in response to ischemic pre- (Chou & Messing, 2005; Liu et al., 1999; Ytrehus et al., 1994) and postconditioning (Penna et al., 2006a; Philipp et al., 2006; Zatta et al., 2006), in which brief episodes of ischemia reduce the adverse effects of subsequent or preceding myocardial ischemia, respectively. As the function of multiple proteins may be affected by εPKC, delineation of the isoform-specific regulation of downstream targets, e.g. Cx43Hc, is indeed important to improve our understanding of the pathogenesis of ischemic heart disease and to identify new opportunities for drug development.

5.2 Cx43 mimetic peptide protects heart against myocardial infarction

In this context, another important finding was the rapid depression of Cx43Hc conductance in response to the application of the Cx43 mimetic peptide Gap26. To date, the involvement of unequivocally identified unapposed Hc in CxMPs-mediated phenomena, such as regulation of ATP release and calcium propagation, is still debated (Dahl, 2007). Therefore, we demonstrated here for the first time that superfusion of the ion channel-deficient tsA201 cells, transiently expressing Cx43, with Gap26 readily inhibits Cx43Hc-mediated currents recorded from individual cells. This observation complements with previous studies reporting on the inhibitory effect of Gap26 on the permeability of Cx43Hc (Braet et al., 2003b; Gomes et al., 2005; Leybaert et al., 2003; Pearson et al., 2005), the second major functional characteristic of connexin channels besides conductance. Although not surprisingly, this result represents the most direct evidence reported so far for the Gap26 inhibitory effect on Cx43Hc. Curiously, this inhibition occurred using a peptide concentration that is 1,000 times lower than what has previously been utilized to block Hc currents (0.5 μM in this study versus 500 μM in (Romanov et al., 2007)). Occasionally, the specificity of CxMPs toward Hc has been challenged (Wang et al., 2007). Therefore, we tested the effect of Gap26 on Hc of Cx40 and Cx45 which are also present in the heart. Importantly, Gap26 did not affect currents from Cx40Hc or Cx45Hc.

The most important finding however was the protection that Gap26 conferred to intact rat heart against regional ischemia induced by LAD coronary occlusion. We showed that administration of Gap26 prior to LAD occlusion resulted in more than 48% reduction of infarct size compared to untreated hearts. Similarly, Gap26 reduced infarct size by 55% when administered during ischemia. We also showed that the salutary effect of Gap26 extends to heart function by increasing the MPF during reperfusion by nearly 37% and 32% when the peptide was administered before or during LAD occlusion, respectively, in comparison to untreated hearts. These results indicate that whereas Gap26 can confer resistance to "normal" hearts against subsequent ischemia, it also has the capability to salvage injured hearts when administered after the occurrence of ischemia. Hypothetically, we ascribe these effects to the presumable Gap26-mediated inhibition of cardiomyocytic Cx43Hc opened by ischemic stress. Indeed, Gap26 is also known to inhibit Cx43 GJCs when used at relatively high concentrations and/or following prolonged exposure (Evans et al., 2006). Nonetheless, all experiments in this study were performed using low concentration of Gap26 (0.5 μM) previously shown to selectively inhibit Hc without directly affecting GJCs (Clarke et al., 2009; Verma et al., 2009). Therefore, we consider that neither the peptide concentration nor the duration of exposure to Gap26 (which varied depending on protocols between ~3 and 4 h) was sufficient to modulate GJCs in the studied hearts. In concordance with the fact that death of cardiomyocytes, and therefore myocardial injury, principally occurs during reperfusion (Gottlieb et al., 1994; Shintani-Ishida et al., 2007; Zhao et al., 2000), both structural and functional improvements in intact hearts did not differ significantly whether Gap26 was introduced before occlusion or before reperfusion.

To investigate the cellular basis of the protection of intact hearts, we assessed the effect of Gap26 on isolated cardiomyocytes subjected to simulated ischemia–reperfusion. We found a nearly twofold increase in the number of surviving cells when Gap26 was administered either before or during the simulated ischemia. A similar increase was previously noted in isolated neonatal rat cardiomyocytes treated with Gap26 prior to simulated ischemia (Shintani-Ishida et al., 2007). Clearly, both observations underscore the capability of Gap26 to confer protection to cardiomyocytes in the absence of direct intercellular communication, precisely through GJC, and therefore point to the inhibition of unapposed Hc as the underlying mechanism of cardioprotection. Altogether, these results strongly suggest that the observed cardioprotection conferred by Gap26 is most likely mediated by the specific inhibition of Cx43Hc opened by the ischemic stress.

6. Perspective

The non-junctional Cx43 have previously been associated with ischemic preconditioning-mediated cardioprotection (Li et al., 2004; Padilla et al., 2003). This effect has been related to increase in Cx43 phosphorylation (Hatanaka et al., 2004; Hund et al., 2007; Miura et al., 2004; Schulz et al., 2003). Interestingly, different studies pointed to the isozyme εPKC as a principal mediator of ischemic preconditioning-mediated cardioprotection (Gray et al., 1997; Hund et al., 2007; Inagaki et al., 2003; Liu et al., 1999; Ping et al., 1997; Saurin et al., 2002). Here, we showed using a unique set of PKC isozyme-specific modulator peptides that εPKC, among other PKC isozymes, selectively inhibits the conductance of Cx43Hc. These data prompt us to believe that inhibition of Cx43Hc represents a fundamental basis for the cardioprotection conferred by ischemic preconditioning. In the light of our findings using Cx43 mimetic peptide Gap26 and given the ubiquitous expression of PKC and the abundance of its substrates within cells and throughout tissues, we put forth that the selective inhibition of the abnormally open Cx43Hc, which we believe are solely localized in the ischemic region of the heart, would be more suitable to mimic pharmacologically the cardioprotection conferred by ischemic preconditioning than to modulate PKC isozymes as previously proposed (Chen et al., 2001a; Chen et al., 2001b). The accessibility of CxMP binding sites from extracellular space, which circumvents the need of conjugating the peptides with transmembrane carriers and the limitations deriving from their use, is indeed another therapeutic advantage over the use of intracellular modulators. Certainly, studies using more elaborated experimental models are needed to substantiate the therapeutic potentials of Gap26.

7. Conclusion

In conclusion, we demonstrate for the first time that administration of Gap26 prior to ischemia prevents injury by making intact heart more resistant to ischemic stress. Moreover, usage of Gap26 as a treatment following occurrence of ischemia reduces cardiac tissue damage and improves intact heart function. The discovery of new agents capable to make heart more resistant to ischemia and/or to improve its recovery after injury caused by ischemia will certainly be promising tools to fight ischemic heart disease.

8. Acknowledgements

This work was supported by grants from Heart and Stroke Foundation of Québec [G-07-BA-2924], the Fonds de Recherche en Santé du Québec [13836], and the Natural Science and Engineering Research Council [341794-07]. Dr. G. Baroudi is a research scholar of the FRSQ.

9. References

Armstrong, S., Downey, J.M., & Ganote, C.E. (1994). Preconditioning of isolated rabbit cardiomyocytes: induction by metabolic stress and blockade by the adenosine antagonist SPT and calphostin C, a protein kinase C inhibitor. *Cardiovasc.Res.*, Vol.28, No. 1, pp. (72-77).

Armstrong, S.C., Kao, R., Gao, W., Shivell, L.C., Downey, J.M., Honkanen, R.E., & Ganote, C.E. (1997). Comparison of in vitro preconditioning responses of isolated pig and rabbit cardiomyocytes: effects of a protein phosphatase inhibitor, fostriecin. *J Mol.Cell Cardiol.*, Vol.29, No. 11, pp. (3009-3024).

Avkiran, M. (1999). Protection of the myocardium during ischemia and reperfusion : Na(+)/H(+) exchange inhibition versus ischemic preconditioning. *Circulation*, Vol.100, No. 25, pp. (2469-2472).

Bao, X., Altenberg, G.A., & Reuss, L. (2004a). Mechanism of regulation of the gap junction protein connexin 43 by protein kinase C-mediated phosphorylation. *Am.J Physiol Cell Physiol*, Vol.286, No. 3, pp. (C647-C654).

Bao, X., Lee, S.C., Reuss, L., & Altenberg, G.A. (2007). Change in permeant size selectivity by phosphorylation of connexin 43 gap-junctional hemichannels by PKC. *Proc.Natl.Acad.Sci.U.S.A*,

Bao, X., Reuss, L., & Altenberg, G.A. (2004b). Regulation of purified and reconstituted connexin 43 hemichannels by protein kinase C-mediated phosphorylation of Serine 368. *J.Biol.Chem.*, Vol.279, No. 19, pp. (20058-20066).

Bar-Am, O., Amit, T., & Youdim, M.B. (2007). Aminoindan and hydroxyaminoindan, metabolites of rasagiline and ladostigil, respectively, exert neuroprotective properties in vitro. *J.Neurochem.*, Vol.103, No. 2, pp. (500-508).

Baroudi, G., Qu, Y., Ramadan, O., Chahine, M., & Boutjdir, M. (2006). Protein kinase C activation inhibits Cav1.3 calcium channel at NH2-terminal serine 81 phosphorylation site. *Am.J Physiol Heart Circ.Physiol*, Vol.291, No. 4, pp. (H1614-H1622).

Barry, W.H. & Bridge, J.H. (1993). Intracellular calcium homeostasis in cardiac myocytes. *Circulation*, Vol.87, No. 6, pp. (1806-1815).

Beardslee, M.A., Lerner, D.L., Tadros, P.N., Laing, J.G., Beyer, E.C., Yamada, K.A., Kleber, A.G., Schuessler, R.B., & Saffitz, J.E. (2000). Dephosphorylation and intracellular redistribution of ventricular connexin43 during electrical uncoupling induced by ischemia. *Circ.Res.*, Vol.87, No. 8, pp. (656-662).

Bennett, M.V., Contreras, J.E., Bukauskas, F.F., & Saez, J.C. (2003). New roles for astrocytes: gap junction hemichannels have something to communicate. *Trends Neurosci.*, Vol.26, No. 11, pp. (610-617).

Beyer, E.C., Paul, D.L., & Goodenough, D.A. (1987). Connexin43: a protein from rat heart homologous to a gap junction protein from liver. *J Cell Biol*, Vol.105, No. 6 Pt 1, pp. (2621-2629).

Bowling, N., Huang, X., Sandusky, G.E., Fouts, R.L., Mintze, K., Esterman, M., Allen, P.D., Maddi, R., McCall, E., & Vlahos, C.J. (2001). Protein kinase C-alpha and -epsilon modulate connexin-43 phosphorylation in human heart. *J.Mol.Cell Cardiol.*, Vol.33, No. 4, pp. (789-798).

Braet, K., Aspeslagh, S., Vandamme, W., Willecke, K., Martin, P.E., Evans, W.H., & Leybaert, L. (2003a). Pharmacological sensitivity of ATP release triggered by photoliberation of inositol-1,4,5-trisphosphate and zero extracellular calcium in brain endothelial cells. *J Cell Physiol*, Vol.197, No. 2, pp. (205-213).

Braet, K., Vandamme, W., Martin, P.E., Evans, W.H., & Leybaert, L. (2003b). Photoliberating inositol-1,4,5-trisphosphate triggers ATP release that is blocked by the connexin mimetic peptide gap 26. *Cell Calcium*, Vol.33, No. 1, pp. (37-48).

Bruzzone, S., Guida, L., Zocchi, E., Franco, L., & De Flora, A. (2001). Connexin 43 hemi channels mediate Ca2+-regulated transmembrane NAD+ fluxes in intact cells. *FASEB J*, Vol.15, No. 1, pp. (10-12).

Bukauskas, F.F., Kreuzberg, M.M., Rackauskas, M., Bukauskiene, A., Bennett, M.V., Verselis, V.K., & Willecke, K. (2006). Properties of mouse connexin 30.2 and human connexin 31.9 hemichannels: Implications for atrioventricular conduction in the heart. *Proc.Natl.Acad.Sci.U.S.A*, Vol.103, No. 25, pp. (9726-9731).

Burt, J.M. & Spray, D.C. (1988). Inotropic agents modulate gap junctional conductance between cardiac myocytes. *Am.J Physiol*, Vol.254, No. 6 Pt 2, pp. (H1206-H1210).

Casellini, C.M., Barlow, P.M., Rice, A.L., Casey, M., Simmons, K., Pittenger, G., Bastyr, E.J., III, Wolka, A.M., & Vinik, A.I. (2007). A 6-month, randomized, double-masked, placebo-controlled study evaluating the effects of the protein kinase C-beta inhibitor ruboxistaurin on skin microvascular blood flow and other measures of diabetic peripheral neuropathy. *Diabetes Care*, Vol.30, No. 4, pp. (896-902).

Chan, E.K., Di Donato, F., Hamel, J.C., Tseng, C.E., & Buyon, J.P. (1995). 52-kD SS-A/Ro: genomic structure and identification of an alternatively spliced transcript encoding a novel leucine zipper-minus autoantigen expressed in fetal and adult heart. *J.Exp.Med.*, Vol.182, No. 4, pp. (983-992).

Chen, B.P., Mao, H.J., Fan, F.Y., Bruce, I.C., & Xia, Q. (2005). Delayed uncoupling contributes to the protective effect of heptanol against ischaemia in the rat isolated heart. *Clin.Exp.Pharmacol.Physiol*, Vol.32, No. 8, pp. (655-662).

Chen, C.H., Gray, M.O., & Mochly-Rosen, D. (1999). Cardioprotection from ischemia by a brief exposure to physiological levels of ethanol: role of epsilon protein kinase C. *Proc.Natl.Acad.Sci.U.S.A*, Vol.96, No. 22, pp. (12784-12789).

Chen, L., Hahn, H., Wu, G., Chen, C.H., Liron, T., Schechtman, D., Cavallaro, G., Banci, L., Guo, Y., Bolli, R., Dorn, G.W., & Mochly-Rosen, D. (2001a). Opposing cardioprotective actions and parallel hypertrophic effects of delta PKC and epsilon PKC. *Proc.Natl.Acad.Sci.U.S.A*, Vol.98, No. 20, pp. (11114-11119).

Chen, L., Wright, L.R., Chen, C.H., Oliver, S.F., Wender, P.A., & Mochly-Rosen, D. (2001b). Molecular transporters for peptides: delivery of a cardioprotective epsilonPKC agonist peptide into cells and intact ischemic heart using a transport system, R(7). *Chem Biol*, Vol.8, No. 12, pp. (1123-1129).

Chou, W.H. & Messing, R.O. (2005). Protein kinase C isozymes in stroke. *Trends Cardiovasc.Med.*, Vol.15, No. 2, pp. (47-51).

Clarke, T.C., Williams, O.J., Martin, P.E., & Evans, W.H. (2009). ATP release by cardiac myocytes in a simulated ischaemia model: inhibition by a connexin mimetic and enhancement by an antiarrhythmic peptide. *Eur.J.Pharmacol.*, Vol.605, No. 1-3, pp. (9-14).

Clerk, A., Bogoyevitch, M.A., Anderson, M.B., & Sugden, P.H. (1994). Differential activation of protein kinase C isoforms by endothelin-1 and phenylephrine and subsequent stimulation of p42 and p44 mitogen-activated protein kinases in ventricular myocytes cultured from neonatal rat hearts. *J Biol Chem*, Vol.269, No. 52, pp. (32848-32857).

Clerk, A. & Sugden, P.H. (2001). Untangling the Web: specific signaling from PKC isoforms to MAPK cascades. *Circ.Res.*, Vol.89, No. 10, pp. (847-849).

Cohen, M.V., Liu, G.S., & Downey, J.M. (1991). Preconditioning causes improved wall motion as well as smaller infarcts after transient coronary occlusion in rabbits. *Circulation*, Vol.84, No. 1, pp. (341-349).

Contreras, J.E., Saez, J.C., Bukauskas, F.F., & Bennett, M.V. (2003). Gating and regulation of connexin 43 (Cx43) hemichannels. *Proc.Natl.Acad.Sci.U.S.A*, Vol.100, No. 20, pp. (11388-11393).

Contreras, J.E., Sanchez, H.A., Eugenin, E.A., Speidel, D., Theis, M., Willecke, K., Bukauskas, F.F., Bennett, M.V., & Saez, J.C. (2002). Metabolic inhibition induces opening of unapposed connexin 43 gap junction hemichannels and reduces gap junctional communication in cortical astrocytes in culture. *Proc.Natl.Acad.Sci.U.S.A*, Vol.99, No. 1, pp. (495-500).

Cotrina, M.L., Lin, J.H., Alves-Rodrigues, A., Liu, S., Li, J., Azmi-Ghadimi, H., Kang, J., Naus, C.C., & Nedergaard, M. (1998). Connexins regulate calcium signaling by controlling ATP release. *Proc.Natl.Acad.Sci.U.S.A*, Vol.95, No. 26, pp. (15735-15740).

Cottrell, G.T., Lin, R., Warn-Cramer, B.J., Lau, A.F., & Burt, J.M. (2003). Mechanism of v-Src- and mitogen-activated protein kinase-induced reduction of gap junction communication. *Am.J Physiol Cell Physiol*, Vol.284, No. 2, pp. (C511-C520).

Dahl, G. (2007). Gap junction-mimetic peptides do work, but in unexpected ways. *Cell Commun.Adhes.*, Vol.14, No. 6, pp. (259-264).

Dahl, G., Nonner, W., & Werner, R. (1994). Attempts to define functional domains of gap junction proteins with synthetic peptides. *Biophys.J*, Vol.67, No. 5, pp. (1816-1822).

Dahl, G., Werner, R., Levine, E., & Rabadan-Diehl, C. (1992). Mutational analysis of gap junction formation. *Biophys.J*, Vol.62, No. 1, pp. (172-180).

De Vuyst, E., Decrock, E., Cabooter, L., Dubyak, G.R., Naus, C.C., Evans, W.H., & Leybaert, L. (2006). Intracellular calcium changes trigger connexin 32 hemichannel opening. *EMBO J*, Vol.25, No. 1, pp. (34-44).

DeVries, S.H. & Schwartz, E.A. (1992). Hemi-gap-junction channels in solitary horizontal cells of the catfish retina. *J Physiol*, Vol.445, pp. (201-230).

Doble, B.W., Ping, P., & Kardami, E. (2000). The epsilon subtype of protein kinase C is required for cardiomyocyte connexin-43 phosphorylation. *Circ.Res.*, Vol.86, No. 3, pp. (293-301).

Dorn, G.W., Souroujon, M.C., Liron, T., Chen, C.H., Gray, M.O., Zhou, H.Z., Csukai, M., Wu, G., Lorenz, J.N., & Mochly-Rosen, D. (1999). Sustained in vivo cardiac protection by a rationally designed peptide that causes epsilon protein kinase C translocation. *Proc.Natl.Acad.Sci.U.S.A*, Vol.96, No. 22, pp. (12798-12803).

Duncan, J.C. & Fletcher, W.H. (2002). alpha 1 Connexin (connexin43) gap junctions and activities of cAMP-dependent protein kinase and protein kinase C in developing mouse heart. *Dev.Dyn.*, Vol.223, No. 1, pp. (96-107).

Ebihara, L. & Steiner, E. (1993). Properties of a nonjunctional current expressed from a rat connexin46 cDNA in Xenopus oocytes. *J Gen.Physiol*, Vol.102, No. 1, pp. (59-74).

Ek-Vitorin, J.F., Calero, G., Morley, G.E., Coombs, W., Taffet, S.M., & Delmar, M. (1996). PH regulation of connexin43: molecular analysis of the gating particle. *Biophys.J*, Vol.71, No. 3, pp. (1273-1284).

Evans, W.H., De Vuyst, E., & Leybaert, L. (2006). The gap junction cellular internet: connexin hemichannels enter the signalling limelight. *Biochem.J*, Vol.397, No. 1, pp. (1-14).

Garcia-Dorado, D., Inserte, J., Ruiz-Meana, M., Gonzalez, M.A., Solares, J., Julia, M., Barrabes, J.A., & Soler-Soler, J. (1997). Gap junction uncoupler heptanol prevents cell-to-cell progression of hypercontracture and limits necrosis during myocardial reperfusion. *Circulation*, Vol.96, No. 10, pp. (3579-3586).

Garcia-Dorado, D., Rodriguez-Sinovas, A., & Ruiz-Meana, M. (2004). Gap junction-mediated spread of cell injury and death during myocardial ischemia-reperfusion. *Cardiovasc.Res.*, Vol.61, No. 3, pp. (386-401).

Gomes, P., Srinivas, S.P., Van Driessche, W., Vereecke, J., & Himpens, B. (2005). ATP release through connexin hemichannels in corneal endothelial cells. *Invest Ophthalmol.Vis.Sci.*, Vol.46, No. 4, pp. (1208-1218).

Gomez-Hernandez, J.M., de Miguel, M., Larrosa, B., Gonzalez, D., & Barrio, L.C. (2003). Molecular basis of calcium regulation in connexin-32 hemichannels. *Proc.Natl.Acad.Sci.U.S.A*, Vol.100, No. 26, pp. (16030-16035).

Goodenough, D.A. & Paul, D.L. (2003). Beyond the gap: functions of unpaired connexon channels. *Nat.Rev.Mol.Cell Biol.*, Vol.4, No. 4, pp. (285-294).

Gottlieb, R.A., Burleson, K.O., Kloner, R.A., Babior, B.M., & Engler, R.L. (1994). Reperfusion injury induces apoptosis in rabbit cardiomyocytes. *J.Clin.Invest*, Vol.94, No. 4, pp. (1621-1628).

Gray, M.O., Karliner, J.S., & Mochly-Rosen, D. (1997). A selective epsilon-protein kinase C antagonist inhibits protection of cardiac myocytes from hypoxia-induced cell death. *J.Biol.Chem.*, Vol.272, No. 49, pp. (30945-30951).

Gross, G.J. & Fryer, R.M. (1999). Sarcolemmal versus mitochondrial ATP-sensitive K+ channels and myocardial preconditioning. *Circ.Res.*, Vol.84, No. 9, pp. (973-979).

Gupta, V.K., Berthoud, V.M., Atal, N., Jarillo, J.A., Barrio, L.C., & Beyer, E.C. (1994). Bovine connexin44, a lens gap junction protein: molecular cloning, immunologic characterization, and functional expression. *Invest Ophthalmol.Vis.Sci.*, Vol.35, No. 10, pp. (3747-3758).

Hahn, H.S., Yussman, M.G., Toyokawa, T., Marreez, Y., Barrett, T.J., Hilty, K.C., Osinska, H., Robbins, J., & Dorn, G.W. (2002). Ischemic protection and myofibrillar cardiomyopathy: dose-dependent effects of in vivo deltaPKC inhibition. *Circ.Res.*, Vol.91, No. 8, pp. (741-748).

Hatanaka, K., Kawata, H., Toyofuku, T., & Yoshida, K. (2004). Down-regulation of connexin43 in early myocardial ischemia and protective effect by ischemic preconditioning in rat hearts in vivo. *Jpn.Heart J.*, Vol.45, No. 6, pp. (1007-1019).

Hausenloy, D.J., Maddock, H.L., Baxter, G.F., & Yellon, D.M. (2002). Inhibiting mitochondrial permeability transition pore opening: a new paradigm for myocardial preconditioning? *Cardiovasc.Res.*, Vol.55, No. 3, pp. (534-543).

Hawat, G. & Baroudi, G. (2008). Differential modulation of unapposed connexin 43 hemichannel electrical conductance by protein kinase C isoforms. *Pflugers Arch.*, Vol.456, No. 3, pp. (519-527).

Hawat, G., Benderdour, M., Rousseau, G., & Baroudi, G. (2010). Connexin 43 mimetic peptide Gap26 confers protection to intact heart against myocardial ischemia injury. *Pflugers Arch.*, Vol.460, No. 3, pp. (583-592).

Hertzberg, E.L., Saez, J.C., Corpina, R.A., Roy, C., & Kessler, J.A. (2000). Use of antibodies in the analysis of connexin 43 turnover and phosphorylation. *Methods*, Vol.20, No. 2, pp. (129-139).

Hofer, A. & Dermietzel, R. (1998). Visualization and functional blocking of gap junction hemichannels (connexons) with antibodies against external loop domains in astrocytes. *Glia*, Vol.24, No. 1, pp. (141-154).

Hu, K., Mochly-Rosen, D., & Boutjdir, M. (2000). Evidence for functional role of epsilonPKC isozyme in the regulation of cardiac Ca(2+) channels. *Am.J.Physiol Heart Circ.Physiol*, Vol.279, No. 6, pp. (H2658-H2664).

Hund, T.J., Lerner, D.L., Yamada, K.A., Schuessler, R.B., & Saffitz, J.E. (2007). Protein kinase Cepsilon mediates salutary effects on electrical coupling induced by ischemic preconditioning. *Heart Rhythm.*, Vol.4, No. 9, pp. (1183-1193).

Inagaki, K., Begley, R., Ikeno, F., & Mochly-Rosen, D. (2005). Cardioprotection by epsilon-protein kinase C activation from ischemia: continuous delivery and antiarrhythmic effect of an epsilon-protein kinase C-activating peptide. *Circulation*, Vol.111, No. 1, pp. (44-50).

Inagaki, K., Hahn, H.S., Dorn, G.W., & Mochly-Rosen, D. (2003). Additive protection of the ischemic heart ex vivo by combined treatment with delta-protein kinase C inhibitor and epsilon-protein kinase C activator. *Circulation*, Vol.108, No. 7, pp. (869-875).

Isakson, B.E., Damon, D.N., Day, K.H., Liao, Y., & Duling, B.R. (2006). Connexin40 and connexin43 in mouse aortic endothelium: evidence for coordinated regulation. *Am.J Physiol Heart Circ.Physiol*, Vol.290, No. 3, pp. (H1199-H1205).

Jain, S.K., Schuessler, R.B., & Saffitz, J.E. (2003). Mechanisms of delayed electrical uncoupling induced by ischemic preconditioning. *Circ.Res.*, Vol.92, No. 10, pp. (1138-1144).

Javadov, S.A., Clarke, S., Das, M., Griffiths, E.J., Lim, K.H., & Halestrap, A.P. (2003). Ischaemic preconditioning inhibits opening of mitochondrial permeability transition pores in the reperfused rat heart. *J Physiol*, Vol.549, No. Pt 2, pp. (513-524).

Jennings, R.B., Reimer, K.A., & Steenbergen, C. (1986). Myocardial ischemia revisited. The osmolar load, membrane damage, and reperfusion. *J Mol.Cell Cardiol.*, Vol.18, No. 8, pp. (769-780).

Jeyaraman, M., Tanguy, S., Fandrich, R.R., Lukas, A., & Kardami, E. (2003). Ischemia-induced dephosphorylation of cardiomyocyte connexin-43 is reduced by okadaic acid and calyculin A but not fostriecin. *Mol.Cell Biochem.*, Vol.242, No. 1-2, pp. (129-134).

John, G.R., Scemes, E., Suadicani, S.O., Liu, J.S., Charles, P.C., Lee, S.C., Spray, D.C., & Brosnan, C.F. (1999a). IL-1beta differentially regulates calcium wave propagation between primary human fetal astrocytes via pathways involving P2 receptors and gap junction channels. *Proc.Natl.Acad.Sci.U.S.A*, Vol.96, No. 20, pp. (11613-11618).

John, S.A., Kondo, R., Wang, S.Y., Goldhaber, J.I., & Weiss, J.N. (1999b). Connexin-43 hemichannels opened by metabolic inhibition. *J Biol Chem*, Vol.274, No. 1, pp. (236-240).

Kandasamy, R.A., Yu, F.H., Harris, R., Boucher, A., Hanrahan, J.W., & Orlowski, J. (1995). Plasma membrane Na+/H+ exchanger isoforms (NHE-1, -2, and -3) are differentially responsive to second messenger agonists of the protein kinase A and C pathways. *J Biol Chem*, Vol.270, No. 49, pp. (29209-29216).

Kondo, R.P., Wang, S.Y., John, S.A., Weiss, J.N., & Goldhaber, J.I. (2000). Metabolic inhibition activates a non-selective current through connexin hemichannels in isolated ventricular myocytes. *J Mol.Cell Cardiol.*, Vol.32, No. 10, pp. (1859-1872).

Kwak, B.R. & Jongsma, H.J. (1996). Regulation of cardiac gap junction channel permeability and conductance by several phosphorylating conditions. *Mol.Cell Biochem.*, Vol.157, No. 1-2, pp. (93-99).

Lampe, P.D. & Lau, A.F. (2000). Regulation of gap junctions by phosphorylation of connexins. *Arch.Biochem.Biophys.*, Vol.384, No. 2, pp. (205-215).

Lampe, P.D., TenBroek, E.M., Burt, J.M., Kurata, W.E., Johnson, R.G., & Lau, A.F. (2000). Phosphorylation of connexin43 on serine368 by protein kinase C regulates gap junctional communication. *J.Cell Biol.*, Vol.149, No. 7, pp. (1503-1512).

Lau, A.F., Hatch-Pigott, V., & Crow, D.S. (1991). Evidence that heart connexin43 is a phosphoprotein. *J Mol.Cell Cardiol.*, Vol.23, No. 6, pp. (659-663).

Leaney, J.L., Dekker, L.V., & Tinker, A. (2001). Regulation of a G protein-gated inwardly rectifying K+ channel by a Ca(2+)-independent protein kinase C. *J.Physiol*, Vol.534, No. Pt. 2, pp. (367-379).

Leybaert, L., Braet, K., Vandamme, W., Cabooter, L., Martin, P.E., & Evans, W.H. (2003). Connexin channels, connexin mimetic peptides and ATP release. *Cell Commun.Adhes.*, Vol.10, No. 4-6, pp. (251-257).

Li, F., Sugishita, K., Su, Z., Ueda, I., & Barry, W.H. (2001). Activation of connexin-43 hemichannels can elevate [Ca(2+)]i and [Na(+)]i in rabbit ventricular myocytes during metabolic inhibition. *J Mol.Cell Cardiol.*, Vol.33, No. 12, pp. (2145-2155).

Li, G., Whittaker, P., Yao, M., Kloner, R.A., & Przyklenk, K. (2002). The gap junction uncoupler heptanol abrogates infarct size reduction with preconditioning in mouse hearts. *Cardiovasc.Pathol.*, Vol.11, No. 3, pp. (158-165).

Li, H., Liu, T.F., Lazrak, A., Peracchia, C., Goldberg, G.S., Lampe, P.D., & Johnson, R.G. (1996). Properties and regulation of gap junctional hemichannels in the plasma membranes of cultured cells. *J Cell Biol*, Vol.134, No. 4, pp. (1019-1030).

Li, X., Heinzel, F.R., Boengler, K., Schulz, R., & Heusch, G. (2004). Role of connexin 43 in ischemic preconditioning does not involve intercellular communication through gap junctions. *J Mol.Cell Cardiol.*, Vol.36, No. 1, pp. (161-163).

Liu, G.S., Cohen, M.V., Mochly-Rosen, D., & Downey, J.M. (1999). Protein kinase C-epsilon is responsible for the protection of preconditioning in rabbit cardiomyocytes. *J.Mol.Cell Cardiol.*, Vol.31, No. 10, pp. (1937-1948).

Liu, Y. & O'Rourke, B. (2001). Opening of mitochondrial K(ATP) channels triggers cardioprotection. Are reactive oxygen species involved? *Circ.Res.*, Vol.88, No. 8, pp. (750-752).

Martin, P.E., Wall, C., & Griffith, T.M. (2005). Effects of connexin-mimetic peptides on gap junction functionality and connexin expression in cultured vascular cells. *Br.J Pharmacol.*, Vol.144, No. 5, pp. (617-627).

McDonald, T.F., Pelzer, S., Trautwein, W., & Pelzer, D.J. (1994). Regulation and modulation of calcium channels in cardiac, skeletal, and smooth muscle cells. *Physiol Rev.*, Vol.74, No. 2, pp. (365-507).

Miura, T., Ohnuma, Y., Kuno, A., Tanno, M., Ichikawa, Y., Nakamura, Y., Yano, T., Miki, T., Sakamoto, J., & Shimamoto, K. (2004). Protective role of gap junctions in preconditioning against myocardial infarction. *Am.J Physiol Heart Circ.Physiol*, Vol.286, No. 1, pp. (H214-H221).

Mochly-Rosen, D. & Gordon, A.S. (1998). Anchoring proteins for protein kinase C: a means for isozyme selectivity. *FASEB J.*, Vol.12, No. 1, pp. (35-42).

Morley, G.E., Ek-Vitorin, J.F., Taffet, S.M., & Delmar, M. (1997). Structure of connexin43 and its regulation by pHi. *J Cardiovasc.Electrophysiol.*, Vol.8, No. 8, pp. (939-951).

Murry, C.E., Jennings, R.B., & Reimer, K.A. (1986). Preconditioning with ischemia: a delay of lethal cell injury in ischemic myocardium. *Circulation*, Vol.74, No. 5, pp. (1124-1136).

Musil, L.S., Cunningham, B.A., Edelman, G.M., & Goodenough, D.A. (1990). Differential phosphorylation of the gap junction protein connexin43 in junctional communication-competent and -deficient cell lines. *J Cell Biol*, Vol.111, No. 5 Pt 1, pp. (2077-2088).

Nishizuka, Y. (1988). The molecular heterogeneity of protein kinase C and its implications for cellular regulation. *Nature*, Vol.334, No. 6184, pp. (661-665).

Osada, S., Mizuno, K., Saido, T.C., Suzuki, K., Kuroki, T., & Ohno, S. (1992). A new member of the protein kinase C family, nPKC theta, predominantly expressed in skeletal muscle. *Mol.Cell Biol.*, Vol.12, No. 9, pp. (3930-3938).

Padilla, F., Garcia-Dorado, D., Rodriguez-Sinovas, A., Ruiz-Meana, M., Inserte, J., & Soler-Soler, J. (2003). Protection afforded by ischemic preconditioning is not mediated by effects on cell-to-cell electrical coupling during myocardial ischemia-reperfusion. *Am.J.Physiol Heart Circ.Physiol*, Vol.285, No. 5, pp. (H1909-H1916).

Paul, D.L., Ebihara, L., Takemoto, L.J., Swenson, K.I., & Goodenough, D.A. (1991). Connexin46, a novel lens gap junction protein, induces voltage-gated currents in nonjunctional plasma membrane of Xenopus oocytes. *J Cell Biol*, Vol.115, No. 4, pp. (1077-1089).

Pearson, R.A., Dale, N., Llaudet, E., & Mobbs, P. (2005). ATP released via gap junction hemichannels from the pigment epithelium regulates neural retinal progenitor proliferation. *Neuron*, Vol.46, No. 5, pp. (731-744).

Penna, C., Cappello, S., Mancardi, D., Raimondo, S., Rastaldo, R., Gattullo, D., Losano, G., & Pagliaro, P. (2006a). Post-conditioning reduces infarct size in the isolated rat heart: role of coronary flow and pressure and the nitric oxide/cGMP pathway. *Basic Res.Cardiol.*, Vol.101, No. 2, pp. (168-179).

Penna, C., Rastaldo, R., Mancardi, D., Raimondo, S., Cappello, S., Gattullo, D., Losano, G., & Pagliaro, P. (2006b). Post-conditioning induced cardioprotection requires signaling through a redox-sensitive mechanism, mitochondrial ATP-sensitive K+ channel and protein kinase C activation. *Basic Res.Cardiol.*, Vol.101, No. 2, pp. (180-189).

Pfahnl, A. & Dahl, G. (1999). Gating of cx46 gap junction hemichannels by calcium and voltage. *Pflugers Arch.*, Vol.437, No. 3, pp. (345-353).

Pfahnl, A., Zhou, X.W., Werner, R., & Dahl, G. (1997). A chimeric connexin forming gap junction hemichannels. *Pflugers Arch.*, Vol.433, No. 6, pp. (773-779).

Philipp, S., Yang, X.M., Cui, L., Davis, A.M., Downey, J.M., & Cohen, M.V. (2006). Postconditioning protects rabbit hearts through a protein kinase C-adenosine A2b receptor cascade. *Cardiovasc.Res.*, Vol.70, No. 2, pp. (308-314).

Ping, P., Zhang, J., Pierce, W.M., Jr., & Bolli, R. (2001). Functional proteomic analysis of protein kinase C epsilon signaling complexes in the normal heart and during cardioprotection. *Circ.Res.*, Vol.88, No. 1, pp. (59-62).

Ping, P., Zhang, J., Qiu, Y., Tang, X.L., Manchikalapudi, S., Cao, X., & Bolli, R. (1997). Ischemic preconditioning induces selective translocation of protein kinase C isoforms epsilon and eta in the heart of conscious rabbits without subcellular redistribution of total protein kinase C activity. *Circ.Res.*, Vol.81, No. 3, pp. (404-414).

Plotkin, L.I., Manolagas, S.C., & Bellido, T. (2002). Transduction of cell survival signals by connexin-43 hemichannels. *J Biol Chem*, Vol.277, No. 10, pp. (8648-8657).

Quist, A.P., Rhee, S.K., Lin, H., & Lal, R. (2000). Physiological role of gap-junctional hemichannels. Extracellular calcium-dependent isosmotic volume regulation. *J Cell Biol*, Vol.148, No. 5, pp. (1063-1074).

Rodriguez-Sinovas, A., Boengler, K., Cabestrero, A., Gres, P., Morente, M., Ruiz-Meana, M., Konietzka, I., Miro, E., Totzeck, A., Heusch, G., Schulz, R., & Garcia-Dorado, D. (2006). Translocation of Connexin 43 to the Inner Mitochondrial Membrane of Cardiomyocytes Through the Heat Shock Protein 90-Dependent TOM Pathway and Its Importance for Cardioprotection. *Circ.Res.*,

Romanov, R.A., Rogachevskaja, O.A., Bystrova, M.F., Jiang, P., Margolskee, R.F., & Kolesnikov, S.S. (2007). Afferent neurotransmission mediated by hemichannels in mammalian taste cells. *EMBO J.*, Vol.26, No. 3, pp. (657-667).

Rybin, V.O., Xu, X., & Steinberg, S.F. (1999). Activated protein kinase C isoforms target to cardiomyocyte caveolae : stimulation of local protein phosphorylation. *Circ.Res.*, Vol.84, No. 9, pp. (980-988).

Saez, J.C., Berthoud, V.M., Branes, M.C., Martinez, A.D., & Beyer, E.C. (2003). Plasma membrane channels formed by connexins: their regulation and functions. *Physiol Rev.*, Vol.83, No. 4, pp. (1359-1400).

Saez, J.C., Nairn, A.C., Czernik, A.J., Fishman, G.I., Spray, D.C., & Hertzberg, E.L. (1997). Phosphorylation of connexin43 and the regulation of neonatal rat cardiac myocyte gap junctions. *J.Mol.Cell Cardiol.*, Vol.29, No. 8, pp. (2131-2145).

Saez, J.C., Retamal, M.A., Basilio, D., Bukauskas, F.F., & Bennett, M.V. (2005). Connexin-based gap junction hemichannels: gating mechanisms. *Biochim.Biophys.Acta*, Vol.1711, No. 2, pp. (215-224).

Saez, J.C., Spray, D.C., Nairn, A.C., Hertzberg, E., Greengard, P., & Bennett, M.V. (1986). cAMP increases junctional conductance and stimulates phosphorylation of the 27-kDa principal gap junction polypeptide. *Proc.Natl.Acad.Sci.U.S.A*, Vol.83, No. 8, pp. (2473-2477).

Sato, T. & Marban, E. (2000). The role of mitochondrial K(ATP) channels in cardioprotection. *Basic Res.Cardiol.*, Vol.95, No. 4, pp. (285-289).

Saurin, A.T., Pennington, D.J., Raat, N.J., Latchman, D.S., Owen, M.J., & Marber, M.S. (2002). Targeted disruption of the protein kinase C epsilon gene abolishes the infarct size reduction that follows ischaemic preconditioning of isolated buffer-perfused mouse hearts. *Cardiovasc.Res.*, Vol.55, No. 3, pp. (672-680).

Schulz, R., Gres, P., Skyschally, A., Duschin, A., Belosjorow, S., Konietzka, I., & Heusch, G. (2003). Ischemic preconditioning preserves connexin 43 phosphorylation during sustained ischemia in pig hearts in vivo. *FASEB J*, Vol.17, No. 10, pp. (1355-1357).

Schwanke, U., Konietzka, I., Duschin, A., Li, X., Schulz, R., & Heusch, G. (2002). No ischemic preconditioning in heterozygous connexin43-deficient mice. *Am.J Physiol Heart Circ.Physiol*, Vol.283, No. 4, pp. (H1740-H1742).

Schwanke, U., Li, X., Schulz, R., & Heusch, G. (2003). No ischemic preconditioning in heterozygous connexin 43-deficient mice--a further in vivo study. *Basic Res.Cardiol.*, Vol.98, No. 3, pp. (181-182).

Serova, M., Ghoul, A., Benhadji, K.A., Cvitkovic, E., Faivre, S., Calvo, F., Lokiec, F., & Raymond, E. (2006). Preclinical and clinical development of novel agents that target the protein kinase C family. *Semin.Oncol.*, Vol.33, No. 4, pp. (466-478).

Shi, X., Potvin, B., Huang, T., Hilgard, P., Spray, D.C., Suadicani, S.O., Wolkoff, A.W., Stanley, P., & Stockert, R.J. (2001). A novel casein kinase 2 alpha-subunit regulates membrane protein traffic in the human hepatoma cell line HuH-7. *J Biol Chem*, Vol.276, No. 3, pp. (2075-2082).

Shiki, K. & Hearse, D.J. (1987). Preconditioning of ischemic myocardium: reperfusion-induced arrhythmias. *Am.J Physiol*, Vol.253, No. 6 Pt 2, pp. (H1470-H1476).

Shintani-Ishida, K., Uemura, K., & Yoshida, K. (2007). Hemichannels in cardiomyocytes open transiently during ischemia and contribute to reperfusion injury following brief ischemia. *Am.J.Physiol Heart Circ.Physiol*, Vol.293, No. 3, pp. (H1714-H1720).

Silverman, H.S. & Stern, M.D. (1994). Ionic basis of ischaemic cardiac injury: insights from cellular studies. *Cardiovasc.Res.*, Vol.28, No. 5, pp. (581-597).

Souroujon, M.C. & Mochly-Rosen, D. (1998). Peptide modulators of protein-protein interactions in intracellular signaling. *Nat.Biotechnol.*, Vol.16, No. 10, pp. (919-924).

Spray, D.C. & Burt, J.M. (1990). Structure-activity relations of the cardiac gap junction channel. *Am.J.Physiol*, Vol.258, No. 2 Pt 1, pp. (C195-C205).

Spray, D.C., White, R.L., Mazet, F., & Bennett, M.V. (1985). Regulation of gap junctional conductance. *Am.J Physiol*, Vol.248, No. 6 Pt 2, pp. (H753-H764).

Steenbergen, C., Hill, M.L., & Jennings, R.B. (1985). Volume regulation and plasma membrane injury in aerobic, anaerobic, and ischemic myocardium in vitro. Effects of osmotic cell swelling on plasma membrane integrity. *Circ.Res.*, Vol.57, No. 6, pp. (864-875).

Stout, CE., Costantin, JL., Naus, CC., & Charles, AC. (2002). Intercellular calcium signaling in astrocytes via ATP release through connexin hemichannels. *J Biol Chem*, Vol.277, No. 12, pp. (10482-10488).

Tanaka, M., Gunawan, F., Terry, R.D., Inagaki, K., Caffarelli, A.D., Hoyt, G., Tsao, P.S., Mochly-Rosen, D., & Robbins, R.C. (2005). Inhibition of heart transplant injury and graft coronary artery disease after prolonged organ ischemia by selective protein kinase C regulators. *J Thorac.Cardiovasc.Surg.*, Vol.129, No. 5, pp. (1160-1167).

Tanaka, M., Terry, R.D., Mokhtari, G.K., Inagaki, K., Koyanagi, T., Kofidis, T., Mochly-Rosen, D., & Robbins, R.C. (2004). Suppression of graft coronary artery disease by a brief treatment with a selective epsilonPKC activator and a deltaPKC inhibitor in murine cardiac allografts. *Circulation*, Vol.110, No. 11 Suppl 1, pp. (II194-II199).

Tani, M. & Neely, J.R. (1989). Role of intracellular Na+ in Ca2+ overload and depressed recovery of ventricular function of reperfused ischemic rat hearts. Possible involvement of H+-Na+ and Na+-Ca2+ exchange. *Circ.Res.*, Vol.65, No. 4, pp. (1045-1056).

TenBroek, E.M., Lampe, P.D., Solan, J.L., Reynhout, J.K., & Johnson, R.G. (2001). Ser364 of connexin43 and the upregulation of gap junction assembly by cAMP. *J Cell Biol*, Vol.155, No. 7, pp. (1307-1318).

Tranum-Jensen, J., Janse, M.J., Fiolet, W.T., Krieger, W.J., D'Alnoncourt, C.N., & Durrer, D. (1981). Tissue osmolality, cell swelling, and reperfusion in acute regional myocardial ischemia in the isolated porcine heart. *Circ.Res.*, Vol.49, No. 2, pp. (364-381).

Trexler, E.B., Bennett, M.V., Bargiello, T.A., & Verselis, V.K. (1996). Voltage gating and permeation in a gap junction hemichannel. *Proc.Natl.Acad.Sci.U.S.A*, Vol.93, No. 12, pp. (5836-5841).

Valiunas, V. (2002). Biophysical properties of connexin-45 gap junction hemichannels studied in vertebrate cells. *J Gen.Physiol*, Vol.119, No. 2, pp. (147-164).

van Veen, A.A., van Rijen, H.V., & Opthof, T. (2001). Cardiac gap junction channels: modulation of expression and channel properties. *Cardiovasc.Res.*, Vol.51, No. 2, pp. (217-229).

VanSlyke, J.K. & Musil, L.S. (2000). Analysis of connexin intracellular transport and assembly. *Methods*, Vol.20, No. 2, pp. (156-164).

Vergara, L., Bao, X., Cooper, M., Bello-Reuss, E., & Reuss, L. (2003). Gap-junctional hemichannels are activated by ATP depletion in human renal proximal tubule cells. *J Membr.Biol*, Vol.196, No. 3, pp. (173-184).

Verma, V., Hallett, M.B., Leybaert, L., Martin, P.E., & Evans, W.H. (2009). Perturbing plasma membrane hemichannels attenuates calcium signalling in cardiac cells and HeLa cells expressing connexins. *Eur.J.Cell Biol.*, Vol.88, No. 2, pp. (79-90).

Wang, J., Ma, M., Locovei, S., Keane, R.W., & Dahl, G. (2007). Modulation of membrane channel currents by gap junction protein mimetic peptides: size matters. *Am.J.Physiol Cell Physiol*, Vol.293, No. 3, pp. (C1112-C1119).

Wang, Y. & Ashraf, M. (1999). Role of protein kinase C in mitochondrial KATP channel-mediated protection against Ca2+ overload injury in rat myocardium. *Circ.Res.*, Vol.84, No. 10, pp. (1156-1165).

Warn-Cramer, B.J., Cottrell, G.T., Burt, J.M., & Lau, A.F. (1998). Regulation of connexin-43 gap junctional intercellular communication by mitogen-activated protein kinase. *J Biol Chem*, Vol.273, No. 15, pp. (9188-9196).

Warner, A., Clements, D.K., Parikh, S., Evans, W.H., & DeHaan, R.L. (1995). Specific motifs in the external loops of connexin proteins can determine gap junction formation between chick heart myocytes. *J Physiol*, Vol.488 (Pt 3), pp. (721-728).

Weiss, J.N., Korge, P., Honda, H.M., & Ping, P. (2003). Role of the mitochondrial permeability transition in myocardial disease. *Circ.Res.*, Vol.93, No. 4, pp. (292-301).

White, T.W., Deans, M.R., O'Brien, J., Al Ubaidi, M.R., Goodenough, D.A., Ripps, H., & Bruzzone, R. (1999). Functional characteristics of skate connexin35, a member of the gamma subfamily of connexins expressed in the vertebrate retina. *Eur.J Neurosci.*, Vol.11, No. 6, pp. (1883-1890).

Willecke, K., Eiberger, J., Degen, J., Eckardt, D., Romualdi, A., Guldenagel, M., Deutsch, U., & Sohl, G. (2002). Structural and functional diversity of connexin genes in the mouse and human genome. *Biol.Chem.*, Vol.383, No. 5, pp. (725-737).

Xiao, G.Q., Mochly-Rosen, D., & Boutjdir, M. (2003). PKC isozyme selective regulation of cloned human cardiac delayed slow rectifier K current. *Biochem.Biophys.Res.Commun.*, Vol.306, No. 4, pp. (1019-1025).

Xiao, G.Q., Qu, Y., Sun, Z.Q., Mochly-Rosen, D., & Boutjdir, M. (2001). Evidence for functional role of epsilonPKC isozyme in the regulation of cardiac Na(+) channels. *Am.J.Physiol Cell Physiol*, Vol.281, No. 5, pp. (C1477-C1486).

Xiao, X.H. & Allen, D.G. (2000). Activity of the Na(+)/H(+) exchanger is critical to reperfusion damage and preconditioning in the isolated rat heart. *Cardiovasc.Res.*, Vol.48, No. 2, pp. (244-253).

Ytrehus, K., Liu, Y., & Downey, J.M. (1994). Preconditioning protects ischemic rabbit heart by protein kinase C activation. *Am.J.Physiol*, Vol.266, No. 3 Pt 2, pp. (H1145-H1152).

Zatta, A.J., Kin, H., Lee, G., Wang, N., Jiang, R., Lust, R., Reeves, J.G., Mykytenko, J., Guyton, R.A., Zhao, Z.Q., & Vinten-Johansen, J. (2006). Infarct-sparing effect of myocardial postconditioning is dependent on protein kinase C signalling. *Cardiovasc.Res.*, Vol.70, No. 2, pp. (315-324).

Zhao, Z.Q., Nakamura, M., Wang, N.P., Wilcox, J.N., Shearer, S., Ronson, R.S., Guyton, R.A., & Vinten-Johansen, J. (2000). Reperfusion induces myocardial apoptotic cell death. *Cardiovasc.Res.*, Vol.45, No. 3, pp. (651-660).

Zipes , D.P. & Jalife , J. (2004). Gap junction distribution and regulation in the heart. *Cardiac Electrophysiology: From Cell to Bedside.Fourth Edition.Philadelphia: WB Saunders.*, pp. (181-191).

Zoidl, G., Bruzzone, R., Weickert, S., Kremer, M., Zoidl, C., Mitropoulou, G., Srinivas, M., Spray, D.C., & Dermietzel, R. (2004). Molecular cloning and functional expression of zfCx52.6: a novel connexin with hemichannel-forming properties expressed in horizontal cells of the zebrafish retina. *J Biol Chem*, Vol.279, No. 4, pp. (2913-2921).

Zorko, M. & Langel, U. (2005). Cell-penetrating peptides: mechanism and kinetics of cargo delivery. *Adv.Drug Deliv.Rev.*, Vol.57, No. 4, pp. (529-545).

11

Myocardial Ischemia: Alterations in Myocardial Cellular Energy and Diastolic Function, a Potential Role for D-Ribose

Linda M. Shecterle and J. A. St. Cyr
Jacqmar, Inc., Minneapolis, MN
USA

1. Introduction

Cardiovascular disease still remains the leading cause of deaths worldwide in both males and females. A variety of factors have been associated to play a role in the development of this disease, such as an individual's genetic background and continual life style factors. Life style factors (including diet) have greatly influenced the occurrence and progression of this disease. The medical profession has made great efforts to adequately address and to continually stress to their patients an altered life style to confront the non-genetic factors, in order to potentially minimize their risk for cardiovascular disease. This campaign has centered on a continual direction for refinements in diet, regular exercise, smoking cessation, and to control blood pressure to lower their risk for cardiovascular disease.

The World Health Organization has reported that approximately 17 million people die of cardiovascular diseases, including myocardial infarcts and strokes, every year. [1] The most common type of cardiovascular disease is atherosclerosis, which has shown to progress overtime. This progression involves the narrowing of our arteries, which ultimately limits the delivery of oxygen to viable tissue beds. [2] Atherosclerosis is not confined to a sole anatomic region; for it can eventually progress to involve many arterial vessels in our circulation, producing not only heart disease, but cerebrovascular and peripheral vascular devastating pathological sequelae. Financially, cardiovascular diseases have taxed economies and current trends have shown its continued burden on healthcare dollars worldwide.

The progression of coronary arterial atherosclerosis has the potential to eventually produce myocardial ischemia, reflected in clinical symptoms of angina or chest pain. This atherosclerotic state produces a decrease in blood flow to the myocardium, producing a decrease availability of oxygenated blood to these muscular regions of the heart. Clinically, patients afflicted with coronary artery disease/myocardial ischemia can experience symptoms of angina or chest pain, commonly during and following stressful situations; however, some unfortunately can even have episodes at rest. Furthermore, with the progression of coronary artery disease and the development of significant coronary arterial atherosclerosis, patients are susceptible of sustaining an acute myocardial infarction or live with a chronic, debilitating condition, which has the potential of advancing into the development of heart failure.

Along with significant myocardial ischemic coronary arterial disease, many patients can experience functional abnormalities, such as diastolic dysfunction or an abnormality in ventricular relaxation. This ventricular dysfunctional condition has continued to be a challenging clinical problem for physicians because as of today, there is not yet an approved effective, solely directed therapy for myocardial diastolic dysfunction. Current medical investigations have found that left ventricular diastolic dysfunction is more prevalent than expected. Redfield et al. reported in 2042 randomly selected adults over the age of 45 that 21% had mild and 7% had at least moderate diastolic dysfunction. Six percent had moderate or severe diastolic dysfunction with a normal ejection fraction. [3] This has been supported by additional published studies that have shown that diastolic dysfunction exists with its prevalence varying with age. Fischer et al. found diastolic dysfunction in 2.8% of individuals between 25-35 years of age and increasing to 15.8% among those older than 65 years of age. Compared to women, men had a higher rate of diastolic abnormalities (13.8% vs. 8.6%). Factors associated with diastolic abnormalities have included arterial hypertension, evidence of left ventricular hypertrophy and coronary artery disease. Additionally, diastolic dysfunction has been related to a higher body mass index, high body fat and diabetes mellitus. [4] Unfortunately, when diastolic dysfunction develops early in the post myocardial infarction clinical period, these patients tend to have a poorer outcome.

Myocardial ischemia is a common entity in the development of congestive heart failure (CHF) and many of these patients will have a component of diastolic dysfunction. Clinically, at least half of patients diagnosed with CHF will have a degree of diastolic dysfunction solely or in combination with systolic dysfunction. These CHF patients with diastolic dysfunction can have a challenging therapeutic course and a less favorable clinical outlook. Ingwall and Weiss proposed that the failing heart is energy starved. However, this theory is not novel. This theory was previously proposed, but was not actively pursued because it was unclear whether ATP levels really decreased and if these levels did decrease in the failing heart, then the remaining pool of ATP compounds should be sufficient to satisfy myocardial ATP-requiring reactions. [5] Currently, there appears to be renewed interest in this hypothesis; that the failing heart is energy starved. The advancement in biophysical tools, such as nuclear magnetic resonance (NMR) spectroscopy and positron emission tomography (PET) scans have aided in providing a better understanding of this myocardial energy/functional relationship.

2. Cellular energy and function during and following myocardial ischemia: A potential role for D-ribose

2.1 Pre-clinical investigations

All cells require high energy phosphates, predominantly ATP, to maintain their integrity and function. Normally, the cellular supply of ATP meets tissue demands. Glycolysis and the tricarboxylic acid cycle pathways produce ATP compounds with glucose as the starting substrate. However, cells can also rely on alternative pathways, such as the hexose monophosphate shunt or pentose phosphate pathway for the production of energy molecules. [6] As stated, the supply of ATP is essential to preserve cellular cardiac energy and function; and without these levels of ATP, a myocyte's integrity and function is jeopardized. When myocytes are subjected to ischemia, there is a depletion in energy stores, which can potentially decrease intracellular reactions, including cellular function. Obviously, if this ischemic insult is severe enough, viability can be affected. Besides this assumed immediate depletion in ATP levels, numerous studies have shown that this depletion in myocardial ATP levels from ischemia lasts for a considerable time period due to slow adenine nucleotide synthesis, of which this delay in ATP recovery is reflected in abnormal function. [7] Because of these published findings, future developed methods directed at enhancing the recovery of this energy deficiency due to ischemia should strongly be considered in the therapeutic management of myocardial ischemic diseases.

There is a direct interaction between adequate myocardial ATP levels and the development of ventricular dysfunction, predominantly diastolic dysfunction. Calcium plays a major role in this interaction, which is an energy dependent process. Adenosine triphosphate provides the energy for this interaction between cytosolic calcium and the sarcoplasmic reticulum. Depleted ATP levels can result in calcium remaining fixed to troponin longer in diastole, producing a state of diastolic dysfunction or altered ventricular compliance. Following ischemia, a return in diastolic function may be limited by the availability of the high energy phosphate, ATP. [8] Theoretically, efforts to maximize the recovery of myocardial ATP levels during and following ischemia could aid in minimizing the functional untoward effects following ischemia.

Research over decades has explored the relationship of myocardial ATP levels during and following ischemia. Most of these initial myocardial ischemic studies involved acute isolated heart models, mainly Langendorff or Neely preparations. Reibel and Rovetto reported in isolated perfused rat hearts that a moderate ischemic insult (10-30 minutes) resulted in a 50-70% decrease in myocardial ATP levels. [9] The recovery of myocardial ATP levels following ischemia is not prompt with reperfusion. Hours to days are required for substantial recovery, depending upon the degree of the ischemic insult. Kloner et al. found that the recovery of ATP compounds after 15 minutes of coronary occlusion in the healthy canine heart was only 75% restored after three days with one week required for full recovery. [10] Likewise, Zimmer concurred that an extended time period is required for the recovery of depressed myocardial energy levels, as well as a measured improvement in the alteration in mechanical function following ischemia. [11] Even though these isolated myocardial experimental models have provided important findings, they have limitations due to the nature of the isolated heart preparation. Therefore, experiments involving an intact animal model would be essential to support these initial isolated heart preparation findings. Short term investigations involving an intact animal model found similar findings in measured myocardial adenine nucleotide levels following ischemia. Twelve to 30 minutes of myocardial ischemia produced a substantial drop in ATP levels with a significant decrease in total adenine nucleotides, and days were required for total recovery. [12]

However, to fully appreciate this important energy-functional relationship, a chronic animal model to measure both myocardial energy levels and function would be ideal to better understand the long term effects of ischemia. A chronic canine animal model was developed to provide the means for long term assessment of myocardial energy levels and function during and following ischemia. [13-15] Using this chronic model, 20 minutes of normothermic myocardial ischemia produced a significant decrease (approximately 50%) in ATP levels, which was accompanied with a state of left ventricular diastolic dysfunction. Furthermore, the data from this chronic animal study confirmed that the effects of myocardial ischemia have a long term effect. Researchers reported that there was a substantial delay, over one week, in myocardial energy levels and functional recovery following a moderate, reversible ischemic insult. [13-15]

Ward et al. reported that myocardial precursor availability is an important limiting factor in the recovery of myocardial ATP molecules following an ischemic insult. [15] Many researchers have investigated various substrates and methods in replenishing depressed levels of ATP following ischemia. Investigations with adenine nucleotide precursor substrates have included adenosine, 5-amino-4-imidazolecarboxamide riboside, inosine, adenine, D-ribose, as well as an adenine degradative enzymatic inhibitor (erythro-9-(2-hydroxy-3-nonyladenine hydrochloride). However, these studies have reported mixed results in the recovery of energy molecules and function following ischemia. The majority of these precursors have at best shown a minimal improvement in both ATP recovery and function. However, this was not the case when investigating the effects of D-ribose during and following myocardial ischemia. D-ribose, a natural occurring pentose carbohydrate, supplementation demonstrated in numerous animal studies its significant benefit in enhancing the return in ATP levels and improved function following global and regional myocardial ischemia. Zimmer and Gerlach reported that supplementation with D-ribose in adult, isolated rat hearts resulted in an increase rate of adenine nucleotide synthesis. [16] Pasque et al. found similar results in isolated, perfused, working rat hearts subjected to 15 minutes of ischemia, followed by 2-15 minutes of myocardial work. D-ribose supplementation improved the recovery in myocardial ATP levels along with a mean percent improvement in functional recovery. [17] St. Cyr et al. also observed the benefits of D-ribose and adenine in a chronic animal model. Supplementation with D-ribose and adenine following 20 minutes of global ischemia resulted in 85% return in ATP levels as compared to no ATP recovery without D-ribose and adenine. [18]

In the same chronic canine model design described by St.Cyr et al. with additional functional instrumentation, Schneider et al. reported similar ATP benefits with D-ribose and adenine, as well as improvements in left ventricular non-compliance/diastolic dysfunction following 20 minutes of global myocardial ischemia. [13,19] Further investigations revealed the sole benefits of D-ribose during and following ischemia. Tveter et al. investigated the benefits of D-ribose alone in a chronic canine model, in which hearts were subjected to a moderate (20 minutes) global myocardial ischemic insult. They found that D-ribose solely produced similar benefits in both myocardial energy levels and functional recovery following global ischemia, as was previously reported with D-ribose and adenine. [20] D-ribose appeared to solely enhance the recovery of myocardial adenine nucleotide levels, improve diastolic dysfunction and the adenine nucleotide pool following ischemia.

A significant restrictive or narrowing of a coronary arter(ies) can potentially result in an acute occlusion or an acute myocardial infarct, for which myocardial dysfunction post infarct can be present. Following infarction, some of these hearts can experience a continual decline in function, leading to the development of heart failure. The remote myocardium not involved in the infarcted tissue is subjected to an increased workload, which can severely tax its myocardial energy supply, which over time can affect remodeling. Zimmer et al. reported in adult rats that a decline in left ventricular hemodynamics occurs following myocardial infarction. They observed a progressive decline in left ventricular systolic pressure, a decline in left ventricular dP/dt_{max}, elevated left ventricular end diastolic pressure, and lower cardiac outputs and stroke volume indices post infarction. Upon supplying the substrate D-ribose, there was an improvement in the above measured left ventricular hemodynamic parameters with stimulation in adenine nucleotide synthesis. [21] Likewise, Befera et al. observed similar findings with the supplementation of D-ribose following acute myocardial infarction in adult rats. They found an improvement in left ventricular function in the remote left ventricular areas when supplying D-ribose. There was increased contractility and myocardial wall thickness with less ventricular dilatation with D-ribose supplementation. [22]

These two pre-clinical, animal studies reported that D-ribose prevented or delayed the development of left ventricular dysfunction following acute myocardial infarction. Hence, the question posed is: might D-ribose offer an additional benefit, if supplemented prior to a myocardial infarction? When D-ribose was supplied pre-infarction, Gonzalez et al. reported that providing D-ribose in adult rats resulted in a significant reduction in the created left ventricular infarct area and a significant improvement in left ventricular function when assessed at 6 hours post infarct. Left ventricular systolic pressure and contractility were restored to normal levels with a significant improvement in measured parameters of left ventricular relaxation with supplemental D-ribose. [23]

2.2 Clinical D-ribose evaluation

The observed positive energy enhancing and functional benefits associated with D-ribose in the pre-clinical investigations initiated subsequent clinical studies to further assess its potential in patients afflicted with cardiovascular diseases. Because of the benefits of D-ribose during and following ischemia, researchers investigated this potential in enhancing the identification of hibernating myocardium. Hibernating myocardium represents regional areas of myocardial dysfunction due to prolonged hypoperfusion or ischemia. This condition can be reversed upon restoration of a more adequate level of blood flow to these regions. Theoretically, efforts to aid in the identification of these regions can help in the management strategies for revascularization. Current methods in identifying these regions include Thallium-201 scans, dobutamine stress echocardiography, PET, and magnetic resonance imagery. Hibernating myocardium is likely to be associated with lower levels of myocardial ATP; and therefore, supplementation with an adenine nucleotide agent might aid in further identifying these viable regions. D-ribose has demonstrated a benefit in this identification process. Before undertaking clinical investigations, pre-clinical animal studies demonstrated the identification benefit of D-ribose in hibernating myocardium. In the clinical realm, Perlmutter et al. reported that D-ribose identified more reversible defects using Thalium-201 scans. [24] Other clinical studies have supported this finding. Hegewald et al. found that D-ribose also increased the detection of viable ischemic myocardial regions using SPECT Thallium imaging. [25] More recently, Sawada et al. demonstrated that the supplementation of D-ribose provided anti-ischemic effects with improving the identification of wall motion dysfunctional abnormalities during dobutamine stress echocardiography. [26]

Previously reported positive pre-clinical animal studies demonstrating the benefits of D-ribose during and following ischemia generated additional clinical investigative interest. Since D-ribose has shown in animal studies to enhance the recovery in ATP levels and improve function following myocardial ischemia, Pliml et al. argued that there is significant impairment in ATP levels in the ischemic myocardium. The current lack of therap(ies) directed to the restoration or preventing further decrease in these myocardial energy compounds lead the researchers to design a study in which patients with stable coronary artery disease underwent serial treadmill exercise testing while supplementing with D-ribose. D-ribose demonstrated significant benefits in increasing treadmill exercise time before the onset of angina and/or ischemic electrocardiographic changes. [27]

Myocardial ischemia is an etiological factor in the development of CHF and reports have proposed that the failing heart is energy starved. [5] Because of D-ribose's ability to enhance the recovery of myocardial ATP levels and improve diastolic dysfunction following ischemic, Omran et al. investigated the role of D-ribose in class II-III CHF patients. They reported both objective and subjective benefits with D-ribose. There was an improvement in diastolic dysfunctional parameters, as assessed by serial echocardiographic examinations; and subjectively, the patients experienced an improved quality of life and physical function. [28]

Commonly, CHF patients complain of shortness of breath and fatigue. As their failure progresses, patients have a decrease in their ventilatory efficiency. Carter et al. found that supplementation with D-ribose enabled class II-III CHF study patients with left ventricular dysfunction to maintain their VO_{2max}, improve their ventilatory efficiency and experience a positive trend in their daily quality of life assessment. [29] Vijay et al. concurred in a separate clinical study the positive benefits of D-ribose in class II-IV CHF patients. They observed significant improvements in ventilatory efficiency in class III-IV patients with a positive, but not statistically significant, .trend in improved ventilator efficiency in class II patients. [30]

The use of D-ribose has also been explored in cardiovascular surgery. Alterations in myocardial function have been observed in the post-ischemic interval following surgery. Wyatt et al. found that the use of a cardioplegic solution containing adenosine, hypoxanthine and D-ribose during intra-operative ischemia maintained myocardial energy levels during ischemia and with reperfusion resulted in enhanced functional recovery post operatively. [31] Vance et al. reported that parenteral use of D-ribose in patients undergoing elective aortic valve replacement with or without accompanying coronary arterial bypass grafting resulted in the maintenance in ejection fraction postoperatively, unlike the decline in ejection fraction observed in the patients not receiving D-ribose. They concluded that the treatment regimen of D-ribose preserved left ventricular function peri-operatively. [32] More recently, oral D-ribose was added to a metabolic designed protocol for patients undergoing off pump coronary artery bypass revascularization procedures. Perkowski et al. found that this D-ribose metabolic protocol resulted in lower mortality and morbidities, along with a significant early postoperative improvement in cardiac index in patients undergoing "off pump" coronary artery revascularization. [33]

3. Summary

Even with the advances in cardiovascular medical technologies over decades, cardiovascular disease still ranks as the leading cause of death worldwide for both males and females. Myocardial ischemia, a factor in cardiovascular disease, has continued to be a leading cause of deaths in middle to elderly aged individuals. With continued current aggressive education, there have been strides in addressing the cardiovascular risk factors in this disease, including refinements in diet, regular exercise, smoking cessation, and blood pressure control. However, the underlying metabolic energy deficiency found with myocardial ischemia still requires further attention.

Every cell requires adequate levels of high energy phosphates, i.e. ATP, to maintain its integrity and function. Myocardial ischemia lowers myocardial ATP levels, which has shown to reflect functional abnormalities. Relaxation of the myocardium, occurring during diastole, requires adequate ATP levels for the normal flux of calcium interacting with the sarcoplasmic reticulum. Without adequate levels of myocardial ATP, a state of ventricular diastolic dysfunction or non-compliance develops. Over decades research has centered on developing strategies in replenishing deficient levels of ATP during and following myocardial ischemia. The abundance of research has entertained on providing metabolic substrates to regenerate ATP compounds following ischemia. The results of these numerous investigations have been mixed; however, supplementation with D-ribose, a natural occurring pentose carbohydrate, has been found to not only to enhance the recovery of ATP levels, but to aid in improving the state of ventricular diastolic dysfunction following myocardial ischemia. D-ribose has shown to improve ventricular compliance following ischemia, for which there is not an approved marketed device or pharmaceutical that can offer this functional benefit.

The clinical therapeutic cardiovascular uses of D-ribose continue to expand. Published studies have reported its potential benefits, such as in acute and chronic myocardial ischemic conditions, identifying hibernating myocardium, in CHF patients, and its use in the peri-operative cardiovascular surgical patient. The literature has provided support that supplemental D-ribose may offer the means to enhance the recovery of myocardial cellular energy with functional benefits in patients afflicted with ischemic cardiovascular disease.

4. References

[1] Cardiovascular disease. The atlas of heart disease and stroke. World Health Organization. http://www.who.int/cardiovascular_diseases/resources/atlas/en/

[2] Heart disease overview, incidence and prevalence of heart disease. http://www.healthcommunities.com/heart-disease/heart-disease-overview.sh
[3] Redfield MM, Jacobson SJ, Burnett JC, Mahoney DW, Bailey KR, Rodenheffer RJ. Burden of systolic and diastolic ventricular dysfunction in the community. Appreciating the scope of the heart failure epidemic. JAMA 2003;289(2):194-202.
[4] Fischer M, Baessler A, Hense HW, Hengstenberg C, Muscholl M, Holmer S, Doring A, Broeckel U, Reigger G, Schunkert H. Prevalence of left ventricular diastolic dysfunction in the community. Results from a Doppler echocardiographic-based survey of a population sample. Eur Heart J 2003;24(4):320-328.
[5] Ingwall JS and Weiss RG. Is the failing heart energy starved? On using chemical energy to support cardiac function. Circ Res 2004;95:135-145.
[6] Pauly DF, Johnson CA, St.Cyr JA. The benefits of ribose in cardiovascular disease. Med Hypoth 2003;60(2):149-151.
[7] Mahoney JR. Recovery of post ischemic myocardial ATP levels and hexosemonophosphate shunt activity. Med Hypoth 1990;31:21-23.
[8] Pauly DF and Pepine CJ. D-riobse as a supplement for cardiac energy metabolism. J Cardiovasc Pharmacol Therapeut 2000;5(4):249-258.
[9] Reibel DK and Rovetto MJ. Myocardial ATP synthesis and mechanical function following oxygen deficiency. Am J Physiol 1978;243:H620.
[10] Kloner RA, DEBoer LW, Darsee JR, Ingwall JS, Braunwald E. Recovery from prolonged abnormalities of canine myocardium salvaged from ischemic necrosis by coronary reperfusion. Proc Natl Acad Sci USA 1981;78(11):7152-7156.
[11] Zimmer HG. Normalization of depressed heart function in rats by ribose. Science 1983;220:81-82.
[12] Reimer KA, Hill ML, Jennings RB. Prolonged depletion of ATP and of the adenine nucleotide pool due to delayed resynthesis of adenine nucleotides following reversible myocardial ischemic injury in dogs. J Mol CellCardiol 1981;13:229-239.
[13] St.Cyr J, Ward H, Kriett J, Alyono D, Einzig S, Bianco R, Anderson R, Foker J.Long term model term model for evaluation of myocardial metabolic recovery following global ischemia. In: Brautbar, N(ed), Myocardial and Skeletal Muscle Bioenergetics, AEMB series. New York, NY, Plenum Publishing 194:401, 1986.
[14] Ward HB, Kriett J, St.Cyr JA, Alyono D, Einzig S, Bianco RW, Anderson R, Foker JE. Relationship between recovery of myocardial ATP levels and cardiac function following ischemia. J AM Coll Cardiol 1984;3(2):544.
[15] Ward HB, St.Cyr JA, Cogordan JA, Alyono D, Bianco RW, Kriett JM, Foker JE. Recovery of adenine nucleotide levels after global myocardial ischemia in dogs. Surg 1984;96(2):248-255.
[16] Zimmer HG and Gerlach E. Stimulation of myocardial adenine nucleotide biosynthesis by pentoses and penitols. Pflugers Arch 1978;376:223-227.
[17] Pasque MK, Spray TL, Pellom GL Van Trigt P, Peyton RB, Currie WD, Wechsler AS. Ribose-enhanced myocardial recovery following ischemia in the isolated working rat heart. J Thorac Cardiovasc Surg 1982;83:390-398.

[18] St.Cyr J, Bianco RW, Schneider JR, Mahoney JR, Tveter K, Einzig S, Foker J. Enhanced high energy phosphate recovery with ribose infusion after global myocardial ischemia in a canine model. J Surg Res 1989;46(2):157-162.

[19] Schneider JR, St.Cyr JA, Mahoney JR, Bianco RW, Ring WS, Foker JE: Recovery of ATP and return of function after global ischemia. Circ (Part II), 72(4):III_298, 1985.

[20] Tveter K, St.Cyr JA, Schneider J, Bianco R, Foker J. Enhanced recovery of diastolic function after global myocardial ischemia in the intact animal. Pediatr Res 1988;23:226A.

[21] Zimmer HG, Martius PA, Marschner G. Myocardial infarction in rats: effects of metabolic and pharmacologic interventions. Basic Res Cardiol 1989;84:332-343.

[22] Befera N, Rivard A, Gatlin D, Zhang J, Foker JE. Ribose treatment helps preserve function of the remote myocardium after myocardial infarction. J Surg Res 2007;137(2):156.

[23] Gonzalez GE, Rabald S, Briest W, Gelpi RJ, Seropian I, Zimmer HG, Deten A. Ribose treatment reduced the infarct size and improved heart function after myocardial infarction in rats. Cell Physiol Biochem 2009;24:211-218.

[24] Perlmutter NS, Wilson RA, Angello DA, Palac RT, Lin J, Brown BG. Ribose facilitates Thallium-201 redistribution in patients with coronary artery disease. J Nucl Med 1991;32:193-200.

[25] Hegewald MG, Palac RT, Angello DA, Perlmutter NS, Wilson RA. Ribose Infusion accelerates Thallium redistribution with early imaging compared with late 24 hour imaging without ribose. J Am Coll Cardiol 1991;18:1671-1681.

[26] Sawada SG, Lewis S, Kovacs R, Khouri S, Gradus-Pizlo I, St. Cyr J, Feigenbaum H. Evaluation of the anti-ischemic effects of D-ribose during dobutamine stress echocardiography: a pilot study. Cardiovasc Ultrasound 2009;7(5):7120-7127.

[27] Pliml W, Von Arnim T, Stablein A, Hofmann H, Zimmer HG, Erdmann E. Effects of ribose on exercise-induced ischaemia in stable coronary artery disease. Lancet 1992;340:507-510.

[28] Omran H, Illien S, MacCarter D, St. Cyr J, Luderitz B. D-ribose improves diastolic function and quality of life in congestive heart failure patients: a prospective feasibility study. Eur J Heart Fail 2003;5(5):615-619.

[29] Carter O, MacCarter D, Mannebach S, Biskupiak J, Stoddard G, Gilbert EM, Munger MA. D-ribose improves peak exercise capacity and ventilatory efficiency in heart failure patients. J Am Coll Cardiol 2005;45 (3 Suppl A):185A.

[30] Vijay N, MacCarter D, Washam M, Munger M, St.Cyr J. D-ribose improves ventilatory efficiency in congestive heart failure NYHA class II-IV patients. HFSA 2005;suppl 1:S-95.

[31] Wyatt DA, Ely SW, Lasley RD, Walsh R, Mainwarning R, Berne RM, Mentzer RM. Purine-enriched asanguineous cardioplegia retards adenosine triphosphate degradation during ischemia and improves postischemic ventricular function. J Thorac Cardiovasc Surg 1989;97:771-778.

[32] Vance RA, Einzig S, Kreisler K, St. Cyr J. D-ribose maintained ejection fraction following aortic valve surgery. FASEB J 2000;14(4):A419.

[33] Perkowski DJ, Wagner S, Schneider JR, St. Cyr JA. A targeted metabolic protocol with D-ribose for off-pump coronary artery bypass procedures: a retrospective analysis. Ther Adv Cardiovasc Dis 2011;5:185-192.

12

Two Novel Approaches Providing Cardiac Protection Against Oxidative Stress

Howard Prentice[1,2,3,*] and Herbert Weissbach[3]
[1]*College of Medicine,*
[2]*Center for Complex Systems and Brain Sciences,*
[3]*Center for Molecular Biology and Biotechnology,*
Florida Atlantic University, Florida,
USA

1. Introduction

Coronary artery disease is the highest contributor to morbidity and premature death in the developed world (Nabel, 2003; Fuster et al., 1992; Melo et al., 2004). Cardiac function is compromised in patients that survive an initial ischemic event and this progressive myocardial impairment leads to heart failure (Liu et al., 2007; Sugamura and Keaney, 2011; Jessup and Brozena, 2003). High levels of reactive oxygen species (ROS) contribute to the process of disease progression in both myocardial ischemia and in models of heart failure. ROS play a role in short term responses (stunning and arrhythmias) as well as long term responses (infarction) to ischemia with reperfusion. The primary source of ROS in myocardial ischemia is from mitochondria of cardiac cells with additional ROS arising from neutrophils that infiltrate ischemic regions (Sugamura and Keaney, 2011). There have been promising preclinical studies employing some antioxidant enzymes but there are no currently accepted clinical applications of these enzymes for myocardial ischemia (Downey, 1990; Zweier et al., 1987, Otani et al., 1986; Papaharalambus and Griendling, 2007; Vivekananthan et al., 2003). It is likely that the responses in the ischemic heart are more complicated than was initially realized and other antioxidant based strategies have to be developed. Our work has focused on two protective agents that act to prevent the detrimental effects of oxidative stress in the ischemic heart. The first cardio-protectant is methionine methionine sulfoxide reductase A (MsrA), a member of the Msr family of enzymes. The other major enzyme in the Msr family is MsrB and these two enzymes differ in their substrate stereo-specificity. The Msr family of enzymes can protect cells in two ways: 1) by repairing oxidative damage to critical methionine (Met) residues in proteins which have been oxidized to methionine sulfoxide (met(o)), and 2) by functioning as part of an ROS scavenger system in which Met residues in proteins function as catalytic antioxidants. MsrA has been studied in most detail and shown to protect bacterial and animal cells against oxidative damage (for review see Weissbach et al., 2005). The studies with MsrA led to investigations with the drug sulindac, a known non-steroidal anti-

*Corresponding Author

inflammatory drug (NSAID), that is a substrate for the Msr system (Etienne et al. 2003; Brunell et al. 2011). Sulindac protects the heart against ischemic infarction through a newly described activity as a pharmacological preconditioning agent (Moench et al., 2009).

2. Antioxidant therapies and oxidative stress in heart disease

ROS normally produced as a by-product of the electron transport chain are now considered to be a major factor in aging and age related diseases (Bokov et al., 2004). In the heart high levels of ROS have been implicated in both ischemic damage and in the progression of heart failure (Giordano, 2005). Preclinical studies for ischemic heart disease employing antioxidants although still at an early stage have shown some promise (Sugamura and Keaney, 2011; Bolli et al., 2004; Cannon, 2005). For example heme oxygenase -1 (HO-1) based gene therapy has been proposed as a therapeutic strategy for ischemic heart disease because the enzyme has a clear antioxidant capacity (Liu et al., 2007). In addition, the products of heme metabolism, carbon monoxide and bilirubin have been reported to possess cyto-protective properties (Poss and Tonegawa, 1997; Stocker et al., 1987). Cardiac expression of HO-1 increased Akt phosphorylation and decreased infarct size in a mouse model of ischemia/reperfusion. Knockdown of the bilirubin producing enzyme biliverdin reductase increases apoptosis of cardiac cells subjected to hypoxia /re-oxygenation and decreases Akt phosphorylation. Thus the protection afforded by HO-1 involves activation of Akt that is dependent upon biliverdin reductase (Pachori et al., 2007).

Other antioxidant enzymes that have shown potential for protection against ischemic damage include extracellular superoxide dismutase (EC-SOD-1), thioredoxin (Trx), and glutathione peroxidase (GSHPx) (Agrawal et al., 2004; Yoshida et al., 1996; Turoczi et al., 2003; Maulik et al., 1999). Gene transfer of EC-SOD-1 by direct intra myocardial injection using an AAV vector resulted in high level cardio-protection in rats at 7 days following ischemia and reperfusion injury (Agrawal et al., 2004). Using the rat working heart model of transient global ischemia it has been shown that thioredoxin is substantially decreased, whereas preconditioning by non-lethal ischemia elicited up-regulation of Trx expression and induced tolerance against severe ischemic stress (Turoczi et al., 2003). Likewise Trx-1 overexpressing mice were found to have reduced myocardial infarct size after a prolonged ischemia episode (Turoczi et al., 2003). Glutathione peroxidase (GSHPx) knockout mice have been shown to be more susceptible to ischemic damage than wild type mice, whereas GSHPx overexpressing mice are protected against myocardial ischemic damage (Maulik et al., 1999).

In models of heart failure the contribution of ROS has been demonstrated to contribute to hypertrophic adaptations and to apoptosis (Li et al., 2002; Kwon et al., 2003; Giordano, 2005). Cardiac hypertrophy can be either a physiological adaptation or part of the pathology that ultimately progresses to heart failure (Giordano, 2005). ROS signaling has been implicated in hypertrophic growth associated activation of MAPKs (Sabri et al., 2003; Ghosh et al., 2003). For example, inhibition of ROS by chemical antioxidants prevents A-II induced hypertrophy (Nakamura et al., 1998; Delbosc et al., 2002). ROS induced alterations in transcription factor activation has been reported in cardiac hypertrophy and several studies point to a role for ROS in the induced chromatin remodeling in the failing heart (Giordano,

2005). ASK-1 provides a link between oxidative stress and hypertrophy since following activation by ROS, Ask1 induces activation of p38-MAPK and JNK causing apoptosis (Izumiya et al., 2003). The apoptotic process is central to heart failure and the effect of ROS on apoptosis is dependent upon the levels of ROS produced (Kwon et al., 2003). It is clear that high levels of ROS will elicit apoptosis via JNK and p38-MAPKs, whereas low levels of ROS can function as signaling molecules and help to protect cells under certain physiological conditions, as is the case with ischemic preconditioning discussed below (Kwon et al., 2003; Das, 2001; Hool, 2006; Murry et al., 1986; Yellon and Downey, 2002; Bolli, 2000).

3. MsrA and cellular protection

Of the amino acids in proteins that can be oxidized by ROS, Met is one of the most sensitive, being converted to methionine sulfoxide (Met(o)) (Weissbach et al., 2005). Since the sulfur in Met(o) has a chiral center this chemical oxidation yields a mixture of the R and S epimers, Met-R-(o) and Met-S-(o), as shown in Figure 1.

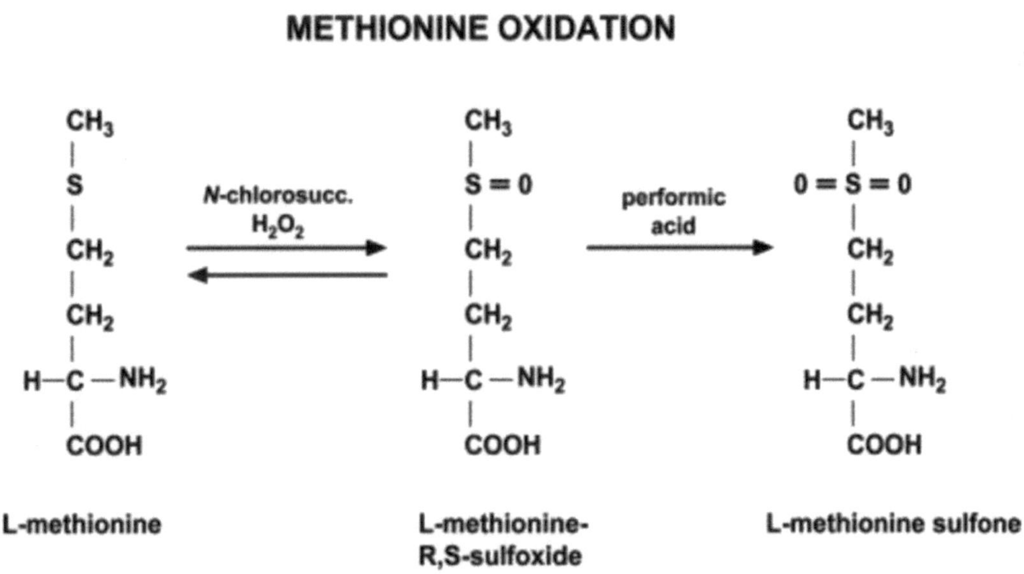

Fig. 1. Products of methionine oxidation.

Further oxidation of Met(o), leads to the formation of methionine sulfone, which has been detected in proteins at very low levels and its significance is not known. As also shown in Figure 1 Met(o) in proteins can be reduced back to Met by the Msr enzymes. The two main members are MsrA and MsrB, which reduce the S epimer and R epimer of Met(o), respectively. It is now known that there is one msrA gene in mammalian cells and three msrB genes, the latter referred to as MsrB1, 2 and 3 (Vougier et al., 2003; Kim and Gladyshev, 2004; Hansel et al., 2005).

Although MsrA was first discovered more than 30 years ago in studies on protein synthesis in bacteria (Brot et al.,1981), its important role in protecting cells against oxidative damage only became apparent in the early 1990's after the MsrA gene was cloned from both Escherichia coli and bovine liver (Rahman et al., 1992; Moskovitz et al., 1996). When MsrA was knocked out in E. coli the organism grew normally, but was extremely sensitive to oxidizing agents (Moskovitz et al., 1996, St. John et al., 2001). Since then there have been several studies demonstrating that over-expressing MsrA in animal cells can protect them against oxidative damage (Moskovitz et al., 1998; Kantorow et al., 2004; Yermolaieva et al., 2000) and lead to extended life span in both flies and yeast (Ruan et al., 2002, Koc et al., 2004) . As one example in cells in culture, over-expression of MsrA by transfection of PC12 cells with an adenovirus vector encoding MsrA resulted in a greater tolerance for oxidative stress following hypoxia with re-oxygenation (Yermolaieva et al., 2004). MsrA overexpressing cells showed significantly lower levels of ROS and apoptosis than cells infected with no virus or control plain virus. In Drosophila, overexpression of MsrA was protective against oxidative stress. When the MsrA transgene was over-expressed the flies were found to be more resistant to paraquat induced oxidative stress and when the MsrA was predominantly expressed in the nervous system there was a dramatic increase in lifespan (Ruan et al., 2002) (Figure 2).

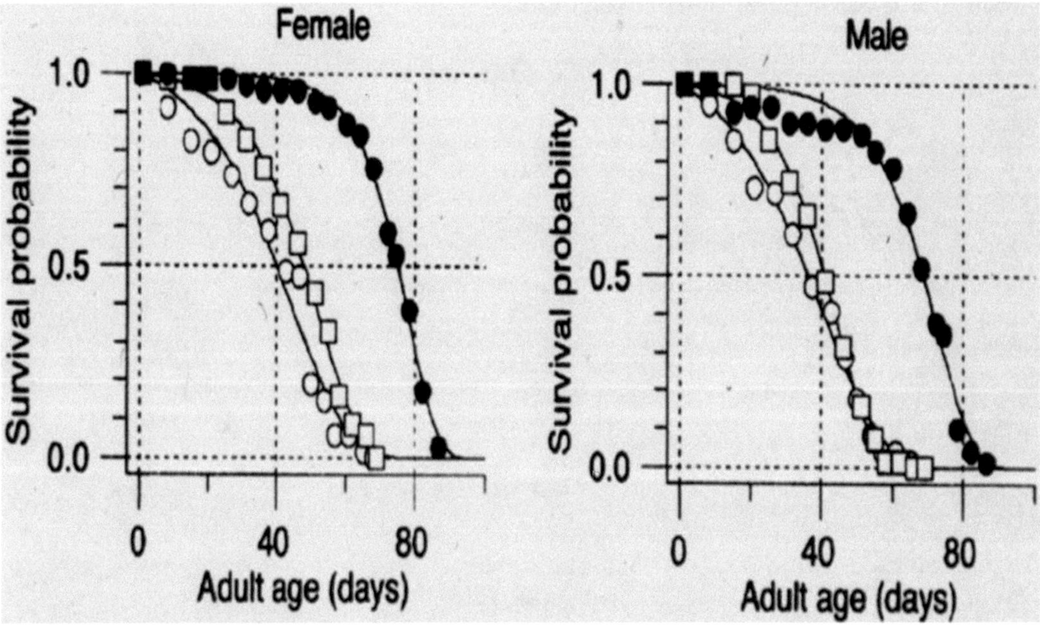

Fig. 2. Extension of life span of flies by neuronal expression of MsrA. □—□ and O-O, control flies; ●—● MsrA overexpressing flies. From Ruan et al., 2001.

To determine the effect of MsrA in protecting against hypoxia/re-oxygenation damage in cardiac cells we transduced primary rat cardiac myocytes with an MsrA encoding adenovirus (Prentice et al., 2008). In cells over-expressing MsrA, apoptotic cell death resulting from hypoxia/re-oxygenation was decreased by greater than 45% relative to cells expressing control virus (Figure 3).

The protection of cardiac myocytes in culture against hypoxia/re-oxygenation stress by MsrA over-expression points to MsrA as a potential therapeutic agent for treatment of ischemic heart disease (Prentice et al., 2008).

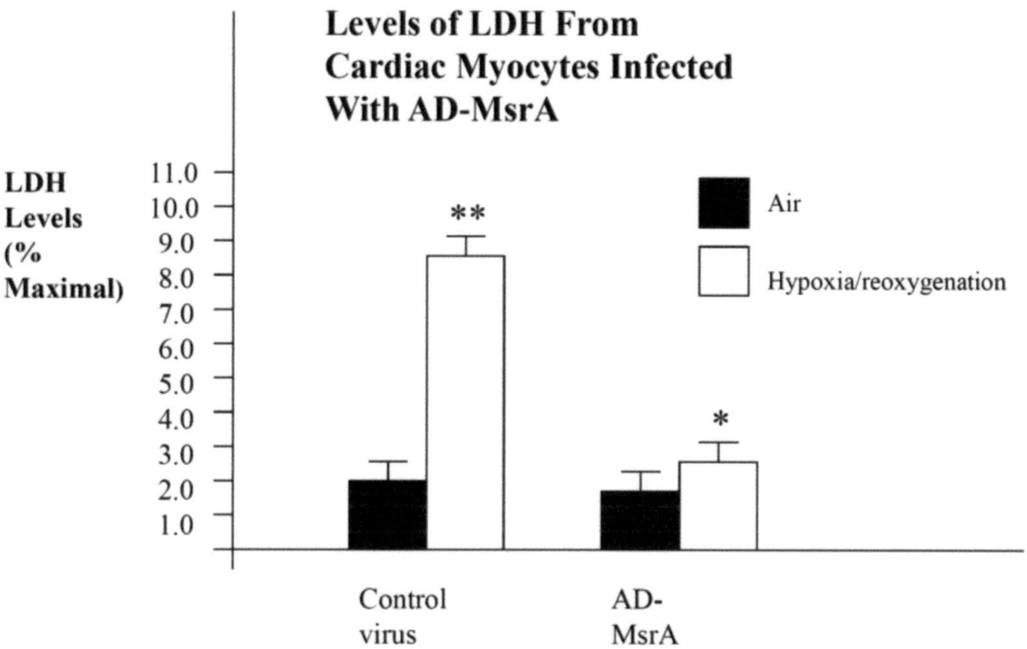

Fig. 3. Protection of cardiac myocytes following hypoxia /reoxygenation by sulindac as measured by levels of LDH released. **$p<0.01$ vs air control virus (N=6). *$p<0.01$ vs hypoxia/reoxygenation control virus (N=6). From Prentice et al. 2008

In contrast, knocking out MsrA makes mammalian cells more sensitive to oxidative stress. MsrA and MsrB knockout in lens and retinal cells make these cells more sensitive to oxidation (Marchetti et al., 2006; Kantorow et al., 2004). There have been reports on MsrA knockout mice in which it is clear that these animals are very sensitive to increased oxygen tension, although there is conflicting data on their life span and the presence of a neurological defect (Moskovitz et al., 2001, Salmon et al., 2009). The MsrA knockout mice also have been reported to contain increased brain dopamine levels at 6 and 12 months of age perhaps because of enhanced dopamine synthesis, but at 16 months the mice showed reduced dopamine levels compared to younger animals (Oien et al., 2008). Experiments addressing physiological alterations in the heart resulting from a loss of MsrA have been carried out using the MsrA-/- knock-out mouse model (Nan et al., 2010). Under normal non-stressed conditions cellular contractility and cardiac function are not altered in the MsrA-/- mice. However when cardiac cells are stressed with high stimulation frequencies (2Hz) or with hydrogen peroxide a significant modulation in cardiac contractility is seen (Figure 4).

There were corresponding changes in calcium transients in MsrA-/- cardiac myocytes treated with 2 Hz stimulation or with hydrogen peroxide. EM analysis also showed significant swelling of the mitochondria in MsrA-/-mouse hearts and protein oxidation levels in MsrA-/- mouse hearts were higher than those of wild type controls (Nan et al., 2010). Similar morphological changes in mitochondria have previously been reported in diseased hearts either from dilated cardiomyopathy or from myocardial ischemia and such ultrastructural changes have been associated with aging and senescence (Trillo et al., 1978; Schaper et al., 1991; Scholz et al., 1994; Terman et al., 2004) . This study indicates that there is a serious defect in mitochondrial function in the hearts of MsrA-/- mice resulting in compromised contractility and cellular dysfunction, especially under stress (Nan et al., 2010).

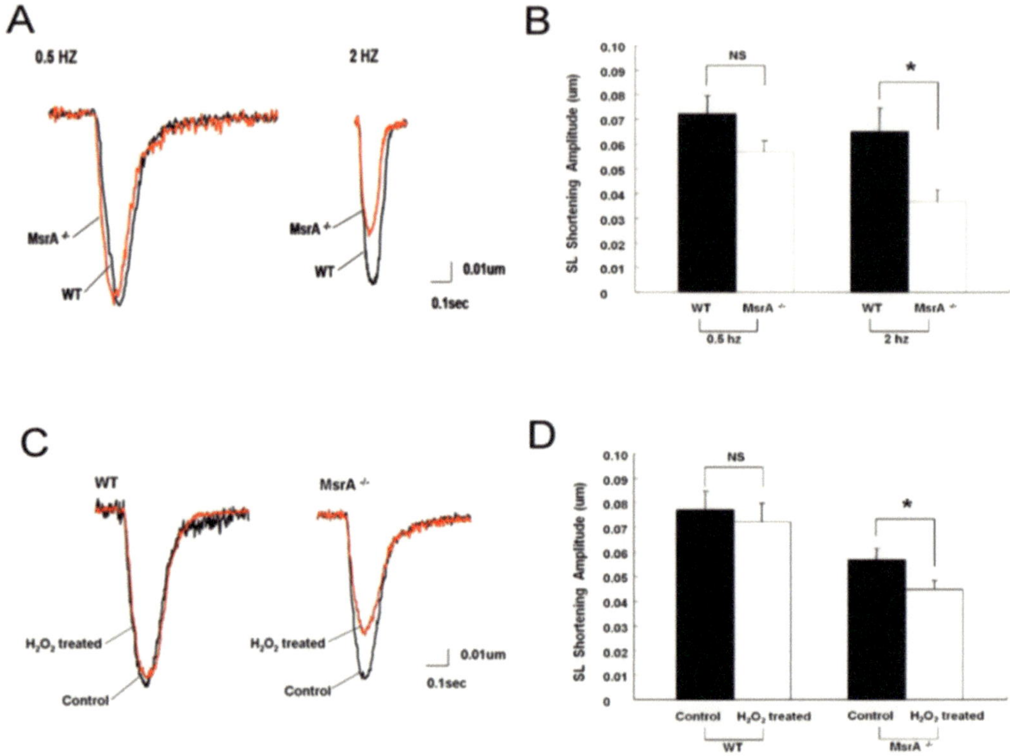

Fig. 4. MsrA knockout (MsrA -/-) mice show decreased contractility when stressed by high frequency (2Hz) or with hydrogen peroxide treatment. (a) Raw traces of sarcomere contraction under 0.5 Hz or 2 Hz stimulation. (b) Shortening amplitude with 0.5Hz and 2 Hz. (c) Raw traces of sarcomere contraction with or without H2O2 treatment. (d) Shortening amplitude in cardiomycytes with or without H2O2 treatment. Data are presented as mean+/- SD and obtained from 25-30 cells (3 mice per group); *p<0.05. From Nan et al.,2010

Previous studies had demonstrated that approximately 75% of MsrA was targeted to the cytosol and 25% to the mitochondria (Kim et al., 2010; Vougier et al., 2003). A recent study by Zhao et al., (2011) examined the role of MsrA in different cellular compartments and assessed whether the enzyme would protect against ischemia reperfusion damage in the Langendorff heart. The investigators employed transgenic mice that overexpressed MsrA either in the myocardium or in the cytosol. A surprising finding was that mitochondrial targeted MsrA was not protective in the Langendorff model against ischemia/reperfusion. By contrast the cytoplasmic form of MsrA was protective, but the effect was dependent on myristoylation of the enzymes. It was proposed that myristoylation may facilitate targeting of MsrA to its protein targets to elicit myocardial protection.

4. Dual function of the Msr system

It was initially thought that the main role of the Msr system was to repair oxidative damage to proteins in which critical met residues were oxidized to met(o). There has been ample evidence that this is an important function of the Msr system. Once again most of the studies have been done with MsrA. There are now a long list of proteins and peptides whose activities are altered by Met oxidation in vitro (Brot and Weissbach, 2000) and many examples of how the activity can be restored in part by MsrA. One of the first examples was the oxidation of Met 358 in alpha one proteinase inhibitor. This enzyme, which may play a role in emphysema, loses its protease inhibitor activity when this Met is oxidized and the activity can be restored by MsrA (Abrams et al., 1981). More recently, oxidation of met residues in proteins has been reported to cause a major change in function of a number of proteins. As examples, in a shaker ShC/B voltage gated potassium channel, when a key methionine residue in the inactivation ball is oxidized, the channel activation is slowed down, but this process is reversed by MsrA (Ciorba et al., 1997). A methionine in the C terminus of calmodulin is selectively oxidized by hydrogen peroxide (Yao et al., 1996). The extent of oxidative modification was found to correlate with loss of CaM dependent activation of the plasma membrane Ca-ATPase. The protein calcium/calmodulin (Ca2+ CaM) dependent protein kinase II (CamKII) links increases in intracellular calcium to activation of ion channels, transcriptional responses and cell fate decisions. A recent study analyzing the role of CaMKII in heart demonstrated that CamKII is a common signaling point for increased apoptosis regulated by ROS, catecholamine signaling and angiotensin-II (Ang-II) (Erickson et al., 2008). MsrA was found to be essential for reversing CaMKII methionine oxidation in the ischemic heart in vivo.

However, Levine et al. (1996), in their studies on glutamine synthetase, first introduced the important concept that the Msr system could be part of a ROS scavenger mechanism. In this mechanism, Met residues in proteins, even when not at an active site, can be oxidized to Met(o) and in the process destroy a ROS molecule. The Msr system could then regenerate the Met which could once again be oxidized by an ROS molecule. Thus, the Met residues in proteins could function as catalytic anti-oxidants dependent on the Msr system. There are now several cell culture studies to support this mechanism. In PC12 cells over-expression of MsrA lowers the level of ROS in the cells and in lens and retinal cells knocking out of MsrA leads to higher ROS levels (Yermolaieva et al., 2004; Marchetti et al., 2006).

5. Sulindac is a substrate for the Msr enzymes

If Met residues in proteins could function as catalytic anti-oxidants based on the Msr system it seemed reasonable that other substrates of the Msr enzymes might function in cells as catalytic anti-oxidants. One such compound that was shown to be a substrate for MsrA was sulindac, a known NSAID (Duggan et al., 1977). The structure of sulindac and its metabolites is shown in Figure 5. Sulindac is a prodrug that must be reduced to sulindac sulfide which is the active NSAID. Since sulindac is also a mixture of the R and S epimers the metabolism of both epimers has been recently elucidated as shown in Figure 5 (Brunell et al., 2011).

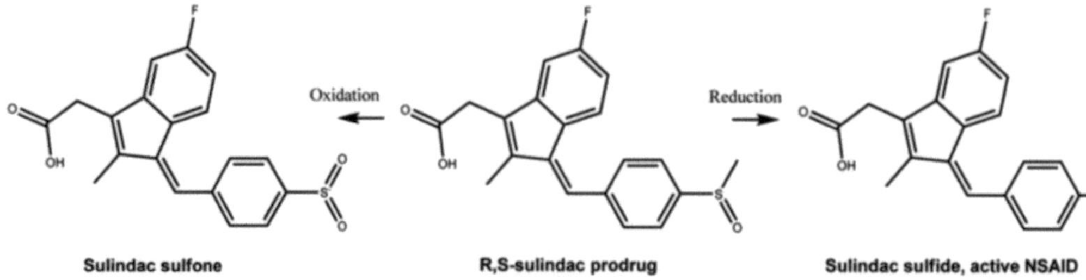

Fig. 5. Metabolism of the sulindac epimers. The R and S epimers of sulindac can be oxidized to sulindac sulfone and reduced to sulindac sulfide. From Brunell et al. 2011.

The reduction of the S epimer is catalyzed by MsrA and as seen in Figure 6, the R epimer is reduced by an enzyme in liver that has the properties of MsrB (Brunell et al., 2011). Sulindac can also induce the P450 system and be oxidized by the P450 system to sulindac sulfone (Ciolino et al., 2008; Brunell et al., 2011). Sulindac sulfone is not an NSAID and is not a substrate for the Msr system. It seemed reasonable to see whether sulindac might function as a catalytic anti-oxidant and protect cells against oxidative damage. In our preliminary experiments several normal cells were not protected by sulindac after exposure to oxidative stress, but normal lung cells were (Marchetti et al., 2009). An unexpected finding was that under similar conditions colon and lung cancer cell lines, that were pretreated with sulindac, showed enhanced killing of these cells when exposed to oxidative stress. The protective effect of sulindac with normal lung cells and the enhanced killing with the cancer cell lines was not due to the NSAID activity of sulindac or did it involve the Msr system since sulindac sulfone gave a similar effect as sulindac (Marchetti et al., 2009). As will be shown below, using cardiac cells, the protection seen against oxidative damage by sulindac is by an ischemic preconditioning mechanism (Moench et al., 2009).

6. Sulindac causes cardiac protection by ischemic preconditioning

Pharmacological preconditioning has been reported to occur in response to certain drugs that mimic the effects of ischemic preconditioning, a process known to elicit protective responses against myocardial stunning and infarction. Ischemic preconditioning has been reported to elicit an early phase of protection from 0-2 hours after the initial stimulus as well as a late phase of preconditioning from 1 -7 days after ischemia (Kuzuya et al., 1993; Marber et al., 1993; Bolli, 2000). A number of pharmacological agents can induce preconditioning include cytokines, opioids, adenosine, nitric oxide donors and bradykinin although these agents may differ in their capacity to protect against infarction, stunning or both infarction and stunning (Bolli, 2000).

The mechanisms of early preconditioning have been shown to involve NO activation of soluble guanylyl cyclase (GC), activation of PKG and opening of mitochondrial ATP dependent potassium channels (K-ATP channels) (Costa et al., 2008). Subsequent generation of ROS from the mitochondrion results in activation of PKC (Costa et al., 2008; Baines et al., 1997; Tritto et al., 1997). The mediation events of early preconditioning have been shown to involve inhibition of the formation of the mitochondrial permeability transition pore, and in some cases, such as with protection by adenosine, this mediation involves PKC activation and PKG activation (Costa et al., 2008).

Late preconditioning is triggered through the action of NO as well as through ROS release (Bolli, 2001; Bolli et al., 1997). PKC epsilon translocates to the membrane fraction which is then followed by activation of the MAPK signaling cascade (Xuan et al., 2007). Downstream events include phosphorylation of STAT1/3 and activation of STAT dependent genes which include the COX-2 gene. Other events that mediate late preconditioning include NO release (through a PKG dependent mechanisms and opening of mitochondrial K(ATP) channels (Bernardo et al., 1999; Ockaili et al., 1999). It has been reported that the NO that mediates late preconditioning is derived from inducible NOS (iNOS). Some of the components involved in ischemic preconditioning are summarized in Figure 6.

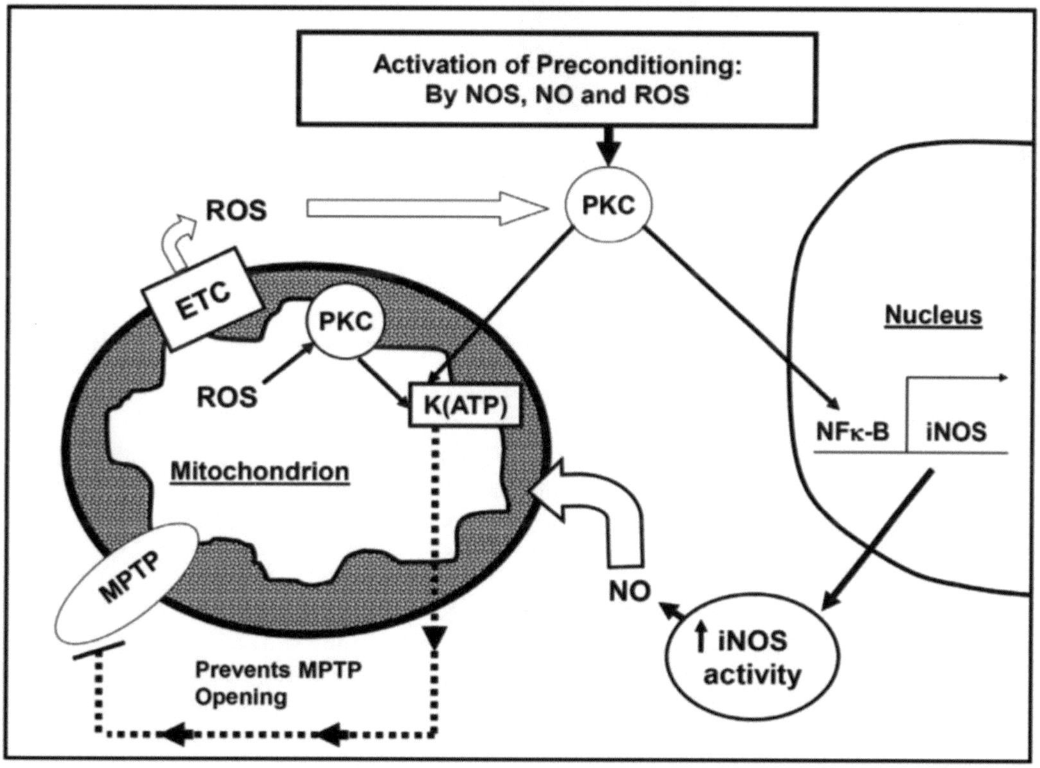

Fig. 6. Overview of mechanisms of preconditioning involving PKC, iNOS and mitochondrial pro-survival events.

In investigating the role of sulindac as a protective agent we examined the effect of sulindac treatment on neonatal rat cardiac myocytes subjected to hypoxia and re-oxygenation and in an ex vivo Langendorff model of myocardial ischemia (Moench et al., 2009). We demonstrated that sulindac (<100uM) afforded high level protection of cardiac myocytes subjected to hypoxia and re-oxygenation (Figure 7).

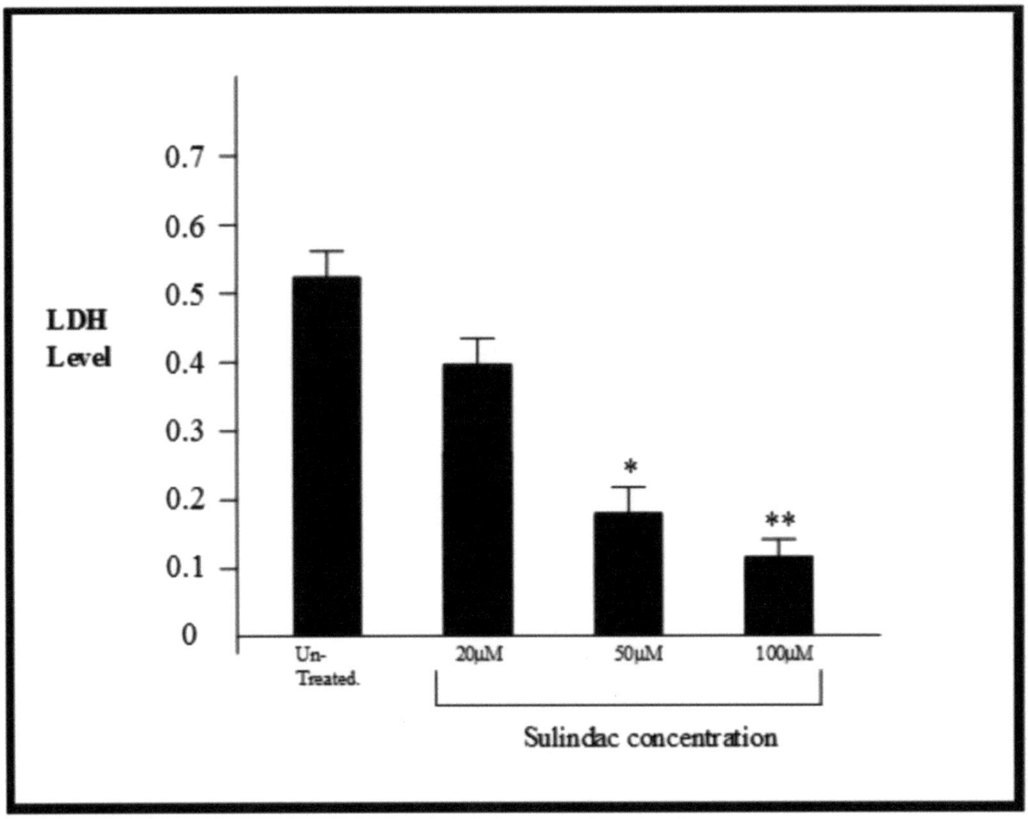

Fig. 7. Sulindac protects cardiac myocytes against oxidative damage. Cardiac myocytes were exposed to hypoxia for 24 h and reoxygenation for 20 h to elicit oxidative stress in the presence or absence of sulindac. Lactate dehydrogenase (LDH) levels (shown as absorbance units) were measured in the media as an index of cell death and levels were compared to those for untreated myocytes (*,$P<0.05$ vs. no drug; n=6, **, $p<0.01$ vs. no drug; n=6). From Moench et al., 2009.

In the Langendorff experiments rats were fed sulindac for 2 days prior to removal of the heart which was then subjected to 45 minutes of ischemia followed by 2 hours of reperfusion with oxygenated buffer (Figure 8). Sulindac was highly protective against myocardial ischemia through mechanisms that did not involve Cox inhibition or its anti-inflammatory capacity.

As an example, the NSAID ibuprofen was not capable of protecting against no flow ischemia in the Langendorff model. Furthermore the oxidized form of sulindac, sulindac sulfone, which as mentioned, is not an NSAID was found to give significant protection against ischemic damage. Through the use of a PKC inhibitor and a ROS scavenging agent we have demonstrated that sulindac protects the heart from ischemic stress by acting as a pharmacological preconditioning agent. PKC is known to mediate preconditioning either by ischemia or by pharmacological agents and in our studies daily administration of the PKC blocker chelerytherine removed the protection provided by sulindac (Figure 8). The

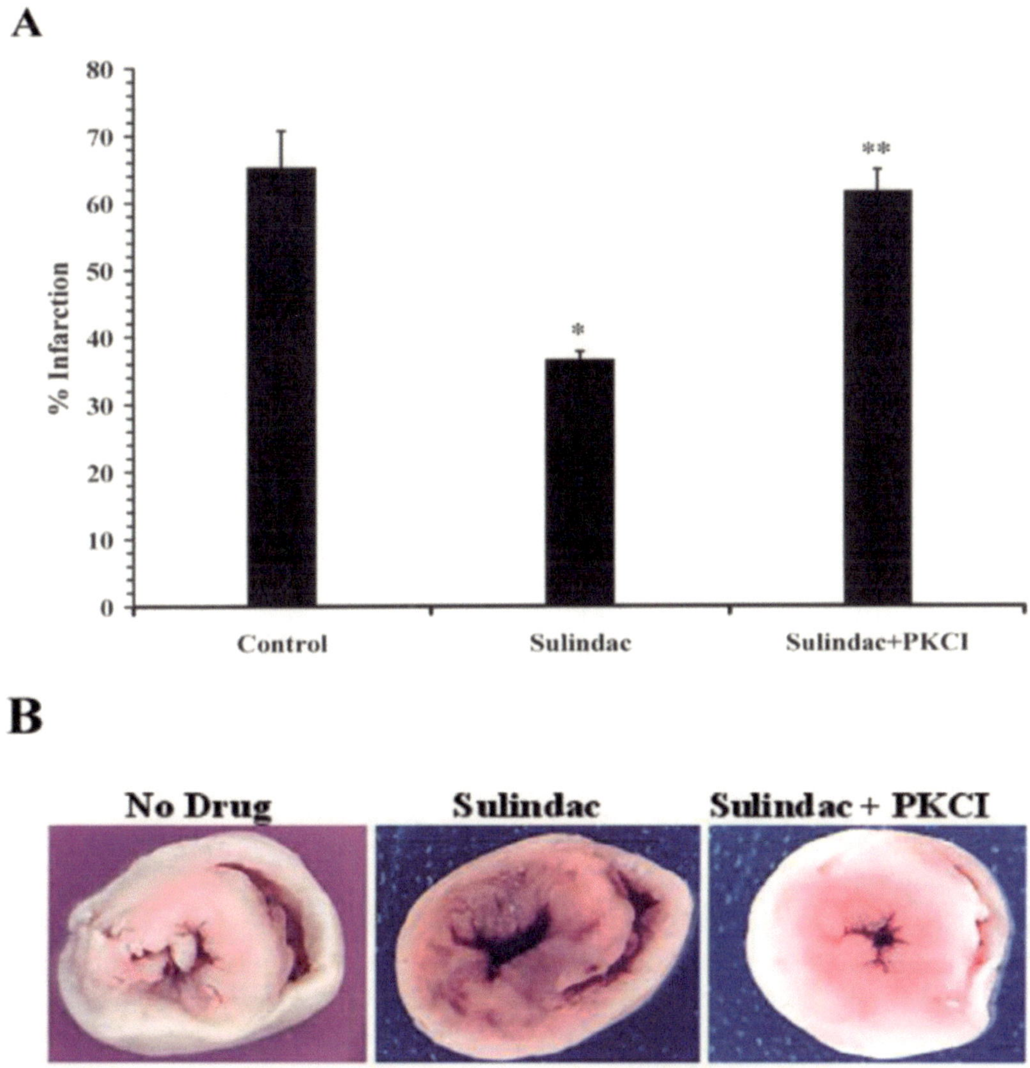

Fig. 8. Effect of feeding sulindac on infarct size after ischemia and reperfusion as measured by TTC staining. Where indicated the PKC inhibitor chelerythrine was administered to the animals. (A) Graph represents percent of heart that was infarcted (*, P<0.01 compared to no-drug control; n=4, **., P<0.01 compared to sulindac treated hearts; n=4). (B) Representative sections from langendorff hearts subjected to 45 min ischemia and 2h reperfusion showing viable tissue (red) and infarcted tissue (white). From Moench et al. 2009.

mechanism of sulindac protection appear to involve the following steps: 1) ROS increase as a trigger for subsequent signaling, 2) signaling through PKC, 3) induction of expression of downstream gene products including iNOS and Hsp27. Ongoing experiments are addressing more specifically the PKC isoforms involved in the protective action of sulindac, in addition to identifying mitochondrial signals that may contribute to the pro-survival response.

As noted above, a remarkable property of sulindac is its ability to kill cancer cells in the presence of an oxidant while being able to protect certain normal cells through pharmacological preconditioning (Marchetti et al., 2009; Moench et al., 2009). It is notable that a similar phenomenon has recently been reported for the PDE-5 inhibitor sildenafil (Das et al., 2010). This drug was found to enhance the doxorubicin induced killing of prostate cancer cells while also protecting cardiac cells from doxorubicin induced cardiomyopathy. The mechanisms of doxorubicin induced killing of cancer cells involved enhanced generation of ROS (Das et al., 2010). It will be important in future studies to determine the ways by which sulindac and sildenafil are capable of modifying the effects of increased ROS in cardiac cells leading to cell survival while also sensitizing cancer cells to oxidative stress resulting in killing of these cells.

7. Final thoughts

Antioxidant based approaches have already shown potential as strategies for the treatment of heart disease and interventions that increase intracellular MsrA have been protective in cardiac cells either through preventing an increase in ROS levels or through modifying important protein targets. Future therapies that are likely to be successful using the MsrA system may need to focus on activation of endogenous MsrA through applying pharmacological activators of MsrA identified from library screening procedures. A recent study by Minniti and colleagues (Minniti et al., 2009) noted that the MsrA promoter is activated by FOXO3A (De Luca et al., 2010). On the basis of this finding a potentially powerful strategy for increasing MsrA expression would involve transfer of FOXO3A protein into cells as a highly permeable TAT-FOXO3A-fusion protein which in turn would translocate to the nucleus and activate the MsrA gene. A simpler and more direct avenue for increasing MsrA levels would be to transfer a TAT-MsrA fusion protein directly into cells.

Regarding sulindac, although there has been serious concern that NSAIDs cause cardiac damage, here we demonstrate that at the concentrations used sulindac can, in fact, afford cardiac protection through preconditioning mechanisms. This is very likely due to the fact that a substantially lower dose is needed for preconditioning than was previously employed for anti-inflammatory applications. Future approaches based on the preconditioning properties of sulindac may involve metabolites or derivatives that are not NSAIDs and do not inhibit COX 1 or COX2. One such metabolite, sulindac sulfone, has been shown to be lacking in NSAID activity but has the cardiac protectant activity (Moench et al., 2009). As there is a very significant need clinically for effective cardioprotective agents our recent studies on cell culture and in vivo models showing high level cardiac protection by MsrA and by sulindac may point to the future application of these agents as important therapeutic breakthroughs for heart disease.

8. Acknowledgements

The research was funded in part by a Grant in Aid from the American Heart Association (to H.P.) and a Florida State University Research Commercialization Assistance Grant (to H.W.).

9. References

Abrams WR, Weinbaum G, Weissbach L, Weissbach H, Brot N. Enzymatic reduction of oxidized alpha-1-proteinase inhibitor restores biological activity. Proc Natl Acad Sci U S A. 1981;78(12):7483-6.

Agrawal RS, Muangman S, Layne MD, Melo L, Perrella MA, Lee RT, Zhang L, Lopez-Ilasaca M, Dzau VJ. Pre-emptive gene therapy using recombinant adeno-associated virus delivery of extracellular superoxide dismutase protects heart against ischemic reperfusion injury, improves ventricular function and prolongs survival. Gene Ther. 2004;11(12):962-9.

Baines CP, Goto M, Downey JM. Oxygen radicals released during ischemic preconditioning contribute to cardioprotection in the rabbit myocardium. J Mol Cell Cardiol. 1997;29(1):207-16.

Bernardo NL, D'Angelo M, Okubo S, Joy A, Kukreja RC. Delayed ischemic preconditioning is mediated by opening of ATP-sensitive potassium channels in the rabbit heart. Am J Physiol. 1999;276(4 Pt 2):H1323-30.

Bokov A, Chaudhuri A, Richardson A. The role of oxidative damage and stress in aging. Mech Ageing Dev. 2004;125(10-11):811-26.

Bolli R. The late phase of preconditioning. Circ Res. 2000;87(11):972-83.

Bolli R. Cardioprotective function of inducible nitric oxide synthase and role of nitric oxide in myocardial ischemia and preconditioning: an overview of a decade of research. J Mol Cell Cardiol. 2001;33(11):1897-918.

Bolli R, Becker L, Gross G, Mentzer R Jr, Balshaw D, Lathrop DA; NHLBI Working Group on the Translation of Therapies for Protecting the Heart from Ischemia. Myocardial protection at a crossroads: the need for translation into clinical therapy. Circ Res. 2004;95(2):125-34.

Bolli R, Bhatti ZA, Tang XL, Qiu Y, Zhang Q, Guo Y, Jadoon AK. Evidence that late preconditioning against myocardial stunning in conscious rabbits is triggered by the generation of nitric oxide. Circ Res. 1997;81(1):42-52.

Brot N, Weissbach L, Werth J, Weissbach H. Enzymatic reduction of protein-bound methionine sulfoxide. Proc Natl Acad Sci U S A. 1981;78(4):2155-8.

Brot N, Weissbach H. Peptide methionine sulfoxide reductase: biochemistry and physiological role. Biopolymers. 2000;55(4):288-96.

Brunell D, Sagher D, Kesaraju S, Brot N, Weissbach H. Studies on the metabolism and biological activity of the epimers of sulindac. Drug Metab Dispos. 2011;39(6):1014-21. Epub 2011 Mar 7.

Cannon RO 3rd. Mechanisms, management and future directions for reperfusion injury after acute myocardial infarction. Nat Clin Pract Cardiovasc Med. 2005;2(2):88-94.

Ciorba MA, Heinemann SH, Weissbach H, Brot N, Hoshi T. Modulation of potassium channel function by methionine oxidation and reduction. Proc Natl Acad Sci U S A. 1997;94(18):9932-7.

Ciolino HP, Bass SE, MacDonald CJ, Cheng RY, Yeh GC. Sulindac and its metabolites induce carcinogen metabolizing enzymes in human colon cancer cells. Int J Cancer. 2008;122(5):990-8.

Costa AD, Pierre SV, Cohen MV, Downey JM, Garlid KD. cGMP signalling in pre- and post-conditioning: the role of mitochondria. Cardiovasc Res. 2008;77(2):344-52.

Das DK. Redox regulation of cardiomyocyte survival and death. Antioxid Redox Signal. 2001;3(1):23-37.

Das A, Durrant D, Mitchell C, Mayton E, Hoke NN, Salloum FN, Park MA, Qureshi I, Lee R, Dent P, Kukreja RC. Sildenafil increases chemotherapeutic efficacy of doxorubicin in prostate cancer and ameliorates cardiac dysfunction. Proc Natl Acad Sci U S A. 2010;107(42):18202-7.

De Luca A, Sanna F, Sallese M, Ruggiero C, Grossi M, Sacchetta P, Rossi C, De Laurenzi V, Di Ilio C, Favaloro B. Methionine sulfoxide reductase A down-regulation in human breast cancer cells results in a more aggressive phenotype. Proc Natl Acad Sci U S A. 2010;107(43):18628-33.

Delbosc S, Cristol JP, Descomps B, Mimran A, Jover B. Simvastatin prevents angiotensin II-induced cardiac alteration and oxidative stress. Hypertension. 2002 Aug;40(2):142-7.

Downey JM. Free radicals and their involvement during long-term myocardial ischemia and reperfusion. Annu Rev Physiol. 1990;52:487-504.

Duggan DE, Hooke KF, Risley EA, Shen TY, Arman CG. Identification of the biologically active form of sulindac. J Pharmacol Exp Ther. 1977;201(1):8-13.

Erickson JR, Joiner ML, Guan X, Kutschke W, Yang J, Oddis CV, Bartlett RK, Lowe JS, O'Donnell SE, Aykin-Burns N, Zimmerman MC, Zimmerman K, Ham AJ, Weiss RM, Spitz DR, Shea MA, Colbran RJ, Mohler PJ, Anderson ME. A dynamic pathway for calcium-independent activation of CaMKII by methionine oxidation. Cell. 2008;133(3):462-74.

Fuster V, Badimon L, Badimon JJ, Chesebro JH. The pathogenesis of coronary artery disease and the acute coronary syndromes (1). N Engl J Med. 1992;326(4):242-50.

Ghosh MC, Wang X, Li S, Klee C. Regulation of calcineurin by oxidative stress. Methods Enzymol. 2003;366:289-304.

Giordano FJ. Oxygen, oxidative stress, hypoxia, and heart failure. J Clin Invest. 2005;115(3):500-8.

Hansel A, Heinemann SH, Hoshi T. Heterogeneity and function of mammalian MSRs: enzymes for repair, protection and regulation. Biochim Biophys Acta. 2005;1703(2):239-47.

Hool LC. Reactive oxygen species in cardiac signalling: from mitochondria to plasma membrane ion channels. Clin Exp Pharmacol Physiol. 2006;33(1-2):146-51.

Izumiya Y, Kim S, Izumi Y, Yoshida K, Yoshiyama M, Matsuzawa A, Ichijo H, Iwao H. Apoptosis signal-regulating kinase 1 plays a pivotal role in angiotensin II-induced cardiac hypertrophy and remodeling. Circ Res. 2003;93(9):874-83.

Jessup M, Brozena S. Heart failure. N Engl J Med. 2003;348(20):2007-18.

Kantorow M, Hawse JR, Cowell TL, Benhamed S, Pizarro GO, Reddy VN, Hejtmancik JF. Methionine sulfoxide reductase A is important for lens cell viability and resistance to oxidative stress. Proc Natl Acad Sci U S A. 2004;101(26):9654-9.

Kim G, Cole NB, Lim JC, Zhao H, Levine RL. Dual sites of protein initiation control the localization and myristoylation of methionine sulfoxide reductase A. J Biol Chem. 2010;285(23):18085-94.

Kim HY, Gladyshev VN. Methionine sulfoxide reduction in mammals: characterization of methionine-R-sulfoxide reductases. Mol Biol Cell. 2004;15(3):1055-64.

Koc A, Gasch AP, Rutherford JC, Kim HY, Gladyshev VN. Methionine sulfoxide reductase regulation of yeast lifespan reveals reactive oxygen species-dependent and -independent components of aging. Proc Natl Acad Sci U S A. 2004;101(21):7999-8004.

Kuzuya T, Hoshida S, Yamashita N, Fuji H, Oe H, Hori M, Kamada T, Tada M. Delayed effects of sublethal ischemia on the acquisition of tolerance to ischemia. Circ Res. 1993;72(6):1293-9.

Kwon SH, Pimentel DR, Remondino A, Sawyer DB, Colucci WS. H(2)O(2) regulates cardiac myocyte phenotype via concentration-dependent activation of distinct kinase pathways. J Mol Cell Cardiol. 2003;35(6):615-21.

Levine RL, Mosoni L, Berlett BS, Stadtman ER. Methionine residues as endogenous antioxidants in proteins. Proc Natl Acad Sci U S A. 1996;93(26):15036-40.

Li JM, Gall NP, Grieve DJ, Chen M, Shah AM. Activation of NADPH oxidase during progression of cardiac hypertrophy to failure. Hypertension. 2002;40(4):477-84.

Liu X, Simpson JA, Brunt KR, Ward CA, Hall SR, Kinobe RT, Barrette V, Tse MY, Pang SC, Pachori AS, Dzau VJ, Ogunyankin KO, Melo LG. Preemptive heme oxygenase-1 gene delivery reveals reduced mortality and preservation of left ventricular function 1 yr after acute myocardial infarction. Am J Physiol Heart Circ Physiol. 2007;293(1):H48-59.

Marber MS, Latchman DS, Walker JM, Yellon DM. Cardiac stress protein elevation 24 hours after brief ischemia or heat stress is associated with resistance to myocardial infarction. Circulation. 1993;88(3):1264-72.

Marchetti MA, Lee W, Cowell TL, Wells TM, Weissbach H, Kantorow M. Silencing of the methionine sulfoxide reductase A gene results in loss of mitochondrial membrane potential and increased ROS production in human lens cells. Exp Eye Res. 2006;83(5):1281-6.

Marchetti M, Resnick L, Gamliel E, Kesaraju S, Weissbach H, Binninger D. Sulindac enhances the killing of cancer cells exposed to oxidative stress. PLoS One. 2009;4(6):e5804.

Maulik N, Yoshida T, Das DK. Regulation of cardiomyocyte apoptosis in ischemic reperfused mouse heart by glutathione peroxidase. Mol Cell Biochem. 1999;196(1-2):13-21.

Melo LG, Pachori AS, Kong D, Gnecchi M, Wang K, Pratt RE, Dzau VJ. Gene and cell-based therapies for heart disease. FASEB J. 2004;18(6):648-63.

Moench I, Prentice H, Rickaway Z, Weissbach H. Sulindac confers high level ischemic protection to the heart through late preconditioning mechanisms. Proc Natl Acad Sci U S A. 2009;106(46):19611-6.

Moskovitz J, Bar-Noy S, Williams WM, Requena J, Berlett BS, Stadtman ER. Methionine sulfoxide reductase (MsrA) is a regulator of antioxidant defense and lifespan in mammals. Proc Natl Acad Sci U S A. 2001;98(23):12920-5.

Moskovitz J, Flescher E, Berlett BS, Azare J, Poston JM, Stadtman ER. Overexpression of peptide-methionine sulfoxide reductase in Saccharomyces cerevisiae and human T cells provides them with high resistance to oxidative stress. Proc Natl Acad Sci U S A. 1998;95(24):14071-5.

Moskovitz J, Weissbach H, Brot N. Cloning and expression of a mammalian gene involved in the reduction of methionine sulfoxide residues in proteins. Proc Natl Acad Sci U S A. 1996;93(5):2095-9.

Murry CE, Jennings RB, Reimer KA. Preconditioning with ischemia: a delay of lethal cell injury in ischemic myocardium. Circulation. 1986;74(5):1124-36.

Nabel EG. Cardiovascular disease. N Engl J Med. 2003;349(1):60-72.

Nakamura K, Fushimi K, Kouchi H, Mihara K, Miyazaki M, Ohe T, Namba M. Inhibitory effects of antioxidants on neonatal rat cardiac myocyte hypertrophy induced by tumor necrosis factor-alpha and angiotensin II. Circulation. 1998;98(8):794-9.

Nan C, Li Y, Jean-Charles PY, Chen G, Kreymerman A, Prentice H, Weissbach H, Huang X. Deficiency of methionine sulfoxide reductase A causes cellular dysfunction and mitochondrial damage in cardiac myocytes under physical and oxidative stresses. Biochem Biophys Res Commun. 2010;402(4):608-13.

Ockaili R, Emani VR, Okubo S, Brown M, Krottapalli K, Kukreja RC. Opening of mitochondrial KATP channel induces early and delayed cardioprotective effect: role of nitric oxide. Am J Physiol. 1999;277(6 Pt 2):H2425-34.

Oien DB, Osterhaus GL, Latif SA, Pinkston JW, Fulks J, Johnson M, Fowler SC, Moskovitz J. MsrA knockout mouse exhibits abnormal behavior and brain dopamine levels. Free Radic Biol Med. 2008;45(2):193-200.

Otani H, Umemoto M, Kagawa K, Nakamura Y, Omoto K, Tanaka K, Sato T, Nonoyama A, Kagawa T. Protection against oxygen-induced reperfusion injury of the isolated canine heart by superoxide dismutase and catalase. J Surg Res. 1986;41(2):126-33.

Pachori AS, Smith A, McDonald P, Zhang L, Dzau VJ, Melo LG. Heme-oxygenase-1-induced protection against hypoxia/reoxygenation is dependent on biliverdin reductase and its interaction with PI3K/Akt pathway. J Mol Cell Cardiol. 2007;43(5):580-92.

Papaharalambus CA, Griendling KK. Basic mechanisms of oxidative stress and reactive oxygen species in cardiovascular injury. Trends Cardiovasc Med. 2007;17(2):48-54.

Poss KD, Tonegawa S. Reduced stress defense in heme oxygenase 1-deficient cells. Proc Natl Acad Sci U S A. 1997;94(20):10925-30.

Prentice HM, Moench IA, Rickaway ZT, Dougherty CJ, Webster KA, Weissbach H. MsrA protects cardiac myocytes against hypoxia/reoxygenation induced cell death. Biochem Biophys Res Commun. 2008;366(3):775-8.

Rahman MA, Nelson H, Weissbach H, Brot N. Cloning, sequencing, and expression of the Escherichia coli peptide methionine sulfoxide reductase gene. J Biol Chem. 1992;267(22):15549-51.

Ruan H, Tang XD, Chen ML, Joiner ML, Sun G, Brot N, Weissbach H, Heinemann SH, Iverson L, Wu CF, Hoshi T. High-quality life extension by the enzyme peptide methionine sulfoxide reductase. Proc Natl Acad Sci U S A. 2002;99(5):2748-53.

Sabri A, Hughie HH, Lucchesi PA. Regulation of hypertrophic and apoptotic signaling pathways by reactive oxygen species in cardiac myocytes. Antioxid Redox Signal. 2003;5(6):731-40.

Salmon AB, Pérez VI, Bokov A, Jernigan A, Kim G, Zhao H, Levine RL, Richardson A. Lack of methionine sulfoxide reductase A in mice increases sensitivity to oxidative stress but does not diminish life span. FASEB J. 2009;23(10):3601-8.

Schaper J, Froede R, Hein S, Buck A, Hashizume H, Speiser B, Friedl A, Bleese N. Impairment of the myocardial ultrastructure and changes of the cytoskeleton in dilated cardiomyopathy. Circulation. 1991;83(2):504-14.

Scholz D, Diener W, Schaper J. Altered nucleus/cytoplasm relationship and degenerative structural changes in human dilated cardiomyopathy. Cardioscience. 1994;5(2):127-38.

St John G, Brot N, Ruan J, Erdjument-Bromage H, Tempst P, Weissbach H, Nathan C. Peptide methionine sulfoxide reductase from Escherichia coli and Mycobacterium tuberculosis protects bacteria against oxidative damage from reactive nitrogen intermediates. Proc Natl Acad Sci U S A. 2001;98(17):9901-6.

Stocker R, Yamamoto Y, McDonagh AF, Glazer AN, Ames BN. Bilirubin is an antioxidant of possible physiological importance. Science. 1987;235(4792):1043-6.

Sugamura K, Keaney JF Jr. Reactive oxygen species in cardiovascular disease. Free Radic Biol Med. 2011;51(5):978-92.

Terman A, Dalen H, Eaton JW, Neuzil J, Brunk UT. Aging of cardiac myocytes in culture: oxidative stress, lipofuscin accumulation, and mitochondrial turnover. Ann N Y Acad Sci. 2004;1019:70-7.

Trillo AA, Holleman IL, White JT. Presence of satellite cells in a cardiac rhabdomyoma. Histopathology. 1978;2(3):215-23.

Tritto I, D'Andrea D, Eramo N, Scognamiglio A, De Simone C, Violante A, Esposito A, Chiariello M, Ambrosio G. Oxygen radicals can induce preconditioning in rabbit hearts. Circ Res. 1997;80(5):743-8.

Turoczi T, Chang VW, Engelman RM, Maulik N, Ho YS, Das DK. Thioredoxin redox signaling in the ischemic heart: an insight with transgenic mice overexpressing Trx1. J Mol Cell Cardiol. 2003;35(6):695-704.

Vivekananthan DP, Penn MS, Sapp SK, Hsu A, Topol EJ. Use of antioxidant vitamins for the prevention of cardiovascular disease: meta-analysis of randomised trials. Lancet. 2003;361(9374):2017-23.

Vougier S, Mary J, Friguet B. Subcellular localization of methionine sulphoxide reductase A (MsrA): evidence for mitochondrial and cytosolic isoforms in rat liver cells. Biochem J. 2003;373(Pt 2):531-7.

Weissbach H, Resnick L, Brot N. Methionine sulfoxide reductases: history and cellular role in protecting against oxidative damage. Biochim Biophys Acta. 2005;1703(2):203-12.

Xuan YT, Guo Y, Zhu Y, Wang OL, Rokosh G, Bolli R. Endothelial nitric oxide synthase plays an obligatory role in the late phase of ischemic preconditioning by activating the protein kinase C epsilon p44/42 mitogen-activated protein kinase pSer-signal transducers and activators of transcription1/3 pathway. Circulation. 2007;116(5):535-44.

Yao Y, Yin D, Jas GS, Kuczer K, Williams TD, Schöneich C, Squier TC. Oxidative modification of a carboxyl-terminal vicinal methionine in calmodulin by hydrogen peroxide inhibits calmodulin-dependent activation of the plasma membrane Ca-ATPase. Biochemistry. 1996;35(8):2767-87.

Yellon DM, Downey JM. Spotlight on preconditioning. Cardiovasc Res. 2002;55(3):425-8.

Yermolaieva O, Brot N, Weissbach H, Heinemann SH, Hoshi T. Reactive oxygen species and nitric oxide mediate plasticity of neuronal calcium signaling. Proc Natl Acad Sci U S A. 2000;97(1):448-53.

Yermolaieva O, Xu R, Schinstock C, Brot N, Weissbach H, Heinemann SH, Hoshi T. Methionine sulfoxide reductase A protects neuronal cells against brief hypoxia/reoxygenation.Proc Natl Acad Sci U S A. 2004;101(5):1159-64.

Yoshida T, Watanabe M, Engelman DT, Engelman RM, Schley JA, Maulik N, Ho YS, Oberley TD, Das DK. Transgenic mice overexpressing glutathione peroxidase are resistant to myocardial ischemia reperfusion injury. J Mol Cell Cardiol. 1996;28(8):1759-67.

Zhao H, Sun J, Deschamps AM, Kim G, Liu C, Murphy E, Levine RL. Myristoylated Methionine Sulfoxide Reductase A Protects the Heart from Ischemia-Reperfusion Injury. Am J Physiol Heart Circ Physiol. 2011. [Epub ahead of print]

Zweier JL, Flaherty JT, Weisfeldt ML. Direct measurement of free radical generation following reperfusion of ischemic myocardium. Proc Natl Acad Sci U S A. 1987;84(5):1404-7.

13

Hepatic Lipid Accumulation by High Cholesterol Diet is Inhibited by the Low Dose Fish Oil in Male C57BL/6J Mice

Satoshi Hirako, Miki Harada, Hyoun-Ju Kim*,
Hiroshige Chiba and Akiyo Matsumoto
Josai University
Japan

1. Introduction

Atherosclerotic diseases such as ischemic heart disease and cerebral infarction account for the major causes of death in many countries. It is well known that hyperlipidemia is closely associated with these diseases (Kodama, 1990). Fish oil consumption reduces lipogenesis and induces fatty acid oxidation in liver(Rustan, 1990; Halminski, 1991), and ameliorates plasma and hepatic lipid levels (Nestel, 1990). These effects of fish are greatly attributed to the action of n-3 polyunsaturated fatty acids, such as eicosapentaenoic acid (EPA) or docosahexaenoic acid (DHA). Several studies have reported that n-3 PUFA decreases the expression of genes coding for lipogenesis enzymes such as fatty acid synthase (FAS), acetyl-CoA carboxylase (ACC), and stearoyl-CoA desaturase (SCD) through the lowering of sterol regulatory element binding protein-1 (SREBP-1) (Kim, 1999; Shimano, 1999; Nakatani, 2002). In addition, n-3 PUFA activates the peroxisome proliferator-activated receptor α (PPARα) (Krey, 1997). PPARα is a ligand-activated transcription factor that regulates the expression of genes involved in triglyceride hydrolysis and fatty acid oxidation (Latruffe, 1997; Nakatani, 2002; Schoonjans, 1996), such as acyl-CoA oxidase (AOX), lipoprotein lipase (LPL), medium-chain acyl-CoA dehydrogenase (MCAD), acyl-CoA synthetase (ACS), and uncoupling protein-2 (UCP-2).

Cholesterol is crucial for the components of animal cell membranes, and for the synthesis of bile acid and steroid hormone. Cholesterol in the inner cavity of the small intestine are entered in to epithelial cells by Niemann-Pick C1 like-1 (NPC1L1) protein on the brush border of epithelial cells of the small intestine (Davis, 2004), and cholesterol is released into the lymph duct. It is well known that cholesterols, including 22- and 24-hydroxy cholesterol, act as ligands for liver X receptor (LXR) α (Schultz, 2000). LXRα, a nuclear receptor, forms a heterodimer together with the retinoid X receptor (RXR) and combines with LXR element (LXRE) at the promoter of target genes to control transcription. LXR target genes include cholesterol 7α-hydroxylase (CYP7A1), ATP-binding cassette transporter (ABC)A1, ABCG1, and SREBPs, which are highly involved in cholesterol metabolism (Repa, 2000; Peet, 1998).

We previously indicated that 20en% fish oil diet dramatically inhibited hepatic lipids accumulation in female C57BL/6J mice fed 2% cholesterol (Hirako, 2010). In this study, we determined whether 2 or 5en% fish oil, eqivalent to 10 or 25% of the total fat energy, improves lipid metabolism in high cholesterol diet fed male C57BL/6J mice. Mice were given SO diet consisted of 20en% safflower oil, 2FO diet consisted of 2en% fish oil plus 18en% safflower oil, 5FO diet consisted of 5en% fish oil plus 15en% safflower oil, and SO/CH, 2FO/CH, 5FO/CH are consisted of SO, 2FO, 5FO with 2%cholesterol. The body fat composition of mice was examined radiographically using an X-ray CT for experimental animals. Blood parameter and hepatic lipids were measured using enzymatic methods. Hepatic mRNA expression levels were measured by real-time RT-PCR.

2. Results and discussion

2.1 Body weight and tissue weight did not change with the low dose fish oil feeding in male C57BL/6J mice

Final body weights were not significantly different among the groups. No large difference in weights of the white adipose tissue around the uterus and brown adipose tissue from the interscapular region between the groups was observed. In previous study, we reported that body weight gain was significantly decreased in female C57BL/6J mice fed 20 en% fish oil (Hirako, 2010). However, our study observed that 5 en% fish oil feeding in female C57BL/6J mice did not modify body weights (data not shown). These results revealed that 2 and 5 en% fish oil feeding in male C57BL/6J mice did not modify body weight and adipose tissue weight

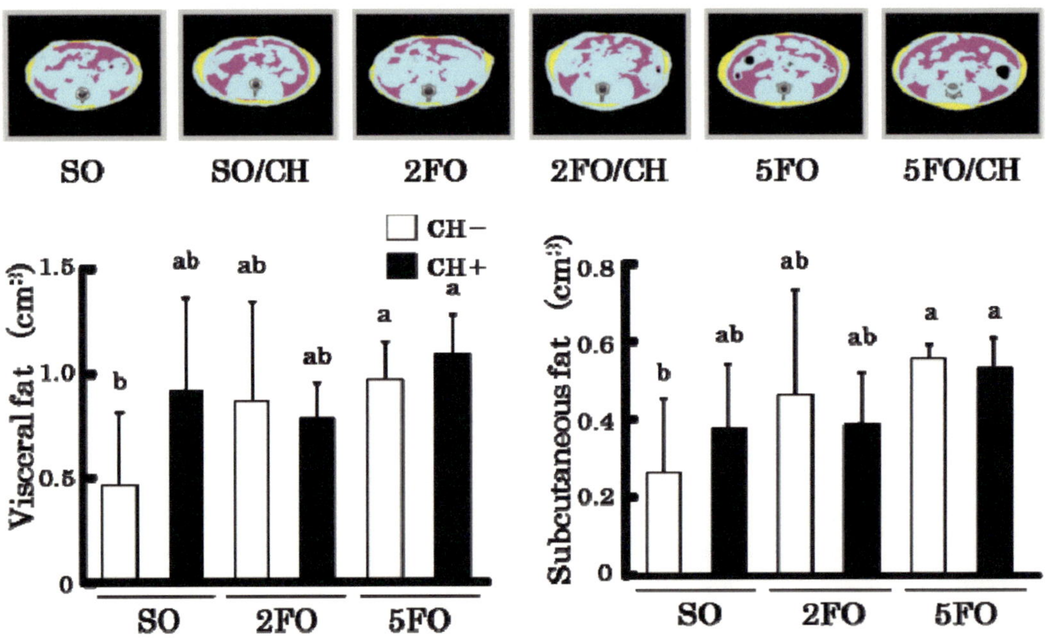

Representative X-ray CT images of mice fed SO, SO/CH, 2FO, 2FO/CH, 5FO, and 5FO/CH for 8 weeks, at the L3 level (upper). The areas indicated with pink, yellow, and light-blue are visceral fat, subcutaneous fat, and muscle, respectively. CT-estimated amounts of visceral fat and subcutaneous fat in the abdominal area of L2–L4(bottom). Values represent means ± S.D. (n=5). Means with different letters are different at the $p<0.05$ level by Fisher's protected least significant difference (PLSD) test.

Fig. 1. CT-based fat tissues composition analysis of 16-week-old male C57BL/6J mice.

as well as female C57BL/6J mice. CT scan analysis showed that visceral and subcutaneous fat mass were significantly increased in the 5FO and 5FO/CH groups, but not changed by cholesterol feeding (Figure 1). Meanwhile, these levels were high in all group compared with the fat mass in the female C57BL/6J mice (0.45±0.28cm^3 visceral fat in male C57BL/6J mice fed the SO diet and 0.24±0.13 cm^3 visceral fat in female C57BL/6J mice fed the SO diet).

2.2 Hepatic tissue histology and lipid levels modified with the low dose fish oil feeding in male C57BL/6J mice

Although the liver weight significantly increased in the SO/CH group compared with the SO group, there was no difference in the fish oil groups compared with the SO group (SO: 0.96 ± 0.10, SO/CH: 1.31 ± 1.2, 2FO: 1.00 ± 0.13, 2FO/CH: 1.11 ± 0.12, 5FO: 0.92 ± 0.08, 5FO/CH: 1.12 ± 0.12, $p<0.05$). The liver size in the SO/CH group had enlarged, and the entire surface had a pale color, suggestive of increased lipid storage. In contrast, the livers of the 2FO/CH and 5FO/CH groups were less pale and had a normal reddish appearance (data not shown). The hepatic tissues showed numerous lipid droplets in the livers of SO/CH group. However, these lipid droplets were markedly decreased in the 2FO/CH and 5FO/CH groups (Figure 2A). These results in the microscopic images of hepatic tissue were confirmed in hepatic lipid content reductions. Hepatic TG levels in both 2FO/CH and 5FO/CH group significantly decreased to about 50% of that in the SO/CH group. Hepatic TC levels also decreased by about 40% in both 2FO/CH and 5FO/CH group compared with the SO/CH group(Figure 2B). Fabbrini suggested that hepatic lipid accumulation is considered a risk factor for fatty liver and steatohepatitis, which promote the development

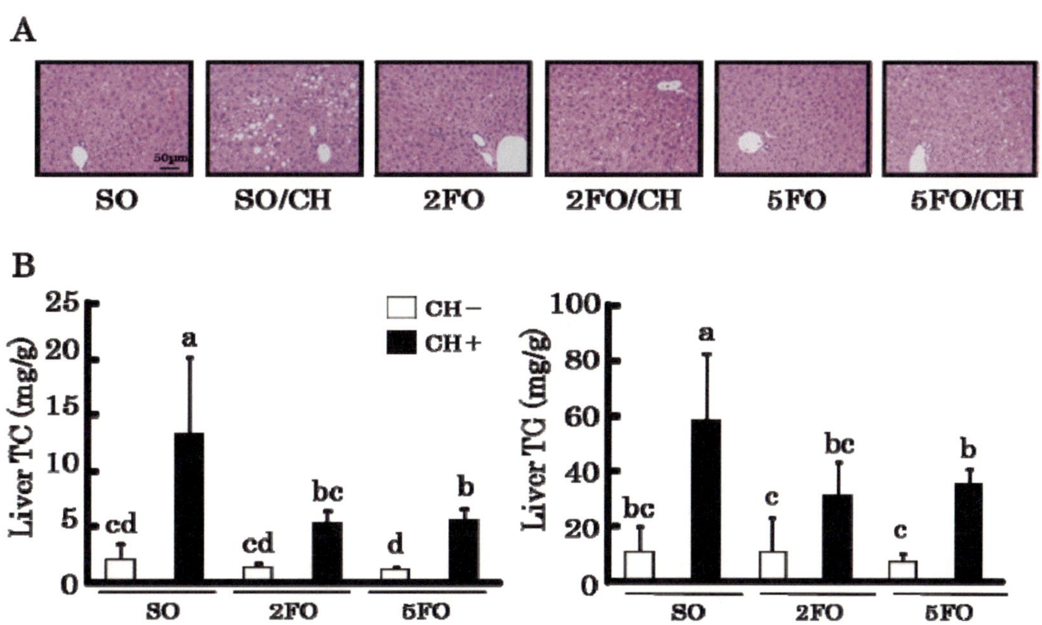

H&E-stained liver sections (A), total cholesterol (TC) and triglycerides (TG) (B) in mice fed SO, SO/CH, 2FO, 2FO/CH, 5FO, and 5FO/CH for 8. Values represent means ± S.D. (n=5). Means with different letters are different at the $p<0.05$ level by Fisher's protected least significant difference (PLSD) test.

Fig. 2. Liver tissue histology and lipid levels of 16-week-old male C57BL/6J mice.

of insulin resistance, dyslipidemia, and cardiovascular disease (Fabbrini, 2010). In this study, lipid deposition caused by high cholesterol feeding significantly decreased in the 2FO/CH and 5FO/CH groups, in which low dose fish oil was used as the lipid source. We confirmed that the 2 en% fish oil exerts ameliorating effects on hepatic lipid accumulation due to dietary cholesterol consumption in male C57BL/6J mice.

2.3 The hepatic mRNA levels of lipid metabolism-regulating genes modfied with the fish oil or cholesterol feeding in male C57BL/6J mice

The hepatic mRNA levels of lipid metabolism-regulating genes are shown in Table 1. The mRNA levels of SREBP-1c, which is transcription factor of genes related to lipogenesis, were not significantly changed in all groups. Low dose fish oil or cholesterol feeding did not particularly affect in FAS mRNA. However, SCD1 mRNA levels significantly decreased in the fish oil groups regardless of the addition the addition of cholesterol, compared with the SO/CH group. Previous studies showed that fish oil feeding decreases SREBP1c mRNA expression and/or mature protein production and results in the inhibition of SREBP1 target genes, such as ACC, FAS, and SCD-1 (Kim, 1999; Nakatani, 2002). In this study, different results were observed, suggesting that the inhibitory effect of fish oil on fatty acid biosynthesis is more clear at high dose fish oil.

	SO	SO/CH	2FO	2FO/CH	5FO	5FO/CH
SREBPs						
SREBP-1c	1.00 ± 0.31	1.27 ± 0.45	0.96 ± 0.56	1.21 ± 0.99	0.88 ± 0.29	0.81 ± 0.55
SREBP-2	1.00 ± 0.51^{c}	0.95 ± 0.06^{c}	1.88 ± 0.19^{a}	0.93 ± 0.14^{c}	1.41 ± 0.32^{b}	0.71 ± 0.12^{c}
Insig-1	1.00 ± 0.76^{bc}	1.44 ± 0.75^{abc}	2.42 ± 1.50^{a}	0.89 ± 0.52^{bc}	1.87 ± 0.57^{ab}	0.61 ± 0.20^{c}
Fatty acid biosynthesis						
FAS	1.00 ± 0.84^{a}	0.81 ± 0.58^{ab}	0.98 ± 0.39^{a}	0.58 ± 0.24^{ab}	0.85 ± 0.23^{ab}	0.32 ± 0.19^{b}
SCD1	1.00 ± 0.33^{ab}	1.46 ± 0.73^{a}	0.43 ± 0.32^{c}	0.82 ± 0.38^{bc}	0.35 ± 0.08^{c}	0.63 ± 0.19^{bc}
Cholesterol homeostasis						
HMGCo(A) Reductase	1.00 ± 0.30^{a}	0.67 ± 0.15^{bc}	0.85 ± 0.37^{ab}	0.66 ± 0.03^{bc}	1.07 ± 0.23^{a}	0.54 ± 0.10^{c}
ABCG5	1.00 ± 0.57^{c}	2.61 ± 0.29^{a}	0.94 ± 0.15^{c}	1.68 ± 0.25^{b}	0.81 ± 0.13^{c}	1.41 ± 0.18^{b}
ABCG8	1.00 ± 0.32^{d}	1.54 ± 0.32^{a}	1.25 ± 0.29^{cd}	2.18 ± 0.72^{ab}	0.95 ± 0.15^{d}	1.95 ± 0.43^{bc}
Fatty acid β-oxidation						
PPARα	1.00 ± 0.30^{b}	1.74 ± 0.74^{ab}	2.51 ± 1.03^{a}	2.32 ± 0.68^{a}	1.93 ± 0.49^{a}	1.97 ± 0.77^{a}
AOX	1.00 ± 0.49^{c}	1.54 ± 0.61^{bc}	1.66 ± 0.39^{b}	1.79 ± 0.43^{abc}	1.82 ± 0.33^{ab}	2.42 ± 0.66^{a}
UCP2	1.00 ± 0.32^{ab}	1.54 ± 0.32^{a}	0.99 ± 0.74^{ab}	$1.19 \pm 0.68a^{b}$	0.70 ± 0.13^{b}	1.05 ± 0.38^{ab}
Bile acid bioynthesis						
CYP7A1	1.00 ± 0.57^{c}	3.12 ± 0.79^{ab}	1.27 ± 1.17^{c}	1.96 ± 0.80^{bc}	1.43 ± 0.81^{c}	3.63 ± 1.01^{a}
CYP8B1	1.00 ± 0.45^{b}	1.26 ± 0.29^{ab}	1.12 ± 0.47^{ab}	1.33 ± 0.32^{ab}	1.01 ± 0.19^{b}	1.55 ± 0.58^{a}

The mRNA expression levels in liver of male C57BL/6J mice fed SO, SO/CH, 2FO, 2FO/CH, 5FO, and 5FO/CH for 8 weeks. Values represent means ± S.D. (n=4-5). Means with different letters are different at the $p<0.05$ level by Fisher's protected least significant difference (PLSD) test.

Table 1. Expression of genes associated with lipid metabolism in the liver

The mRNA levels of PPARα and AOX, genes involved in fatty acid oxidation, were significantly higher in the fish oil groups regardless of the addition of cholesterol. However, the mRNA levels of UCP-2, which is involved in heat production, were unaffected by low dose fish oil or cholesterol feeding. The mRNA levels of ABCG5 and ABCG8, genes involved in cholesterol transport into the bile, were significantly induced with the cholesterol addition . Biliary cholesterol excretion increases due to the upregulation of these genes (Repa, 2002). These increases in ABCG5 and ABCG8 mRNA by cholesterol feeding are crucial for the maintenance of cholesterol homeostasis. Indeed, the mRNA levels of CYP7A1, the rate-limiting gene in bile acid synthesis, were significantly increased in all cholesterol-supplemented groups. However, no such increases were observed in the expression of CYP8B1 mRNA. The synthesis of bile acid in the liver is important in the catabolic pathway of cholesterol. The bile acid systhesis is controlled by CYP7A1 (Berge, 2000). In this study, the mRNA levels of CYP7A1 were not significantly affected by fish oil feeding, but its levels significantly increased when cholesterol was added. This is consistent with previous observation that CYP7A1 mRNA level is increased on the addition of cholesterol to maintain the homeostasis of cholesterol.

3. Conclusion

Body weight gains and adipose tissue weights did not change with the low dose fish oil feeding in male C57BL/6J mice. Hepatic triglyceride and total cholesterol levels of the SO/CH group were dramatically increased compared to the SO group. However, in 2FO/CH and 5FO/CH groups, the hepatic lipids were significantly decreased compared to the SO/CH group. Low dose fish oil or cholesterol feeding did not particularly affect in SREBP-1C and FAS mRNA levels. But, PPARα and AOX mRNA levels were significantly higher in the fish oil groups regardless of the cholesterol addition. The present study indicates that low dose fish oil obviously improved the hepatic lipid accumulation by high cholesterol diet. And, this improving effect is partly due to the fatty acid degradation, which was facilitated by increased expression of fatty acid oxidation-related genes, such as AOX.

4. Acknowledgments

We would like to thank NOF Corporation (Tokyo, Japan) for providing FO.

5. References

Berge KE, Tian H, Graf GA, Yu L, Grishin NV, Schultz J, Kwiterovich P, Shan B, Barnes R, Hobbs HH. Accumulation of dietary cholesterol in sitosterolemia caused by mutations in adjacent ABC transporters. Science 2000; 290: 1771-1775

Davis HR Jr, Zhu LJ, Hoos LM, Tetzloff G, Maguire M, Liu J, Yao X, Iyer SP, Lam MH, Lund EG, Detmers PA, Graziano MP, Altmann SW. Niemann-Pick C1 Like 1 (NPC1L1) is the intestinal phytosterol and cholesterol transporter and a key modulator of whole-body cholesterol homeostasis. J Biol Chem 2004; 279: 33586-33592

Fabbrini E, Sullivan S, Klein S. Obesity and nonalcoholic fatty liver disease: biochemical, metabolic, and clinical implications. Hepatology 2010; 51: 679-689

Halminski MA, Marsh JB, and Harrison EH: Differential effects of fish oil, safflower oil and palm oil on fatty acid oxidation and glycerolipid synthesis in rat liver. J Nutr, 1991; 121: 1554-1561

Hirako S, Kim HJ, Arai T, Chiba H, Matsumoto A. Effect of concomitantly used fish oil and cholesterol on lipid metabolism. J Nutr Biochem 2010; 21: 573-579

Kim HJ, Takahashi M, Ezaki O: Fish oil feeding decreases mature sterol regulatory element-binding protein 1 (SREBP-1) by down-regulation of SREBP-1c mRNA in mouse liver. A possible mechanism for down-regulation of lipogenic enzyme mRNAs. J Biol Chem, 1999; 274: 25892-25898

Kodama K, Sasaki H, Shimizu Y. Trend of coronary heart disease and its relationship to risk factors in a Japanese population: a 26-year follow-up, Hiroshima/Nagasaki study. Circ J, 1990; 54: 414-421

Krey G, Braissant O, L'Horset F, Kalkhoven E, Perroud M, Parker MG, Wahli W: Fatty acids, eicosanoids, and hypolipidemic agents identified as ligands of peroxisome proliferator-activated receptors by coactivator-dependent receptor ligand assay. Mol Endocrinol, 1997; 11: 779–791

Latruffe N, Vamecq J: Peroxisome proliferators and peroxisome proliferator activated receptors (PPARs) as regulators of lipid metabolism. Biochimie, 1997; 79: 81–94

Nakatani T, Tsuboyama-Kasaoka N, Takahashi M, Miura S, Ezaki O; Mechanism for peroxisome proliferator-activated receptor-alpha activator-induced up-regulation of UCP2 mRNA in rodent hepatocytes. J Biol Chem, 2002; 277: 9562–9569

Nestel PJ. Effects of N-3 fatty acids on lipid metabolism. Annu Rev Nutr, 1990; 10:149-167

Peet DJ, Turley SD, Ma W, Janowski BA, Lobaccaro JM, Hammer RE, Mangelsdorf DJ. Cholesterol and Bile Acid Metabolism Are Impaired in Mice Lacking the Nuclear Oxysterol Receptor LXRα. Cell 1998; 93: 693-704

Repa JJ, Berge KE, Pomajzl C, Richardson JA, Hobbs H, Mangelsdorf DJ. Regulation of ATP-binding cassette sterol transporters ABCG5 and ABCG8 by the liver X receptors alpha and beta. J Biol Chem 2002 ; 277: 18793-18800

Repa JJ, Liang G, Ou J, Bashmakov Y, Lobaccaro JM, Shimomura I, Shan B, Brown MS, Goldstein JL, Mangelsdorf DJ. Regulation of mouse sterol regulatory element-binding protein-1c gene （SREBP-1c） by oxysterol receptor, LXRα and LXRβ. Genes Dev 2000; 14: 2819-2830

Rustan AC, Nossen JO, Christiansen EN, and Drevon CA: Eicosapentaenoic acid reduces hepatic synthesis and secretion of triacylglycerol by decreasing the activity of acyl-coenzyme A:1,2- diacylglycerol acyltransferase. J Lipid Res, 1988; 29: 1417-1426

Schoonjans K, Staels B, Auwerx J: The peroxisome proliferator activated receptors (PPARS) and their effects on lipid metabolism and adipocyte differentiation. Biochim Biophys Acta, 1996; 1302: 93–109

Schultz JR, Tu H, Luk A, Repa JJ, Medina JC, Li L, Schwendner S, Wang S, Thoolen M, Mangelsdorf DJ, Lustig KD, Shan B.Role of LXRs in control of lipogenesis. Genes Dev 2000; 14: 2831-2838

Shimano H, Yahagi N, Amemiya-Kudo M, Hasty AH, Osuga J, Tamura Y, Shionoiri F, Iizuka Y, Ohashi K, Harada K, Gotoda T, Ishibashi S, Yamada N. Sterol regulatory element-binding protein-1 as a key transcription factor for nutritional induction of lipogenic enzyme genes. J Biol Chem 1999; 274: 35832-35829

14

Cardiac Protection with Targeted Drug Delivery to Ischemic-Reperfused Myocardium

Michael Galagudza
V. A. Almazov Federal Heart, Blood and Endocrinology Centre
Russian Federation

1. Introduction

The concept of targeted drug delivery implies selective accumulation of the drug in the tissue affected by the pathological process after systemic administration of the drug and its carrier with minimal effect of the former on the intact organs and tissues (Lammers et al., 2010). The idea of targeted delivery has been first suggested by Paul Erhlich in 1906 when he introduced the concept of «magic bullet» which is directed against target cells only without any damage to healthy tissue (Erhlich, 1906). In the current medical practice, most of the drugs are administered orally or parenterally, resulting in natural biodistribution and systemic effect on the organism. This type of distribution is justified for the drugs which act on the systemic mechanisms of disease development and progression. At the same time, in case of focal pathological processes such as tumor growth, inflammation and ischemia it may be more clinically attractive to ensure the local rise in the drug concentration within the pathological area thus avoiding the putative side effects on neighboring tissues. This point can be illustrated by several examples. It is known that the administration of antitumor drug doxorubicin is associated with severe cardiomyopathy, suppression of myelo- and megakaryopoiesis, nausea, vomiting, and development of alopecia (Carvalho et al., 2009). Encapsulation of doxorubicin into liposomes resulted in dramatic reduction of these dose-limiting side effects (Leonard et al., 2009). The implementation of site-specific drug delivery may also benefit female patients receiving estrogens for treatment of osteoporosis. Along with desirable effect on the bone, estrogens may cause some unwanted effects, especially increased risk of uterine bleeding and development of endometrial cancer (Romer, 2006). One might suggest that bone-targeted delivery of estrogens will decrease the probability of these side effects. The application of nano-sized particles for drug transport may offer a new means of delivering drugs selectively into the affected tissue.

Typical nanoparticulate carrier for targeted drug delivery comprises several functional elements. The major part of the carrier is drug-loaded nanoparticle. An important step in nanocarrier fabrication is the functionalization of its surface which implies binding of the targeting ligands to the nanoparticle surface. Targeting ligand ensures specific interaction of the nanoparticle with the complementary molecules on the surface membrane of the target cell. In order to facilitate the process of functionalization and prevent rapid clearance of nanoparticles by the reticulo-endothelial system, the surface of the nanoparticle is often covered with biocompatible coating such as polyethylene glycol. The nanoparticles can be additionally labeled with radioactive isotopes or fluorescent dyes which allows visualization of their accumulation in the damaged tissue. Successful targeted drug delivery with use of nanoparticulate carriers can bring solutions to several serious problems. In particular, it may result in reduced toxicity, increased solubility and stability of the drugs.

To date, the research on targeted drug delivery has been mostly concentrated on the development of tumor-targeted nanomedicines (Ali et al., 2011). It might be hypothesized that targeted drug delivery strategy approved in oncology can be applied in other clinical fields, now not for destruction but for the sake of salvage of reversibly injured cells, in particular of those destined otherwise to die within the area of myocardial ischemia-reperfusion. One reasonable approach to the problem may be targeted intramyocardial delivery of the agents (i.e., certain angiogenic growth factors, erythropoietin, ATP-sensitive potassium channel openers, etc.), either covalently and/or non-covalently bound to the nanoparticulate carriers. Thus, the purpose of this chapter is to provide an account of acquired knowledge on nanoparticle-based targeted drug delivery with particular emphasis on heart targeting. Besides, the original experimental data on the fabrication of silica nanoparticles which can be used as prototype carriers for cardioprotective drugs are presented. We also present the data on silica nanoparticle biodistribution, biodegradation, and acute toxicity. Finally, the preliminary evidence for enhanced infarct size limitation with use of silica nanoparticle-bound adenosine is provided.

2. Major types of nanocarriers for targeted drug delivery

The various types of nano-sized particles can be utilized for transport of drugs into the diseased tissues. Liposomes, drug-polymer conjugates, polymeric micelles, dendrimers, nanoshells, and nucleic acid-based carriers can all be used as nanocarriers for drugs (Wang et al., 2008). Among them, drug-polymer conjugates and liposomes are currently most commonly used for drug delivery in the clinical settings and collectively amount to at least 80% of all nanopharmaceuticals available on the market. The choice of the material for nanocarrier fabrication mainly depends on the chemical structure of the drug to be transported, characteristics of the target tissue and the route of nanocarrier administration into the organism (Ganta et al., 2008). It is generally accepted that the properties of ideal nanocarrier should include biocompatibility, biodegradability, and evasion of rapid uptake by the macrophages.

2.1 Liposomes

Liposomes are spherical membrane structures that consist of a phospholipid bilayer which can entrap aqueous solutions. In the past decade, considerable information has been accumulated on the therapeutic applications of liposomes (Fenske & Cullis, 2008). By now, there are 9 liposomal drugs approved for clinical use. Liposomal doxorubicin and daunomycin are successfully used for treatment of cancer while liposomal amphotericin remains to be a cornerstone for the treatment of some fungal infections.

2.2 Polymer-drug conjugates

Peptides and the drugs with low molecular weight are often characterized by the short half-life in the circulation thus requiring repeated administration and, furthermore, can exhibit non-specific adverse effect on organs and tissues. Binding of the drugs with polymer nanocarriers may reduce these negative effects. Despite the fact that a great number of diverse polymers have been initially considered for drug delivery, the very few of them have been finally approved for clinical applications. Polyethylene glycol is the most universal polymer drug carrier. It has been introduced in the clinical practice in the early 90s and has rapidly become popular as drug vehicle because of its capability to increase the stability of drugs in the plasma, improve solubility of hydrophobic drugs and reduce their immunogenicity. Apart from polyethylene glycol, gamma-polyglutamic acid, N-(2-hydroxypropyl) methacrylamide and certain polysaccharides with linear structure are currently viewed as promising polymeric drug carriers (Sanchis et al., 2010). Tissue-recognition ligands engrafted on the polyethylene glycol chain conjugated with the drug may facilitate targeted delivery of the entire complex into the tissue of interest.

2.3 Dendrimers

Dendrimers represent three-dimensional highly branched polymeric macromolecules with the diameter varying from 2.5 to 10 nm. Dendrimers can be synthesized from both synthetic and natural monomers, e. g. amino acids, monosaccharides and nucleotides. High surface area, narrow range of polydispersity and abundance of functional groups on the outer shell of dendrimers make them an attractive tool for targeted drug delivery (for review, see Cheng et al., 2008). Two classes of dendrimers are most commonly used for biomedical applications - polyamidoamines and polypropyleneimines. Although polycationic macromolecules such as dendrimers were shown to be moderately toxic for living cells, the attachment of polyethylene glycol (PEGylation) to the dendrimer can overcome this limitation. The methods of drug binding to the surface of dendrimer include covalent conjugation and electrostatic adsorption. Besides, low molecular weight drugs can be placed into the cavities within the dendrimer molecules being temporarily immobilized there with hydrophobic forces, hydrogen and covalent bonds.

2.4 Polymeric nanoparticles

Biodegradable polymeric nanoparticles were extensively studied as drug carriers. This type of nanocarriers is usually synthesized by means of self-assembly of copolymers consisting of two or more blocks with different hydrophobicity. In the aqueous environment, these copolymers spontaneously form micellar structures with hydrophilic shell and hydrophobic core (Torchilin, 2007). Hydrophobic core may serve as an ideal container for water-insoluble drugs while the hydrophilic shell can be additionally modified for attachment of water-soluble drugs. Polymeric nanoparticles can in principle transport not only low molecular weight hydrophilic and hydrophobic drugs but also the macromolecules such as proteins and nucleic acids (Perez et al., 2001). The kinetics of the release of nanoparticle-bound drug depends on the duration of nanoparticles residence in the organism and characteristics of their microenvironment. Polylactide, polyglycolide and poly(ε–caprolactone) as well as their diblock copolymers with polyethylene glycol at different molar ratios are most commonly used for fabrication of biodegradable nanoparticles. In general, biodegradable polymeric nanoparticles maintain therapeutic drug concentration in the tissue of interest for a longer period of time than other nanocarriers. This feature makes them suitable platforms for transport of highly toxic, water insoluble and unstable drugs.

2.5 Metallic nanoshells

Metallic nanoshells typically consist of dielectric core and thin metallic shell which increases their biocompatibility and optical absorption. The resonance frequency at which the nanoshells demonstrate maximal absorption of energy and its minimal dissipation strongly depends on the ratio between the diameter of the core and the thickness of the metallic layer on the surface of the particle. Gold nanoshells heated with use of near-infrared light were successfully used for photothermal destruction of tumors *in vivo* (Hirsch et al., 2003). Similarly, thermosensitive polymer hydrogels and optically active nanoshells may be used for targeted delivery of drugs. For instance, Arias et al. (2006) developed nanoshells consisting of magnetic core (carbonyl iron) and biodegradable coating (polybutylcyanacrylate) designed for controlled release of 5–fluorouracil in the tumor tissue.

2.6 Nucleic acid-based nanoparticles

RNA and DNA can also play a role of macromolecular carriers for delivery of the drugs. For fabrication of nucleic acid nanoparticles, modified chains of RNA or DNA with non-linear shape are utilized. One of the studies on this topic provided the description of 100 nm multifunctional complex on the basis of DNA designed for consecutive targeted delivery of the drug, visualization of the pathologic focus and gene therapy (Li et al., 2004). The effects of RNA nanoparticles (25-40 nm) containing inactive RNA within the core, RNA aptamers as targeting ligands and small interfering RNA for inhibition of tumor cells were investigated in another recent study (Khaled et al., 2005).

3. Passive and active targeting

Two main strategies currently utilized for site-specific drug delivery are passive and active tissue targeting. In passive targeting, nanoparticles of specific size and charge are nonspecifically accumulated within the affected tissue because of the special characteristics of its vascular bed. Good example of passive targeting is selective accumulation of PEGylated nanoparticles within the tumor tissue after their intravenous administration. This phenomenon is explained by the increased permeability of the tumor microvessels which, in turn, is due to defective endothelial lining and local fenestrations of basement membrane. These observations were first made by Matsumura & Maeda (1986) in the murine solid tumors and are usually referred to as enhanced permeability and retention phenomenon.

Due to the enhanced permeability and retention phenomenon, systemic administration of polymer-drug conjugates results in 10-100-fold higher concentration of the drug in the tumor tissue than after administration of aqueous solution of the drug. Enhanced permeability and retention effect has been observed not only in tumors but also in chronic inflammation and infection. Furthermore, it is well established that nanoparticles without polymer coating are rapidly eliminated from the circulation because of the uptake by the reticulo-endothelial system elements. This fact provides a rationale for passive targeting of liver and spleen in chronic inflammatory diseases associated with prolonged persistence of pathogens within the macrophages (e.g.candidiasis , listeriosis, leishmaniasis, brucellosis, etc.). Stimuli-responsive nanoparticles have recently emerged as another feasible approach to passive targeting (Ganta et al., 2008).

It has been shown that nanoparticles diameter and charge can have a significant impact on their ability to accumulate in the damaged tissue. For instance, van Vlerken et al. (2007) suppose that the most intensive and prolonged accumulation within the tumor is typical for positively charged nanoparticles with diameter of less than 200 nm.

Active targeting employs nanoparticles with specific targeting ligands which selectively bind to biomarkers on target cells. These biomarkers include integrins $\alpha_V\beta_5$ and $\alpha_V\beta_3$ which are expressed on the tumor cells and endothelial cells of the tumor vessels. It is documented that integrins $\alpha_V\beta_5$ and $\alpha_V\beta_3$ specifically interact with arginine-glysine-aspartic acid (RGD) tripeptide sequence. It follows, therefore, that the attachment of RGD peptide to the surface of antitumor drug-loaded nanoparticles may result in their targeted delivery to the tumor tissue. Other variants of targeting ligands are considered in the following section.

4. Tissue-recognition ligands

Monoclonal antibodies and their fragments, aptamers, peptides and low molecular weight compounds may function as tissue-recognition ligands. Considerable efforts have been directed towards developing targeted drug delivery systems with use of monoclonal antibodies. Synthetic monoclonal antibodies are most commonly used for this purpose. For example, the conjugation of fluorescent polystyrene nanoparticles with monoclonal antibodies against platelet endothelial cell adhesion molecule-1 resulted in efficient internalization of the entire complex into the endothelial cells (Garnacho et al., 2008). It was shown in this study that the fate of the nanoparticle (presence of endocytosis, intracellular trafficking, and fusion of vesicles with lysosomes) was dependent on the type of the monoclonal antibody epitope against platelet endothelial cell adhesion molecule-1. On the basis of these data, one might suggest that the drugs can be delivered not only in the affected cells but also in the specific intracellular compartments.

The use of native monoclonal antibodies for tissue targeting is limited by their considerable immunogenicity. In this connection, the development of chimeric and humanized monoclonal antibodies is of importance. The use of monoclonal antibodies as targeting ligands has several other disadvantages such as high cost of monoclonal antibodies fabrication and significant variability of their specificity from batch to batch. Antigen recognition fragments such as Fab fragments, single-chain variable fragments, minibodies, diabodies, and nanobodies may become an alternative to antibodies. Nanobodies are the smallest antibody-derived structures which are produced from the variable domain of the heavy chain of single-domain immunoglobulins and retain the ability to recognize specific antigen. Nanobodies seem to be optimal tissue recognition ligands since they have small size and low immunogenicity. Qiu et al. (2007) produced low-molecular weight antibody mimetics by virtue of fusion between two complementarily-determining regions of the prototype antibodies. Obtained mimetics with molecular weight of 3 kDa were characterized by the better distribution pattern than corresponding antibodies, suggesting that these mimetics may be used as highly specific targeting ligands.

Aptamers are small nucleic acid molecules which may function as specific receptors for low-molecular weight organic substances. The selection of aptamers specific for certain molecular target is a laborious and complicated procedure consisting of several stages. One of the major stages is the enrichment of combinatorial oligonucleotide libraries including up to 10^{15} random sequences resulting in the identification of aptamers specifically interacting with target molecule. The advantages of aptamers include low molecular weight (around 15 kDa) and low immunogenicity leading to improved pattern of tissue distribution (Zhou & Rossi, 2011). It is worth noting that the technology of aptamer synthesis can be easily scaled to industrial production, as opposed to synthesis of monoclonal antibodies. It has been shown that RNA aptamers for recognition of vascular endothelial growth factor can cause regression of tumor microvessels and demonstrate high stability in plasma of the monkey (Ruckman et al., 1998). Anti-vascular endothelial growth factor aptamer pegaptanib has been approved by the American Food and Drug Administration in 2004 for clinical use in the patients with age-related macular degeneration. This fact underscores rapid advancement of aptamers from the bench to clinical applications.

In the last years, with the advent of combinatorial peptide libraries, the peptide targeting ligands are becoming more and more widespread. The peptides can bind to target molecule with very high specificity and affinity. For instance, cyclic peptide cilengitide, an integrin-targeting RGD peptide, is currently being tested in the phase I/II clinical trial for therapy of recurrent and/or metastatic squamous cell cancer of the head and neck (Vermorken et al., 2011).

Low-molecular weight compounds may also serve as efficient tissue-recognition ligands because of their low cost and negligible immunogenicity. One of the most intensively studied molecules within this group is folic acid. Folate is especially helpful for tumor targeting since tumor cells are over-expressing folate receptor on their surface. Folic acid has been used for tumor-targeted delivery of cytostatics immobilized on different types of nanoparticulate carriers (e. g., polymeric nanoparticles, liposomes, dendrimers, etc.).

Various methods of binding targeting ligand with the nanoparticle surface have been suggested, which can be generally divided into covalent and non-covalent techniques. Covalent binding has been suggested more than 25 years ago for immobilization of proteins on the surface of liposomes. Protein conjugation with the nanoparticle is usually mediated through the bifunctional polyethylene glycol which contains hydrophobic anchor for fixation in the liposomal coating and molecular spacer with amino or sulfhydryl moieties for drug binding. Specific interaction between protein A and Fc-fragments of monoclonal antibodies as well as the biotinylation of the nanoparticles and their subsequent conjugation with ligand-streptavidin complex can both be used for non-covalent binding of nanoparticle with targeting ligand.

5. Heart targeting with nanoparticulate carriers

Much of the work on targeted drug delivery has focused on cancer treatment. The reasons for this include high morbidity and mortality due to cancer as well as focal tumor growth associated with severe alterations in tumor molecular phenotype, thus making possible the design of highly selective targeting ligands. However, it can be hypothesized that the concepts of passive and active targeted drug delivery can be applied efficiently to any type of focal pathological process including ischemia-reperfusion and inflammation. Ischemic heart disease is generally thought to be a major cause of morbidity and mortality worldwide. It follows, therefore, that prevention and/or alleviation of myocardial ischemia-reperfusion injury remains to be among the most important goals of the medical care. One solution to the problem might be direct delivery of cardioprotective drugs into the ischemic myocardium.

At present, there is some, albeit limited, published evidence that the ischemic heart can be actively and passively targeted with drug-loaded liposomes. In particular, anti-myosin monoclonal antibody-doped liposomes containing ATP were administered to the isolated rat heart prior to global ischemia-reperfusion (Verma et al., 2006), which was associated with better postischemic contractile recovery. Intracoronary infusion of non-targeted ATP-loaded liposomes before regional ischemia-reperfusion resulted in significant reduction in infarct size as compared to controls in rabbit model (Verma et al., 2005). One possible limitation of these studies is that drug-loaded nanocarriers were administered prior to ischemia instead of administering at the end of ischemia or at the early stage of reperfusion. It seems justified that myocardial nanoparticle accumulation is most intensive at the time of reperfusion. Therefore, one can also expect to get the best result as to the extent of myocardial protection when infusing nanoparticle-loaded drug at this time. There are several lines of evidence in support of this notion. First, myocardial cell injury associated with exposure/expression of injury markers required for active targeting becomes more pronounced after reperfusion. Second, myocardial reperfusion initiates the inflammatory response associated with increased microvascular permeability, the latter being a major prerequisite of passive targeting. Third, reperfusion is accompanied by reactive hyperemia which may contribute to better delivery of nanocarriers to the area of interest. Fourth, early stage of reperfusion itself strongly contributes to the formation of irreversible myocardial injury (Yellon & Hausenloy, 2007). Hence, the release of nanoparticle payload at this narrow time interval may prevent or block some of the mechanisms of lethal reperfusion injury. Thus, in order to optimize the pharmacokinetic profile of the heart-targeted drug delivery system, it should be administered at the final stage of ischemia or at the very beginning of reperfusion. In conclusion, the timing of nanoparticle-loaded cardioprotective drug administration is crucial for successful heart targeting.

In the study of Scott et al. (2009), the vascular endothelial growth factor-loaded liposomes functionalized with monoclonal antibodies against P-selectin were administered intravenously to the rats after permanent coronary artery ligation. The authors showed increased density of capillaries within the infarct area 4 weeks after infarction and better post-infarct left ventricular function. Despite positive findings, it is difficult to extrapolate the results of this study to the current clinical practice since it was performed with use of permanent ischemia model without reperfusion. At the same time, current gold standard for treatment of acute coronary syndrome is prompt myocardial revascularization. Besides, the benefits of applied treatment regimen might be explained rather by the improved neovascularizarion of peri-infarct area, and not by the direct prevention of cardiac myocyte death within the ischemic area.

Important results were obtained in a landmark study by Takahama et al. (2009) who used liposomal adenosine for treatment of myocardial ischemia-reperfusion in rats. Adenosine-loaded liposomes were infused intravenously for 10 minutes starting 5 minutes prior to myocardial reperfusion. Selective accumulation of liposomes within the ischemic-reperfused area was verified with electron microscopy, optical fluorescence, and radionuclide imaging. Besides, liposomal adenosine administration was associated with more significant infarct size limitation and less severe arterial hypotension as compared to free adenosine treatment.

The research of our group working at the Institute of Experimental Medicine, V.A. Almazov Federal Heart, Blood and Endocrinology Centre is focused on the development of both active and passive techniques of heart targeting. We hypothesized that local accumulation of drug-loaded nanoparticles within the ischemic area of the heart may be achieved by selective binding of the annexin V to the nanoparticle surface (Fig. 1).

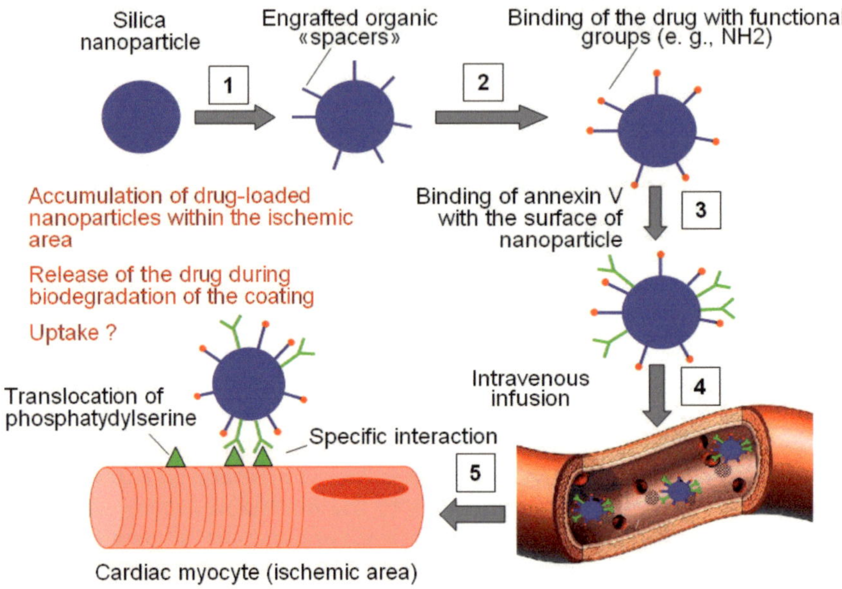

Fig. 1. Proposed algorithm of active targeted drug delivery into the ischemic cardiac muscle

Annexin V is a naturally expressed protein that binds to phosphatidylserine in a calcium-dependent fashion. Phosphatidylserine is normally localized on the inner surface of the plasmalemma, but it is translocated on the exterior cell surface when sublethal cell injury occurs (Vance & Steenbergen, 2005). Annexin V is widely used as one of the marker proteins for cell injury and apoptotic cell death *in vitro*. Besides, the intravenous administration of annexin V conjugated with fluorescent probe to the dogs subjected to 1 hour regional ischemia and 1 hour reperfusion resulted in bright fluorescence of ischemic area indicative of site-specific conjugate accumulation (Ohnishi et al., 2006). Specific interaction of the nanoparticle-anchored annexin V with phosphatidylserine would potentially result in the binding of nanoparticles to the cardiomyocyte membrane with their subsequent accumulation in the area of interest.

Apart from active heart targeting with use of annexin V as a tissue-recognition ligand, we also feel that ischemic-reperfused myocardium may offer an advantage of passive targeting. The basic idea is that the nanoparticulate carriers, if administered in proper time (see above), can be retained within the ischemic-reperfused area of the heart owing to local inflammatory response and severely increased microvascular permeability. In this regard, the functional characteristics of myocardial microvessels are more or less similar to those of the tumor. Therefore, it seems not unlikely that drug-loaded nanoparticles can tend to accumulate within the ischemic-reperfused area of the heart just because of the raised permeability of myocardial capillaries.

5.1 Fabrication, characterization, and surface modification of silica nanoparticles

Among inorganic drug carriers, nanodisperse silica, titania, zirconia, and iron oxide as well as fullerenes and carbon nanotubes have been considered to be the most promising. In our studies, the prototype carriers for antiischemic drugs are suggested to be nanodispersed silica particles. It has been shown before that silica nanomaterials are characterized by fairly good biocompatibility and biodegradability (Slowing *et al.*, 2008). Chemical modification of silica nanoparticle surface can be performed with use of two different synthetic approaches, namely, immobilization and chemical assembly. In immobilization strategy, the modifier is attached to the carrier surface with use of a single-stage reaction. Chemical assembly represents another approach toward synthesis of engrafted surface compounds that has recently emerged as a promising alternative to immobilization strategy. Chemical assembly is based on multistage synthesis of engrafted chemical compounds on the surface of solid phase particles which play a role of matrices. The major advantage of chemical assembly in comparison to immobilization is the larger diversity of functional groups that can be applied to the matrix surface.

Taking into account the above considerations, we suppose that nanodisperse silica of the Aerosil type may be a perspective drug carrier for biomedical applications. In our studies, the standard pyrogenic highly dispersed silica (Aerosil A380 mark obtained from Vekton, Russia) was used throughout experiments. Surface area of silica nanoparticles was determined with use of Brunauer-Emmett-Teller (BET) method and averaged from 170 to 380 m^2/g (Galagudza et al., 2010). The mean particle diameter varied from 6 to 13 nm. The technique of silica nanoparticle functionalization included three sequential steps: modification of silica nanoparticles with (3-aminopropyl)triethoxysilane, hydrolysis of unreacted alkoxysilane groups, and binding of fluorescein. Chemosorption of (3-aminopropyl)triethoxysilane was performed from the gaseous phase with use of dried nitrogen as a carrier gas. The synthesis was done in the vertical quartz flow reactor at 220°C during 2 hours. Hydrolysis of the unreacted alkoxysilane groups was achieved with water vapor at 150°C during 1 hour. The covalent binding of fluorescein to the aminated silica was done using carbodiimide technique during 1 hour. The surface reactions were controlled with infrared spectroscopy. The amount of fluorescein bound to the surface of silica nanoparticles was determined spectrophotometrically at λ=490 nm. Fluorescein content within the samples of modified silica nanoparticles varied from 0.01 to 0.02 mmol/g. Another fluorescent dye that can be used for labeling of silica nanoparticles is considered to be indocyanine green. This fluorophore has an absorption band in the near-infrared region (λ=780 nm). We have developed the technique of indocyanine green immobilization on the surface of aminated silica. Then, fluorescently labeled silica nanoparticles were used for biodistribution studies.

The above-described techniques of matrix synthesis of engrafted surface compounds can be easily applied for Aerosil modification. Combination of the molecular layering method with chemical assembly of engrafted organic compounds is especially promising for development of targeted nanopharmaceuticals. With use of this approach, thin layers of inorganic substances possessing magnetic properties can be laid on the Aerosil surface with subsequent modification of the latter by the organic compounds containing active centers crucial for immobilization of drug molecules. We believe that the use of chemically modified silica as a prototype carrier for targeted drug delivery holds great promise because of several advantages, such as biocompatibility and biodegradation, low cost, and detailed account on the techniques of surface immobilization of drugs, fluorophores, and targeting ligands.

5.2 Acute toxicity, biodistribution and biodegradation of silica nanoparticles

To investigate the acute toxicity of silica nanoparticles experimentally, we studied the acute hemodynamic effects of nanoparticle formulations in the rat model. For this purpose, the suspensions of silica and fluorescein-doped silica nanoparticles in 0,9% sodium hydrochloride solution were prepared and administered intravenously 3 times with 20-minute intervals between infusions. Control animals received vehicle. Measurements of heart rate, mean arterial pressure and pulse arterial pressure were done throughout the experiments. In all groups of animals, there were no significant alterations in heart rate over time. The first infusion of any tested nanoparticle formulation had no effect on hemodynamic parameters. Furthermore, there were no statistically significant differences in mean arterial pressure between the baseline time point and the end of the experiment. However, the second and the third infusions of silica nanoparticles evoked transient increases of mean arterial pressure. There were significant increases in pulse arterial pressure in the animals that received silica nanoparticles at the end of the observation. Administration of fluorescein-labeled silica nanoparticles resulted in increase of pulse arterial pressure too, while pulse arterial pressure in controls was unaffected throughout the entire experiment. Thus, intravenous infusion of silica nanoparticle formulations caused mild changes in systemic hemodynamic parameters which appears to be indicative of appropriate biocompatibility of these nanomaterials.

Biodistribution of silica nanoparticles was studied with use of optical fluorescence. Fluorescein and indocyanine green were used for fluorescent labeling of silica nanoparticles. The animals received intravenous infusion of fluorescently labeled nanoparticles suspended in normal saline at a volume of 1 ml for 10 minutes. 20 minutes after the end of infusion, the animals were sacrificed by an overdose of anesthesia, and the following organs were removed for subsequent measurements: heart, brain, liver, spleen, lung, and kidney. Control animals were treated with the vehicle. The registration of fluorescence was performed using FLUM3 setup for fluorescent imaging of small animals and biopsy specimens consisting of the mercury lamp illuminator and TV camera 285. The fluorescence of fluorescein- and indocyanine green-labeled nanoparticles was elicited by the use of band-pass interference filters of 435 and 780 nm, respectively. The images obtained in the experiments with fluorescein-labeled nanoparticles were split into RBG channels. Channel G has been chosen as target channel. The relative change in the level of fluorescence (i. e., percent change from control, ΔG, %) has been calculated as follows: $\Delta G=(G2 - G1)/G1$, where G1 is the level of (auto)fluorescence in controls, G2 – the level of fluorescence in animals treated with fluorescein-labeled silica nanoparticles. In the experiments with indocyanine green-labeled nanoparticles, black-and-white images were obtained, and the relative change in the level of fluorescence (i. e., percent change from control, ΔF, %) was calculated as described above. The biodistribution data are shown in the Table 1. It should be noted that exposure of organ samples to UV light (λ=435 nm) for detection of fluorescein-doped nanoparticles was associated with significant deal of auto fluorescence which may interfere with the desired signal. Despite that, we observed predominant accumulation of fluorescein-labeled nanoparticles within the lung, spleen and liver, that is, in the organs of reticulo-endothelial system. The use of indocyanine green was helpful in avoiding the high level of auto fluorescence because this fluorophore is excited at λ=780 nm. Generally, we found the highest accumulation of indocyanine green-labeled nanoparticles within the liver and kidney. Therefore, we recommend the use of infrared fluorophores for fluorescent labeling of silica nanoparticles and investigation of their biodistribution.

Organ	λ=780 nm			λ=435 nm		
	Control, F1	Indocyanine green-labeled nanoparticles, F2	ΔF, %	Control, G1	Fluorescein-labeled nanoparticles, G2	Δ G,%
Heart	12±0.5	22±0.4	81±3.9	90±13.2	106±7.0	18±9.3
Brain	26±0.5	35±0.5	77±7.0	115±7.1	119±13.4	5±2.8
Liver	14±0.6	1213±193.0	8311±1232.0	95±31.5	113±24.8	22±14.6
Spleen	16±9.9	20±4.2	62±27.0	81±10.2	99±7.1	23±6.8
Lung	29±5.7	127±24.8	357±123.0	88±6.0	113±2.1	30±11.4
Kidney	16±5.7	164±21.2	1018±373.0	76±0.4	82±6.2	9±6.7

Table 1. Distribution of indocyanine green- and fluorescein-labelled silica nanoparticles at the organ level of Wistar rats after 30 min of dose administration

Silica nanoparticle biodegradation was studied both *in vitro* and *in vivo*. When designing the experiments, we speculated that silica nanoparticles are undergoing biodegradation due to gradual erosion of their surface resultant in the formation of water-soluble salts of silicic acid which are excreted from the organism by the kidney (Fig. 2).

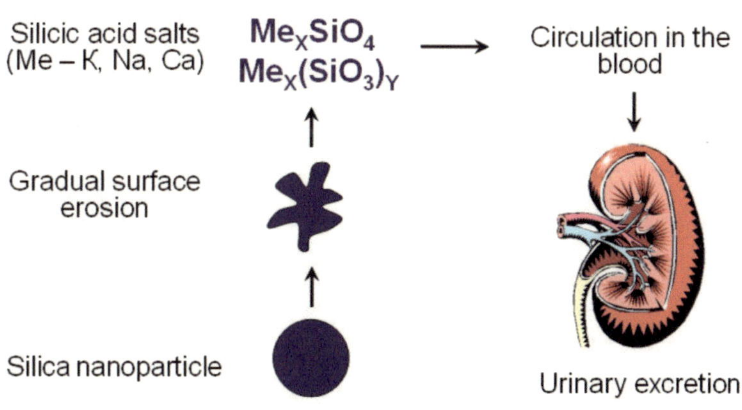

Fig. 2. Hypothetical mechanism of silica nanoparticle biodegradation

The suspension of Aerosil A380 in Krebs-Henseleit buffer having electrolyte composition similar to that of blood plasma with final concentration of silica nanoparticles 2 mg/ml and pH=7,4 was used for investigation of biodegradation *in vitro*. The experiments were performed in the settings of continuous stirring in the polymer 100 ml glass. The temperature of the media was maintained at 37°C by means of water jacketing. The samples were continuously gassed with carbogen (95% O_2 and 5% CO_2). Total incubation time was equal to 15 hours. The samples were taken each 5 hours and analyzed for silicate content spectrophotometrically after reaction with molybdenum blue. The concentration of silicate in samples increased logarithmically with time. With use of mathematical analysis, we derived the value which corresponds to 95% biodegradation of silica and equals to 41 day. These data fit well to the results of Finnie et al. (2009) who studied biodegradation of sol-gel mesoporous silica microparticles. It has been shown in this study that silica microparticles are rapidly degraded in physiological buffer. Besides, the authors demonstrated that the addition of plasma proteins to the buffer retarded biodegradation by 20-30%. It follows, therefore, that *in vivo* biodegradation might be slower than in the *in vitro* settings.

In vivo biodegradation of silica nanoparticles was studied in the male Wistar rats weighting 200-250 g. Silica nanoparticles were infused intravenously at a dose of 2 mg/ml and volume of 1 ml followed by sampling of the liver at 1 h, 10, 20, and 30 days after infusion. The controls were animals received intravenous infusion of 1 ml of vehicle. Liver samples were dried at 90°C during 24 h to obtain constant weight. The liver was chosen for sampling and analyses on the basis of biodistribution experiments which showed maximal accumulation of silica in this organ. Quantitative analysis of silicon content within the samples was performed with atomic absorption spectroscopy. The mineralizat obtained after drying was analyzed on the atomic absorption spectrometer with electrothermic atomization and Zeman correction. Silicon content within the mineralizat was recalculated for the dry sample weight and expressed in µg/g. Silicon content in the liver of the rats according to the results of atomic absorption spectroscopy is shown on the Fig. 3.

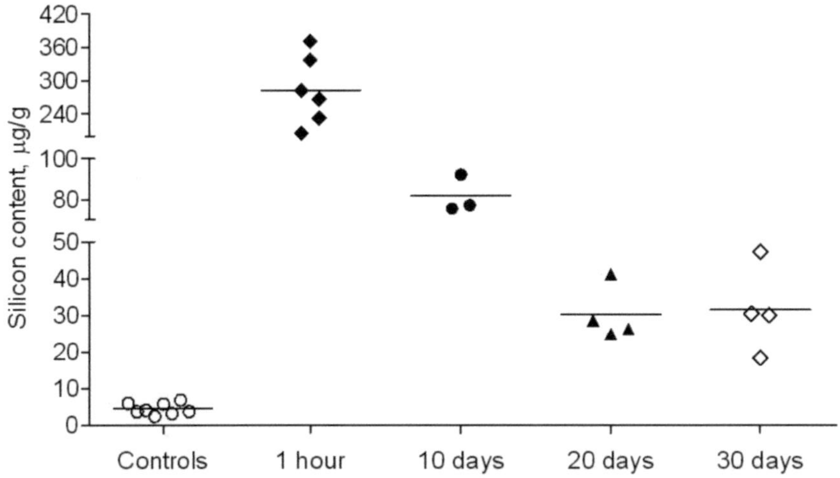

Fig. 3. Biodegradation of silica nanoparticles *in vivo*: silicon content in the liver at different durations after infusion of nanoparticles

Silicon content in the liver of healthy rats averaged 4.4±1.55 µg/g. At 1 hour after silica nanoparticles infusion silicon content was increased up to 282.3±62.65 µg/g. 10 and 20 days after silica nanoparticle infusion silicon content in the liver was significantly lower (81.5±9.25 and 30.2±7.48 µg/g, respectively). This dynamics of silica dissolution is consistent with the data obtained in the *in vitro* model. However, at 30 days after silica nanoparticle administration we failed to see any additional decrease in silicon tissue content (31.5±11.87 μg/g). This fact might be accounted for by the higher stability of the intracellular pool of silica nanoparticles, produced as a result of their phagocytosis by the Kupffer cells and, to a lesser extent, silica nanoparticle internalization into hepatocytes and other liver cells. It remains unclear, however, whether this increased silicon content in the liver cells affects liver function or not.

5.3 Passive heart targeting with silica nanoparticles

For investigation of passive heart-targeted drug delivery with silica nanoparticles, we first studied biodistribution of unmodified nanoparticles in the rats with regional myocardial ischemia-reperfusion. For this purpose, the animals were randomly allocated into one of three groups: 1) controls (these animals received intravenous infusion of saline), 2) silica nanoparticle-treated animals (2 mg/ml, 1 ml intravenously) with sham surgical procedure; 3) silica nanoparticle-treated animals with myocardial ischemia-reperfusion. Regional myocardial ischemia was induced by 30-minute left coronary artery ligation followed by 60 minutes of reperfusion. Silica nanoparticles were infused for 10 minutes starting 5 minutes prior to reperfusion (Fig. 4). The left ventricle of the heart and liver were sampled at the end of the experiments, rinsed and dried at 90°C during 24 h to obtain constant weight. Silicon content in the organ samples was done with atomic absorption spectroscopy as described above.

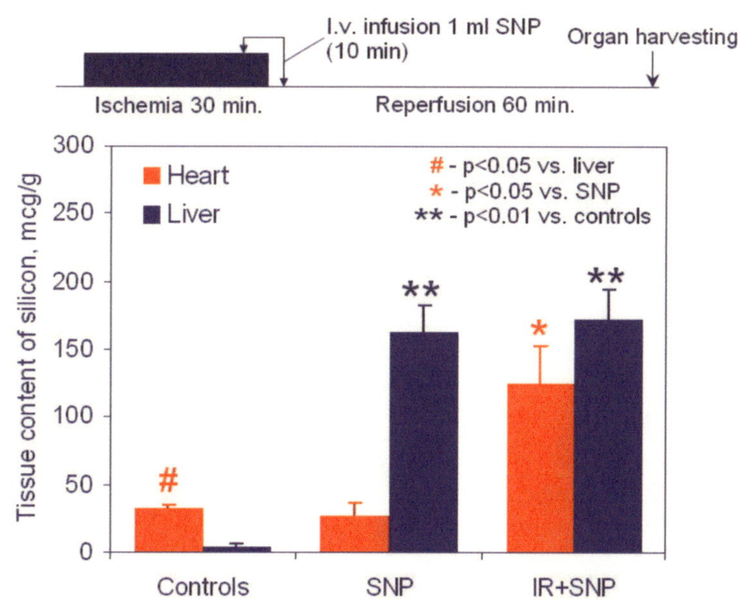

Fig. 4. Biodistribution of non-modified silica nanoparticles in rat model of myocardial ischemia-reperfusion. SNP - silica nanoparticles, IR - ischemia-reperfusion

In controls, silicon content was found to be significantly higher in myocardial tissue then in the liver (32±2.8 vs. 4±2.3 μg/g, respectively, $p<0.05$) (Fig. 4). Of note, physiological role of this fact is currently unknown. Silica nanoparticle administration to sham-operated rats resulted in dramatic rise in liver silicon content as compared to controls (163±19.5 vs. 4±2.3 μg/g, respectively, $p<0.01$), while myocardial silicon concentration remained unaffected (27±9.7 vs. 32±2.8, respectively, $p>0.05$). Administration of silica nanoparticles to the animals with cardiac ischemia-reperfusion was associated with significant increase in myocardial silicon content in comparison to sham-operated animals (125±28.2 vs. 32±2.8 μg/g, respectively, $p<0.05$). Thus, the first evidence that non-modified silica nanoparticles can accumulate within the anatomical area at risk after regional myocardial ischemia-reperfusion was provided in this study.

The next series of experiments was performed to study the hemodynamic effects of nanoparticle-bound and free adenosine. Adenosine adsorption on the surface of silica nanoparticles was achieved by mixing the suspension of silica nanoparticles in 0.9% sodium chloride and adenosine solution in the same vehicle. The samples thus prepared were subjected to 10-minute sonication and left at +4°C overnight. Silica nanoparticle-bound adenosine was administered to the rats intravenously for 10 minutes at a dose of 300 μg/kg×min. Control animals received 10-minute intravenous infusion of adenosine at a dose of 300 μg/kg×min. Mean blood pressure was registered before the beginning of drug infusion, at 5th and 10th minutes of infusion, and at 5th and 10th minutes of recovery. The data on blood pressure values are shown in Table 2. The extent of blood pressure decrease was significantly less marked when adenosine was immobilized on the surface of nanoparticles (Fig. 5).

MBP, mmHg	Baseline	5 min infusion	10 min infusion	5 min recovery	10 min recovery
Free ADO	125±12	82±7	85±9	128±5	119±13
ADO+SNP	131±8	108±14*	113±11*	134±12	130±10

Table 2. Attenuation of adenosine-induced hypotension after its immobilization on the surface of silica nanoparticles. MBP - mean blood pressure, ADO - adenosine, SNP - silica nanoparticles. * - $p<0.05$ vs. free adenosine

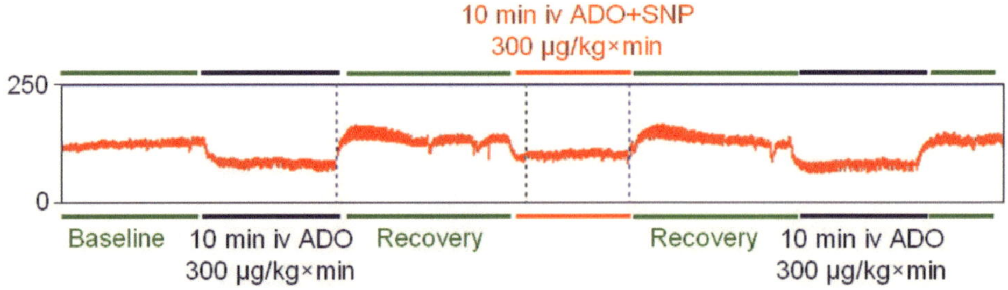

Fig. 5. Representative blood pressure recording showing different blood pressure response to free and silica nanoparticle-bound adenosine. Initial free adenosine infusion was followed by recovery period and infusion of silica-nanoparticle bound adenosine. After recovery, one more episode of adenosine infusion was performed. ADO – adenosine, SNP – silica nanoparticles

The final series of experiments was focused on investigation of the effect of free adenosine and nanoparticle-bound adenosine on infarct size. Five minutes prior to the end of 30-minte ischemia, animals received either 10-minute adenosine infusion at a dose of 300 µg/kg×min or infusion of adenosine adsorbed on silica nanoparticles in the equivalent dose. Control animals were treated with vehicle. Myocardial area at risk and infarct size were determined after 90 minutes of reperfusion with use of Evans blue and triphenyltetrazolium chloride staining, respectively. There were no differences in risk area between groups (Fig. 6).

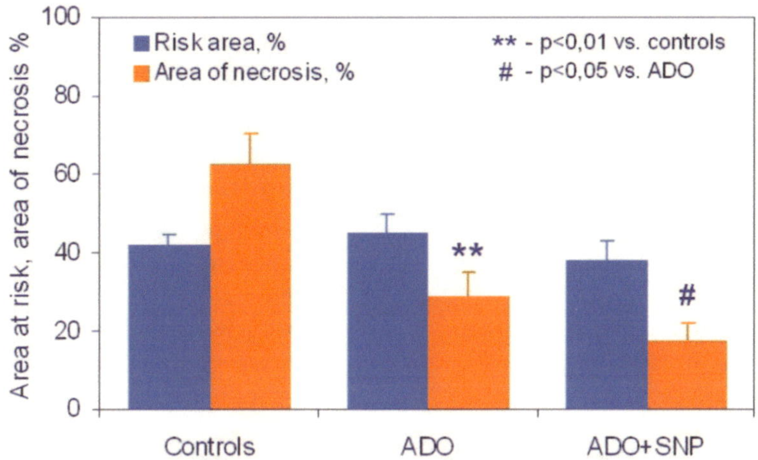

Fig. 6. Increased infarct-limiting effect of adenosine after its immobilization on silica nanoparticles. ADO – adenosine, SNP – silica nanoparticles

Adenosine infusion caused significant reduction in infarct size as compared to controls (29±6,2 vs. 63±7,3%, respectively, $p<0.01$). Administration of adenosine adsorbed on silica nanoparticles resulted in additional significant decrease in infarct size in comparison to free adenosine (18±4.2 vs. 29±6,2, respectively, $p<0.05$).

In conclusion, adsorption of adenosine on silica nanoparticles results in its passive delivery to the ischemic area of the heart which, in turn, leads to more pronounced infarct size limitation and attenuation of hemodynamic side effect typical for the drug used.

5.4 Candidate drugs for heart-targeted delivery

Several groups of drugs with different mechanisms of action might potentially be targeted to the heart with nano-sized carriers (Table 3). One of the most efficient means of myocardial protection known to date is ischemic preconditioning, a phenomenon which describes dramatically increased heart tolerance to prolonged ischemia occurring after one or several brief episodes of ischemia-reperfusion (Galagudza et al., 2008). It is well established that preconditioning can elicit several cardioprotective effects including infarct-limitation, reduction of ischemic and reperfusion arrhythmias, prevention of endothelial dysfunction and attenuation of stunning. The mechanisms of preconditioning include generation of chemical triggers during brief bouts of ischemia, their interaction with corresponding sarcolemmal G-protein-coupled receptors with subsequent activation of multiple intracellular kinases, and, eventually, engagement of putative mitochondrial effectors responsible for initiation of energy-sparing processes. It has been shown that such preconditioning triggers as adenosine, bradykinin, and opioid peptides are all able to mimic the preconditioning response when administered exogenously. However, their clinical use at doses required for preconditioning-like response is hampered by the high risk of dangerous side effects. For example, intravenous administration of adenosine is associated with arterial hypotension and bradycardia (Takahama et al., 2009), while administration of bradykinin might lead to hypotension and bronchial spasm (Homma & Irvin, 1999). It follows, therefore, that targeted delivery of preconditioning mimetics or synthetic agonists of G-protein-coupled receptors might contribute to improved safety and efficacy profile of these compounds, especially taking into account the encouraging results with heart-targeted delivery of adenosine (Takahama et al., 2009).

Mechanism	Drug/ligand
Activation of G-protein-coupled receptors (preconditioning)	Bradykinin, opioids, adenosine and synthetic ligands of corresponding receptors
Activation of tyrosine kinase receptors (angiogenesis, cardiac myocyte proliferation?)	Insulin, insulin-like growth factor-1, transforming growth factor-β1, erythropoietin, vascular endothelial growth factor, etc.
Inhibition of mitochondrial permeability transition pore opening (attenuation of reperfusion injury, antiapoptotic effect)	Cyclosporine
Activation of peroxisome proliferator-activated receptors gamma (reduction of inflammation, improved endothelial function)	Rosiglitazone, pioglitazone
Opening of ATP-sensitive potassium channels (improved mitochondrial function)	Nicorandil
Nitric oxide signaling pathway (preconditioning, vasodilation)	Nitric oxide donors, atorvastatin, atrial natriuretic peptide, etc.

Table 3. Candidate drugs for ischemic heart targeting

Another group of compounds demonstrating cardioprotective effects are growth factors which interact with tyrosine kinase receptors. Such molecules as insulin, insulin-like growth factor-1, transforming growth factor-β1, erythropoietin, vascular endothelial growth factor, and fibroblast growth factor may not only induce cytoprotective effect when administered either prior or just after index ischemia, but also possess late cardioprotective effects due to stimulation of angiogenesis and attenuation of inflammation (Boucher et al., 2008; Ueda et al., 2010). Again, heart-targeted delivery of growth factors may result in better outcome because of local increase in the concentration and reduction of such side effects as hypotension and hypersensitivity reactions.

One more key player in the mechanisms of ischemia-reperfusion myocardial injury is mitochondrial permeability transition pore (mPTP). mPTP represents multiprotein complex localized in the inner mitochondrial membrane which functions as voltage-dependent nonselective channel. The probability of mPTP opening is very low during in both normal and ischemic environment. However, at reperfusion mPTP becomes opened thus making inner mitochondrial membrane permeable for water, ions, and molecules with molecular weight up to 1.5 kDa. Major stimuli for mPTP opening are increased calcium concentration, mitochondrial matrix pH>7.0, increased concentration of reactive oxygen species, and mitochondrial membrane depolarization (Di Lisa et al., 2011). mPTP opening results in immediate complete depolarization of mitochondrial membrane and, therefore, loss of electrochemical gradient. In this situation, ATP synthase starts to degrade ATP in a futile attempt to regenerate membrane potential. Besides, massive swelling of mitochondrial matrix may contribute to mechanical rupture of the organelles with resultant release of several pro-apoptotic molecules normally retained in the intermembrane space. It follows that mPTP opening at the early moments of reperfusion can lead to development of lethal reperfusion injury by means of both necrosis and apoptosis. mPTP inhibitors were shown to be cardioprotective in experimental and clinical settings. Intravenous administration of mPTP inhibitor cyclosporine to the patients with acute ST-elevation myocardial infarction just prior to percutaneous coronary intervention resulted in significant reduction in infarct size as compared to controls (Piot et al., 2008). Cyclosporine is commonly used for immune suppression, and its prolonged use is associated with several serious side effects including renal failure, hepatotoxicity, infection, and increased risk of tumor development. Thus, it is of prime importance to develop the technique of targeted delivery of cyclosporine to the ischemic heart which may help to attenuate its systemic toxicity.

Peroxisome proliferator-activated receptors (PPAR) are nuclear receptors that function as transcription factors for numerous genes. In terms of myocardial ischemia-reperfusion injury, activation of PPARγ with either endogenous ligands or thiazolidinedione derivatives has been shown to be cardioprotective (Di Paola & Cuzzocrea, 2007). Potential mechanisms of PPARγ-mediated cardioprotection include inhibition of the activation of nuclear transcription factor κB, stimulation of endothelial NO-synthase function, and increased expression of heme oxygenase-1. Decreased function of nuclear transcription factor κB in the ischemic-reperfused heart is supposed to be beneficial since this transcription factor positively regulates a battery of proinflammatory genes, all of which contribute to secondary injury in the infarcted area.

ATP-sensitive potassium channels have been believed to be major end effectors of ischemic preconditioning in the late 90s. There are two main populations of ATP-sensitive potassium channels, that is, sarcolemmal and mitochondrial. Currently, the cardioprotective role of sarcolemmal ATP-sensitive potassium channels has been unequivocally proved while there is some debate as to the role of mitochondrial channels (Hanley & Daut, 2005). Several ATP-sensitive potassium channel openers were shown to exert preconditioning-like protective effect in the experimental models. However, the only drug from this group that is approved for use in humans is nicorandil. The results of IONA trial demonstrated reduced incidence of acute coronary syndrome in the patients with stable angina receiving nicorandil. It seems, therefore, that targeted delivery of nicorandil to the heart might further strengthen its cardioprotective effect.

Finally, pharmacological modulation if nitric oxide (NO)-dependent pathway in the heart is also of interest. It has been shown that endogenous NO participation in the mechanisms of cardiac protection if unlikely but exogenous supplementation of the heart with NO can mimic the protective effect of preconditioning (Dawn & Bolli, 2002). NO-dependent mechanisms were also proposed for infarct-limiting effect of atorvastatin (Atar et al., 2006) and atrial natriuretic peptide (Okawa et al., 2003).

In conclusion, the list of cardioprotective drugs which might be delivered to the heart with nanocarriers is incomplete. By now, hundreds of drugs were shown to be cardioprotective in the preclinical models. However, very few of them were proved to be effective in the patients with coronary artery disease. The reasons for this failure are multiple and analyzed elsewhere, but at least one is the fact that many drugs have significant side effects which hinder the process of clinical translation. Recent evidence indicates that some side effects can be substantially reduced when the drug is navigated to the tissue of interest by the nanocarrier. Targeted delivery concept holds promise for development of new efficient and safe therapies for ischemic heart disease.

6. Perspectives and future work

Although the concept of targeted drug delivery to the ischemic heart seems to be generally coherent, it is evident that large questions lie ahead. Systemic administration of multifunctional drug carriers results in their selective accumulation in the target tissues with normal blood flow. It might be problematic to achieve the minimal effective dose of the nanopharmaceutical within the tissue subjected to critical ischemia. This problem may be solved by the increased residence time of nanocarriers within the adjacent to ischemic tissues providing diffusion of the drug into the poorly vascularized area. Alternative solution may involve increased loading of the nanoparticles with payload and/or targeting ligands. On the other hand, intensive functionalization of nanoparticles may result in better recognition by the immune system and faster clearance by the reticulo-endothelial system.

Insufficient evidence is currently available on the clinical effectiveness of nanoparticulate drug carriers. Additional studies are required to elucidate the pharmacokinetics of nanocarriers as well as their biodistribution and putative toxicity. All newly developed nanosystems for targeted delivery possess unique properties requiring individual testing. The refinement of the techniques of nanocarrier fabrication is aimed at ensuring of better uptake of nanoparticles by the target cells, formation of higher gradient of drug between injured and intact tissue, and more complete avoidance of drug toxicity. The accomplishment of these goals will be a major step in development of an ideal tool for targeted delivery of the drug into the tissue of interest.

7. Conclusion

Concepts of passive and active targeting can be applied to the development of targeted drug delivery to the ischemic myocardial tissue. Targeted delivery of various cardioprotective agents to the ischemic cardiac muscle with use of nanoparticles seems to be a challenging approach to treatment of coronary artery disease.

Silica nanoparticles are non-toxic materials that might be potentially used as carriers for heart-targeted drug delivery. Silica nanoparticles can be functionalized with use of the techniques of immobilization and chemical assembly. Immobilization of adenosine on the surface of silica nanoparticles resulted in enhancement of free adenosine-mediated infarct size limitation in the animal model. Furthermore, hypotensive effect of adenosine was attenuated after its adsorption on silica nanoparticles. Additional studies will be required to demonstrate silica nanoparticle biocompatibility in the chronic experiments.

8. References

Ali, I.; Rahis-Uddin; Salim, K.; Rather, M.A.; Wani, W.A. & Haque, A. (2011). Advances in Nano Drugs for Cancer Chemotherapy. *Current Cancer Drug Targets*, Vol.11, No.2, (February 2011), pp. 135-146, ISSN 1568-0096

Arias, J.L.; Gallardo, V.; Linares–Molinero, F. & Delgado, A.V. (2006). Preparation and Characterization of Carbonyl Iron/Poly(butylcyanoacrylate) Core/Shell Nanoparticles. *Journal of Colloid and Interface Science*, Vol.299, No.2, (July 2006), pp. 599–607, ISSN 0021-9797

Atar, S.; Ye, Y.; Lin, Y.; Freeberg, S.Y.; Nishi, S.P.; Rosanio, S.; Huang, M.H.; Uretsky, B.F.; Perez-Polo, J.R. & Birnbaum, Y. (2006). Atorvastatin-Induced Cardioprotection is Mediated by Increasing Inducible Nitric Oxide Synthase and Consequent S-Nitrosylation of Cyclooxygenase-2. *American Journal of Physiology. Heart and Circulatory Physiology*, Vol.290, No.5, (May 2006), pp. H1960-H1968, ISSN 0363-6135

Boucher, M.; Pesant, S.; Lei, Y.H.; Nanton, N.; Most, P.; Eckhart, A.D.; Koch, W.J. & Gao, E. (2008). Simultaneous Administration of Insulin-Like Growth Factor-1 and Darbepoetin Alpha Protects the Rat Myocardium Against Myocardial Infarction and Enhances Angiogenesis. *Clinical and Translational Science*, Vol.1, No.1, (May 2008), pp. 13-20, ISSN 1752-8054

Carvalho, C.; Santos, R.X.; Cardoso, S.; Correia, S.; Oliveira, P.J.; Santos, M.S. & Moreira, P.I. (2009). Doxorubicin: the Good, the Bad and the Ugly Effect. *Current Medicinal Chemistry*, Vol.16, No.25, (September 2009), pp. 3267-3285, ISSN 0929-8673

Cheng, Y.; Wang, J.; Rao, T.; He, X. & Xu, T. (2008). Pharmaceutical Applications of Dendrimers: Promising Nanocarriers for Drug Delivery. *Frontiers in Bioscience*, Vol.13, (January 2008), pp. 1447–1471, ISSN 1093-9946

Dawn, B. & Bolli, R. (2002). Role of Nitric Oxide in Myocardial Preconditioning. *Annals of the New York Academy of Sciences*, Vol.962, (May 2002), pp. 18-41, ISSN 0077-8923

Di Lisa, F.; Carpi, A.; Giorgio, V. & Bernardi, P. (2011). The Mitochondrial Permeability Transition Pore and Cyclophilin D in Cardioprotection. *Biochimica et Biophysica Acta*, Vol.1813, No.7, (July 2011), pp. 1316-1322, ISSN 0006-3002

Di Paola, R. & Cuzzocrea, S. (2007). Peroxisome Proliferator-Activated Receptors Ligands and Ischemia-Reperfusion Injury. *Naunyn-Schmiedeberg's Archives of Pharmacology*, Vol.375, No.3, (May 2007), pp. 157-175, ISSN 0028-1298

Erhlich, P. (1906). *Collected studies on immunity*, John Wiley, New York, USA

Fenske, D.B. & Cullis, P.R. (2008). Liposomal Nanomedicines. *Expert Opinion on Drug Delivery*, Vol.5, No.1, (January 2008), pp. 25-44, ISSN 1742-5247

Finnie, K.S.; Waller, D.J.; Perret, F.L.; Krause-Heuer, A.M.; Lin, H.Q.; Hanna, J.V. & Barbe, C.J. (2009). Biodegradability of Sol–Gel Silica Microparticles for Drug Delivery. *Journal of Sol-Gel Scientific Technology*, Vol.49, No.1, (January 2009), pp. 12-18, ISSN 0928-0707

Galagudza, M.M.; Blokhin, I.O.; Shmonin, A.A. & Mischenko, K.A. (2008). Reduction of Myocardial Ischemia-Reperfusion Injury with Pre- and Postconditioning:

Molecular Mechanisms and Therapeutic Targets. *Cardiovascular & Hematological Disorders Drug Targets*, Vol.8, No.1, (March 2008), pp. 47-65, ISSN 1871-529X

Galagudza, M.M.; Korolev, D.V.; Sonin, D.L.; Postnov, V.N.; Papayan, G.V.; Uskov, I.S.; Belozertseva, A.V. & Shlyakhto, E.V. (2010). Targeted Drug Delivery into Reversibly Injured Myocardium with Silica Nanoparticles: Surface Functionalization, Natural Biodistribution, and Acute Toxicity. *International Journal of Nanomedicine*, Vol.5, (April 2010), pp. 231-237, ISSN 1176-9114

Ganta, S.; Devalapally, H.; Shahiwala, A. & Amiji, M. (2008). A Review of Stimuli-Responsive Nanocarriers for Drug and Gene Delivery. *Journal of Controlled Release*, Vol.126, No.3, (March 2008), pp. 187–204, ISSN 0168-3659

Garnacho, C.; Albelda, S.M.; Muzykantov, V.R. & Muro, S. (2008). Differential Intra-Endothelial Delivery of Polymer Nanocarriers Targeted to Distinct PECAM-1 Epitopes. *Journal of Controlled Release: Official Journal of the Controlled Release Society*, Vol.130, No.3, (September 2008), pp. 226–233, ISSN 0168-3659

Hanley, P.J. & Daut, J. (2005). K(ATP) Channels and Preconditioning: a Re-Examination of the Role of Mitochondrial K(ATP) Channels and an Overview of Alternative Mechanisms. *Journal of Molecular and Cellular Cardiology*, Vol.39, No.1, (July 2005), pp. 17-50, ISSN 0022-2828

Hirsch, L.R.; Stafford, R.J.; Bankson, J.A.; Sershen, S.R.; Rivera, B.; Price, R.E.; Hazle, J.D.; Halas, N.J. & West, J.L. (2003). Nanoshell-Mediated Near-Infrared Thermal Therapy of Tumors under Magnetic Resonance Guidance. *Proceedings of the National Academy of Sciences of the United States of America*, Vol.100, No.23, (November 2003), pp. 13549-13554, ISSN 0027-8424

Homma, T. & Irvin, C.G. (1999). Bradykinin-Induced Bronchospasm in the Rat In Vivo: a Role for Nitric Oxide Modulation. *The European Respiratory Journal: Official Journal of the European Society for Clinical Respiratory Physiology*, Vol.13, No.2, (February 1999), pp. 313-320, ISSN 0903-1936

Khaled, A.; Guo, S.; Li, F. & Guo, P. (2005). Controllable Self–Assembly of Nanoparticles for Specific Delivery of Multiple Therapeutic Molecules to Cancer Cells Using RNA Nanotechnology. *Nano Letters*, Vol.5, No.9, (September 2005), pp. 1797–1808, ISSN 1530-6984

Lammers, T.; Kiessling, F.; Hennink, W.E. & Storm, G. (2010). Nanotheranostics and Image-Guided Drug Delivery: Current Concepts and Future Directions. *Molecular Pharmaceutics*, Vol.7, No.6, (December 2010), pp. 1899-1912, ISSN 1543-8384

Leonard, R.C.; Williams, S.; Tulpule, A.; Levine, A.M. & Oliveros, S. (2009). Improving the Therapeutic Index of Anthracycline Chemotherapy: Focus on Liposomal Doxorubicin (Myocet). *Breast*, Vol.18, No.4, (August 2009), pp. 218-224, ISSN 0960-9776

Li, Y.; Tseng, Y.D.; Kwon, S.Y.; D'Espaux, L.; Bunch, J.S.; McEuen, P.L. & Luo, D. (2004). Controlled Assembly of Dendrimer–Like DNA. *Nature Materials*, Vol.3, No.1, (January 2004), pp. 38–42, ISSN 1476-1122

Matsumura, Y. & Maeda, H. (1986). A New Concept for Macromolecular Therapeutics in Cancer Chemotherapy: Mechanism of Tumoritropic Accumulation of Proteins and the Antitumor Agent Smancs. *Cancer Research*, Vol.46, No.12, (December 1986), pp. 6387–6392, ISSN 0008-5472

Ohnishi, S.; Vanderheyden, J.L.; Tanaka, E.; Patel, B.; De Grand, A.M.; Laurence, R.G.; Yamashita, K. & Frangioni, J.V. (2006). Intraoperative Detection of Cell Injury and Cell Death with an 800 nm Near-Infrared Fluorescent Annexin V Derivative. *American Journal of Transplantation*, Vol.6, No.10, (October 2006), pp. 2321-2331, ISSN 1600-6135

Okawa, H.; Horimoto, H.; Mieno, S.; Nomura, Y.; Yoshida, M. & Shinjiro, S. (2003). Preischemic Infusion of Alpha-Human Atrial Natriuretic Peptide Elicits Myoprotective Effects against Ischemia Reperfusion in Isolated Rat Hearts. *Molecular and Cellular Biochemistry*, Vol.248, No.1-2, (June 2003), pp. 171-177, ISSN 0300-8177

Perez, C.; Sanchez, A.; Putnam, D.; Ting, D.; Langer, R. & Alonso, M.J. (2001). Poly(Lactic Acid)–Poly(Ethylene Glycol) Nanoparticles as New Carriers for the Delivery of Plasmid DNA. *Journal of Controlled Release: Official Journal of the Controlled Release Society*, Vol.75, No.1–2, (July 2001), pp. 211–224, ISSN 0168-3659

Piot, C.; Croisille, P.; Staat, P.; Thibault, H.; Rioufol, G.; Mewton, N.; Elbelghiti, R.; Cung, T.T.; Bonnefoy, E.; Angoulvant, D.; Macia, C.; Raczka, F.; Sportouch, C.; Gahide, G.; Finet, G.; Andre-Fouet, X.; Revel, D.; Kirkorian, G.; Monassier, J.P.; Derumeaux, G. & Ovize, M. (2008). Effect of Cyclosporine on Reperfusion Injury in Acute Myocardial Infarction. *New England Journal of Medicine*, Vol.359, No.5, (July 2008), pp. 473-481, ISSN 0028-4793

Qiu, X.Q.; Wang, H.; Cai, B.; Wang, L.L. & Yue, S.T. (2007). Small Antibody Mimetics Comprising Two Complementarity–Determining Regions and a Framework Region for Tumor Targeting. *Nature Biotechnology*, Vol.25, No.8, (August 2007), pp. 921–929, ISSN 1087-0156

Romer, T. (2006). Hormone Replacement Therapy and Bleeding Disorders. *Gynecological Endocrinology: the Official Journal of the International Society of Gynecological Endocrinology*, Vol.22, No.3, (March 2006), pp. 140-144, ISSN 0951-3590

Ruckman, J.; Green, L.S.; Beeson, J.; Waugh, S.; Gillette, W.L.; Henninger, D.D.; Claesson-Welsh, L. & Janjic, N. (1998). 2′–Fluoropyrimidine RNA–Based Aptamers to the 165–Amino Acid Form of Vascular Endothelial Growth Factor (VEGF165). Inhibition of Receptor Binding and VEGF–Induced Vascular Permeability Through Interactions Requiring the Exon 7–Encoded Domain. *Journal of Biological Chemistry*, Vol.273, No.32, (August 1998), pp. 20556–20567, ISSN 0021-9258

Sanchis, J.; Canal, F.; Lucas, R. & Vicent, M.J. (2010). Polymer-Drug Conjugates for Novel Molecular Targets. *Nanomedicine (London, England)*, Vol.5, No.6, (August 2010), pp. 915-935, ISSN 1743-5889

Scott, R.C.; Rosano, J.M.; Ivanov, Z.; Wang, B.; Chong, P.L.; Issekutz, A.C.; Crabbe, D.L. & Kiani, M.F. (2009). Targeting VEGF-Encapsulated Immunoliposomes to MI Heart Improves Vascularity and Cardiac Function. *The FASEB Journal: Official Publication of the Federation of American Societies for Experimental Biology*, Vol.23, No.10, (October 2009), pp. 3361-3367, ISSN 0892-6638

Slowing, I.I.; Vivero-Escoto, J.L.; Wu, C.W. & Lin, V.S. (2008). Mesoporous Silica Nanoparticles as Controlled Release Drug Delivery and Gene Transfection Carriers. *Advanced Drug Delivery Reviews*, Vol.60, No.11, (August 2008) pp. 1278–1288, ISSN 0169-409X

Takahama, H.; Minamino, T.; Asanuma, H.; Fujita, M.; Asai, T.; Wakeno, M.; Sasaki, H.; Kikuchi, H.; Hashimoto, K.; Oku, N.; Asakura, M.; Kim, J.; Takashima, S.; Komamura, K.; Sugimachi, M.; Mochizuki, N. & Kitakaze, M. (2009). Prolonged Targeting of Ischemic/Reperfused Myocardium by Liposomal Adenosine Augments Cardioprotection in Rats. *Journal of the American College of Cardiology*, Vol.53, No.8, (February 2009), pp. 709-717, ISSN 0735-1097

Torchilin, V.P. (2007). Micellar Nanocarriers: Pharmaceutical Perspectives. *Pharmaceutical Research*, Vol.24, No.1, (January 2007), pp. 1–16, ISSN 0724-8741

Ueda, K.; Takano, H.; Niitsuma, Y.; Hasegawa, H.; Uchiyama, R.; Oka, T.; Miyazaki, M.; Nakaya, H. & Komuro, I. (2010) Sonic Hedgehog is a Critical Mediator of Erythropoietin-Induced Cardiac Protection in Mice. *The Journal of clinical investigation*, Vol.120, No.6, (June 2010), pp. 2016-2029, ISSN 0021-9738

Vance, J.E. & Steenbergen, R. (2005). Metabolism and Functions of Phosphatidylserine. *Progress in Lipid Research*, Vol.44, No.4, (July 2005), pp. 207–234, ISSN 0163-7827

van Vlerken, L.E.; Duan, Z.; Seiden, M.V. & Amiji, M.M. (2007). Modulation of Intracellular Ceramide Using Polymeric Nanoparticles to Overcome Multidrug Resistance in Cancer. *Cancer Research*, Vol.67, No.10, (May 2007), pp. 4843–4850, ISSN 0008-5472

Verma, D.D.; Levchenko, T.S.; Bernstein, E.A.; Mongayt, D. & Torchilin, V.P. (2006) ATP-Loaded Immunoliposomes Specific for Cardiac Myosin Provide Improved Protection of the Mechanical Functions of Myocardium from Global Ischemia in an Isolated Rat Heart Model. *Journal of Drug Targeting*, Vol.14, No.5, (June 2006), pp. 273-280, ISSN 1061-186X

Verma, D.D.; Hartner, W.C.; Levchenko, T.S., Bernstein, E.A. & Torchilin, V.P. (2005) ATP-Loaded Liposomes Effectively Protect the Myocardium in Rabbits with an Acute Experimental Myocardial Infarction. *Pharmaceutical Research*, Vol.22, No.12, (December 2005), pp. 2115-2120, ISSN 0724-8741

Vermorken, J.B.; Guigay, J.; Mesia, R.; Trigo, J.M.; Keilholz, U.; Kerber, A.; Bethe, U.; Picard, M. & Brummendorf, T.H. (2011). Phase I/II Trial of Cilengitide with Cetuximab, Cisplatin and 5-Fluorouracil in Recurrent and/or Metastatic Squamous Cell Cancer of the Head and Neck: Findings of the Phase I Part. *British Journal of Cancer*, Vol.104, No.11, (May 2011), pp. 1691-1696, ISSN 0007-0920

Wang, A.Z.; Gu, F.; Zhang, L.; Chan, J.M.; Radovic-Moreno, A.; Shaikh, M.R. & Farokhzad, O.C. (2008). Biofunctionalized Targeted Nanoparticles for Therapeutic Applications. *Expert Opinion on Biological Therapy*, Vol.8, No.8, (August 2008), pp. 1063–1070, ISSN 1471-2598

Yellon, D.M. & Hausenloy D.J. (2007). Myocardial Reperfusion Injury. *New England Journal of Medicine*, Vol.357, No.11, (September 2007), pp. 1121-1135, ISSN 0028-4793

Zhou, J. & Rossi, J.J. (2011). Cell-Specific Aptamer-Mediated Targeted Drug Delivery. *Oligonucleotides*. Vol.21, No.1, (February 2011), pp. 1-10, ISSN 1545-4576

15

Topical Negative Pressure, Applied onto the Myocardium, a Potential Alternative Treatment for Patients with Coronary Artery Disease in the Future

Sandra Lindstedt[1], Malin Malmsjö[2],
Joanna Hlebowicz[3] and Richard Ingemansson[1]
[1]Department of Cardiothoracic Surgery,
[2]Department of Ophthalmology,
[3]Department of Medicine,
Lund University Hospital, Skane
Sweden

1. Introduction

The majority of patients who require intervention for coronary artery disease are adequately treated by percutaneous coronary interventions (PCI) or coronary artery bypass grafting (CABG). However, a major reason for failure of these treatments is their dependency on luminal size and coronary outflow. Methods stimulating myocardial angiogenesis and new vessel formation that are not dependent on vessel caliber therefore provide an important alternative means of treatment. Topical negative pressure (TNP) has been used in the treatment of chronic and problematic wounds since the beginning of the 1990´s, and has been shown to increase blood flow and stimulate angiogenesis in the underlying tissue. Because of TNP´s stimulating effect on blood flow and angiogenesis TNP has been tried to be applied directly onto the myocardium, referred to as myocardial topical negative pressure (MTNP) to increase myocardial blood flow and reduce myocardial ischemia, and reduce myocardial infarction (Lindstedt et al. 2008a, Lindstedt et al. 2008b, Lindstedt et al. 2007c, Lindstedt et al. 2007a, Lindstedt et al. 2007b, Lindstedt et al. 2008c, Lindstedt et al. 2008d).

2. Development of the topical negative pressure technique

Topical negative pressure (TNP) therapy (also called vacuum-assisted closure (VAC) therapy, vacuum sealing or vacuum therapy) has developed from the standard surgical procedure of vacuum-assisted drainage to remove blood or serous fluid from a wound or surgical site. In essence, the TNP technique is very simple. A piece of foam, with an open structure, is inserted into the wound cavity and a wound drain with lateral perforations is placed on top of it. The entire area is then covered with a transparent adhesive membrane, which is firmly secured to the healthy skin around the wound margin. When the exposed end of the drain tube is connected to a vacuum source, fluid is drawn from the wound through the foam into a reservoir for subsequent disposal. The plastic membrane prevents the ingress of air and allows a partial vacuum to form within the wound, reducing its volume and facilitating the removal of fluid.

The practice of exposing a wound to sub-atmospheric pressure for an extended period of time to promote healing was first described by Fleischmann et al. in 1993, following the successful use of this technique in 15 patients with open fractures. They reported that the treatment resulted in, "efficient cleaning and conditioning of the wound, with marked proliferation of granulation tissue". No bone infections occurred in any of the patients, although one developed a soft tissue infection, which subsequently resolved with further treatment. In two further papers, Fleischmann and his colleagues described the treatment of 25 patients with compartment syndromes of the lower limb and 313 patients with various types of acute and chronic infections. Further success with topical negative pressure treatment in Germany was reported by Muller following the treatment of 300 patients with infected wounds.

In these early studies, negative pressure was achieved by the use of conventional methods such as wall suction equipment or surgical vacuum bottles. Both these systems are associated with practical problems in terms of the delivery, control and maintenance of the required levels of negative pressure, as discussed by Banwell et al. . In 1995, a commercial system for vacuum-assisted closure was introduced in the United States. This equipment, called the VAC®, was designed to overcome some of the problems described by Banwell. The heart of the system is a microprocessor-controlled vacuum unit that is capable of providing controlled levels of continuous or intermittent sub-atmospheric pressure ranging from -25 to -200 mmHg.

In early studies no attempts were made to investigate the physiological mechanisms behind the observed clinical effects, or to determine the optimum level of pressure. A seminal study by Morykwas et al. addressed both these issues using a series of animal studies. Deep circular defects, 2.5 cm in diameter, produced on the backs of pigs were dressed with open-cell polyurethane-ether foam with a pore size ranging from 400-600 μm. In the first series of experiments, a laser Doppler technique was used to measure blood flow in the subcutaneous tissue and muscles surrounding the wounds as these were exposed to increasing levels of negative pressure, applied both continuously and intermittently. Their results indicated that while an increase in blood flow equivalent to four times the baseline value occurred with a negative pressure of -125 mmHg, blood flow was inhibited by the application of negative pressures of -400 mmHg and above. A negative pressure of -125 mmHg was therefore used in subsequent studies. The rate of granulation tissue production under negative pressure was determined using the same model by measuring the reduction in wound volume over time. Compared with control wounds dressed with saline-soaked gauze, significantly increased rates of granulation tissue formation were observed with the application of both continuous (63.3 ± 26.1%) and intermittent (103% ±35.3%) negative pressure.

The observation that intermittent or cycled treatment appeared to be more effective than continuous therapy is interesting, although the reasons for this are not fully understood. Two possible explanations were advanced by Philbeck et al.. They suggested that intermittent pressure application results in rhythmic perfusion of the tissue, which is maintained because the process of capillary autoregulation is not activated. They also suggested that as cells that are undergoing mitosis must go through a cycle of rest, cellular component production and division, constant stimulation may cause the cells to 'ignore' the stimulus. Intermittent stimulation allows the cells time to rest and prepare for the next cycle. For this reason, it has been suggested that cyclical negative pressure should be used clinically, although some authors suggest that this should follow a 48-hour period of continuous vacuum to bring about a rapid initial cleansing effect. Following these investigations, Morykwas and colleagues postulated that multiple mechanisms might be responsible for the effects observed. In particular, they suggested that the removal of interstitial fluid decreased localized oedema and increased blood flow, which in turn decreased bacterial levels in tissue. It has since been proposed that the application of sub-atmospheric pressure produces mechanical deformation or stress within the tissue resulting in protein and matrix molecule synthesis and enhanced angiogenesis. Using the rabbit ear as a model, Fabian et al. provided further evidence of the stimulatory effects of sub-atmospheric pressure on the production of granulation tissue, and also demonstrated a trend towards enhanced epithelialisation. In experimental partial-thickness burns in pigs, sub-atmospheric pressure was shown to prevent progressive tissue damage in the zone of stasis that surrounds the area of the initial injury. This effect was demonstrable within 12 hours of injury, with treatment times as short as six hours being sufficient to exert a measurable effect. The authors proposed that the removal of oedema fluid, containing suspended cellular debris, osmotically active molecules and biochemical mediators released following the initial injury, may lessen the obstruction of blood flow.

Numerous other papers have described the use of TNP in the treatment of a variety of wound types, including extensive degloving injuries, infected sternotomy wounds and various soft tissue injuries prior to surgical closure, and in burn wound management.

3. Physiological basis of TNP

Numerous theories have been advanced to explain the physiological basis of the marked improvement in clinical outcomes achieved with TNP. Two basic, broad mechanisms have been proposed to account for the increased rate of granulation tissue formation and accelerated healing rate: a fluid-based mechanism and a mechanical mechanism. Application of a controlled vacuum to the wound interface facilitates the removal of excess interstitial fluid due to the higher pressure gradient. This physically results in a decrease in interstitial pressure. When the interstitial pressure falls below the capillary pressure, the capillaries reopen and flow to the periwound tissue is restored. This same mechanism is responsible for the success of the vacuum technique for decompression of both muscle compartment and abdominal compartment syndrome. All non-bound soluble factors will also be removed with the fluid, including inhibiting factors and promoting factors. Numerous descriptions have been presented of the change in concentration of various factors over time. Factors measured range from growth factors to metalloproteinases to C-reactive protein. The interactions between the soluble factors related to wound healing, and also those factors and interactions that inhibit or delay healing, are extremely complex. The same factor can both promote and inhibit wound healing, depending on the concentration and timing during the healing process. Moreover, the negative pressure and increase in blood flow to the wound bed have been shown to accelerate the formation of granulation tissue. Interestingly, intermittent application of sub-atmospheric pressure has produced superior results, possibly due to mitigation of the cellular desensitization that occurs with exposure to continuous sub-atmospheric pressure. Although it is likely that each of these factors plays a role in the action of TNP, the application of mechanical forces to the wound site is probably the most significant mechanism of action.

Mechanical force is known to be responsible for the induction of cell proliferation and division. Plastic surgeons use tissue expansion to obtain soft-tissue envelopes in reconstructive surgery, while orthopaedic surgeons and maxillofacial surgeons use distraction osteogenesis to lengthen bones. Ingber et al. have shown that for cells to respond to soluble mitogenic factors and proliferate, they must be extended, leading to isometric tension, either by adherence to a stiff substrate or by external application of mechanical forces. Only stretched cells can divide and proliferate in response to soluble growth factors, whereas cells that are not stretched and assume a more spherical shape are cell-cycle arrested and tend to undergo apoptosis. It has also been shown in vitro that directional growth of capillary sprouts is promoted by the application of tension in three-dimensional angiogenesis models. The applied forces deform the extracellular matrix and, as cells are anchorage-dependent, the cells in the stretched tissue are deformed. Cell deformation has been shown to cause a wide variety of molecular responses, including changes in ion concentration and permeability of membrane ion channels, release of secondary messengers, stimulation of molecular pathways, and alterations in gene expression. Moreover, it is known that vascular endothelial cells express a different array of genes depending on whether they have been exposed to static, laminar or turbulent flow. It is apparent that cells are able to sense mechanical forces and respond through the regulation of specific genes and the induction of cellular programs. The exact mechanisms behind these effects are not fully understood, but are probably related to conformational changes in the cytoskeleton in response to mechanical forces. This behavior provides a natural mechanism for tissue homeostasis, where tissue mass expands, cells are stretched and are thus stimulated to divide.

The application of negative pressure may promote wound angiogenesis by directly stimulating endothelial cells. For example, the application of TNP may cause local wound hypoxia, which is a potent stimulator of vascular endothelial growth factor (VEGF) production, the major endothelial cell mitogen. Alternatively, TNP may activate signal transduction pathways leading to endothelial cell division and growth factor production since endothelial tension causes capillary sprouting, gene expression, and changes in matrix metalloproteinase (MMP) activity. While TNP may directly stimulate endothelial proliferation by local hypoxia or cell deformation, increased wound angiogenesis may be an indirect effect of the TNP-mediated reduction in MMP activity. Although low levels of MMPs have been shown to favour angiogenesis, elevated MMP activity inhibits neovascularization and is associated with chronic wounds. Specifically, the levels of the gelatinases MMP-9 and MMP-2 are significantly higher in nonhealing wounds, but return to normal as wound healing progresses towards closure. In addition, chronic wound exudates that inhibit endothelial activity will instead stimulate angiogenesis after treatment with an MMP inhibitor. A reduction in MMP activity may promote endothelial proliferation by lowering MMP-mediated angiostatin and endostatin production. Alternatively, the inhibition of a MMP-propagated inflammatory cascade may provide an environment more favorable to capillary growth.

Mechanical properties seem to have a greater influence on clinical efficacy than fluid-based properties, according to a recently published article, in which the authors showed that the application of mechanical shear stresses was able to activate the VEGF pathway without any VEGF being present in the culture fluid

4. Application of TNP directly onto the myocardium

It was first described by Lindstedt et al that application of a negative pressure directly onto the myocardium resulted in an increase in blood flow in the underlying myocardium. In this first study microvascular blood flow in the myocardium was measured by laser Doppler flowmetry (LDF). The LDF probes were located 5-6 mm lateral to the middle part of the left anterior descending (LAD) , 5-6 mm down into the myocardial wall, and measurements were made before and after application of a MTNP of -50 mmHg. A significant increase was seen in all the animals when the myocardium was exposed to MTNP of -50 mmHg. The increase in blood flow was seen both in non-ischaemic myocardium (normal myocardium), in ischemic myocardium (after 20 minutes of LAD occlusion), and also in reperfused myocardium (formerly ischaemic myocardium after 20 minutes of reperfusion). In all the settings the increase in microvascular blood flow appeared immediately when MTNP was applied. In another study myocardial blood flow was measured using ultrasonic flow meter probes at the proximal part of the left anterior descending artery (LAD), the circumflex coronary artery (CCX) and the right coronary artery (RCA), before and after application of MTNP of -50 mmHg. Measurements were performed during normal conditions (non ischemic) and after occlusion of the LAD, i.e. ischemic conditions. The results implying that MTNP increases the total amount of coronary blood flow to the myocardium. Interestingly, an increase in myocardial perfusion measured by LDF, when the MTNP was applied, correlated to an increase in coronary blood flow in every animal. A non-uniform or a decrease in the total coronary blood flow might hypothetically cause ischemia in parts of the myocardium not exposed to MTNP. Since the present results shows a significant increase in the total amount of coronary blood flow, the authors believe that ischemic areas are not likely to occur. However, local effects in the myocardium could not be deduced from the study.

When applying different negative pressures to periwound tissues (skeletal muscle and subcutaneous tissue) may causes different changes in blood flow. When the negative pressure exceeds a specific level it seems to constringe the vessels in periwound tissue and a decrease in local blood flow is seen. Morykwas et al has previously reported that the microvascular blood flow to a wound increased to four times the baseline value when a negative pressure of 125 mm Hg was applied, whereas it was inhibited at negative pressures of 400 mm Hg and above. The changes in blood flow is thought to be related to local effects, since the blood flow at a distance of 4.5 cm from the wound edge was not affected by the negative pressure between -50 and -200 mmHg. A zone of relative hypoperfusion has been observed close to the wound edge. Hypoperfusion induced by TNP is thought to depend on tissue density, distance from the negative pressure source, and the amount negative pressure applied. In the myocardium, however, MTNP between -25 and -50 mmHg have been shown to induce a significant increase in blood flow, whereas MTNP between -75 and -150 mmHg have not been shown to induce any significant blood flow changes in the underlying myocardium. The differences in blood flow pattern between periwound tissue and myocardium might be due to the differences in tissue histology, where the myocardium has a higher density than periwound tissue. The absence of increase in blood flow when the myocardium is exposed to pressures between -75 and -150 mmHg might, in part be due to, counteract forces. Hypothetic pressures above -150 mmHg might have led to constringe of the vessels, thus reducing the microvascular blood flow to the exposed myocardium. In a study, comparing the two negative pressures -25 and -50 mmHg, both pressures resulted in a significant increase in myocardial blood flow, and no significant difference could be observed between the two pressures. However, the increase in blood flow was greater in normal myocardium when the pressure of -25 mmHg was used. Furthermore, in ischemic myocardium the increase was greater when using -50 mmHg. The study, however, only contained six animals, and the difference might have been significant in a larger study. The authors believe that the optimal MTNP in clinical perspective might be -50 mmHg, since ischemic conditions would be of greater interest than normal.

As earlier mentioned, a zone of relative hypoperfusion has been observed in studies when TNP is applied on wounds. The zone of hypoperfusion is believed to appear close to the negative pressure source. When MTNP, a large zone of hypoperfusion, would theoretically cause ischemia in the epicardium that would theoretically cause ischemia. In wound healing the effect of hypoperfusion or ischemia close to the negative pressure source might be beneficial to wound healing, since hypoxia has been shown to be a strong factor for stimulating VEGF and new vessel formation. In MTNP however, a zone of hypoperfusion would probably not be desirable. Interestingly, three different studies on animals have shown a significant increase in epicardial blood flow when exposed to MTNP of -50mmHg. MTNP between -75 and -150mmHg did not; in any of the studies induce a significant change in myocardial blood flow. Probably because the amount of negative pressure applied is to large, resulting in an obstruction of the vessels. Consequently, no hypoperfusion could be observed during MTNP in either normal, ischemic, or reperfused myocardium during both normo- and hypo-thermia. The absence of hypoperfusion could possibly be explained by the higher density of myocardium than wound tissue. It could however also possibly be explained by the release of vasodilators close to the negative pressure source. Another possible explanation is that the increase in blood flow is due to a redistribution of the microvascular blood flow to the epicardium caused by natural physiological microvascular mechanisms in the myocardial wall, as seen during for example systolic blood pressure below 50 mmHg. Another possible explanation is that the negative force is greater closer to the vacuum source and subsequently decreases with distance.

Argenta et al. investigated in 2010 if MTNP applied onto the myocardium followed acute myocardial infarction could decrease the size of myocardial infarction in an animal model. They induce ischemia by 75 minutes of left main coronary artery occlusion and thereafter three hours of reperfusion. Animals were assigned to one of three groups: (A) untreated control; treatment of involved myocardium for 180 minutes of MTNP with (B) -50 mmHg, or (C) -125 mmHg. Treatment of the ischemic area with MTNP for 180 minutes significantly reduced infarct size (area of necrosis/area at risk) in both treatment groups compared to control. Total area of cell death was reduced by 65% with -50 mmHg treatment and 55% in the -125 mmHg group. They concluded that treatment of ischemic myocardium with MTR, for a controlled period of time during reperfusion, successfully reduced the extent of myocardial death after acute myocardial infarction.

5. Ischemic heart disease; clinical application of TNP

The majority of patients who require intervention for coronary artery disease are adequately treated by PCI or CABG. However, a major reason for failure of these treatments is their dependency on luminal size and coronary outflow. Methods of stimulating new vessel formation in the myocardium that are not dependent on vessel caliber therefore provide an important alternative treatment. A large group of patients suffer from refractory angina pectoris. Conventional treatment such as PCI and CABG has not been successful in these patients. Various other therapies have been tried, such as percutaneous myocardial laser revascularization, and enhanced external counter-pulsation, with varying success. Even spinal cord stimulation has been used in an attempt to ease their ischaemic pain. However, a satisfactory means of treating these patients has yet to be found. A new form of treatment resulting in new collateral vessel formation would thus be of interest for these patients. Numerous studies have evaluated the efficacy of gene therapy in the treatment of ischemic heart disease for the restoration of myocardial function by stimulation of angiogenesis and collateral vessel formation. VEGF has been found to be one of the most interesting growth factors in therapeutic angiogenesis. Interestingly, the mechanical forces exerted by TNP stimulate the endogenous production of VEGF.

In patients with acute coronary syndrome and coronary vessel occlusion, it is of great importance to improve or, if possible, restore the blood flow to the ischemic myocardium to protect it from ischemic stress and, in some cases, acute coronary infarction. Most patients are successfully treated with conventional methods such as PCI or CABG. However, these procedures do not result in satisfactory results in all patients due to extensive coronary disease or small vessel caliber. Furthermore, the procedure is not suitable for some patients due to their advanced age, renal failure, or other complicating factors. In some cases of acute ST elevation myocardial infarction there is no reflow during PCI. No-reflow situations may also arise during saphenous vein graft intervention, and rotational atherectomy. During no-reflow, epicardial flow is reduced due to obstructions at the microvasculature level. This no-reflow condition is usually transient, but patients with refractory no-reflow are associated with a markedly increased risk of 30-day mortality, compared with patients in whom no-reflow is transient. MTNP of -50 mmHg significantly increased the microvascular blood flow in both the epicardium and the myocardium. Interestingly, MTNP increases both the velocity and volume of blood flow by opening up the capillary beds. Furthermore, the method is not dependent on vessel caliber.

6. Conclusion

In conclusion, MTNP increases blood flow to the heart during normal, ischemic and reperfused conditions during both normo- and hypo-thermia. Interestingly, MTNP increases blood flow both in the endocardium and in the epicardium of the myocardial wall. The authors believe that MTNP may in the future represent an alternative treatment for patients with coronary artery disease and in particular patients with refractory angina pectoris.

7. References

Argenta, L. C. & M. J. Morykwas (1997) Vacuum-assisted closure: a new method for wound control and treatment: clinical experience. *Ann Plast Surg,* 38, 563-76; discussion 577.

Argenta, L. C., M. J. Morykwas, J. J. Mays, E. A. Thompson, J. W. Hammon & J. E. Jordan (2010) Reduction of myocardial ischemia-reperfusion injury by mechanical tissue resuscitation using sub-atmospheric pressure. *J Card Surg,* 25, 247-52.

Armstrong, D. G. & L. A. Lavery (2005) Negative pressure wound therapy after partial diabetic foot amputation: a multicentre, randomised controlled trial. *Lancet,* 366, 1704-10.

Armstrong, D. G., L. A. Lavery, P. Abu-Rumman, E. H. Espensen, J. R. Vazquez, B. P. Nixon & A. J. Boulton (2002) Outcomes of subatmospheric pressure dressing therapy on wounds of the diabetic foot. *Ostomy Wound Manage,* 48, 64-8.

Banwell, P., S. Withey & I. Holten (1998) The use of negative pressure to promote healing. *Br J Plast Surg,* 51, 79.

Banwell, P. E. (1999) Topical negative pressure therapy in wound care. *J Wound Care,* 8, 79-84.

Banwell, P. E. (2004) Topical negative pressure wound therapy: advances in burn wound management. *Ostomy Wound Manage,* 50, 9S-14S.

Banwell, P. E. & L. Teot (2003) Topical negative pressure (TNP): the evolution of a novel wound therapy. *J Wound Care,* 12, 22-8.

Bauer, P., G. Schmidt & B. D. Partecke (1998) [Possibilities of preliminary treatment of infected soft tissue defects by vacuum sealing and PVA foam]. *Handchir Mikrochir Plast Chir,* 30, 20-3.

Biswas, S. S., G. C. Hughes, J. E. Scarborough, P. W. Domkowski, L. Diodato, M. L. Smith, C. Landolfo, J. E. Lowe, B. H. Annex & K. P. Landolfo (2004) Intramyocardial and intracoronary basic fibroblast growth factor in porcine hibernating myocardium: a comparative study. *J Thorac Cardiovasc Surg,* 127, 34-43.

Chen, C., G. S. Schultz, M. Bloch, P. D. Edwards, S. Tebes & B. A. Mast (1999a) Molecular and mechanistic validation of delayed healing rat wounds as a model for human chronic wounds. *Wound Repair Regen,* 7, 486-94.

Chen, C. S., M. Mrksich, S. Huang, G. M. Whitesides & D. E. Ingber (1997) Geometric control of cell life and death. *Science,* 276, 1425-8.

Chen, C. S., M. Mrksich, S. Huang, G. M. Whitesides & D. E. Ingber (1998) Micropatterned surfaces for control of cell shape, position, and function. *Biotechnol Prog,* 14, 356-63.

Chen, K. D., Y. S. Li, M. Kim, S. Li, S. Yuan, S. Chien & J. Y. Shyy (1999b) Mechanotransduction in response to shear stress. Roles of receptor tyrosine kinases, integrins, and Shc. *J Biol Chem,* 274, 18393-400.

Clare, M. P., T. C. Fitzgibbons, S. T. McMullen, R. C. Stice, D. F. Hayes & L. Henkel (2002) Experience with the vacuum assisted closure negative pressure technique in the treatment of non-healing diabetic and dysvascular wounds. *Foot Ankle Int,* 23, 896-901.

Cohn, P. F. (2006) Enhanced external counterpulsation for the treatment of angina pectoris. *Prog Cardiovasc Dis,* 49, 88-97.

Cornelius, L. A., L. C. Nehring, E. Harding, M. Bolanowski, H. G. Welgus, D. K. Kobayashi, R. A. Pierce & S. D. Shapiro (1998) Matrix metalloproteinases generate angiostatin: effects on neovascularization. *J Immunol,* 161, 6845-52.

Deer, T. R. & L. J. Raso (2006) Spinal cord stimulation for refractory angina pectoris and peripheral vascular disease. *Pain Physician,* 9, 347-52.

DeFranzo, A. J., M. W. Marks, L. C. Argenta & D. G. Genecov (1999) Vacuum-assisted closure for the treatment of degloving injuries. *Plast Reconstr Surg,* 104, 2145-8.

Detmar, M., L. F. Brown, B. Berse, R. W. Jackman, B. M. Elicker, H. F. Dvorak & K. P. Claffey (1997) Hypoxia regulates the expression of vascular permeability factor/vascular endothelial growth factor (VPF/VEGF) and its receptors in human skin. *J Invest Dermatol,* 108, 263-8.

Fabian, T. S., H. J. Kaufman, E. D. Lett, J. B. Thomas, D. K. Rawl, P. L. Lewis, J. B. Summitt, J. I. Merryman, T. D. Schaeffer, L. A. Sargent & R. P. Burns (2000) The evaluation of subatmospheric pressure and hyperbaric oxygen in ischemic full-thickness wound healing. *Am Surg,* 66, 1136-43.

Fleischmann, W., E. Lang & L. Kinzl (1996) [Vacuum assisted wound closure after dermatofasciotomy of the lower extremity]. *Unfallchirurg,* 99, 283-7.

Fleischmann, W., E. Lang & M. Russ (1997) [Treatment of infection by vacuum sealing]. *Unfallchirurg,* 100, 301-4.

Fleischmann, W., W. Strecker, M. Bombelli & L. Kinzl (1993) [Vacuum sealing as treatment of soft tissue damage in open fractures]. *Unfallchirurg,* 96, 488-92.

Gimbrone, M. A., Jr., T. Nagel & J. N. Topper (1997) Biomechanical activation: an emerging paradigm in endothelial adhesion biology. *J Clin Invest,* 100, S61-5.

Gowda, R. M., I. A. Khan, G. Punukollu, B. C. Vasavada & C. K. Nair (2005) Treatment of refractory angina pectoris. *Int J Cardiol,* 101, 1-7.

Greene, A. K., M. Puder, R. Roy, S. Kilroy, G. Louis, J. Folkman & M. A. Moses (2004) Urinary matrix metalloproteinases and their endogenous inhibitors predict hepatic regeneration after murine partial hepatectomy. *Transplantation,* 78, 1139-44.

Huang, S., C. S. Chen & D. E. Ingber (1998) Control of cyclin D1, p27(Kip1), and cell cycle progression in human capillary endothelial cells by cell shape and cytoskeletal tension. *Mol Biol Cell,* 9, 3179-93.

Huang, S. & D. E. Ingber (1999) The structural and mechanical complexity of cell-growth control. *Nat Cell Biol,* 1, E131-8.

Ilizarov, G. A. (1989a) The tension-stress effect on the genesis and growth of tissues. Part I. The influence of stability of fixation and soft-tissue preservation. *Clin Orthop Relat Res,* 249-81.

Ilizarov, G. A. (1989b) The tension-stress effect on the genesis and growth of tissues: Part II. The influence of the rate and frequency of distraction. *Clin Orthop Relat Res,* 263-85.

Ingber, D. E. (2002) Mechanical signaling and the cellular response to extracellular matrix in angiogenesis and cardiovascular physiology. *Circ Res,* 91, 877-87.

Kang, S. & Y. Yang (2007) Coronary microvascular reperfusion injury and no-reflow in acute myocardial infarction. *Clin Invest Med,* 30, E133-45.

Korff, T. & H. G. Augustin (1999) Tensional forces in fibrillar extracellular matrices control directional capillary sprouting. *J Cell Sci,* 112 (Pt 19), 3249-58.

Ladwig, G. P., M. C. Robson, R. Liu, M. A. Kuhn, D. F. Muir & G. S. Schultz (2002) Ratios of activated matrix metalloproteinase-9 to tissue inhibitor of matrix metalloproteinase-1 in wound fluids are inversely correlated with healing of pressure ulcers. *Wound Repair Regen,* 10, 26-37.

Leon, M. B., R. Kornowski, W. E. Downey, G. Weisz, D. S. Baim, R. O. Bonow, R. C. Hendel, D. J. Cohen, E. Gervino, R. Laham, N. J. Lembo, J. W. Moses & R. E. Kuntz (2005) A blinded, randomized, placebo-controlled trial of percutaneous laser myocardial revascularization to improve angina symptoms in patients with severe coronary disease. *J Am Coll Cardiol,* 46, 1812-9.

Lerman, O. Z., R. D. Galiano, M. Armour, J. P. Levine & G. C. Gurtner (2003) Cellular dysfunction in the diabetic fibroblast: impairment in migration, vascular endothelial growth factor production, and response to hypoxia. *Am J Pathol,* 162, 303-12.

Lindstedt, S., M. Johansson, J. Hlebowicz, M. Malmsjo & R. Ingemansson (2008a) Myocardial topical negative pressure increases blood flow in hypothermic, ischemic myocardium. *Scand Cardiovasc J,* 1-9.

Lindstedt, S., M. Malmsjo, B. Gesslein & R. Ingemansson (2008b) Topical negative pressure effects on coronary blood flow in a sternal wound model. *Int Wound J.,* 5, 511-529.

Lindstedt, S., M. Malmsjo, B. Gesslein & R. Ingemansson (2008b) Evaluation of continuous and intermittent myocardial topical negative pressure. *J Cardiovasc Med (Hagerstown),* 9, 813-9.

Lindstedt, S., M. Malmsjo & R. Ingemansson (2007a) Blood flow changes in normal and ischemic myocardium during topically applied negative pressure. *Ann Thorac Surg,* 84, 568-73.

Lindstedt, S., M. Malmsjo & R. Ingemansson (2007b) The effect of different topical negative pressures on microvascular blood flow in reperfused myocardium during hypothermia. *Innovations* 2, 231–236.

Lindstedt, S., M. Malmsjo & R. Ingemansson (2007c) No hypoperfusion is produced in the epicardium during application of myocardial topical negative pressure in a porcine model. *J Cardiothorac Surg,* 2, 53.

Lindstedt, S., M. Malmsjo, J. Sjogren, R. Gustafsson & R. Ingemansson (2008c) Impact of different topical negative pressure levels on myocardial microvascular blood flow. *Cardiovasc Revasc Med,* 9, 29-35.

Lindstedt, S., P. Paulsson, A. Mokhtari, B. Gesslein, J. Hlebowicz, M. Malmsjo & R. Ingemansson (2008d) A compare between myocardial topical negative pressure levels of -25 mmHg and -50 mmHg in a porcine model. *BMC Cardiovasc Disord,* 8, 14.

Meara, J. G., L. Guo, J. D. Smith, J. J. Pribaz, K. H. Breuing & D. P. Orgill (1999) Vacuum-assisted closure in the treatment of degloving injuries. *Ann Plast Surg,* 42, 589-94.

Mochitate, K., P. Pawelek & F. Grinnell (1991) Stress relaxation of contracted collagen gels: disruption of actin filament bundles, release of cell surface fibronectin, and down-regulation of DNA and protein synthesis. *Exp Cell Res,* 193, 198-207.

Morykwas, M. J. & L. C. Argenta (1997a) Nonsurgical modalities to enhance healing and care of soft tissue wounds. *J South Orthop Assoc,* 6, 279-88.

Morykwas, M. J., L. C. Argenta, E. I. Shelton-Brown & W. McGuirt (1997b) Vacuum-assisted closure: a new method for wound control and treatment: animal studies and basic foundation. *Ann Plast Surg,* 38, 553-62.

Morykwas, M. J., L. R. David, A. M. Schneider, C. Whang, D. A. Jennings, C. Canty, D. Parker, W. L. White & L. C. Argenta (1999) Use of subatmospheric pressure to prevent progression of partial-thickness burns in a swine model. *J Burn Care Rehabil,* 20, 15-21.

Moses, M. A., M. Marikovsky, J. W. Harper, P. Vogt, E. Eriksson, M. Klagsbrun & R. Langer (1996) Temporal study of the activity of matrix metalloproteinases and their endogenous inhibitors during wound healing. *J Cell Biochem,* 60, 379-86.

Muller, G. (1997) [Vacuum dressing in septic wound treatment]. *Langenbecks Arch Chir Suppl Kongressbd,* 114, 537-41.

Nagel, T., N. Resnick, C. F. Dewey, Jr. & M. A. Gimbrone, Jr. (1999) Vascular endothelial cells respond to spatial gradients in fluid shear stress by enhanced activation of transcription factors. *Arterioscler Thromb Vasc Biol,* 19, 1825-34.

O'Reilly, M. S., D. Wiederschain, W. G. Stetler-Stevenson, J. Folkman & M. A. Moses (1999) Regulation of angiostatin production by matrix metalloproteinase-2 in a model of concomitant resistance. *J Biol Chem,* 274, 29568-71.

Philbeck, T. E., Jr., K. T. Whittington, M. H. Millsap, R. B. Briones, D. G. Wight & W. J. Schroeder (1999) The clinical and cost effectiveness of externally applied negative pressure wound therapy in the treatment of wounds in home healthcare Medicare patients. *Ostomy Wound Manage,* 45, 41-50.

Pozzi, A., W. F. LeVine & H. A. Gardner (2002) Low plasma levels of matrix metalloproteinase 9 permit increased tumor angiogenesis. *Oncogene,* 21, 272-81.

Pozzi, A., P. E. Moberg, L. A. Miles, S. Wagner, P. Soloway & H. A. Gardner (2000) Elevated matrix metalloprotease and angiostatin levels in integrin alpha 1 knockout mice cause reduced tumor vascularization. *Proc Natl Acad Sci U S A,* 97, 2202-7.

Saxena, V., C. W. Hwang, S. Huang, Q. Eichbaum, D. Ingber & D. P. Orgill (2004) Vacuum-assisted closure: microdeformations of wounds and cell proliferation. *Plast Reconstr Surg,* 114, 1086-96; discussion 1097-8.

Silver, F. H. & L. M. Siperko (2003a) Mechanosensing and mechanochemical transduction: how is mechanical energy sensed and converted into chemical energy in an extracellular matrix? *Crit Rev Biomed Eng,* 31, 255-331.

Silver, F. H., L. M. Siperko & G. P. Seehra (2003b) Mechanobiology of force transduction in dermal tissue. *Skin Res Technol,* 9, 3-23.

Tang, A. T. (2003) Vacuum-assisted suction drainage of sternotomy infection: a new paradigm? *Eur J Cardiothorac Surg,* 23, 649-50; author reply 650.

Tang, A. T., S. K. Ohri & M. P. Haw (2000) Novel application of vacuum assisted closure technique to the treatment of sternotomy wound infection. *Eur J Cardiothorac Surg,* 17, 482-4.

Tardy, Y., N. Resnick, T. Nagel, M. A. Gimbrone, Jr. & C. F. Dewey, Jr. (1997) Shear stress gradients remodel endothelial monolayers in vitro via a cell proliferation-migration-loss cycle. *Arterioscler Thromb Vasc Biol,* 17, 3102-6.

Tarlton, J. F., C. J. Vickery, D. J. Leaper & A. J. Bailey (1997) Postsurgical wound progression monitored by temporal changes in the expression of matrix metalloproteinase-9. *Br J Dermatol,* 137, 506-16.

Ulrich, D., F. Lichtenegger, F. Unglaub, R. Smeets & N. Pallua (2005) Effect of chronic wound exudates and MMP-2/-9 inhibitor on angiogenesis in vitro. *Plast Reconstr Surg,* 116, 539-45.

Wackenfors, A., R. Gustafsson, J. Sjogren, L. Algotsson, R. Ingemansson & M. Malmsjo (2005) Blood flow responses in the peristernal thoracic wall during vacuum-assisted closure therapy. *Ann Thorac Surg,* 79, 1724-30; discussion 1730-1.

Wackenfors, A., J. Sjogren, R. Gustafsson, L. Algotsson, R. Ingemansson & M. Malmsjo (2004) Effects of vacuum-assisted closure therapy on inguinal wound edge microvascular blood flow. *Wound Repair Regen,* 12, 600-6.

van Gaal, W. J. & A. P. Banning (2007) Percutaneous coronary intervention and the no-reflow phenomenon. *Expert Rev Cardiovasc Ther,* 5, 715-31.

Webb, L. X. (2002) New techniques in wound management: vacuum-assisted wound closure. *J Am Acad Orthop Surg,* 10, 303-11.

Venturi, M. L., C. E. Attinger, A. N. Mesbahi, C. L. Hess & K. S. Graw (2005) Mechanisms and clinical applications of the vacuum-assisted closure (VAC) Device: a review. *Am J Clin Dermatol,* 6, 185-94.

Yan, L., M. A. Moses, S. Huang & D. E. Ingber (2000) Adhesion-dependent control of matrix metalloproteinase-2 activation in human capillary endothelial cells. *J Cell Sci,* 113 (Pt 22), 3979-87.

Yau, T. M., C. Kim, G. Li, Y. Zhang, S. Fazel, D. Spiegelstein, R. D. Weisel & R. K. Li (2007) Enhanced angiogenesis with multimodal cell-based gene therapy. *Ann Thorac Surg,* 83, 1110-9.

16

Ischemic Heart Disease, Diabetes and Mineralocorticoid Receptors

Anastasia Susie Mihailidou
Department of Cardiology & Kolling Medical Research Institute
Royal North Shore Hospital & University of Sydney
Australia

1. Introduction

Ischemic heart disease continues to be a leading cause of death in most countries, with the death rate in men almost twice as high as that of women. Following an ischemic event, the primary clinical strategy is to quickly restore blood flow to the heart muscle, myocardial reperfusion, using drug therapy (thrombolytics) or percutaneous coronary intervention. The damage that follows ischemia-reperfusion is triggered by increased production of oxygen free radicals at the time of reperfusion when blood flow is restored (Ambrosio et al. 1993; Marczin et al. 2003) and impaired myocardial antioxidant defences, leading to cardiomyocyte apoptosis and increased infarct size.

Hyperglycaemia and high plasma levels of aldosterone are two critical factors that produce poor outcomes following an ischemic event and reperfusion strategies. Diabetes is now the fastest growing disease worldwide, and a public health concern globally given the aging population -currently affecting more than 240 million people worldwide, and the number is predicted to rise to more than 360 million by 2030, according to the World Health Organization. Global health expenditure on diabetes is estimated to rise to USD 490 billion (Zhang et al. 2010) and cardiovascular disease is the major cause of death. In adults with type 2 diabetes, cardiovascular disease is responsible for 65-75% of deaths due to myocardial infarction and end stage renal disease; and the age-adjusted relative risk for cardiovascular complications in type 1 diabetes may exceed that of type 2 (Nadeua et al. 2010). Although first line treatment for diabetes is anti-hyperglycaemic agents, additional therapeutic strategies are needed. In addition, during hypoglycaemia there is an increase in aldosterone production (Adler et al. 2010) and there is emerging evidence of a relationship between aldosterone and insulin resistance.

High plasma aldosterone levels during percutaneous coronary intervention double the risk of mortality and are an independent risk factor for mortality (Beygui et al. 2006). Inappropriately elevated aldosterone levels produce cardiac and vascular inflammation and fibrosis, leading to remodelling and disease via activation of mineralocorticoid receptors (MR) (Brilla et al. 1990; Young et al. 1995). Recent experimental studies (Mihailidou et al. 2009) show that during myocardial ischemia-reperfusion, cardiac damage is aggravated by activation of mineralocorticoid receptors by both aldosterone (Fig.1) and cortisol (Fig. 2).

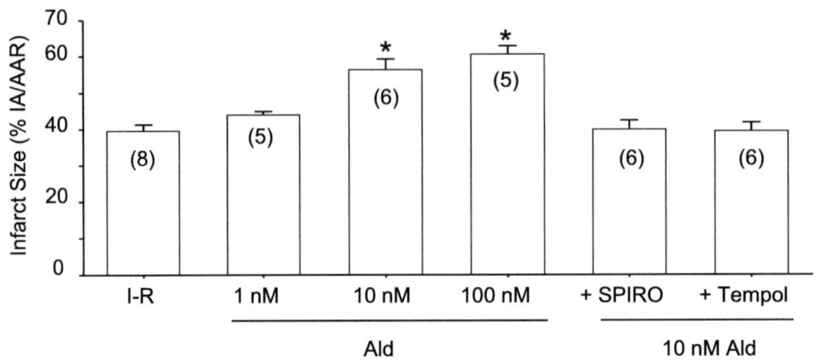

Reproduced from Mihailidou et al. (2009) with permission

Fig. 1.

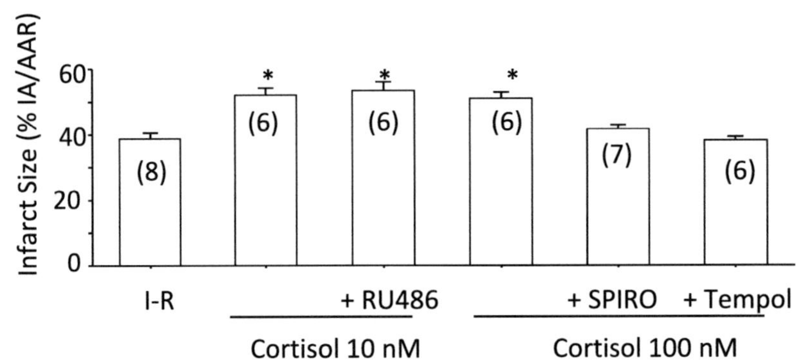

Reproduced from Mihailidou et al. (2009) with permission

Fig. 2.

Current therapies, such as antagonism of the renin-angiotensin-system, mitigate the cardiorenal complications of diabetes but do not suppress aldosterone production. Aldosterone levels increase ("aldosterone breakthrough") in 10-53% patients and recent studies suggest an association between aldosterone production and insulin resistance in normotensive subjects (Balkau et al. 1998), indicating aldosterone is an independent risk factor for myocardial damage. The results from RALES (Randomised ALdactone Evaluation Study, Pitt et al. 1999), EPHESUS (Eplerenone Post acute Myocardial Infarction HEart Failure SUrvival and efficacy Study, Pitt et al. 2003), and recently EMPHASIS-HF (Eplerenone in Mild Patients Hospitalization and Survival Study in Heart Failure, Zannad et al. 2011) provide strong evidence that preventing MR activation increases survival and decreases hospitalization in patients with heart failure and acute myocardial infarction. In these trials 32% of patients were diabetic.

Since patients with diabetes have a 2-3 fold increased risk of ischemic heart disease, any new drug therapy for lowering glucose levels in this population must be evaluated in terms of its safety for use in patients with cardiovascular disease. It would be advantageous if this medication is shown to have cardio-protective effects, and to ensure there isn't aggravated cardiac damage following a heart attack. Glucagon-Like Peptide-1 (GLP-1) agonists are a relatively new class of anti-hyperglycaemic medications for the management of patients with diabetes. These agents also elicit a cytoprotective effect on beta cells leading to preservation and survival of beta-cell mass (Tschen et al. 2009; 2011; Brubaker & Drucker 2004). The impact of these new therapeutic agents on cardiovascular disease remains unclear. Controlled large clinical studies of GLP-1 agonists on cardiovascular outcomes following ischemic heart disease for patients with diabetes are currently in progress. Whether there is added benefit of combining GLP-1 agonists with a mineralocorticoid receptor antagonist has not been examined.

Given the increasing aging populations globally, increased incidence of both type 1 and type 2 diabetes and elevated mortality in patients with high plasma aldosterone levels, this chapter will provide a review of our current understanding of the incidence of ischemic heart disease in both type 1 and type 2 diabetes; mechanisms involved and new treatment strategies. These include the GLP-1 agonists and mineralocorticoid receptor antagonists as potential additional therapeutic strategies to reduce cardiovascular complications of diabetes.

2. Ischemic heart disease and diabetes

Cardiovascular disease is the major cause of disease burden and death globally and along with diabetes and cancer make up two-thirds of all deaths globally, according to the World Health Organization's report for 2011 World Health Statistics. The impact of hyperglycemia in patients with acute myocardial infarction (AMI) varies with age, with higher risk for in-hospital mortality among younger patients (Nicolau et al. 2011). Hyperglycemia was associated with 7.6-fold increased odds for in-hospital death in patients younger than 50 years, compared with a 3.5-fold increased risk in those aged 50-60 years. Worldwide, there is a higher risk of diabetes or cardiovascular disease in rural areas than in urban areas (Wan et al. 2007). The prevalence of type 2 diabetes is increasing dramatically due to the aging population, obesity and physical inactivity. Although Type 1 diabetes is less common and usually has onset in younger subjects, age-adjusted relative risk for cardiovascular complications in type 1 may exceed type 2 diabetes (Nadeau et al. 2010).

Patients with either type 1 or type 2 diabetes have significantly higher mortality and morbidity following acute myocardial infarction than do the rest of the population, with increasing focus on hyperglycemia contributing directly to the excessive cardiovascular risk in patients with diabetes. The hazard ratio for major cardiovascular disease (CVD) was reported to be 3.6 (95% CI 2.9–4.5) in men with type 1 diabetes compared with those without diabetes (Soedamah-Muthu et al. 2006), while men with type 2 diabetes, the hazard ratio was 3.3 (95% CI 2.5- 4.5) and 10.1 (6.7–17.4) in women. (Juutilainen et al. 2008). Clinically, elevated but non-diabetic blood glucose levels increase cardiovascular mortality risk (Balkau et al. 1998). During myocardial reperfusion injury, hyperglycaemia increases cardiomyocyte apoptosis in both human (Frustaci et al.2000) and animal models (Fiordaliso et al. 2000; Sheu et al. 2007) of diabetes. Restoring blood flow to the ischemic myocardium is accompanied be increased oxygen free radicals (Ambrosio et al. 1993; Brown et al. 1988) and impaired myocardial antioxidant defence capacity leading to tissue injury (Leichtweis et al 2001), and therefore additional therapeutic strategies are needed to complement glycemic control.

Inflammation also promotes reperfusion injury (Kawaguchi et al. 2011), and both type 1 and type 2 diabetes include inflammatory components: type 1 diabetes is an auto-immune disease (Atkinson and Eisenbarth, 2001), and more recently type 2 diabetes has also been considered an auto-inflammatory condition (Donath and Shoelson, 2011) leading to an increase production of pro-inflammatory mediators including pro-inflammatory cytokines IL-6 and TNF-α. Activation of TNF-α, activates apoptosis, and amplifies the innate immune response. The innate immune response has been identified to interact with danger associated molecular patterns (DAMPs) found on proteins released by necrotic cells following ischemia-reperfusion that include HMGB1 and heat shock proteins via toll like receptors (TLRs). This interaction activates NF–κβ signalling promoting innate immune cell infiltration into the myocardium, increased cytokine production and increased pro-apoptotic activity through caspase 3/7 and hence further aggravating reperfusion injury (Arslan et al., 2010). Additionally $CD4^+$ T-cells have been identified to infiltrate the myocardium during reperfusion and through the release of cytokine IFN-γ promote infiltration of innate immune cells, in particular macrophages and neutrophils, the effector cells of the immune response to reperfusion injury (Yang et al., 2006). This increase in adaptive and innate immune responses in diabetes promotes activity of the complement system, which also further aggravates reperfusion injury (van der Pals et al., 2010).

3. Mechanisms involved in hyperglycaemia-aggravated ischemic heart disease

During prolonged ischemia ATP levels decrease leading to reduced Na^+/K^+ ATPase and sarcoplasmic reticulum (SR) Ca^{2+} pump activity and cystolic Na^+ and Ca^{2+} retention. Additionally the decreasing oxygen supply during ischemia leads to an increased reliance on anaerobic glycolysis evident in the increased production of anaerobic-glycolysis by-products and hydrogen ions (H^+), thus decreasing cellular pH and lactate in the ischemic myocardium (van der Vusse et al. 1987). The increase in H^+ in the myocardium promotes the activity of the sodium (Na^+)/H^+ exchanger leading to further increase in sodium retention, This is followed by calcium entry through the activity of the Na^+/Ca^{2+} exchanger; increased Ca^{2+} opens the ryanodine receptor further increasing cytosolic Ca^{2+} referred to as Ca^{2+} overload (Cannell et al. 1995) triggering cell death. ROS production also promotes Ca^{2+} overload through its interaction with various Ca^{2+}-related ion channels, including increasing the open probability of the ryanodine receptor found on the sarcoplasmic reticulum via oxidation of key thiol groups within the protein (Boraso & Williams, 1994), Ca^{2+} leakage through lipid perioxidation of phospholipid membranes (Burton et al.1990) and stimulation of the Na^+-Ca^{2+} exchanger (Shi et al. 1989) through both lipid perioxidation and oxidation of thiol groups within the exchanger protein.

Increased production of reactive oxygen species (ROS) (Arroyo et al., 1987; Steenbergen et al., 1987) during reperfusion triggers increased uncoupling of mitochondria complex I (Rolo and Palmeira, 2006, Tanaka et al., 2000). Additionally diabetes is associated with decreased antioxidant capacity measured by both direct enzyme activity by total plasma anti-oxidant capacity (TRAP) assay and indirectly by measures of lipid peroxidation such as lipid hydroperoxides and conjugate dienes (Likidlilid et al., 2007, Marra et al., 2002, Santini et al., 1997; Santos et al., 2011) and calcium overload (Steenbergen et al., 1987), leading to cell death and cardiac damage (Chen et al., 2002). Clinically, the Prevention of REStenosis with Tranilast and its Outcomes (PRESTO) trial found that diabetic patients had increased incidence of mortality and myocardial infarction 9 months after percutaneous coronary intervention (Mathew et al., 2004). Diabetic patients with hypertension were at a greater risk of adverse outcomes following percutaneous coronary intervention (Lingman et al., 2011)

Hyperglycaemia that is not controlled can lead to abnormal cardiac contractile dysfunction, with decreased Ca^{2+} sensitivity of contractile proteins. Animal studies show that there is increased post-translational modification of contractile proteins with phosphorylation of myofilament proteins troponin I and troponin T resulting in decreased Ca^{2+} sensitivity (Akella et al., 1995). Myocardial tissue collected from diabetic and non-diabetic patients undergoing coronary artery bypass surgery showed that the presence of diabetes decreased Ca^{2+} sensitivity (Jweied et al. 2005). Diabetic patients also have a higher risk of developing hypertension than normoglycaemic individuals. Sodium (Na^{+}) retention has been identified as a possible cause of this increased risk of hypertension due to increased Na^{+} -glucose co-transporter activity found in the renal tubules of diabetic patients (Nosadini et al., 1993). Hyperglycaemia and hypertension have an additive effect on long-term cardiovascular risk, and when both are present there is greater risk of microvascular complications, including nephropathy and retinopathy, and macrovascular complications such as atherosclerosis.

During ischemia-reperfusion (refer Fig. 3), there is programmed loss of cardiomyocytes, apoptosis, with rates of 2–12% reported in the border zone of human myocardial infarcts (Ottaviani et al., 1999; Olivetti et al., 1996). This loss of viable tissue leads to structural remodelling of the heart and deteriorating cardiac function. Both acute stress hyperglycaemia (Suleiman et al., 2005) and diabetes (Mathew et al., 2004; Muhlestein et al., 2003) aggravate injury following reperfusion of the ischemic myocardium. Hyperglycaemia increases cardiomyocyte apoptosis, both acutely as shown by recent studies (Wong et al. 2011) as well as after prolonged exposure in diabetic animals (Fiordaliso et al. 2000; Sheu et al. 2007) and human tissue (Frustaci et al. 2000). Aggravated reperfusion injury correlates with increased apoptosis in the area at risk (Crow et al. 2004). Clinically, elevated but non-diabetic blood glucose levels also increase cardiovascular mortality risk (Balkau et al. 1998).

Apoptosis is up-regulated in hyperglycaemic cellular models of ischemia, where cardiac myocytes are deprived of serum and placed in hypoxic conditions (Bonavita, 2003, Aki et al., 2010). Bonavita et al 2003 identified activation of pro-apoptotic mediators of Bid and Bax and down-regulation of anti-apoptotic mediator Bcl-xl in H9c2 rat cardiomyoblast cell line. Further support is provided by Aki et al. (2010) using H9c2 cells in hypoxic hyperglycaemic conditions that showed AIF release through ATP depletion promoting chromatin condensation and DNA fragmentation. Receptor for Advanced Glycation End products (RAGE) expression has been identified to be crucial to the promotion of apoptosis and reperfusion injury via increased c-Jun N-terminal Kinases (JNK) signalling promoting pro-apoptotic caspase-3 activation and cytochrome-c release (Aleshin et al., 2008).

As well as apoptosis, when cells have been exposed to sustained damage, there is necrosis of myocardial tissue, which is aggravated by hyperglycaemia. Hyperglycaemia-activated ROS promote the production of methylgloxal a side product of many metabolic pathways; increase in methygloxal promotes the NF-κβ to bind to the promoter region of RAGE (Yao and Brownlee, 2010). Increased RAGE expression and increased induced nitric oxide synthase (iNOS) expression, increase nitric oxide production (NO) (Bucciarelli et al., 2006). NO and ROS species combine to form peroxynitrate, increasing high mobility group box 1 (HMGB1) release, a marker of necrotic cell death, although mechanisms has not been defined (Loukili et al., 2011).

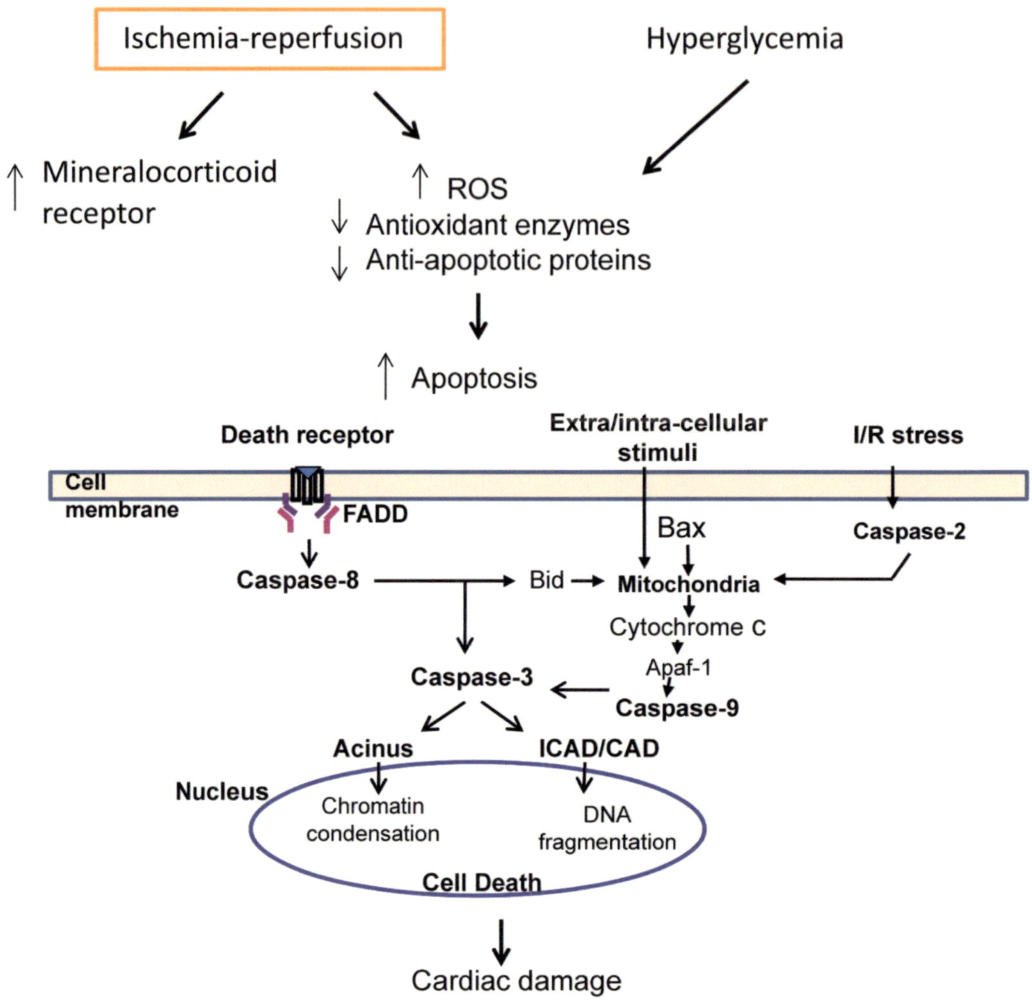

Fig. 3. Ischemia-reperfusion induced signal transduction pathway leading to apoptosis in cardiac myocytes.

4. New treatment strategies during ischemic heart disease

First line treatment for diabetes is anti-hyperglycaemic agents, with insulin the anti-hyperglycaemic agent for type 1 diabetes and in some type 2 diabetes cases. Intensive glycaemic control clinically delayed development of microvascular complications in type 2 diabetic patients in the United Kingdom Prospective Diabetes Study (UKPDS, 1998a), but did not lead to a reduction in cardiovascular events; a subgroup of patients treated with metformin had a 39% reduction in myocardial infarction, although there were only a small number of events. Patients with Type 1 diabetes in the Diabetes Control and Complications Trial/Epidemiology of Diabetes Interventions and Complications (DCCT/EDIC) study only showed a reduction in risk of any cardiovascular complications by 42% only years after recruitment (The Diabetes Control and Complications Trial/Epidemiology of Diabetes

Interventions and Complications Research Group, 2003). In the large randomised clinical trials, ADVANCE (Action in Diabetes and Vascular Disease: Preterax and Diamicron Modified Release Controlled Evaluation) and ACCORD (Action to Control Cardiovascular Risk in Diabetes), intensive glycemic control compared to standard glucose-lowering targets in type 2 diabetes led to a reduction in risk for microvascular complications, although the optimum treatment for minimising the risk of cardiovascular complications was not defined. Metformin is routinely used in type 2 diabetes and has some cardiovascular benefits in obese type 2 diabetic patients (UKPDS, 1998b). In a pre-clinical study, acute stress hyperglycaemia aggravated infarct area and apoptosis following ischemia-reperfusion whereas perfusion with insulin decreased apoptosis and reduced reperfusion injury (Wong et al., 2011).

4.1 GLP-1 agonists

Glucagon-like peptide 1 (GLP-1) agonists are an exciting new class of anti-hyperglycaemic medication that not only lower glucose levels, but also reduce weight and have protective effects on pancreatic islets. Since the insulinotropic and insulinomimetic effects of GLP-1 are mitigated at plasma glucose concentrations of 3.9 mmol/L, this minimizes the risks of hypoglycemia and the need for glucose infusion. Therefore, the pharmacological properties of GLP-1 are attractive as a means to stimulate myocardial glucose uptake during post-ischemic contractile dysfunction. Currently, there are limited clinical studies to confirm the impact of GLP-1 agonists on cardiovascular events in subjects with type 2 diabetes. Glucagon like peptide-1 (GLP-1) agonists, mimic the action of the incretin GLP-1 upon its binding to the GLP-1 receptor, which has been shown to be expressed in cardiomyocytes (Ban et al., 2008). GLP-1 also promotes the release of insulin, whilst inhibiting the release of glucagon, both these effects occur postprandial.

Several animal studies involving murine and canine models have examined the effects of GLP-1 agonists on the ischaemic myocardium (Timmers et al. 2009; Noyan-Ashraf et al. 2009; Kristensen et al. 2009; Ban et al. 2010). Most, but not all of these studies suggest that GLP-1 agonists may have beneficial effects on the myocardium following an ischemic insult. These benefits ranged from reduction in infarct size to improvement in left ventricular function, although the mechanisms for the cardio-protective action are not well understood. In addition, most studies used non-diabetic animal models, where the hearts were subjected to normal glucose levels and transient administration of GLP-1 agonists. In a recent study (Noyan-Ashraf et al. 2009), Liraglutide conferred cardio-protection over Metformin despite equivalent degrees of glycaemic control. In this study, diabetes was induced in mice by using streptozotocin, and therefore a model of Type I diabetes. The cardioprotective properties of GLP-1 agonist are independent of its glycaemic control properties and inactivate a key pro-apoptotic protein BAD mediated via PKB/AKT signalling, thus decreasing apoptosis and reperfusion injury (Timmers et al. 2009). The effects of GLP-1 on outcomes following acute coronary occlusion for subjects with Type 2 diabetes have yet to be defined.

4.2 Mineralocorticoid receptor antagonists

High plasma aldosterone levels during percutaneous coronary intervention double the risk of mortality and are an independent risk factor for mortality (Beygui et al. 2006). Preclinically the administration of aldosterone increased reperfusion injury by promoting apoptosis (Mihailidou et al., 2009). Aldosterone at inappropriate levels promotes inflammation and cardiovascular remodelling via activation of mineralocorticoid receptors (MR). Aldosterone has also been reported to trigger oxidative stress, inflammation, thrombosis and sudden cardiac death (Rajagopalan et al. 2002; Struthers 2001). ACE inhibitors or angiotensin receptor antagonists mitigate the cardiorenal complications of diabetes but do not suppress aldosterone production. Aldosterone levels increase ("aldosterone breakthrough") in 10-53% patients, indicating aldosterone is an independent risk factor for myocardial damage.

Recent studies show aldosterone interferes with insulin signalling pathways and reduces expression of insulin-sensitizing factors adiponectin and peroxisome proliferator activated receptor–γ (Wada et al. 2009; Guo et al. 2008). Blockade of the mineralocorticoid receptor increased adiponectin and peroxisome proliferator-activated receptor-γ in adipose tissue leading to improved insulin sensitivity in obese, diabetic ob/ob and db/db mice (Guo et al. 2008; Hirata et al. 2009). Further confirmation of cross talk between aldosterone and insulin signalling pathways is that insulin resistance improved with treatment in patients with primary hyperaldosteronism (Catena et al. 2006). Spironolactone has also been shown to be effective in decreasing albuminuria in patients with type 2 diabetes with proteinuria who were being treated with ACE inhibitors. (Davidson et al. 2008). Although the mechanism was not defined, an anti-inflammatory action was proposed.

The relationship between aldosterone, glucose metabolism and insulin resistance is poorly explored. The results from RALES (Randomised ALdactone Evaluation Study), EPHESUS (Eplerenone Post acute Myocardial Infarction HEart Failure SUrvival and efficacy Study) [Pitt et al. 2003], and recently EMPHASIS-HF (Eplerenone in Mild Patients Hospitalization and Survival Study in Heart Failure) provide strong evidence that preventing mineralocorticoid receptor activation increases survival and decreases hospitalization in patients with heart failure and acute myocardial infarction. In these trials 32% of patients were diabetic, highlighting a potential benefit of MR antagonist use to minimise cardiovascular complications in diabetic patients in addition to anti-hyperglycaemic treatment. Subgroup analysis of EPHESUS showed the beneficial effects of eplerenone were also found in patients with diabetes (O'Keefe et al. 2008). Diabetic patients treated with eplerenone had a higher rate of absolute risk reduction, compared with patients without diabetes, for both end-point of death from cardiovascular causes or hospitalization for cardiovascular events (5.1 vs. 3.5%).

5. Conclusion

There is an enormous public health problem emerging given the increasing aging population who are at highest risk of having an acute ischemic event and with diabetes the fastest growing disease, the proportion of people at risk of cardiovascular disease is therefore increasing dramatically. Globally health expenditure on diabetes is estimated to rise, with the health burden growing - currently 300 million people with diabetes worldwide, despite preventative strategies. Additional therapies are required and the results from clinical trials to determine the cardiovascular effects of the new anti-hyperglycemic agents, GLP-1 agonists are eagerly anticipated. Mineralocorticoid receptor antagonists, spironolactone and eplerenone have demonstrated specific actions at low doses, preventing end-organ damage. In particular, diabetic patients showed greater absolute cardiovascular risk reduction. Provided there is monitoring of plasma K^+, there is potential for use of MR antagonists in diabetes.

6. References

Adler GK, Bonyhay I, Curren V, Waring E, Freeman R. (2010). *Diabet. Med.* 27: 1250–1255.

Akella AB, Ding XL, Cheng R, Gulati J. (1995). *Circ. Res.* 76: 600-606.

Aki T, Nara A, Funakoshi T, Uemura K. (2010). *Biochem Biophys Res Commun.* 396(3): 614–618.

Aleshin A, Ananthakrishnan R, Li Q, Rosario R, Lu Y, Qu W, et al. (2008). *Am J Physiol Heart Circ Physiol.* 294(4): H1823–32.

Ambrosio G, Zweier JL, Duilio C et al. (1993). *J. Biol. Chem.* 268: 18532-18541.

Arroyo CM, Kramer JH, Dickens BF, Weglicki WB. (1987). *FEBS Lett,* 221: 101-104.

Arslan F, de Kleijn DP, Pasterkamp G. (2011). Nat Rev Cardiol. 8(5): 292–300.

Atkinson MA and Eisenbarth GS. (2001). Lancet 358(9277): 221–229.

Balkau B, Shipley M, Jarrett RJ, Pyorala K, Pyorala M, Forhan A, Eschwege E. (1998). Diabetes Care. 21:21: 360-367.

Balkau B, Shipley M, Jarrett RJ, Pyorala K, Pyorala M, Forhan A, Eschwege E. (1998). Diabetes Care. 21:21: 360-367.

Ban K, Kim KH, Cho CK, Sauvé M, Diamandis EP, Backx PH, Drucker DJ, Husain M (2010). *Endocrinology* 151(4): 1520-1531.

Ban K, Noyan-Ashraf MH, Hoefer J, Bolz SS, Drucker DJ, Husain M (2008). *Circulation.* 117(18):2340-50.

Beygui F, Collet J-P, Benoliel J-J, Vignolles N, Dumaine R, Barthélémy O, Montalescot G (2006) *Circulation* 114:2604-2610.

Bonavita F. (2003). *FEBS Letters.* 536(1-3): 85–91.

Boraso A, Williams AJ. (1994). *Am J Physiol.* 267(3 Pt 2): H1010–1016.

Brilla CG, Pick R, Tan LB, Janicki JS, and Weber KT. (1990). *Circ Res* 67: 1355–1364.

Brubaker PL, Drucker DJ. (2004) *Endocrinology* 145:2653–2659.

Bucciarelli LG, Kaneko M, Ananthakrishnan R, Harja E, Lee LK, Hwang YC, Lerner S, Bakr S, Li Q, Lu Y, Song F, Qu W, Gomez T, Zou YS, Yan SF, Schmidt AM, Ramasamy R. (2006). *Circulation,* 113: 1226-34.

Burton KP, Morris AC, Massey KD, Buja LM, Hagler HK. (1990). *J Mol Cell Cardiol.* 22(9): 1035–1047.

Cannell MB, Cheng H, Lederer WJ. (1995). *Science.* 268(5213): 1045–1049. \

Catena C, Lapenna R, Baroselli S, Nadalini E, Colussi G, NovelloM, Favret G, Melis A, Cavarape A, Sechi LA. (2006). *J Clin. Endocrinol. Metab.* 91: 3457–3463

Chen M, Won DJ, Krajewski S, Gottlieb RA. (2002). *J Biol Chem,* 277: 29181-29186.

Crow, MT, Mani, K, Nam, YJ, Kitsis, RN (2004) *Circ. Res.* 95:957-970.

Davidson MB, Wong A, Hamrahian AH, Stevens M, Siraj ES. (2008). *Endocrine Practice.* 14(8): 985-992.

Donath MY and Shoelson SE. (2011). Nat Rev Immunol. 11(2): 98–107.

Fiordaliso F, Li B, Latini R, Sonnenblick EH, Anversa P, Leri A, and Kajstura J. (2000). *Lab Invest* 80: 513–527, 2000.

Fiordaliso F, Li B, Latini R, Sonnenblick EH, Anversa P, Leri A, and Kajstura J. (2000). *Lab Invest* 80: 513–527, 2000.

Frustaci A, Kajstura J, Chimenti C, Jakoniuk I, Leri A, Maseri A, Nadal-Ginard B, and Anversa P. (2000) *Circ Res* 87: 1123–1132.
Frustaci A, Kajstura J, Chimenti C, Jakoniuk I, Leri A, Maseri A, Nadal-Ginard B, and Anversa P. (2000) *Circ Res* 87: 1123–1132.
Guo C, Ricchiuti V, Lian BQ, Yao TM, Coutinho P, Romero JR, Li J, Williams GH, Adler GK. (2008). *Circulation* 117: 2253–226

Hirata A, Maeda N, Hiuge A, Hibuse T, Fujita K, Okada T, Kihara S, Funahashi T, Shimomura I. (2009). *Cardiovasc Res.* 84: 164–172

Juutilainen A, Lehto S, Ronnemaa T, Pyorala K, Laakso M. (2008). *Diabetes Care* 31:714–719.

Jweied EE, McKinney RD, Walker LA, Brodsky I, Geha AS, Massad MG, et al. (2005). *Am J Physiol Heart Circ Physiol.* 289(6): H2478–2483.

Kawaguchi M, Takahashi M, Hata T, Kashima Y, Usui F, Morimoto H, et al. (2011) *Circulation* 123(6):594–604.

Kristensen J, Mortensen UM, Schmidt M, Nielsen PH, Nielsen TT, Maeng M (2009). *BMC Cardiovasc Disord.* 9: 31.

Leichtweis S, Ji LL (2001). *Acta Physiol. Scand.* 172: 1-10.

Likidlilid A, Patchanans N, Poldee S, Peerapatdit T. (2007). *J Med Assoc Thai.* 90(9): 1759–1767.

Lingman M, Albertsson P, Herlitz J, Bergfeldt L, Lagerqvist B. (2011). *Am J Med.* 124(3): 265–275.

Loukili N, Rosenblatt-Velin N, Li J, Clerc S, Pacher P, Feihl F, Waeber B, Liaudet L. (2011). *Cardiovascular research.* 89: 586-94.

Marczin N, El-Habashi N, Hoare GS, Bundy RE, Yacoub M. (2003). *Archives of Biochemistry and Biophysics* 420: 222–236

Marra G, Cotroneo P, Pitocco D, Manto A, Di Leo MA, Ruotolo V, et al. (2002). *Diabetes Care.* 25(2): 370–375.

Mathew V, Gersh BJ, Williams BA, Laskey WK, Willerson JT, Tilbury RT, Davis BR, Holmes DR, Jr. (2004). *Circ.* 109: 476-480.

Mihailidou AS, Le TYL, Mardini M, Funder JW (2009). *Hypertension* 54:1306-1312.

Muhlestein JB, Anderseon JL, Horne BD, Lavasani F, Allen Maycock CA, Bair TL, Pearson RR, Carlquist JF; Intermountain Heart Collaborative Study Group. (2003). *Am. Heart J,* 146: 351-358.

Nadeua K, Regensteiner JG, Bauer TA, Brown MS, Dorosz JL, Hull A, Zeitler P, Draznin B, Reusch JEB (2010). *J. Clin. Endocrinol. Metab.* 95:513-521.

Nicolau JC, Serrano Jr CV, Rocha Giraldez R, Moreira Baracioli L, Graner Moreira H, Lima F, Franken M, Kalil R, Franchini Ramires JA and Giugliano RP. (2011) *Diabetes Care* doi: 10.2337/dc11-1170.

Nosadini R, Sambataro M, Thomaseth K, Pacini G, Cipollina MR, Brocco E, Solini A, Carraro A, Velussi M, Frigato F, et al. (1993). *Kidney International* 44: 139-146.

Noyan-Ashraf MH, Momen MA, Ban K, Sadi AM, Zhou YQ, Riazi AM, Baggio LL, Henkelman RM, Husain M, Drucker DJ. (2009). *Diabetes,* 58(4): 975-983.

O'Keefe JH, Abuissa H, Pitt B. (2008). *Diabetes, Obesity and Metabolism.* 10: 492–497.

Olivetti G, Quaini F, Sala R, Lagrasta C, Corradi D, Bonacina E, et al. *J Mol Cell Cardiol* 1996;28:2005–16.

Ottaviani G, Lavezzi AM, Rossi L, Matturri L. *Eur J Histochem* 1999;43:7– 14.

Pitt B, Remme W, Zannad F, Neaton J, Martinez F, Roniker B, Bittman R, Hurley S, Kleiman J, Gatlin M, for the Eplerenone Post–Acute Myocardial Infarction Heart Failure Efficacy and Survival Study Investigators. (2003). N Engl J Med. 348:1309-21.

Pitt B, Zannad F, Remme W, Cody R, Castaigne A, Perez A, Palensky J, Wittes J. for the Randomized Aldactone Evaluation Study Investigators. (1999). *N Engl J Med* 341:709-717.

Rajagopalan S, Duquaine D, King S, Pitt B, Patel P. (2002). Circulation. 105: 2212–2216.

Rolo AP, Palmeira CM. (2006). *Toxicol Appl Pharmacol.* 212(2): 167–178.

Santini SA, Marra G, Giardina B, Cotroneo P, Mordente A, Martorana GE, et al. (1997). *Diabetes.* 46(11): 1853–1858.

Santos CXC, Anilkumar N, Zhang M, Brewer AC, Shah AM. (2011). Free Radic Biol Med. 50(7): 777–793.

Sheu J-J, Chang L-T, Chiang C-H, Sun C-K, Chang N-K, Youssef AA, Wu C-J, Lee F-Y, Yip H-K. (2007) *Int Heart J.* 48: 233-245.

Sheu J-J, Chang L-T, Chiang C-H, Sun C-K, Chang N-K, Youssef AA, Wu C-J, Lee F-Y, Yip H-K. (2007) *Int Heart J.* 48: 233-245.

Shi ZQ, Davison AJ, Tibbits GF. (1989). *J Mol Cell Cardiol.* 21(10): 1009–1016.

Soedamah-Muthu SS, Fuller JH, Mulnier HE, Raleigh VS, Lawrenson RA, Colhoun HM. (2006). *Diabetes Care* 29:798–804.

Steenbergen C, Murphy E, Levy L, London RE. (1987). *Circ. Res.* 60: 700-707.

Struthers AD (2001). J Renin Angiotensin Aldosterone Syst. 2: 211–214.

Suleiman M, Hammerman H, Boulos M, Kapeliovich MR, Suleiman A, Agmon Y, Markiewicz W, Aronosn D. (2005). *Circulation* 111: 754-760.

Tanaka N, Yonekura H, Yamagishi S, Fujimori H, Yamamoto Y, Yamamoto H. (2000). *J Biol Chem.* 275(33): 25781–25790.

The Diabetes Control and Complications Trial/Epidemiology of Diabetes Interventions and Complications Research Group. (2003). *N Engl J Med.* 348: 2294-2303.

Timmers L, Henriques JP, de Kleijn DP, Devries JH, Kemperman H, Steendijk P, Verlaan CW, Kerver M, Piek JJ, Doevendans PA, Pasterkamp G, Hoefer IE (2009). *J Am Coll Cardiol.* 53(6): 501-510.

Tschen SI, Dhawan S, Gurlo T, Bhushan A. (2009). *Diabetes* 58:1312–1320.

Tschen S-I, Georgia S, Dhawan S, Bhushan A. (2011). *Molecular Endocrinology* 25: 0000- 0000.

UKPDS 33. UK Prospective Diabetes Study (UKPDS) Group. (1998a). *Lancet.* 352(9131): 837–853.

UKPDS 34). UK Prospective Diabetes Study (UKPDS) Group. (1998b). *Lancet.* 12;352(9131):854–865.

van der Pals J, Koul S, Andersson P, Gotberg M, Ubachs JF, Kanski M, et al.(2010). BMC Cardiovasc Disord. 10(1): 45.

van der Vusse GJ, Stam H. (1987). *Basic Res Cardiol.* 82 Suppl 1: 149–153.

Wada T, Ohshima S, Fujisawa E, Koya D, Tsuneki H, Sasaoka T. (2009). *Endocrinology.* 150: 1662–1669

Wan Q, Harris MF, Powell-Davies G, Jayasinghe UW, Flack J, Georgiou A, Burns JR, Penn DL (2007). Aust J Rural Health, 15: 327–333.

Wong V, Mardini M, Cheung W, Mihailidou AS. (2011). *Journal of Diabetes and Its Complications.* 25: 122-128.

World Health Organisation (2011) World Health Statistics Report.

Yang Z, Day Y-J, Toufektsian M-C, Xu Y, Ramos SI, Marshall MA, French BA and Linden J. (2006) *Circulation* 114: 2056-2064.

Yao D, Brownlee M. (2010). *Diabetes,* 59: 249-55.

Young M, Head G, and Funder JW (1995). *Am J Physiol Endocrinol Metab* 269: E657–E662.

Zannad F, McMurray JJV, Krum H, van Veldhuisen DJ, Swedberg K, Shi H, Vincent J, Pocock SJ, & Pitt B,, for the EMPHASIS-HF Study Group. (2011) N Engl J Med. 364:11-21.

Zhang P., Zhang X, Brown J, Vistisen D, Sicree R, Shaw J, Nichols G.(2010) *Diabetes research and clinical practice* 87:293-301.

Part 5

Public Health Importance of Ischemic Heart Disease

17

Cardiology Best Practice – Effective Health Education Meets Biomedical Advances: Reducing the Ultimate Knowledge Translation Gap

Elizabeth Dean[1], Zhenyi Li[2], Wai Pong Wong[3] and Michael E. Bodner[4,5]
[1]*University of British Columbia, Vancouver*
[2]*Royal Roads University, Victoria*
[3]*Singapore General Hospital*
[4]*Duke University, Durham*
[5]*Trinity Western University, Langley*
[1,2,5]*Canada*
[3]*Singapore*
[4]*USA*

1. Introduction

The long-term outcomes of biomedical advances in cardiology and surgery, the focus of this book, fall short of their potential unless coupled with changes in patients' lifestyle behaviors. Within the context of a busy, resource- and time-constrained practice, this chapter presents practical and effective evidence-informed strategies for health education that can be readily implemented by the cardiologist and surgeon. Given the unequivocal link between lifestyle behaviors and ischemic heart disease, 'healthy living' not only promises to augment a patient's health overall and reduce the need for drugs and surgery but, when biomedical interventions are indicated, it can augment their outcomes.

Based on epidemiological indicators this century, effective health education needs to be a clinical competency that is practiced systematically and inter-professionally and whose outcomes are routinely and quantitatively evaluated over time. Strategies that are most amenable to being integrated into cardiology practice involve initiating and supporting such education rather than the cardiologist or surgeon necessarily being the primary educator. Clinicians need practical effective strategies; these include expedient means of assessing the patient's needs, targeting and tailoring health education to these needs, identifying patient learning outcomes, and following-up systematically.

2. The ultimate knowledge translation gap

Although the associations among lifestyle behaviors (primarily smoking, nutrition and exercise) and health and ischemic heart disease are well documented (see reviews Dean et al. 2009a; Dean et al. 2009b; Joint WHO/FAO Expert Consultation, 2002; Neuhouser et al. 2002; World Health Organization, 2002, & 2011; Yusuf et al. 2004; Yusuf et al. 2005), most adults and many children have one or more risk factors for ischemic heart disease. In the adult population, risk factors are often coupled with one or more manifestations of the condition. This trend is projected to reduce life expectancy this century for the first time in recorded history (Olshansky et al. 2005). The persisting gap between the scientific community's knowledge about the associations between lifestyle and health, and the prevalence of chronic lifestyle-related conditions is not acceptable (Glasgow et al. 2004), nor socially and economically sustainable (World Health Organization, www.who.int/mediacentre/factsheets/fs172/en/). Health education that is effective and seamlessly supported by an inter-professional team is needed to bridge this ultimate knowledge translation gap.

The pandemic of lifestyle-related conditions reflects multiple influences ranging from the capacity of health professionals to educate patients effectively, and the adherence of patients to health recommendations. Patient adherence to the most fundamental evidence-based lifestyle and health knowledge appears marginal at best even when they are confronted by the proverbial wake-up call (Blanchard et al. 2008). Of interest is that adverse lifestyle practices such as smoking, suboptimal nutrition, overweight and obesity, sedentary behavior, lack of regular physical activity, suboptimal sleep and undue stress now contribute to several of the ten leading causes of premature death in North America and in other high-income countries. With westernization this trend is appearing increasingly in middle- and low-income countries (Beaglehole & Yach, 2003; Mortality Country Fact Sheets, 2006) that stand to benefit from the western experience. Given the common lifestyle behavior pathway and associated low-level inflammation associated with a western lifestyle and related conditions (Bruunsgaard, 2005), effectively educating patients about lifestyle changes related to health risks and the risk of ischemic heart disease or its manifestations would help to reduce the prevalence of other chronic lifestyle-related conditions such as hypertension, stroke, type 2 diabetes mellitus, obesity, and even cancer (Dean et al. 2011). Although health professionals have a major role in promoting public health policy, this topic extends beyond the scope of this chapter, hence, is addressed elsewhere.

2.1 Lifestyle behaviors associated with ischemic heart disease

All of the most deleterious health risk lifestyle behaviors, namely, smoking, suboptimal nutrition, obesity, inactivity, sleep deprivation and excess stress, are implicated in the pathoetiology of ischemic heart disease (Soler et al. 2010). Smoking has been described as the leading cause of preventable premature death (Mokdad et al. 2004). About twenty percent of American adults continue to smoke despite widespread public health campaigns and health policy legislation (Dube et al. 2010). Further, two thirds of the population is overweight or obese. And, although physical inactivity has long been known to be deleterious to health and claimed to be the leading public health priority this century (Blair, 2009; Thompson et al. 2003), prolonged periods of being sedentary has been identified as an independent risk factor for lifestyle-related conditions (Healy et al. 2008; Jakes et al. 2003; Stannard & Johnson, 2004; Biddle et al. 2010; Thorpe et al. 2010). Lastly, many North Americans have been reported to be chronically sleep deprived (Coren, 2009), and have stress levels long been known to be deleterious to health (DeLongis, 1988). One or more of these risk factors in combination can contribute to ischemic heart disease.

Although the literature has focused on adults, the pandemic of lifestyle risk factors for ischemic heart disease in children is also well documented (Berenson et al. 1998). Children with adverse lifestyle practices constitute the new wave of adults with this condition who will manifest signs and symptoms at an earlier age; a trend that is changing priorities in pediatric practice. This trend has implications for health education involving the family given the shared lifestyle of adults and their children (Gidding et al. 1999) as well as the need for the health care community to support public health initiatives related to smoking cessation, healthy eating and active living.

2.2 Health living is the best revenge

Few clinicians would argue the benefits of a healthy lifestyle to overall health and wellbeing, and risk factor reduction for ischemic heart disease and its prevention. What appears to be less well appreciated however are the effect sizes of healthy living practices. Small changes in weight and physical activity for example can reap appreciable benefits with respect to risk reduction of lifestyle-related conditions, reversing pathology in some cases, as well as managing these conditions (Dean, 2009a; Dean, 2009b; World Health Organization, 2003). Knowledge of these relative effects sizes can provide powerful incentives to clinicians in motivating their patients and to the patients themselves.

In one exemplary study of over 23,000 people between 35 and 65 years old, Ford and colleagues (Ford et al. 2009) reported that over an eight year period, people who did not smoke; had a body mass index of less than 30; were physically active for a minimum of 3.5 hours a week; and ate healthily had an 81% lower risk of myocardial infarction; an outcome few medical advances could achieve. Further, by following these non-stringent lifestyle practices, type 2 diabetes mellitus was reduced by 93%, stroke by 50% and cancer by 36%. Even if not all four health factors were present, risk of developing a chronic lifestyle-related condition decreased commensurate with an increase in the number of positive lifestyle factors.

Health behavior change with respect to diet and exercise has also long been known to normalize blood pressure and blood lipids, and help reverse atherosclerosis (American College of Sports Medicine, 2009 and 2010; American Heart Association, 2003; Ornish, 1998; Ornish et al. 1998). Nutritional regimens such as Mediterranean type diets and the DASH diet (Dietary Approaches to Stop Hypertension) are highly evidence based in terms of their capacity to control risk factors for ischemic heart disease and type 2 diabetes mellitus (Sofi et al, 2008; Sacks et al, 1995; Appel et al, 1997). Given these compelling findings that few if any drugs can replicate systematically, health behavior change needs to be viewed and expediently practiced with the same rigor and precision as the prescription of drugs or conducting a surgical procedure.

Hypertension is a major contributing factor in ischemic heart disease for which diet and exercise can address in many cases (Task Force for the Management of Arterial Hypertension, 2007). Even reducing daily salt intake as little as one-third has been projected to reduce the cases of hypertension in the United States by 11 million cases annually (25% reduction), and associated health care costs by $1.7 billion (Report of the Institute of Medicine of the National Academy of Sciences, 2010).

Obesity is a strong independent risk factor for hypertension (Shaper, 1996), and both conditions are strongly associated with ischemic heart disease. Strategies for sustained weight management and control have shifted from calorie restriction to good nutrition.

2.3 Health education as a clinical competency

Effective patient health education is aimed at not only reducing a patient's need for drug therapy, surgery, or both, but minimizing the social and economic burdens of ischemic heart disease to his or her family and community. Promoting healthy lifestyle behaviors targets the causes or principal factors that contribute to ischemic heart disease, which is distinct to a primary focus on reducing its signs and symptoms. Further, 'healthy living' minimizes the indications for drugs and surgery and the degree of their invasiveness and, if indicated, may augment their outcomes.

2.4 Cardiologists as health educators

Medical curricula are overwhelmed and replete with the need to assimilate the exponential growth of biomedical knowledge. Despite the evidence supporting the unequivocal benefits of healthy lifestyle practices on health and curbing chronic lifestyle-related conditions, attention to patient education as a competency pales in comparison with other topics in medical curricula.

Notwithstanding, cardiologists and surgeons are pre-eminently qualified to prescribe drugs or perform surgery. They and the public are bombarded continuously with a dizzying array of new advances. Such advances include that heralded in the popular press recently to announce a new drug class that blocks cholesterol protein, 'Drugmakers are racing to develop a new class of medicines they believe could be the biggest weapon against heart disease since statins were introduced in the 1980s' (Pierson, 2011). Despite the potential contribution of such advances, the unequivocal potency of lifestyle behavior change and inarguably its superior effects, should not be minimized nor lost sight of in the face of such news headlines. However, the discordance between the efficacy of healthy lifestyle behaviors to prevent, in some cases reverse, as well as manage lifestyle-related conditions such as ischemic heart disease, and the effectiveness of people actually changing their lifestyles when fully aware of the detrimental effect of unhealthy lifestyles, is well known to every clinician. This supports the need for health professionals to develop competency in advising and educating patients with respect to long-term multiple health behavior change. Their effectively practicing collectively and seamlessly will help maximize the outcomes of 'healthy living'.

Health professionals practicing in the third millennia remain committed to the Hippocratic tenets of 'first, do no harm', and 'the function of protecting and developing health must rank even above that of restoring it when it is impaired'. To meld the two, that is, practice health promotion within the context of contemporary biomedical practice, elevates health education to a bone fide clinical competency in the interest of best practice. Best practice in cardiology can be described as effective health education coupled with biomedical advances. The goal of the cardiologist and the surgeon is to maximize the outcomes of medical and surgical procedures and prevent recurrences of cardiac episodes, as well as promote the patient's overall health and wellbeing.

Cardiologists and surgeons have become gatekeepers to a substantial proportion of society in need of lifestyle behavior modification. Although patients are often perceived by physicians and surgeons as viewing lifestyle behavior change as arduous, requiring discipline and deprivation, some patients are quite motivated to change (Alegrante et al. 2008), e.g., 70% of smokers have been reported wanting to quit (Centers for Disease Control, 2002). Some physicians believe that if their patients simply adhere to their medications most of the time, this will have the greatest chance of reducing their complaints. However, even with the proverbial wake-up call with a diagnosis of a chronic lifestyle-related life-threatening condition, adherence of patients to 'healthy living' practices is alarmingly low (Blanchard et al. 2008). A major step toward enabling patients to effect sustained health behavior change is for clinicians to understand their own perceived and actual barriers to successfully educating their patients, as well as those of the patients to changing.

To effect sustained lifestyle behavior changes in their patients, clinicians need basic knowledge about the processes of teaching and learning. Even brief advice by health professionals that is targeted and tailored can be effective in terms of its priming effect on health behavior change (Kreuter et al. 2000). With respect to smoking cessation, brief advice can augment quit rates (Bodner & Dean, 2009). Additional benefits can be achieved when the cardiologist or surgeon has rapport with the patient, personalizes the health education messages, and most importantly follows up (Shah et al. 2008). Further, clinicians who adopt 'healthy living' practices themselves not only are more inclined to advise their patients about lifestyle behavior change, but serve as powerful role models whose advice is viewed by patients as being more credible (Frank et al. 2000; Paice et al. 2002; Watts, 1990).

When viewed as a clinical competency, the elements of health behavior change parallel those of invasive biomedical intervention, and can be applied as systematically and stringently. Thus, comparable to assessing, evaluating and following up with a patient following biomedical intervention, the cardiologist or surgeon can ask questions such as the following to establish whether a health education intervention is making a difference:

- What outcomes can I quantify and chart to monitor the patient's short- and long-term improvements?
- Given changes in the targeted health behaviors can be outcomes themselves, how can I quantify changes over time with respect to smoking, diet, weight, sedentary activity, physical activity and exercise?
- How have the outcomes of my medical/surgical management been augmented by the patient's health behavior changes?
- How might my medical and/or future surgical management need to be modified given improvements in a patient's health behaviors and health outcomes?

3. Elements of health education as a clinical competency

Clinical competencies are described and evaluated under the categories of knowledge and skills.

3.1 Health promotion practice as a clinical competence: Knowledge

With respect to health behavior change, cardiologists and surgeons as educators need to be knowledgeable about and capable of assessing and evaluating health and health behaviors (in addition to the usual risk factor assessment/evaluations of ischemic heart disease and its manifestations) (Table 1). Also, effective health educators have specific attributes such as rapport with the learner and have the learner's trust. Effective educators also assess their learners so they can target and tailor the information to be learned to their unique needs (Rollnick et al. 1999).

Knowledge of Health Definition of the World Health Organization: 'A complete state of physical, emotional and social wellbeing' (WHO, 1948) International Classification of Functioning, Disability and Health, 2002) 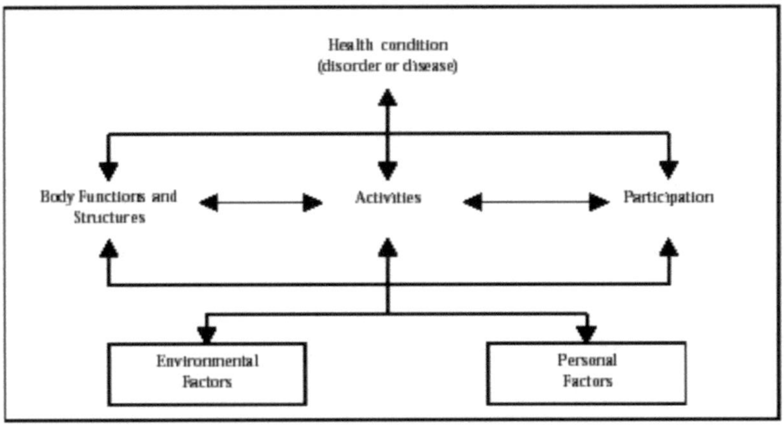 Tools: Standardized outcomes measures (questionnaires, e g, health-related quality of life and life satisfaction)
Knowledge of Health-related Behavior Assessment/Evaluation Tools: Health behaviors including smoking questionnaires such as WISDOM and The Why Test, nutrition logs and physical activity logs in accordance with nutrition and activity pyramids that describe optimal serving sizes and parameters of acceptable activity for health, sleep questionnaires and stress questionnaires
Knowledge of Risk Factor Assessment/Evaluation for the Lifestyle-related Conditions **Tools** (according to usual clinical practice): Ischemic heart disease risk factor assessments such as Grundy, et al. (2002) and Harvard School of Public Health (2011)
Knowledge of the Assessment/Evaluation of the Manifestations of Lifestyle-related Conditions Tools (according to usual clinical practice): Established medical and surgical history taking, assessment and evaluation methods often related to cardiovascular dysfunction and impairments

Table 1. Health promotion practice as a clinical competency: knowledge.

3.2 Health promotion practice as a clinical competence: Health behavior change skills

Health education interventions and skills that promote 'healthy living' can be implemented readily within the context of cardiology practice appear in Table 2. The focus of such approaches to health education of patients within a biomedical framework have evolved from the leading behavior change theories. Emphasis is given to efficient strategies that require minimal time and resources, yet have the potential for substantial benefit to the patient. Behavioral change theories include Reasoned Action and Planned Behavior

(Achterberg et al. 2010; Elder et al. 1999), Social Cognitive Theory (Bandura, 1977; Bandura, 1995), and the Transtheoretical Model (Prochaska and DiClemente, 1982). Attention is paid to the patient's stage of readiness to change behavior so the education can be tailored to this stage, motivational interviewing which views motivation as dynamic and capable of being augmented, and the tenets of giving meaningful feedback and reinforcement. Although the table identifies health education strategies that frequently appear in the literature because of their clinical feasibility, we do not suggest that one strategy is superior to another. Rather, like medical and surgical interventions, the patient and context are considered.

Physician as Role Model • Exploit in a professional manner: • Position of authority • Credibility in delivery health message	Frank et al. 2000 Paice et al. 2002 Watts, 1990
Physician-Patient Relationship • Respect • Rapport • Trust • Active listening • Personal	Clark et al. 1995 Shah et al. 2008 Stott & Pill, 1990
Assessment/Evaluation of Patient's Health Behavior Related Knowledge and Behaviors (quantitatively, for ease of comparison with the patient over time) • Baseline (objective tests and outcome measures; patient logs, diaries and graphs) • Serial measurements (of variables above) • Follow-up (of variables above)	Tulloch et al. 2006
Motivational Interviewing (culturally modified as indicated) • Identify resistance to change • Understand the patient's motivation (e.g., decision balance analysis) • Listen to the patient • Empower the patient	Poirier et al. 2004 Lee et al. 2011 Rosengren, 2009 Stewart & Fox, 2011
Stages of Readiness to Change • Pre-contemplative: not thinking about changing • Contemplative: thinking about changing • Preparation: preparing to change • Action: implementing behavioral change • Maintenance: maintaining behavioral change • (Relapse: reverted to negative behavior change)	Prochaska & DiClemente, 1982 Steptoe et al. 2001
The 5 A's of Behavioral Change • **Assess**: Evaluate behavior change status (and progress) • **Advise**: Personally relevant behavioral recommendations • **Agree**: Set specific collaborative, feasible goals • **Assist**: Anticipate barriers, problem-solve solutions, and complete action plan • **Arrange:** Schedule follow-up, contacts and resources	World Health Organization, 2004

<table>
<tr><td>Decision Balance Analysis

<table><tr><td></td><td>Of Changing Behavior</td><td>Of Not Changing Behavior</td></tr><tr><td>Pros</td><td></td><td></td></tr><tr><td>Cons</td><td></td><td></td></tr></table>
Goal: Identify Barriers and Facilitators
• Reduce the barriers to health behavior change
• Increase the facilitators</td><td>Seymour et al. 2011</td></tr>
<tr><td>Feedback
Objective, timely, and regular, e.g., body weight, step counts with pedometers, tests, charts, lab and test reports
Positive Reinforcement
• Clear
• Direct
• Specific</td><td>Burke et al. 2011
Tudor-Locke & Bassett, 2004
<5000 steps/day: sedentary lifestyle
7500 to 9999 steps/day: somewhat active lifestyle
10000 steps/day: active lifestyle
>12500 steps/day: highly active lifestyle</td></tr>
<tr><td>Social Contagion Health Effect
Framingham Study database:
If your friends are overweight you are likely to be overweight, therefore recommend enjoying activities of 'healthy living' with likeminded friends</td><td>Christakis & Fowler, 2007</td></tr>
<tr><td>Assessing the Learner
• Socioeconomic status
• Literacy and numeracy
• Culture, ethnicity, language, attitudes and beliefs about lifestyle-related health behaviors such as smoking, healthy eating, weight, sedentary behavior, physical activity, sleep and stress</td><td>Lantz et al. 1998
Rollnick et al. 1999</td></tr>
<tr><td>Learner-oriented Teaching and Education
Preferred learning styles often one or more:
• Auditory
• Visual
• Experiential
• Demonstrational
• Interactive, e.g., web-based instructional material and sources</td><td>Rollnick et al. 1999</td></tr>
</table>

Table 2. Health promotion practice as a clinical competency: Health behavior change skills.

3.3 Decision-making tree to augment patient health and outcomes with health education

The role and skills required by cardiologists and surgeons to be health educators are somewhat distinct to those of professionally trained health educators given health promotion is practiced within the context of biomedical care. Clinicians need to be able to readily assess a patient's lifestyle practices, specifically, what needs to change, and then decide how to effect such change most expediently. The extent of health education required and engagement of the cardiologist or surgeon varies from patient to patient.

A schematic of a decision-making tree to augment patient health and outcomes with health education is shown in Figure 1. Health education is effected at two levels: initiated and supported/reinforced or both. After the health education assessment, if education needs to be initiated, the practitioner establishes the degree to which he or she takes responsibility for this and for referring to other professionals who can implement a targeted program. Even if the patient is referred or has been receiving health education, the practitioner supports or reinforces this initiative. He or she continues to monitor the educational strategies that have been implemented, and provides essential follow-up. Such follow-up may be as simple as asking the patient about changes that have been made to requisitioning laboratory testing/imaging to assess its outcomes, comparable to following up drug and surgical interventions.

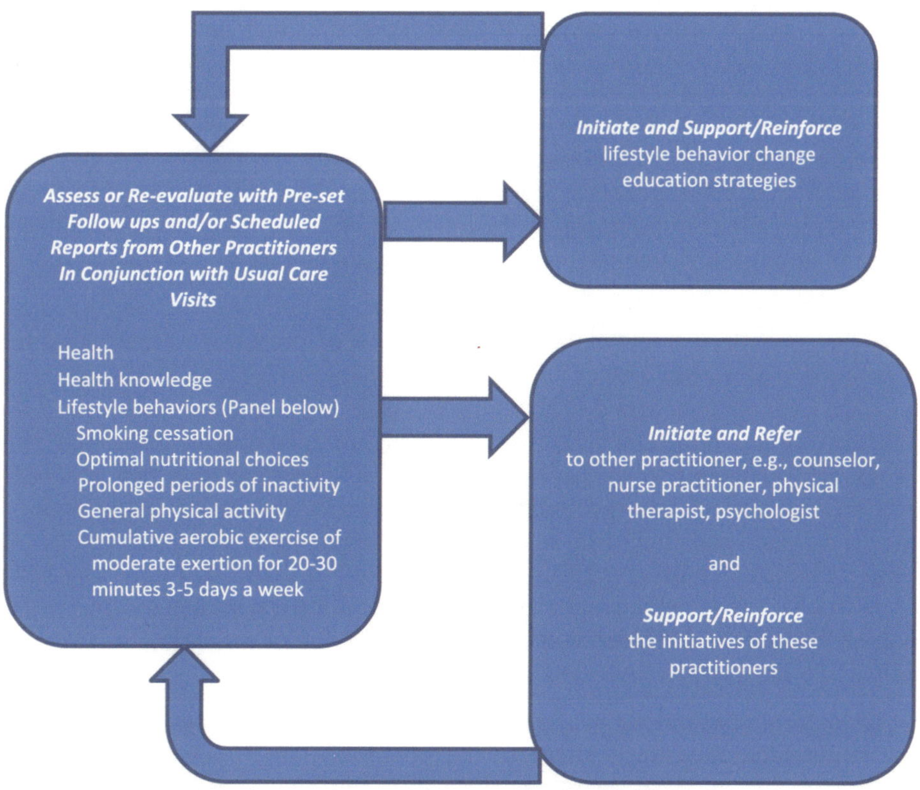

Fig. 1. Decision making tree for cardiologists and surgeons to augment their patient outcomes by initiating and supporting lifestyle-related health behavior changes.

3.4 The patient, the strategy, and their interface

Countries where ischemic heart disease is most prevalent tend to be high income. These countries are increasingly multicultural. This dimension influences a patient's perception about his or her heart disease, beliefs about its origins and its management. Interventions that a patient believes in will inevitably have greater benefit due to a placebo effect. Western biomedical interventions may be subject to being both over and undervalued depending on culture and ethnicity as well as individual personal factors. People from collectivisitic cultures for example may not perceive they have as much control over the management of their signs and symptoms as someone from an individualistic culture (Hofstede, 2001). Patients who believe that the 'will of God' is paramount may experience less self efficacy in determining the outcome of his or her ischemic heart disease, and potentially less receptive to health education. Cultures vary widely with respect to attitudes about smoking and its social acceptability, food, and physical activity. In addition, cultures vary on the acceptability of sleep deprivation and high stress. These differences are not insurmountable. Rather, knowledge of these individual patient distinctions will better able the health educator including the clinician to tailor and target the educational content consistent with the patient's needs.

Other determinants of learning that inform the type of teaching that is indicated include language, literacy, age, and potentially gender (Glanz et al. 2002). Learners also vary with respect to such preferences as reading to learn, experiencing, having someone provide feedback, and interactive learning, or some combination. Thus, a brochure or web-based material even if translated to a patient's native language, may be ineffective due to these other factors. Although it may appear time consuming to evaluate the learner to such a degree, benefits of a teaching moment may be considerably compromised without taking a few moments to evaluate the learner specifically and the learner's preferred learning style. Across all learning preferences however the follow up that is conducted systematically and predictably is important if learning and behavior change is to be effective and sustained over time.

Because of the specialized care that cardiologists and cardiac surgeons provide, the teaching learning process realistically cannot be initiated, implemented and followed up by a single person. Other team members need to partner seamlessly with medical and surgical teams to ensure that health and health behaviors are assessed, and health behavior change strategies that are targeted and tailored to the individual, are followed up. For some patients, little time will be required of the cardiologist or surgeon to ensure the appropriate health education is in place and follow up is conducted over the time the patient is being seen, because of the input of other appropriately qualified support. Patients can readily be referred to well qualified network of professionals including counselors, nutritionists, nurse practitioners, and physical therapists who report back to the referring practitioner to ensure continuity and follow up are sustained.

Some patients from some ethnic groups may prefer practitioners from their cultural group who speak the same language. This may be preferable for not only ensuring accurate information for the medical or surgical history and examination but also for the effectiveness of health education. Without common language, the effectiveness of health education can be compromised significantly.

4. Other factors that influence the provision of best practices

Time, resources and reimbursement are often cited as reasons perceived by physicians and surgeons for not being able to implement new innovations and practice patterns outside the conventional biomedical model. The interview and dialogue conducted systematically between the physician or surgeon and patient can set the stage for effective health education leading to 'healthy living'.

Motivational interviewing is a patient-centered communication tool that has received considerable attention at the clinical level in terms of serving as a basis for health behavior change. The overarching philosophy of motivational interviewing is the partnership between the patient and clinician. Patient behavior change is viewed as a collaboration or shared endeavor between patient and clinician. The patient's internal motivations for change are identified at the outset (Martins & McNeil, 2009; Pollak et al. 2011; Rollnick et al. 2008). Patients are often resistant or ambivalent to change. For example, a patient with ischemic heart disease who smokes may be fearful about his condition yet feels he cannot or will not give up smoking, despite his awareness that smoking is endangering his health. For this patient, a health education message delivered using an 'expert-recipient' style may strengthen his resistance to quit smoking. Clinicians using motivational interviewing are empathetic; they anticipate and recognize their patients' ambivalence about and resistance to quit smoking. Where inconsistencies exist between a patient's values and behavior (e.g., my health is important to me, but I want to continue to smoke), the clinician acknowledges the inconsistency and enables the patient to articulate, explore and resolve such inconsistency. This can be achieved by evoking the patient's internal motivations pertaining to his personal goals and values, and link these to changing health behavior (Britt et al. 2004, Rollnick et al. 2008; Pollak et al. 2011). For example, the clinician may question the patient about how motivated he is to quit smoking, followed by how confident he feels about succeeding. If the clinician determines that her patient is highly motivated but lacks confidence, she may ask him what might explain his high motivation to quit, yet lack of confidence to do so. She can follow up by asking him how she can help to increase his confidence. The autonomy of the patient is acknowledged and respected throughout the interaction, i.e., the patient is free to make his own choices, including whether or not to change his behavior and, if he chooses to do so, how he can (Rollnick et al. 2008; Pollak et al. 2011). Finally, the skills of motivational interviewing can substantially increase the confidence of medical students to effect patient's health behavior change and provide counseling to patients (Poirier et al. 2004).

Although knowledge per se is not a strong predicted of health behavior change, credible reading materials have a role in effectively educating some patients. Simple inexpensive props such as the nutrition and physical activity pyramids (United States Department of Health and Human Services, 2011) can be mounted on the wall in the office and discussed with the patient. Colorful oversized copies for hanging on the wall or refrigerator can be sent home. Personal attention and personalizing of the health messages can be highly effective communication attributes of clinicians.

Reimbursement and fee for service is a concern in some countries. Although best practice is hailed as a priority in most countries, health promotion practice needs to be a central component given it can prevent cardiac events, and augment medical and surgical outcomes. If the power of 'healthy living' and its promotion are neglected, best practice is forfeited. The health professional community needs to ensure that evidence-based best practices are available to all patients; these extend well beyond drugs and surgery.

5. Conclusion

Within the context of busy, resource and time constrained cardiology practices, this chapter presents evidence-informed strategies for effective patient health education. Outcomes of the biomedical advances in cardiology and cardiac surgery, the focus of this book, fall short of their potential unless patients are able to effect long-term lifestyle behavior changes. Given the unequivocal link between lifestyle behaviors and ischemic heart disease, 'healthy living' not only augments a patient's overall health but, in turn, reduces the need for drugs and surgery. When these interventions are indicated, health behavior change may augment their outcomes. Ischemic heart disease is less a pathology and more a physiological response to lifestyle practices. In this century, it behooves health professionals including cardiologists and surgeons to support each other in addressing the underlying causes of ischemic heart disease in addition to addressing the resulting impairments. Clinicians can work with other team members to better solidify their efforts and improve their individual outcomes. Finally, because the lifestyle-related risk factors of ischemic heart disease are common to other leading chronic conditions such as hypertension, stroke, renal dysfunction, type 2 diabetes mellitus, obesity and cancer, cardiologists and surgeons who systematically and aggressively integrate health promotion into their practices, can also reduce the risk factors and potential manifestations of these other prevalent conditions.

6. References

Achterberg, T.V., Huisma-De Waal, G.G.J., Ketelaar, N.A.B., Oostendorp, R.A., Jacobs, J.E., Wolldersheim, H.C.H. (2010). How to promote healthy behaviours in patients? An overview of evidence for behaviour change techniques. Health Promotion International doi: 10.1093/heapro/daq050.

Alegrante, J.P., Perterson, J.C., Boutin-Foster, C., Ogedegbe, G.,Charleson, M.E. (2008). Multiple health-risk behavior in a chronic disease population: what behaviors do people choose to change? Preventive Medicine 46:247-251.

American College of Sports Medicine. (2009). ACSM's Resource Manual for Guidelines for Exercise Testing and Prescription, ed 6. Philadelphia: Lippincott Williams & Wilkins.

American College of Sports Medicine. (2010). ACSM's guidelines for exercise testing and prescription, ed 8. Philadelphia: Lippincott Williams & Wilkins.

American Heart Association. (2003). Exercise and physical activity in the prevention and treatment of atherosclerotic cardiovascular disease. Circulation 107:3109-3116.

Appel, L.J., Moore, T.J., Obarzanek, E., Vollmer, W.M., Svetkey, L.P., Sacks, F.M., Bray, G.A., Vogt, T.M., Cutler, J.A., Windhauser, M.M., Lin, P.H., & Karanja, N. (1997). A clinical trial of the effects of dietary patterns on blood pressure. DASH Collaborative Research Group. New England Journal of Medicine 336:1117-1124.

Bandura, A. (1977). Towards a unifying theory of behavioral change. Psychological Review 84:191-215.

Bandura, A. (1995). Moving into forward gear in health promotion and disease prevention. Keynote address. Society of Behavioral Medicine, San Diego, CA.

Beaglehole, R; Yach, D. (2003). Globalisation and the prevention and control of non-communicable disease: the neglected chronic diseases of adults. The Lancet 362:7903-7908.

Berenson, G.S., Srinivasan, S.R., Bao, W., Newman 3rd, W.P., Tracy, R.E., & Wattigney, W.A. (1998). Association between multiple cardiovascular risk factors and atherosclerosis in children and young adults. The Bogalusa Heart Study. New England Journal of Medicine 338:1650-1656.

Biddle, S.J.H., Pearson, N., Ross, G.M., & Braithwaite, R. (2010). Tracking of sedentary behaviors of young people: a systematic review. Preventive Medicine 51:345-351.

Blair, S.N. (2009). Physical inactivity: the biggest public health problem of the 21st century. British Journal of Sports Medicine 43:1-2.

Blanchard, C.M., Courneya, K.S., & Stein, K. (2008). Cancer survivors' adherence to lifestyle behavior recommendations and associations with health-related quality of life: Results from the American Cancer Society's SCS-II. Journal Clinical Oncology 26: 2198-2204.

Bodner, M.E., & Dean, E. (2009). Brief advice as a smoking cessation strategy: A systematic review and implications for physical therapists. Physiotherapy Theory and Practice 25:369-407.

Bodner, M.E., Miller, W.C., Rhodes, R.E., & Dean, E. (2011). Smoking cessation and counseling: Practices of Canadian physical therapists. Physical Therapy 91:1051-1062.

Britt, E., Hudson, S.M., & Blampied, N.M. (2004). Motivational interviewing in health settings: a review. Patient Education and Counseling 53:147-155.

Bruunsgaard, H. (2005). Physical activity and modulation of systemic low-level inflammation. Journal of Leukocyte Biology 78:819-835.

Burke, L.E., Wang, J., Sevick, M.A. (2011). Self-monitoring in weight loss: a systematic review of the literature. Journal of the American Dietetic Association 111:92-102.

Centers for Disease Control and Prevention. (2002). Cigarette Smoking Among Adults—United States, 2000. Morbidity and Mortality Weekly Report 51:642–5.

Christakis, N.A., & Fowler, J.H. (2007). The spread of obesity in a large social network over 32 years. New England Journal of Medicine 357:370-379.

Clark, N. M., Nothwehr, F., Gong, M., Evans, D., Maiman, L. A., Hurwitz, M. E., Roloff, D., & Mellins, R. B. (1995). Physician-patient partnership in managing chronic illness. Academic Medicine, 70:957-959.

Conway, T.L., & Cronan, T.A. (1990). Smoking, exercise, and physical fitness. Preventive Medicine 21:723-734.

Coren, S. (2009). Sleep health and its assessment and management in physical therapy practice: The evidence. Physiotherapy Theory and Practice 25:442-452.

Dean, E. (2009). Physical therapy in the 21st century (Part II): Evidence-based practice within the context of evidence-informed practice. Physiotherapy Theory and Practice 25:354-368.

Dean, E. (2009). Physical therapy in the 21st century (Part I): Toward practice informed by epidemiology and the crisis of lifestyle conditions. Physiotherapy Theory and Practice 25:330-353.

Dean, E., Lom,i C., Bruno, S., Awad, H., & O'Donoghue, G. (2011). Addressing the common pathway underlying hypertension and diabetes in people who are obese: The ultimate knowledge translation gap. International Journal of Hypertension doi:10.4061/2011/835805.

DeLongis, A., Folkman, S., Lazarus, R.S. (1988). The impact of daily stress on health and mood: Psychological and social resources as mediators. Journal of Personality and Social Psychology 54:486-495.

Dube, S.R., McClave, A., James, C., Caraballo, R., Kaufmann, R., & Pechacek, T. (2010). Vital signs: current cigarette smoking among adults aged ≥18 years – United States, 2009. MMWR 59(35): 1135-1140, 2010.

Elder, J.P., Ayala, G.X., Harris, S. (1999). Theories and intervention approaches to health-behavior change in primary care. American Journal of Preventive Medicine 17:275-284.

Ford, E.S., Bergmann, M.M., Kroger, J., Schienbkiewitz, A., Weikert, C., & Boeing, H. (2009). Healthy living is the best revenge. Archives of Internal Medicine 169:1355-1362.

Frank, E., Breyan, J., & Elon, L. (2000). Physician disclosure of healthy personal behaviors improves credibility and ability to motivate. Archives of Family Medicine 9:287-290.

Gidding, S.S. (1999). Preventive pediatric cardiology: tobacco, cholesterol, obesity, and physical activity. Pediatric Clinics of North America 46:253-262.

Glanz, K., Rimer, B.K., Lewis F.M. (2002). Health behavior and health education (3rd ed). San Francisco:CA: Jossey-Bass.

Glasgow, R.E., Klesges, L.M., Dzewaltowski, D.A;, Bull, S.S., Estabrooks, P. (2004). The future of health behavior change research: What is needed to improve translation of research into health promotion practice? Annals of Behavioral Medicine 27:3-12.

Harvard School of Public Health. Your disease risk. www.yourdiseaserisk.harvard.edu; retrieved August 2011.

Grundy, S.M., Pasternak, R., Greenland, P., Smith, S., Luster, V. (1999). Assessment of cardiovascular risk by use of multiple-risk-factor assessment equations: A statement for healthcare professionals from the American Heart Association and the American College of Cardiology. Circulation 100: 1481-1492

Healy, G.N., Dunstan, D.W., Salmon, J., Cerin, E., Shaw, J.F., Zimmet, P.Z., & Own, N. (2008). Breaks in sedentary time. Beneficial associations with metabolic risk. Diabetes Care 31:661-666.

Hofstede, G. (2001). Culture's consequences: comparing values, behaviors, institutions, and organizations across nations (2nd ed.). Thousand Oaks, CA: SAGE Publications.

Jakes, R.W., Day, N.E., Khaw, K.T., Luben, R., Oakes, S., Welch, A., Bingham, S., Wareham, N.J. (2003). Television viewing and low participation in vigorous recreation are independently associated with obesity and markers of cardiovascular disease risk: EPIC-Norfolk population-based study. European Journal of Clinical Nutrition 57:1089-1096.

Kreuter, M.W., Chheda, S.G., & Bull, F.C. (2000). How does physician advice influence patient behavior? Evidence for a priming effect. Archives of Family Medicine 9:426-433.

Lantz, P.M., House, J.S., Lepkowski J.M., Williams, D.R., Mero, R.P., & Chen, L. (1998). Socioeconomic factors, health behaviors, and mortality. Journal of the American Medical Association 279:1703-1708.

Lee, C.S., López, S.R., Hernández, L., Colby, S.M., Caetano, R., Borrelli, B., Rohsenow, D. (2011). A cultural adaptation of motivational interviewing to address heavy drinking among Hispanics. Cultural Diversity and Ethnic Minority Psychology 17:317-324.

Martins, R.K., & McNeil, D.W. (2009). Review of motivational interviewing in promoting health behaviors. Clinical Psychology Review 29: 283-293.

Mokdad, A. H., Ford, E.S., Bowman, B.A., Dietz, W.H., Vinicor, F., Bales, V.S., & Marks, J.S. Prevalence of obesity, diabetes, and obesity-related health risk factors, 2001. (2004). Journal of the American Medical Association 289:76-79.

Mortality Country Fact Sheets 2006. www.who.int/whosis/mort/profiles/en/; retrieved August 2011.

Neuhouser, M.L., Miller, D.L., Kristal, A.R., Barnett, M.J., & Cheskin, L.J. (2002). Diet and exercise habits of patients with diabetes, dyslipidemia, cardiovascular disease or hypertension. Journal of the American College of Nutrition 21:394-401.

Olshansky, S.J., Passaro, D.J., Hershow, R.C., Layden, J., Carnes, B.A., Brody, J., Hayflick, L., Butler, R.N., Allison, D.B., and Ludwig, D.S. (2005). A potential decline in life expectancy in the United States in the 21st century. New England Journal of Medicine 352:1138-1145.

Ornish, D. (1998). Avoiding revascularisation with lifestyle changes: The Multicenter Lifestyle Demonstration Project. American Journal of Cardiology 82:72-76

Ornish, D., Scherwitz, L.W., Billings, J.H. et al. (1998). Intensive lifestyle change for reversal of coronary heart disease. Journal of the American Medical Association 280:2001-2007.

Paice, E., Heard, S., & Moss, F. (2002). How important are role models in making good doctors? British Medical Journal 707 doi: 10.1136/bmj.325.7366.707.

Pierson, R. New drug class may aid heart disease fight. Vancouver Sun, Vancouver, BC, Canada; Saturday, August 27, 2011.

Poirier, M.K., Clark, M.M., Cerhan, J.H., Pruthi, S., Geda, Y.E., & Dale, L.C. (2004). Teaching motivational interviewing to first-year medical students to improve counseling skills in health behavior change. Mayo Clinic Proceedings 79:327-331.

Pollak, K.I., Childers, J.W., & Arnold, R.M. (2011). Applying motivational interviewing techniques to palliative care communication. Journal of Palliative Medicine 14: 587-592.

Prochaska, J.O., & DiClemente, C.C. (1982). Transtheoretical therapy: Towards a more integrative model of change. Psychother: Theory, Research and Practice 19:276-288.

Report of the Institute of Medicine of the National Academy of Sciences. IOM report declares high blood pressure a neglected disease, calls for strategies to change Americans' lifestyles and diets to curb hypertension. February 22th, 2010.

Rollnick, S., Mason, P., & Butler, C. (1999). Health behavior change. A guide for practitioners. New York: Churchill Livingstone.

Rollnick, S., Miller, W.R., & Butler, C.C. (2008). Motivational interviewing in health care: helping patients change behavior. New York: The Guildford Press.

Rosengren, D.B. (2009). Building motivational interviewing skills: a practitioner workbook. New York: The Guildford Press, 2009.

Sacks, F.M., Obarzanek ,E., Windhauser, M.M., Svetkey, L.P., Vollmer, W.M., McCullough, M., Karanja, N., Lin, P.H., Steele, P., Proschan, M.A., Evans, M.A., Appel, L.J., Bray, G.A., Vogt, T.M., Moore, T.J. and DASH Investigators (1995). Rationale and design for the Dietary Approaches to Stop Hypertension trial (DASH). A multicentered controlled-feeding study of dietary patterns to lower blood pressure. Annals of Epidemiology 5:108-118.

Seymour, R.B., Hughes, S.L., Ory, M.G., Elliot, D.L., Kirby, K.C., Migneault, J., Patrick, H., Roll, J.M., Williams, G. (2010). A lexicon for measuring maintenance of behavior change. American Journal of Health Behavior 34:660-668.

Shah, A., Cabeza, Y., Ostfeld, R.J. (2008). Prevention information: Patient perceptions regarding general and race-based instruction. International Journal of Cardiology 130:72- 74.

Shaper, A.G. (1996). Obesity and cardiovascular disease. Ciba Foundation Symposium 201:90-103.

Sofi, F., Cesari, F., Abbate, R., Gensini, G.F., Casini, A. (2008). Adherence to Mediterranean diet and health status: meta-analysis. BMJ 337:a1344.

Soler, E.P., & Ruiz, V.C. (2010). Epidemiology and risk factors of cerebral ischemia and ischemic heart diseases: similarities and differences. Current Cardiology Reviews 6: 138-149.

Stannard, S.R., & Johnson, N.A. (2004). Insulin resistance and elevated triglyceride in muscle: more important for survival than 'thrifty' genes? Journal of Physiology 554:595-607.

Steptoe, A., Kerry, S., Rink, E., & Hilton, S. (2001). The impact of behavioural counseling on stage of change in fat intake, physical activity, and cigarette smoking in adults at increased risk of coronary heart disease. American Journal of Public Health 91:265–269.

Stewart, E.E., Fox, C.H. (2011). Encouraging patients to change unhealthy behaviors with motivational interviewing. Family Practice Management 18:21-25.

Stott, N.C.H., & Pill, R.M. (1990). 'Advise yes, dictate no'. Patients' views on health promotion in the consultation. Family Practice 7:125-131.

Task Force Guidelines for the Management of Arterial Hypertension. (2007). European Heart Journal 28:1462-1536.

Thorpe, A.A., Healy, G.N., Owen, N., Salmon, J., Ball, K., Shaw, J.F., Zimmet, P.Z., & Dunstand, D.W. (2010). Deleterious associations of sitting time and television viewing time with cardiometabolic risk biomarkers. Diabetes Care 33:327-334.

Thompson, P.D., Buchner, D., Piña, I.L. et al. (2003). Exercise and Physical Activity in the Prevention and Treatment of Atherosclerotic Cardiovascular Disease A Statement from the Council on Clinical Cardiology (Subcommittee on Exercise, Rehabilitation, and Prevention) and the Council on Nutrition, Physical Activity, and Metabolism (Subcommittee on Physical Activity). Circulation 107:3109-3116.

Tudor-Locke, C., & Bassett D.R. Jr. (2004). How many steps/day are enough? Preliminary pedometer indices for public health. Sports Medicine 34:1-8.

Tulloch, H., Fortier, M., & Hogg, W. (2006). Physical activity counseling in primary care: Who has and who should be counseling? Patient Education and Counseling 64:6-20.

United States Department of Health and Human Services, Consumer Information Center. The food guide pyramid. www.usda.gov; retrieved August 2011.

Watts, M.S. Physicians as role models in society. (1990). Western Journal of Medicine 152:292.

World Health Organization (2002). Physical inactivity leading cause of disease and disability. www.who.int/mediacentre/news/releases/release23/en/index.html; retrieved August 2011.

World Health Organization (WHO)/International Society of Hypertension (ISH) statement on management of hypertension. (2003). Journal of Hypertension 21:1983-1992.

World Health Organization. Definition of Health (1948). www.who.int/about/definition; retrieved December 2010.

World Health Organization. International Classification of Functioning, Disability and Health. (2002). www.sustainable-design.ie/arch/ICIDH-2PFDec-2000.pdf; retrieved August 2011.

World Health Organization. Integrating prevention into health care. Fact sheet 172. www.who.int/mediacentre/factsheets/fs172/en/; retrieved August 2011.

World Health Organization. (2004). The 5 A's Cycle. http: //www.who.int/diabetesactiononline/about/WHO%205A%20ppt.pdf; retrieved August 2011.

World Health Organization. Priority noncommunicable diseases and conditions. Prioritynoncommunicablediseasesanddisorders.pdf; www.wpro.who.int/NR/rdonlyres/E72A001F-E6E1-4AB7-B33C-1C77F4FEF8FC/0/13_Chapter8; retrieved August 2011.

Joint WHO/FAO Expert Consultation on Diet, Nutrition and the Prevention of Chronic Diseases Geneva, 28 January--1 February 2002. www.who.int/hpr/NPH/docs/who_fao_expert_report.pdf; retrieved August 2011.

Yusuf, S., Hawken, S., Ôunpuu, S, Bautista, L, Grazia Franzosi, M., Commerford, P., Lang, C.C., Rumboldt, Z., Onen, C.L., Lisheng. L., Tanomsup, S., Wangai, P., Razak, F., Sharma, A.M., Anand, S.S. and on behalf of the INTERHEART Study Investigators.

(2005). Obesity and the risk of myocardial infarction in 27 000 participants from 52 countries: a case-control study The Lancet 366:1640-1649.

Yusuf, S., Hawken, S., Ounpuu, S., Dans, T., Avezum, A., Lanas, F., McQuee,n M., Budaj, A., Pais, P., Varigos, J., Lisheng, L. (2004). Effect of potentially modifiable risk factors associated with myocardial infarction in 52 countries (the INTERHEART study): case-control study. Lancet 11-17;364(9438):937-952.

18

Inpatient Costs Associated with Ischemic Heart Disease Among Adults Aged 18-64 Years in the United States

Guijing Wang, Zefeng Zhang, Carma Ayala, Diane Dunet and Jing Fang
Division for Heart Disease and Stroke Prevention
Centers for Disease Control and Prevention, Atlanta, Georgia
USA

1. Introduction

Ischemic heart disease (IHD) is both the most common and the most costly form of cardiovascular disease (CVD) in the United States (US).[1-2] In 2010, the estimated prevalence of IHD among American adults aged ≥20 years was 7.9% (9.1% in men and 7.0% in women),[1] and the aging of the US population should drive prevalence even higher in the future. Fortunately, the IHD death rate has declined in recent decades, but it remains the leading cause of hospital admissions and the single largest killer of American men and women, causing 1 of every 6 deaths.[1-3] Not surprisingly, spending to treat IHD has increased more than 40% over the past 25 years.[4] For 2010, the total economic burden of IHD was estimated to be $177 billion, $96 billion in direct medical costs and $81 billion in indirect costs. Well over half of the direct costs ($57 billion) were for inpatient care.[1] Thus, information on the costs of hospitalizations involving IHD may be helpful in developing strategies to contain the growth in the disease's economic burden.

To date, researchers have used a variety of approaches in investigating the health care costs of IHD.[4-15] For example, in the US, Hodgson and Cohen used a prevalence-based approach to demonstrate that IHD accounted for just over one half of health care expenditures for heart disease in 1995 ($38.7 billion of $75.9 billion.)[5] Russell et al., using a variety of data sources and a Markov model, estimated incidence-based first-year treatment costs of IHD in the US for that same year at $5.54 billion.[6] More recently, Menzin and coworkers estimated the average cost (in 2005 dollars) of initial hospitalization for acute coronary syndromes to be $22,921, and their estimate for re-hospitalization for IHD was $28,637.[7] In other industrialized countries, the economic burden of IHD has also been very high. For example, in the United Kingdom (UK), Liu and associates estimated the total 1-year cost (1999) of IHD to be £7.06 billion, the highest of any disease in the UK. The total direct health care costs of IHD were £1.73 billion, of which £917 million (53%) was for inpatient care.[8] Unfortunately, these earlier studies either did not use detailed diagnostic codes for IHD, did not address diagnostic status and issues of comorbidity, or focused exclusively on older population. Thus, their results have limited implications for deciding how to allocate resources and, similarly, for evaluating the cost-effectiveness of prevention programs at the community level.

To address these gaps, we used a large administrative dataset to explore the cost of hospitalization for patients with IHD; to make this a valuable exercise we classified the patients in several different ways by IHD diagnosis and also examined the apparent effects of sex, age, and a variety of comorbidities as well as 2 procedures. The estimated costs of hospitalization should provide some insights on why the inpatient costs of IHD have been so high and how the increases in costs can be contained.

2. Methods

The study population was selected from the 2005 MarketScan Commercial Claims and Encounters inpatient dataset, which contains over 1 million records for patients aged 64 or younger from self-insured employers, including state governments. The advantages of using data from MarketScan are the large samples, the detailed diagnostic codes for medical services, and the listings of hospitalization costs that are based on payment to providers.[16] The MarketScan dataset has been used by many other researchers investigating the health and economic burden of CVD.[7, 17-21]

Using codes from the International Classification of Diseases, 9th revision (ICD-9) (Table 1), we identified hospitalizations with a primary or secondary diagnosis of IHD among patients aged 18 to 64 years enrolled in non-capitated health insurance plans. We excluded patients younger than 18 because of the low prevalence of IHD in that age group. We excluded patients in capitated health insurance plans because their costs of hospitalization would not reflect the medical services provided to them. To limit the influence of extreme values for hospitalization costs we also excluded those hospitalizations with costs below the 1st or above the 99th percentile.

IHD Classification, Comorbidity, or Procedure	ICD-9 code
Ischemic heart disease, all	410.xx - 414.xx
Acute myocardial infarction	410.xx
Other coronary heart disease	411.xx - 414.xx
Heart failure	40201, 40211, 40291, 40401, 40403, 40411, 40413, 40491, 40493, 4280, 4281, 4289, 42820, 42821, 42822, 42823, 42830, 42831, 42832, 42833, 42840, 42841, 42842, 42843
Stroke	430.xx - 438.xx
Diabetes	250.xx
Symptoms involving respiratory system and other chest symptoms	786.xx
Cardiac dysrhythmias	427.xx
Hypertension	401.xx, 402.xx, 403.xx, 404.xx, 405.xx
Hyperlipidemia	272.xx
Percutaneous coronary intervention	00.66, 36.01–36.09 plus CPT-4 codes 92980–92982, 92984, 92995, 92996
Coronary artery bypass graft	36.10–36.19 plus CPT-4 codes 33510–33519, 33521–33523, 33533–33536

IHD: ischemic heart disease; ICD-9, International Classification of Diseases, Ninth Revision; CPT: Current Procedural Terminology.

Table 1. Diagnostic codes for ischemic heart disease and selected comorbidities and procedures

For all the hospitalizations in the study we further identified whether the IHD was an acute myocardial infarction (AMI) or not (non-AMI). The comorbidities used for our analyses (expressed as diagnoses in Tables 2 and 3) were heart failure, stroke, diabetes, cardiac dysrhythmias, hypertension, hyperlipidemia, and symptoms involving the respiratory system and other chest symptoms. In addition to these health conditions, we identified hospitalizations with a percutaneous coronary intervention (PCI) or a coronary artery bypass graft (CABG) because these procedures were (and remain) quite expensive.

We analyzed the costs for 3 groups of hospitalizations: 1) those with either a primary or secondary diagnosis of IHD; 2) those with a primary diagnosis of IHD, including those in which there was also a secondary diagnosis of IHD; and 3) hospitalizations with a secondary diagnosis of IHD in which the primary diagnosis was not IHD. For each study sample, we calculated the costs by various diagnosis classifications in four subgroups: men, women, patients aged 18-44, and patients aged 45-64.

Hospitalization costs were considered to be total payments to providers rather than hospital charges to reflect the true economic burden of hospitalizations. In this study we included all costs for physician services, all diagnostic tests, therapeutics, supplies, and room fees.

For cost comparisons, we used the Wilcoxon 2-sample test for the analysis, and a Bonferroni correction to protect against inflation of the type I error rate due to multiple testing was made for costs. Significance was assumed when the 2-tailed probability value was <0.001. For the regression analysis, we used the PROC GLM (General linear model) procedure for the cost regression model and PROC GENMOD (General model) for logit estimation. The regression model was run for the 3 groups of hospitalizations previously defined: 1) those with either a primary or secondary diagnosis of IHD; 2) those with a primary diagnosis of IHD, including those in which there was also a secondary diagnosis of IHD; and 3) hospitalizations with a secondary diagnosis of IHD in which the primary diagnosis was not IHD. We also ran a logit regression for IHD as the primary diagnosis versus IHD as the secondary diagnosis. The logit model was used to investigate the factors potentially influencing the probability of having a primary diagnosis of IHD (versus a secondary diagnosis of IHD). All the statistical analyses were performed using SAS, version 9.2.

3. Results

Among the 63,864 cases of IHD we identified, 33,316 (52%) hospitalizations had a primary diagnosis of IHD and their average costs were $24,079, 30,548 cases (48%) had a secondary diagnosis of IHD (their primary diagnosis was not IHD) and their average costs were $16,113 (Table 2 and Table 3). In both of these major diagnostic status groups, the costs were higher for AMI than for non-AMI, higher for men than for women, and increased with age.

Overall, 31% (n=10,261) of the hospitalizations in which the primary diagnosis was IHD were AMI, with the costs averaging $27,507 (Table 2). This cost was $4,954 higher (p <0.001) than the average for non-AMI cases ($22,553). The cost differences between the AMI and non-AMI cases were similar among each of the 4 subgroups defined by sex or age. For both AMI and non-AMI cases the costs were $4.1-4.5 thousand higher in men than in women. Costs increased with age, but the increase was small for AMI cases.

Among the hospitalizations with a primary diagnosis of IHD, 82.5% also had a secondary diagnosis of IHD; 58.4% had symptoms involving the respiratory system and other chest

Classification (n)	Overall	Men	Women	Age 18-44	Age 45-64
Total IHD (33,316)	24,079.1 ± 19,774.6	25,371.8 ± 20,148.9	20,876.4 ± 18,429.6	22,373.6 ± 19,347.5	24,225.1 ± 19,804.2
AMI (10,261)	27,507.3 ± 21,055.9	28,622.0 ± 21,408.1	24,541.4 ± 19,788.9	27,109.1 ± 20,749.2	27,553.1 ± 21,091.6
Non-AMI (23,055)	22,553.4 ± 18,979.2	23,882.7 ± 19,364.1	19,360.6 ± 17,617.1	19,175.3 ± 17,641.6	22,799.9 ± 19,050.0
Secondary diagnosis					
IHD					
Yes (27,487)	25,466.0 ± 20,295.2	26,633.1 ± 20,632.7	22,447.6 ± 19,068.3	24,545.8 ± 20,043.0	25,543.1 ± 20,314.7
No (5,829)	17,539.4 ± 15,519.7	18,983.8 ± 16,039.6	14,587.4 ± 13,944.9	13,156.1 ± 12,387.1	17,951.6 ± 15,720.6
Symptoms involving respiratory system and other chest symptoms					
Yes (19,451)	23,249.7 ± 20,312.6	24,857.3 ±20,899.5	19,752.9 ± 18,498.7	21,626.4 ± 19,677.7	23,417.3 ± 20,370.2
No (13,865)	25,242.8 ± 18,933.7	26,030.3 ±19,126.0	22,869.1 ± 18,138.6	24,058.9 ± 18,482.5	25,315.9 ± 18,959.5
Cardiac dysrhythmias					
Yes (4,660)	31,259.1 ± 23,890.2	32,268.7 ± 23,850.7	27,535.7 ± 23,677.8	29,263.1 ± 24,127.4	31,408.3 ± 23,868.5
No (28,656)	22 911.5 ±18,763.8	24 112.0 ±19,130.5	20 105.5 ± 17,561.3	21 404.4 ±18,376.9	23 043.3 ± 18,791.9
Heart failure					
Yes (2,750)	32,076.2 ± 25,616.2	34,404.3 ± 26,437.6	27,593.4 ± 23,322.6	34,363.9 ± 27,188.6	31,961.8 ± 25,535.1
No (30,566)	23,359.7 ± 18,998.1	24,626.1 ± 19,352.8	20,145.6 ± 17,664.6	21,744.3 ± 18,641.8	23,503.3 ± 19,023.1
Stroke					
Yes (1,334)	34,977.5 ±25,870.1	37, 228.6 ± 26,078.1	29,721.0 ±24,619.4	34,306.5 ± 25,772.7	34,999.8 ± 25,883.0
No (31,982)	23,624.6 ± 19,346.5	24,886.1 ± 19,717.6	20,491.0 ± 18,015.1	22,175.0 ± 19,166.3	23,752.0 ± 19,357.4
Diabetes					
Yes (5,283)	28,342.2 ± 22,410.2	29,612.4 ±22,916.8	25,577.1 ± 21,008.3	25,607.7 ± 20,614.9	28,549.3 ± 22,528.7
No (28,033)	23,275.7 ± 19,131.9	24,608.7 ± 19,512.4	19,889.0 ± 17,683.9	21,840.1 ± 19,082.5	23,401.3 ± 19,131.4

Classification (n)	Overall	Men	Women	Age 18-44	Age 45-64
Hypertension					
Yes (10,841)	26,049.1 ± 20,883.6	27,513.0 ± 21,382.4	22,294.1 ± 19,041.5	24,166.9 ± 20,508.9	26,195.2 ± 20,906.3
No (22,475)	23,128.9 ± 19,144.9	24,323.8 ± 19,431.6	20, 217.1 ± 18,101.6	21,614.9 ± 18,788.9	23,264.4 ± 19,171.1
Hyperlipidemia					
Yes (8,723)	26,111.3 ± 19,182.2	27,800.9 ± 20,381.2	22,904.6 ± 18,464.6	24,855.3 ± 19,093.2	26 807.6 ± 20,133.8
No (24,593)	22,553.6 ± 18,495.0	24,429.9 ± 19,979.4	20,310.1 ± 18,381.1	21,275.2 ± 19,362.8	23,327.3 ± 19,609.2
PCI					
Yes (17,444)	24,596.8 ± 16,125.4	24,890.3 ± 16,309.2	23,22.9 ± 15,534.1	27,269.3 ± 17,312.0	24,379.3 ± 16,005.8
No (15,872)	23,510.2 ± 23,117.6	25,960.5 ± 24,012.0	18,472.8 ± 20,251.7	17,481.6 ± 20,031.4	24,054.4 ± 23,300.1
CABG					
Yes (5,472)	46,757.2 ± 21,858.9	46,801.0 ± 21,848.1	46,559.1 ± 21,907.8	49,378.4 ± 22,220.7	46,636.4 ± 21,836.7
No (27,844)	19,622.4 ± 15,907.8	20,601.9 ± 16,282.1	17,365.9 ± 14,765.9	19,646.0 ± 16,772.9	19,620.2 ± 15,824.7

Data are means expressed in U.S. dollars +/- standard deviation. N = 33,316. IHD: ischemic heart disease; AMI: acute myocardial infarction; PCI: percutaneous coronary intervention; CABG: coronary artery bypass graft surgery.

Table 2. Mean costs of hospitalizations for patients with primary diagnosis of ischemic heart disease, by sex and age

Classification (n)	Overall	Men	Women	Age 18-44	Age 45-64
Total IHD (30,548)	16,112.9 ± 19,735.1	17,016.6 ± 20,554.8	14,753.3 ± 18,350.6	13,059.5 ± 17,449.8	16,433.5 ± 19,933.1
AMI (2,435)	24,280.9 ± 27,298.5	24,866.8 ± 27,509.5	23,438.7 ± 26,983.7	20,211.1 ± 25,183.3	24,881.2 ± 27,551.5
Non-AMI (28,113)	15,405.4 ± 18,772.6	16,350.1 ± 19,710.1	13,978.4 ± 17,162.8	12,195.2 ± 16,060.8	15,731.2 ± 18,996.2
Primary diagnosis					
Symptoms involving respiratory system and other chest symptoms					
Yes (6,588)	7,452.3 ± 6,52.5	7,423.3 ± 6,381.5	7,481.9 ± 5,911.0	7,640.1 ± 7,002.4	7,413.2 ± 5,959.9
No (23,960)	18,494.2 ± 21,444.5	19,138.6 ± 21,956.6	17,410.1 ± 20,509.9	16,548.6 ± 20,928.1	18 649.0 ± 21,478.0

Classification (n)	Overall	Men	Women	Age 18-44	Age 45-64
Cardiac dysrhythmias					
Yes (1,840)	18,124.4 ± 22,317.4	18,717.3 ± 23,145.7	16,544.0 ± 19,877.5	15,102.2 ± 21,319.11	18,342.8 ± 22,377.9
No (28,708)	15,984.0 ± 19,551.4	16,882.8 ± 20,331.7	14,676.4 ± 18,279.2	12,968.3 ± 17,255.9	16,307.2 ± 19,754.6
Heart failure					
Yes (2,084)	21,762.3 ± 25,688.6	22,823.3 ± 26,615.2	19,739.4 ± 23,709.1	20,527.8 ±23,046.3	21,829.1 ± 25,827.5
No (28,464)	15,699.3 ± 19,162.2	16,549.2 ± 19,914.7	14,441.9 ± 17,918.3	12,773.7 ± 17,140.3	16,018.0 ±19,343.3
Stroke					
Yes (1,383)	15,425.7 ± 17,204.0	14,920.7 ± 16,102.0	16,309.3 ± 18,963.1	14,997.5 ± 16,269.7	15,443.5 ± 17,247.1
No (29,165)	16,145.5 ± 19,846.8	17,122.2 ± 20,748.6	14,686.4 ± 18,321.7	13,022.0 ± 17,472.3	16,483.5 ± 20,058.1
Diabetes					
Yes (559)	17,980.1 ± 23,291.7	18,973.5 ± 23,901.0	16,569.4 ± 22,373.6	14,960.6 ± 25,210.6	18,356.7 ± 23,040.6
No (29,989)	16,078.1 ± 19,661.5	16,981.0 ± 20,487.8	14,718.2 ± 18,263.6	13,018.0 ± 17,245.6	16,398.3 ± 19,870.5
Hypertension					
Yes (652)	13,559.3 ± 17,880.3	15,454.2 ± 20,077.9	11,010.1 ± 14,041.7	8,683.1 ± 6,657.4	14,090.1 ± 18,626.1
No (29,896)	16,168.6 ± 19,770.3	17,049.1 ± 20,563.9	14,840.6 ± 1,8 430.5	13,158.1 ± 17, 605.0	16,484.5 ± 19,957.8
Hyperlipidemia					
Yes (13)	20,917.9 ±19,047.4	24,389.9 ± 20,399.4	9344.7 ± 6,559.5	32,121.5 ± 34,424.1	18,880.9 ± 16,946.8
No (30,535)	16,110.9 ± 19,735.5	17,012.6 ± 20,554.7	14, 754.6 ±18 352.5	13,046.3 ± 17,436.9	16,432.6 ±19,934.4
PCI					
Yes (909)	28,966.3 ± 23,297.8	29,823.0 ± 23,887.1	27,286.4 ± 22,038.1	28,777.8 ± 23,750.8	28,980.8 ± 23,276.8
No (29,638)	15,718.7 ± 19,482.5	16,582.2 ± 20,291.8	14,429.7 ± 18,132.3	12,699.5 ± 17,115.9	16,038.4 ± 19,689.7
CABG					
Yes (402)	60,281.3 ± 29 757.2	59,987.2 ± 29,250.9	60,972.4 ± 31,028.9	51,054.4 ± 41, 641.3	60,764.4 ±28,996.5
No (30,146)	15,523.9 ± 18,882.0	16,345.9 ± 19,660.0	14,294.0 ± 17,583.1	12,795.9 ±16,884.6	15,12.4 ± 19,058.4

Data are means expressed in U.S. dollars +/- standard deviation. N = 30,548. IHD:ischemic heart disease; AMI: acute myocardial infarction; PCI: percutaneous coronary intervention; CABG: coronary artery bypass graft

Table 3. Mean costs of hospitalizations for patients with ischemic heart disease as a secondary but not a primary diagnosis, by sex and age

symptoms; 32.5%, hypertension; 26.2%, hyperlipidemia; 15.9%, diabetes; 14.0%, cardiac dysrhythmias; 8.3%, heart failure; and 4.0%, stroke (Table 2). All the co-morbidities except symptoms involving the respiratory system/chest were associated with increased inpatient costs. Among these 6 secondary diagnoses (comorbidities) the cost was the highest for stroke ($34,978) and lowest for hypertension ($26,049). This pattern held for the male and female groups and for those aged 45-64, but in the 18-44 group the cost for heart failure was marginally higher than that for stroke.

Overall, a hospitalization with PCI had a cost approximately $1,100 greater than one without that procedure, but there were large differences in cost between the PCI and "no PCI" groups for women and the younger age group (18-44). The costs of hospitalizations with CABG averaged $46,757, more than twice the average for stays without CABG ($19,622). This pattern held true for all groups delimited by sex or age.

Among hospitalizations with a secondary but not a primary diagnosis of IHD (Table 3), the mean cost was about $8,900 higher for an AMI stay ($24,281) than for a non-AMI hospitalization ($15,405). Similar patterns were seen for the 4 groups defined by sex or age, and the costs were higher for men and those aged 45-64 than for women and the younger group, respectively. Among the 8 subgroups defined by AMI status and either sex or age, the highest costs were $24,881(45-64, AMI) and $24,867 (men, AMI), and the lowest was $12,195 (18-44, non-AMI).

Overall, having a primary diagnosis of cardiac dysrhythmias, heart failure, or diabetes increased costs (Table 3), while primary diagnoses of hypertension, respiratory/chest symptoms, and stroke were associated with lower costs. Stroke, however, was associated with higher costs in women and the younger population. The cost of hospitalization with PCI averaged $28,966, almost twice the cost of cases without PCI ($15,719). Hospitalizations with CABG cost $60,281, essentially 4 times the cost of hospitalizations without CABG. The cost differences between CABG and no CABG were similar across all 4 groups defined by sex or age.

The regression analysis indicated that the cost of hospitalization increased significantly with age ($p = 0.01$ for age 18-39, $p < 0.001$ for age 40-54) for IHD as a secondary diagnosis, but analyses of IHD as either the primary or secondary diagnosis or as the primary diagnosis did not find a significant age gradient ($p > 0.01$) (Table 4). Costs were always higher for men than for women ($p < 0.001$), especially for hospitalizations with a primary diagnosis of IHD with a cost difference of $4,822. After controlling for age, sex, urbanization, geographic region, and the Charlson Comorbidity Index, the cost of hospitalizations with the primary diagnosis of IHD was $7,319 higher than for those with a secondary diagnosis of IHD. For hospitalizations with a primary diagnosis of IHD, all the comorbidities increased the costs except for respiratory/chest symptoms, albeit the findings for diabetes and heart failure were not statistically significance at the 0.001 level.

Cardiac dysrhythmias and stroke were the most expensive comorbidities for hospitalizations with the primary diagnosis of IHD, and heart failure was the most expensive for hospitalizations when IHD was listed as a secondary diagnosis. Both PCI and CABG were associated with higher costs, especially CABG, which was the largest contributor to costs for both IHD as the primary and as a secondary diagnosis. The logit results revealed that after controlling for Charlson comorbidity index and region, in a comparison with patients aged 55-64 years, patients aged 18-39 were less likely and those aged 40-54 more likely to have a primary diagnosis of IHD rather than a secondary diagnosis of that disease. Men had a higher probability than women of having the diagnosis of IHD be primary (last column of table 4).

Characteristic	Primary or Secondary Diagnosis N=63,864	Primary Diagnosis N=33,316	Secondary Diagnosis N=30,548	Primary Diagnosis Versus IHD as the Secondary Diagnosis N=63,864
Age (years)				
18-39	-2,802.4 (0.0678)	-2,513.7 (0.0617)	-2,650.7 (0.0178)	-0.5393 (<0.0001)
40-54	-1,097.5 (0.0502)	-251.8 (0.5582)	-1,807.9 (<0.0001)	0.0832 (<0.0001)
55-64	Ref	Ref	Ref	Ref
Male	3,326.5 (<0.001)	4,822.2 (<0.001)	2,110.5 (<0.001)	0.5367 (<0.0001)
Urban	-189.9 (0.7537)	-83.1 (0.8573)	566.94 (0.2595)	-0.1511 (<0.0001)
Region				
Northeast	-3,229.4 (<0.0189)	-4,204.17 (<0.0001)	-1,784.6 (0.1137)	0.0081 (0.8546)
North Central	-3,570.6 (0.0004)	-3,584.5 (<0.0001)	-3,324.9 (<.0001)	0.0243 (0.4515)
South	-1,443.9 (0.1353)	-821.7 (0.2730)	-2,006.1 (0.0110)	-0.0164 (0.5947)
West	Ref	Ref	Ref	Ref
Charlson Comorbidity Index	2,065.2 (<0.0001)	2,850.4 (<0.0001)	1,749.7 (<0.0001)	-0.0893 (<0.001)
IHD primary vs. secondary	7,318.8 (<0.0001)	-	-	-
Secondary IHD	-	5,926.2 (<0.0001)	-	-
Heart failure	-	1,747.0 (0.0246)	5,127.7 (<0.0001)	-
Stroke	-	7,054.2 (<0.0001)	2,698.0 (0.0091)	-

Characteristic	Primary or Secondary Diagnosis N=63,864	Primary Diagnosis N=33,316	Secondary Diagnosis N=30,548	Primary Diagnosis Versus IHD as the Secondary Diagnosis N=63,864
Diabetes	-	306.2 (0.6758)	291.1 (0.8559)	-
Hypertension	-	1,294.3 (0.0036)	3,252.8 (0.0275)	-
Symptoms involving respiratory system and other chest symptoms	-	-3.015.7 (<0.0001)	-10,016.0 (<0.0001)	-
Cardiac dysrhythmias	-	7,583.9 (<0.0001)	2,571.2 (0.0044)	-
Hyperlipidem ia	-	2,471.1 (<0.0001)	2,142.2 (<0.0001)	-
PCI	-	1,527.3 (0.0002)	13,140.0 (0.0002)	-
CABG	-	26,164.0 (<0.0001)	44,053.0 (<0.0001)	-

Values in parentheses are p values. IHD: ischemic heart disease; PCI: percutaneous coronary intervention; CABG; coronary artery bypass graft; Ref: reference; All the comorbidities (heart failure, stroke, diabetes, hypertension, symptoms involving respiratory system and other chest symptoms, cardiac dysrhythmias, and hyperlipidemia) refer to the secondary diagnosis for hospitalizations with the primary diagnosis of IHD, and refer to the primary or secondary diagnosis for hospitalizations with a secondary diagnosis of IHD.

Table 4. Coefficient estimates of hospitalization costs and diagnosis status for patients with a diagnosis of ischemic heart disease

4. Discussion

Using a large administrative dataset, we analyzed the costs of hospitalizations in patients diagnosed with IHD and obtained detailed information on a variety of measures. Our cost information on IHD classified by AMI, primary and secondary diagnosis statuses, and comorbidities is the first of its kind to be reported. More important, while many authors have detailed the costs of CABG and PCI procedures over the years, our study is unique in reporting the costs of hospitalization for IHD patients who underwent these procedures by age, sex, and diagnostic status and controlling several major comorbidities of IHD.

We used ICD-9 codes to define IHD; earlier investigations by other researchers were hampered by not clearly defining this disease, and few considered IHD as a secondary diagnosis. We found, as expected, that the hospitalizations in which IHD was the primary diagnosis were far more expensive, on average, than the cases in which IHD was only a secondary diagnosis, but we found that the latter accounted for 48% of the hospital stays of interest. Thus, there is considerable merit in examining these hospitalizations in terms of their economics. More broadly, the information set forth in the present report should be valuable for identifying with greater precision the drivers of costs incurred by patients hospitalized with IHD.

Our cost estimates for hospitalizations with a primary diagnosis of IHD ($24,079 on average, $27,507 for AMI and $22,553 for non-AMI) are comparable to those in the literature. In a study that used data from 1995, Russell and associates estimated the cost of fatal AMI at $17,532 and nonfatal AMI at $15,540.[6] More recently, Menzin and coworkers estimated the cost of IHD at just under $23 thousand for initial hospitalization but about $5,700 higher for re-hospitalization in 2005.[7] Our finding that costs were higher for AMI hospitalizations than for those classified as non-AMI, while expected, adds further to the literature; of additional interest was the fact that the cost gap between AMI and non-AMI hospitalizations when IHD was the primary diagnosis was much larger for those aged 18-44 than it was for the other major subgroups (men, women, and those aged 45-64).

Our findings that stroke, heart failure, and cardiac dysrhythmias drive up the costs of hospitalization when IHD is the primary diagnosis are consistent with the literature but still of great interest. We also found that hyperlipidemia was associated with higher costs as expected. Patients with hyperlipidemia were often referred for lipid-lowering therapy, which incurred costs from medication, clinical visits, and lab tests. As for diabetes, in a study in the UK, Currie and coworkers found that 16.9% of IHD admissions (primary diagnosis) had a secondary diagnosis of diabetes and accounted for 16% of the costs of the disease.[10] Our results were somewhat similar: 15.9% of IHD admissions (primary diagnosis) had diabetes; we also found that those with diabetes had costs $5,067 higher than those who did not. Perhaps surprisingly, in our regression analysis, diabetes did not drive up the cost of IHD hospitalization significantly when IHD was a secondary diagnosis or even when it was the primary diagnosis. This finding deserves more exploration, as diabetes is a risk factor for many kinds of vascular disease and a known predictor of poorer outcomes for CABG surgery.

Nichols and Brown, who also explored the costs associated with a combination of CVD and diabetes, found higher costs in patients with diabetes than in those without that disease, and they reported that diabetes patients with CVD incurred more costs earlier in life than patients with diabetes but no CVD.[22] Elsewhere, Rosen and colleagues found that for patients with IHD in 2000-2002, costs when they also had hypertension were an additional $1,900 (our result was $2,920 for 2005), and when they had diabetes in addition to IHD they were $3,300 more (our result was $5,067 for 2005). These authors also found that the annual costs attributable to IHD were an additional $30,000 in the year an AMI occurred, and $4,000 in each subsequent year (in large part due to revascularization procedures).[4]

In our study, PCI increased the costs dramatically for patients with a secondary (but not a primary) diagnosis of IHD, and CABG increased the costs by 10s of thousands of dollars regardless of whether the IHD diagnosis was primary or secondary. Our mean cost for IHD as a primary diagnosis was $46,757 when there was CABG surgery, $19,622 when there was not. Wittels and coworkers, reporting more than 2 decades ago, found that the 5-year cost per case was $32,465 for CABG surgery and $26,916 for angioplasty. Researchers have investigated the factors influencing the high costs of CABG and have concluded that length of stays, race, age, prescription are the major factors.[23-25] Given the high cost of CABG surgery, reducing the number of procedures and/or lowering the unit costs might be cost-effective strategies in containing the overall costs associated with IHD.

Our finding in the logit model that men were more likely than women and patients aged 40-54 more likely than those either 18-39 or 55-64 to have IHD as the primary diagnosis rather than a secondary diagnosis is of great interest and adds to the literature on IHD among American adults. We found that the economic burden of IHD was higher among men than women, and this finding about the likelihood of primary versus secondary diagnosis would be consistent with that. Further, because men and persons aged 40-54 are major participants in the workforce, these results may suggest high indirect costs associated with IHD for these subpopulations.

The variety of new findings from the present study notwithstanding, several limitations should be considered in interpreting the results. First, the costs reported for IHD with a specific comorbidity could not be allocated explicitly into the cost of IHD and the cost of the comorbidity, and the causal relationships between IHD and its comorbidities were unknown. Thus, the estimated costs for IHD with a comorbidity should be interpreted as the costs associated with IHD when that comorbidity was present rather than the costs of IHD plus the costs of that comorbidity. Fortunately, researchers have proposed ways of attributing hospitalization costs to specific diseases when the comorbidity issues are significant,[26] and such research in the case of IHD should be conducted.

Second, our sample population was of patients aged 18-64 years, while most previous studies focused on persons aged 65 years or older because of the higher prevalence of IHD and the greater costs for this age group. However, our results showed that although there was a tendency toward increased costs with greater age, the cost differences between age groups were not large, and our cost estimates were comparable with those in the literature. Third, the hospitalization costs were direct medical costs only, while the literature has shown that about half of the total economic burden of IHD is represented by indirect costs such as those for informal care and loss of productivity. Thus, the hospitalization costs were very conservative estimates of the total economic burden of IHD. Quantifying the costs of informal care and productivity loss associated with IHD is needed to have a better understanding of the full economic burden of IHD. Fourth, our data did not allow us to identify the hospitalizations as an initial admission or a readmission. Thus, we were unable to investigate the cost relationship between IHD initial admissions and readmissions. Finally, all of the patients had insurance coverage and thus were not representative of the broad US population, a good portion of which has no health insurance. All of these factors may limit the generalization of our results to the general population.

5. Conclusions

Inpatient costs for IHD in the US are high, especially for hospitalizations among patients who had an AMI. Cardiac dysrhythmias, heart failure, and stroke are major factors associated with increased costs for patients with IHD. CABG surgery greatly increases the cost of IHD hospitalization, as does PCI if IHD is a secondary diagnosis only. The high costs we report here provide economic justifications for the development of more effective programs to prevent CVD. New strategies for the comprehensive prevention and control of IHD and its associated comorbidities such as cardiac dysrhythmias, heart failure, and stroke could curb hospitalizations and decrease the use of cardiac procedures for IHD and thereby control the associated medical costs.

6. Acknowledgement

The findings and conclusions in this chapter are those of the authors and do not necessarily represent the official position of the U.S. Centers for Disease Control and Prevention (CDC). Partial results of this chapter were presented at the Annual Meeting of the Society for Medical Decision Making, Toronto, Canada, 20-24 October 2010.

7. References

[1] American Heart Association. Heart and Stroke Statistics – 2010 Update, Dallas, TX: American Heart Association, 2010.

[2] Mensah GA, Brown DW. An overview of cardiovascular disease burden in the United States. *Health Aff (Millwood)* 2007;26:38-48.

[3] Fang J, Alderman MH, Keenan NL, Ayala C. Acute myocardial infarction hospitalization in the United States, 1979 to 2005. *Am J Med* 2010;123:259-266.

[4] Rosen AB, Cutler DM, Norton DM, Hu HM, Vijan S. The value of coronary heart disease care for the elderly: 1987-2002. *Health Aff (Millwood)* 2007;26:111-123.

[5] Hodgson TA, Cohen AJ. Medical care expenditures for selected circulatory diseases: opportunities for reducing national health expenditures. *Med Care* 1999;37:994-1012.

[6] Russell MW, Huse DM, Drowns S, Hamel EC, Hartz SC. Direct medical costs of coronary artery disease in the United States. *Am J Cardiol* 1998;81:1110-1115.

[7] Menzin J, Wygant G, Hauch O, Jackel J, Friedman M. One-year costs of ischemic heart disease among patients with acute coronary syndromes: findings from a multi-employer claims database. *Curr Med Res Opin* 2008;24:461-468.

[8] Liu JL, Maniadakis N, Gray A, Rayner M. The economic burden of coronary heart disease in the UK. *Heart* 2002;88:597-603.

[9] Nichols GA, Bell TJ, Pedula KL, O'Keeffe-Rosetti M. Medical care costs among patients with established cardiovascular disease. *Am J Manag Care* 2010;16:e86-e93.

[10] Currie CJ, Morgan CL, Peters JR. Patterns and costs of hospital care for coronary heart disease related and not related to diabetes. *Heart* 1997;78:544-549.

[11] Wittels EH, Hay JW, Gotto AM Jr. Medical costs of coronary artery disease in the United States. *Am J Cardiol* 1990;65:432-440.

[12] Fidan D, Unal B, Critchley J, Capewell S. Economic analysis of treatments reducing coronary heart disease mortality in England and Wales, 2000-2010. *QJM* 2007;100:277-289.

[13] Luengo-Fernández R, Leal J, Gray A, Petersen S, Rayner M. Cost of cardiovascular diseases in the United Kingdom. *Heart* 2006;92:1384-1389.

[14] McCollam P, Etemad L. Cost of care for new-onset acute coronary syndrome patients who undergo coronary revascularization. *J Invasive Cardiol* 2005;17:307-311.

[15] Etemad LR, McCollam PL. Total first-year costs of acute coronary syndrome in a managed care setting. *J Manag Care Pharm* 2005;11:300-306.

[16] Hansen LG, Chang S. Health research data from the real world: the Thomson Reuters MarketScan databases (January 2011 white paper). Available for request at http://info.thomsonhealthcare.com/forms/HealthResearchWPRequest, Requested May 3, 2011.

[17] Beinart SC, Kolm P, Veledar E, Zhang Z, Mahoney EM, Bouin O, Gabriel S, Jackson J, Chen R, Caro J, Steinhubl S, Topol E, Weintraub WS. Long-term cost-effectiveness of early and sustained dual oral antiplatelet therapy with clopidogrel given for up to one year after percutaneous coronary intervention: results from the Clopidogrel for the Reduction of Events during Observation (CREDO) trial. *J Am Coll Cardiol* 2005;46:761-769.

[18] Kahende JW, Woollery TA, Lee CW. Assessing medical expenditures on 4 smoking-related diseases, 1996-2001. *Am J Health Behav* 2007;31:602-611.

[19] Wang G, Zhang Z, Ayala C. Hospitalization costs associated with hypertension as a secondary diagnosis among insured patients aged 18-64 years. *Am J Hypertens* 2010;23:275-281.

[20] Wang G, Zhang Z, Ayala C, Wall HK, Fang J. Costs of heart failure-related hospitalizations in patients aged 18 to 64 years. *Am J Manag Care* 2010;16: 769-776.

[21] Ye X, Gross CR, Schommer J, Cline R, Xuan J, St Peter WL. Initiation of statins after hospitalization for coronary heart disease. *J Manag Care Pharm* 2007;13:385-396.

[22] Nichols GA, Brown JB. The impact of cardiovascular disease on medical care costs in subjects with and without type 2 diabetes. *Diabetes Care* 2002;25:482-486.

[23] Eisenberg MJ, Filion KB, Azoulay A, Brox AC, Haider S, Pilote L. Outcomes and cost of coronary artery bypass graft surgery in the United States and Canada. *Arch Intern Med* 2005;165:1506-1513.

[24] Liu CF, Subramanian S, Cromwell J. Impact of global bundle payments on hospital costs of coronary artery bypass grafting. *J Health Care Finance* 2001;27:39-54.

[25] Subramanian S, Liu CF, Cromwell J, Thestrup-Nielsen S. Preoperative correlates of the cost of coronary artery bypass graft surgery: Comparison of results from three hospitals. *Am J Med Quality* 2001;16:87-91.

[26] Ward MM, Javitz HS, Smith WM, Bakst A. A comparison of three approaches for attributing hospitalizations to specific diseases in cost analyses. *Int J Technol Assess Health Care* 2000;16:125-136.

19

Post-Myocardial Infarction Depression

Rousseau Guy, Thierno Madjou Bah and Roger Godbout
Université de Montréal
Canada

1. Introduction

Prospective studies show that persons with depression are at increased risk for coronary artery disease, myocardial infarction (MI) and cardiac death (Anda et al. 1993; Barefoot and Schroll 1996; Ferketich et al. 2000; Penninx et al. 2001). This high rate is at least partly related to a greater activation of platelets resulting in an increased risk of thrombosis, which can partly explain the relation between these events (Laghrissi-Thode et al. 1997). Moreover, clinical depression can occur in 30-60% of MI patients and 15-20% develop major depression (Guck et al. 2001; Meneses et al. 2007) following MI. Evidence for a poor prognosis is particularly strong in MI patients with depressive symptoms (Ahern et al. 1990; Forrester et al. 1992; Frasure-Smith et al. 1993; Frasure-Smith et al. 1995; Bush et al. 2001; Lespérance et al. 2002): the risk of cardiac death in the 6 months after acute MI is approximately 4 times greater in patients with depression compared to non-depressed control subjects (Frasure-Smith et al. 1993). A 3.5-fold risk is still present years after MI (Lespérance et al. 2002).

Despite a lower quality of life and poor prognosis for survival, only a few patients with post-MI depression are treated for their affective disorder (Schleifer et al. 1989; Frasure-Smith et al. 1993; Lespérance et al. 1996; Honig and Maes 2000). This unfortunate situation has been attributed either to the fact that symptoms of depression are unrecognized because of the overlap with sequelae of hospitalization for MI (e.g., sleep disturbances, fatigue, feelings of guilt, loss of appetite, preoccupation with death) (Katon and Sullivan 1990; Freedland et al. 1992; Frasure-Smith et al. 1993), or because symptoms of depressive disorder in post-MI patients are not always typical (Honig et al. 1997). It has also been suggested that physicians may hesitate to treat a depression considered to be a normal and transient reaction to a life-threatening event and the associated hospitalization period (Fielding 1991; Littman 1993). Furthermore, some physicians may avoid prescribing antidepressant medication for patients who have sustained an MI, because of the potential interaction or unwarranted adverse cardiac events reported for classic (i.e., tricyclic) antidepressants (Glassman et al. 1993). Still, the mechanisms by which MI is so often followed by depression is little investigated and poorly understood. For this reason, we have undertaken the task to develop an experimental animal model to advance the knowledge on post-MI depression.

2. An experimental model of post-myocardial infarction depression

On a pathophysiological point of view, the occurrence of post-MI depression lead us to search for common threads between the ischemic heart and the brain structures associated with depression. More specifically, we designed our experimental strategy toward documenting biochemical modifications in the brain limbic system as well as the behavioral modifications following an acute MI.

2.1 Myocardial infarction and pro-inflammatory processes

Ischemia occurs when coronary arteries blood flow is interrupted, which leads to reversible changes at the cellular level (swelling of mitochondrial matrix, intracellular fluid accumulation, etc). If ischemia persists, irreversible damage appears: membrane integrity is affected and intracellular substances are released, leading to an inflammatory reaction associated with a significant influx of neutrophils in the ischemic myocardium (Chatelain et al. 1987) and ultimately will be replaced by macrophages (Yu et al. 2003). After a prolonged period of ischemia, almost all the cells present in the ischemic region will die which can lead to heart failure if myocardial damage is extended.

Reperfusion of cardiac ischemic tissue is associated with a massive inflammatory response characterized by the release of chemotactic and inflammatory substances. The accumulation of neutrophils is rapid for the first six hours of reperfusion and diminishes to insignificant levels after 24 hours of reperfusion (de Lorgeril et al. 1990). The inflammatory response observed during the reperfusion period is more intensive that the one observed during the ischemic period (Chatelain et al. 1987). The reperfusion period of ischemic cardiac tissue is also associated with apoptosis, i.e., programmed cell death. This may appear paradoxical at first hand since apoptosis induces cell death without inflammation. It is known, however, that pro-inflammatory substances are released by jeopardized myocardium, which leads to the apoptotic process. Indeed, acute MI is associated with high production of pro-inflammatory cytokines (TNF-α, IL-1β, IL-6 and IL-8) by monocytes, and inflammatory mononuclear cells infiltrate the border zone, cardiomyocytes and endothelial cells (Francis et al. 2004). This represents parts of an intrinsic myocardial stress response system to tissue injury that may contribute not only to wound healing but also to secondary injury (Marx et al. 1997; Gwechenberger et al. 1999; Irwin et al. 1999; Kato et al. 1999; Pudil et al. 1999; Deten and Zimmer 2002; Hillis et al. 2003; Tziakas et al. 2003).

The rapid increase in pro-inflammatory cytokine expression after MI is accompanied by a simultaneous local and systemic increase of catecholamines (Bürger et al. 2001), which can contribute to cytokine expression. Recent confirmation has been obtained with the attenuation of IL-1β mRNA expression in cardiac tissue in presence of propranolol, a β-adrenergic receptor antagonist (Deten et al. 2003). This shows that MI can elicit a quick and intensive inflammatory response that may alter the blood-brain barrier (Wann et al. 2004) or intestinal permeability (Arseneault-Bréard et al. 2011). It has been reported that increased cytokine synthesis (mainly TNF-α) may be observed in the brain following MI, and this could be prevented by the intraperitoneal administration of pentoxifylline (Francis et al. 2004). In parallel, we have observed that MI affects the integrity of the intestinal barrier and this could be prevented by the administration of probiotics, possibly by altering the balance between pro- and anti-inflammatory cytokines (Arseneault-Bréard et al. 2011).

Because reperfusion needs to be performed upon cardiac arrest and since there is an inflammatory response observed early after the onset of reperfusion, we used the reperfused MI as the basis of our model. Smaller infarct size, better survival rate, rapidly recovering animals, and great clinical relevance are among the different advantages of using a short period of ischemia followed rapidly by reperfusion compared to a permanent occlusion.

2.2 Post myocardial infarction depression and apoptosis

Post-mortem brains of depressed patients show DNA fragmentation and neuronal apoptosis, suggesting enhanced neuronal vulnerability in depression (Lucassen et al. 2006). Neuronal loss and reduced neurogenesis have also been observed in animal models of mood disorders (Gould and Tanapat 1999; Czeh et al. 2001; Lucassen et al. 2006). A decrease in the volume of the hippocampus, amygdala and prefrontal cortex is one of the neuropathological signs described in depression in which apoptosis may play a role (Sapolsky 1996; Drevets 2000; Strakowski et al. 2002). Neuronal cell death may occur via 2 mechanisms: a) an acute form, or necrosis, that is rapid; and b) a delayed form, through apoptosis (Yuan and Yankner 2000). The former cannot be prevented efficiently because it tends to be prominent after more extreme conditions, such as ischemic insults or mechanical injury while the later is tightly regulated and dependent of the presence of energy (Yuan and Yankner 2000). Apoptotic cells are characterized by a reduction of volume, cytoplasmic shrinkage, DNA fragmentation, cell rounding and membrane bledding (Kerr et al. 1972). Apoptotic cells can ultimately break into membrane-contained apoptotic bodies, which can be phagocytosed by neighboring cells or phagocytes, which explains the difficulty of documenting apoptosis in vivo (Wyllie et al. 1980).

Clinical evidence has demonstrated the presence of apoptosis in the brain of persons with depression. In one investigation, cell death was observed in the entorhinal cortex, subiculum, dentate gyrus and hippocampus (CA1 and CA4) in 11 out of 15 depressed patients without obvious massive cell loss (Lucassen et al. 2001). An imbalance between neurogenesis and cell death may thus contribute to some extent to the brain volume changes in depression or, alternatively, cell death may be present for a limited time followed by regeneration (Malberg et al. 2000). In another study, the same authors suggested that the contribution of cell death may have been underestimated, since antidepressant treatments are now known to be anti-apoptotic (Lucassen et al. 2004). Since then, 3 investigations have responded to this comment: a) The antidepressant Desipramine is associated with cultured hippocampal neural stem cell neuroprotection against lipopolysaccharide-induced apoptosis by inhibiting inflammatory processes in vitro (Huang et al. 2007); b) Desipramine and Fluoxetine increase Fibroblast Growth Factor-2 activity, a growth factor involved in maturation, synaptic connectivity, neurogenesis and survival of catecholamine neurons in the cortex and hippocampus (Bachis et al. 2008); c) Our own data, showing that Sertraline, an antidepressant with selective serotonin reuptake inhibition properties, blocks early post-MI apoptosis in the limbic system (Wann et al. 2009). The anti-apoptotic effect of antidepressants was also reported in 2 other recent studies in rats (Huang et al. 2007; Bachis et al. 2008). Although apoptosis is difficult to document in human clinical cases (because patients are usually treated with antidepressants), another set of evidence indicates that the lymphocytes (Ivanova et al. 2007) or blood leukocytes (Szuster-Ciesielska et al. 2008) of depressed patients manifest a higher proportion of apoptotic elements compared to healthy controls. It is also observed that proapoptotic serum activity is elevated in depressed patients (Politi et al. 2008), again suggesting a link between apoptosis and depression. Moreover, it has been found that mood-regulating molecules, such as Lithium and Valproate, increase the expression of Bcl_2, an anti-apoptotic cytoprotective protein. Bcl_2 shuts off the apoptotic signal transduction pathway upstream of caspase activation (Chinnaiyan et al. 1996). It is also reported that antidepressant treatments themselves can increase neurogenesis in the rat hippocampus (Malberg et al. 2000) and prevent apoptosis (Lucassen et al. 2004; Nahon et al.). Apoptosis thus holds a key position in our experimental strategic plan to better understand the pathophysiology of post-MI depression.

2.2.1 Intracellular mechanisms of apoptosis

Multiple cellular pathways can trigger apoptosis, involving caspase activation or not (MacFarlane and Williams 2004) and two pathways of caspase activation have been described: extrinsic and intrinsic (figure 1). The extrinsic and intrinsic pathways of caspase activation differ according to the mechanism by which initiator caspases (see below) are activated, whereas effector caspases (caspase-3, -6 and -7) are common in both pathways (Adams 2003).

The extrinsic pathway is initiated by ligand binding to death receptors, such as tumor necrosis factor (TNF), Fas or TNF-related apoptosis-inducing factor receptors (TRAIL) (Thorburn 2004). The formation of death-inducing signaling complexes (DISC) is the key element. These complexes are formed by the activated receptor FAS-associated death domain protein (FADD) or TRAIL-associated death domain protein (TRADD). Pro-caspase-8 is then recruited to the complexes to form DISC, resulting in auto-cleavage and caspase-8 activation (Wang and El-Deiry 2003). Activated caspase-8, in turn, cleaves and activates downstream effector caspases, such as caspase-3, leading to the cleavage of cellular proteins and cell death. Active caspase-8 can cleave Bid, a member of the Bcl-2 family, and cleaved Bid can amplify the death signal by promoting the release of apoptogenic proteins from the mitochondria (Luo et al. 1998).

The intrinsic pathway or mitochondria-dependent pathway can be activated by chemicals, drugs, irradiation and cell stress such as hypoxia (Jeong and Seol 2008). Independently of signals that trigger the intrinsic pathway, mitochondria in the target organelle, resulting in the release of cytochrome c and the loss of mitochondrial membrane potential (Reyland 2007). Cytochrome c, together with apoptotic protease activating factor 1 (Apaf-1), ATP and pro-caspase-9, forms apoptosomes and elicits caspase-9 activation (Jeong and Seol 2008). Apoptosis is suppressed through heterodimerization of anti-apoptotic Bcl_2 proteins, such as Bcl_2 and Bcl-xL, with pro-apoptotic proteins, such as Bak and Bax; thus, the ratio of pro- and anti-apoptotic proteins is an important determinant of cell fate (Reyland 2007). Apoptotic stimuli alleviate the Bcl_2-mediated suppression of pro-apoptotic Bax and Bak, allowing these proteins to oligomerize into transmembrane pores in the mitochondria, induce cytochrome c release and activate caspases.

Caspase activation is also regulated by the release of mitochondrial proteins, such as the inhibitor of apoptosis proteins (cIAP1, cIAP2, XIAP) that suppress activated caspases, and Second Mitochondrial Activator of Caspases SMAC/DIABLO that binds and reduces IAPs (Salvesen and Duckett 2002; Shi 2002). Finally, a group of mitochondrial proteins that induce apoptosis independently of caspase activation has been identified (Lorenzo and Susin 2004; Bras et al. 2005). These include apoptosis-inducing factor (Lorenzo and Susin 2004; Bras et al. 2005) and endonuclease G (Li et al. 2001), which are released from the mitochondria in response to an apoptotic signal and translocate to the nucleus to trigger nuclear condensation and DNA fragmentation (Lorenzo and Susin 2004).

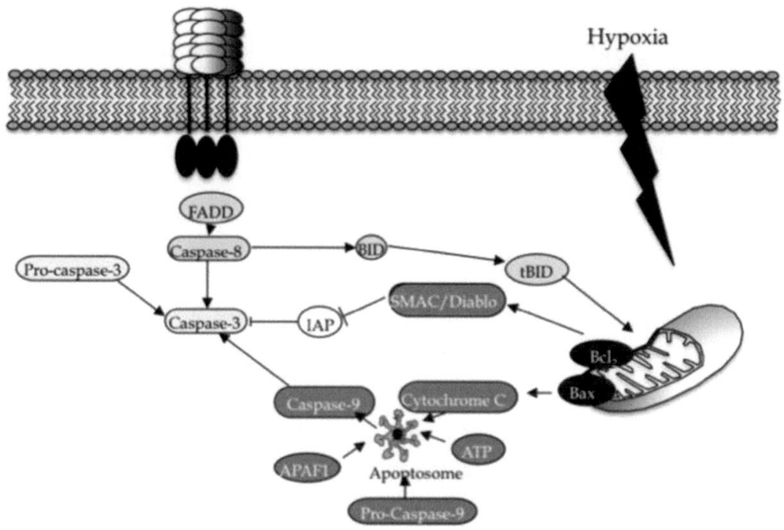

Fig. 1. Intrinsic and Extrinsic pathways of apoptosis. The extrinsic pathway involves receptor-mediated caspase-8 activation with subsequent effector caspase-3 activation. Within the intrinsic apoptosis pathway, caspase-3 is activated after cytochrome c release from the mitochondria and the formation of complexes called apoptosome that consist of caspase-9, Apaf1, ATP and cytochrome C. The release of apoptogenic factors from the mitochondria, such as cytochrome c, is regulated by Bcl_2 family proteins.

2.3 Apoptosis in the limbic system after myocardial infarction

Apoptosis has been observed in the limbic system after myocardial infarction (Wann et al. 2006; Kaloustian et al. 2009). We have documented the presence of apoptotic cells in the limbic system mainly in the amygdala, 3 days after the onset of reperfusion whereas no substantial apoptosis was observed in the sham group. In presence of MI, amygdala presents an increase in the activity of caspase-3 as compared to the sham group, as well as a higher Bax/Bcl2 ratio and a significant number of TUNEL positive cells. In order to be more precise in the localization of the presence of apoptosis at 3 days post-MI, we evaluated the presence of apoptosis in 9 different regions of the brain, using the cerebellum as a control structure (Wann et al. 2009): prefrontal and frontal cortices, CA1, CA3 and dentate gyrus of the hippocampus, lateral and medial amygdala and anterior and posterior hypothalamus. Our data indicate an increase of apoptosis in 7 of these regions (prefrontal and frontal cortices, CA1, dentate gyrus, lateral and medial amygdala and anterior hypothalamus). The next step of our investigation was to determine the kinetic of apoptosis in these regions during the first week after the onset of reperfusion (Kaloustian et al. 2008). Apoptosis was detected in the CA1 region as soon as 15 minutes after the onset of reperfusion, followed 24 hours later by the medial amygdala. Seven days after the onset of reperfusion, the frontal cortex is the only region where apoptosis is present.

As explained above, apoptosis can be triggered via intrinsic and extrinsic pathways. In a series of experiments designed to dissect the respective contribution of these two pathways, we found that caspase-9 activity was increased as soon at 15 minutes after the onset of reperfusion in the CA1, indicating that the intrinsic pathway is rapidly activated in this region (Rondeau et al. 2011). This result can be explain by the sensitivity of this region to hypoxia (Sugawara et al. 1999) which can be induced by MI. However at the same moment, the dentate gyrus presents an activation of caspase-8, (extrinsic pathway) but no activation of caspase-9 or caspase-3, indicating that: 1) intrinsic pathway is not activated in this region; 2) apoptosis is beginning in dentate gyrus at this moment. At three days post-MI, caspase-3 and -8 are activated in the hippocampus and amygdala regions. Overall, these data indicate that apoptosis is rapidly triggered in the CA1 region after the onset of reperfusion by an intrinsic pathway mechanism whereas apoptosis is induced in the other regions, such as dentate gyrus, by an extrinsic pathway mechanism.

An interesting observation from these series of experiments is that apoptosis does not occur at the same time throughout the limbic system. One hypothesis could be that cell death observed in a region can affect other regions later. Indeed, it has been observed that neurons which have no trophic support or electrical activity die by apoptosis (Jacobson et al. 1997). Thus, it can possible that the loss of neurons in a region may affect the neurons in other part by a reduction of trophic support or electrical activity.

Although the characterization of the cells that undergo apoptosis has not been fully completed yet, we have used the fluorojade labeling technique to verify if neurons are affected in the limbic system after myocardial infarction. Positive fluorojade staining cells indicate the presence of degenerating neurons (figure 2).

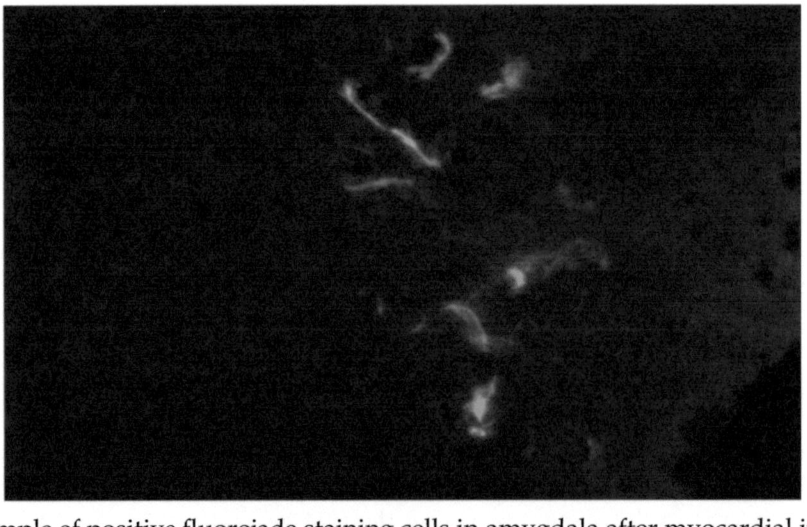

Fig. 2. Example of positive fluorojade staining cells in amygdala after myocardial infarction indicating the presence of degenerating neurons.

2.4 Cytokines, depression and post-myocardial infarction

Since the extrinsic mechanism of apoptosis is activated in the limbic system after MI and because apoptosis can be attenuated by pentoxifylline (Wann et al. 2006), an inhibitor of cytokine synthesis, we hypothesized that pro-inflammatory cytokines could be involved in the pathophysiology of post-MI depression. The following paragraphs summarize some of the supporting evidence.

Cytokines are a heterogeneous group of short-acting soluble proteins, glycoproteins and peptides. These regulatory proteins are secreted by a variety of cell types including white blood cells (lymphocytes and monocytes or macrophages) and somatic cells (O'Brien et al. 2004). Cytokines are multipotent and have pleiotropic effects not only in the immune system but also the CNS (Oprica et al. 2005); they contribute to immune responses of the body, help maintaining homeostasis, and mediate inflammation. Cytokines are associated with the membrane or the extracellular matrix, and toggle between the soluble and membrane forms (Sprague and Khalil 2009). Different cell types can secrete the same cytokine and a single cytokine can act on several cell types (pleiotropy), producing multiple biological activities depending on cell type, time and context (Hirano 1999) or inducing the synthesis of additional cytokines. Cytokines are redundant in their activity, meaning that similar functions might be stimulated by different cytokines (Ozaki and Leonard 2002). Because of the redundancy, the pathophysiological role of cytokines may be difficult to assess. In addition, cytokines are often produced in a cascade of events engaged in diverse modes of action: autocrine (when acting on cells that secrete), paracrine (when acting on cells near those that secrete) and endocrine (when acting on cells far from those that secrete) (Sprague and Khalil 2009). Cytokines can also act synergistically (two or more cytokines acting together) or antagonistically (cytokines causing opposing activities).

Cytokines bind to specific receptors at picomolar to nanomolar concentrations to activate and modulate functions at the cellular and tissular levels. Cytokine receptors are present in different structures of the limbic system. For example, IL-1 receptors are found in the hypothalamus and the hippocampus; IL-6 receptors are located in the hippocampus, hypothalamus, the dentate gyrus and piriform cortex (Vitkovic et al. 2000); TNF receptors are located in the hippocampus, cortex, amygdala, the basal ganglia (Vitkovic et al. 2000) and are also expressed by oligodendrocytes (Tchelingerian et al. 1995).

Recent advances in the field of psychoneuroimmunology suggest that major depression may alter immune function. Conversely, abnormal immune system may play a role in the etiology of depression (Maes et al. 1993). The immune system function in depressed patients involves both the hyperactivity of pro-inflammatory cytokines and anti-inflammatory cytokines (Grippo and Johnson 2002).

The administration of endotoxins in humans increases serum levels of pro-inflammatory cytokines and induces anxiety, mood changes and decreased memory skills, (Reichenberg et al. 2001). In rodents, pro-inflammatory cytokines induce the so-called "sickness behavior", which includes aspects of depression such decreased appetite, weight loss, fatigue, loss of libido, sleep disturbances and reduced social contacts (Krueger et al. 1984; Yirmiya et al. 2000; Dantzer 2001). In humans, the direct administration of pro-inflammatory cytokines such as TNF-α (Spriggs et al. 1988), IFN-γ (Niiranen et al. 1988) and IL-1β (Cunningham and De Souza 1993) leads to symptoms of depression such as irritability, fatigue, lethargy, loss of appetite psychomotor retardation and sleep disturbances. In patients with depression, the activation of the immune system translates into an augmentation in the number of circulating lymphocytes and phagocytic cells, immune cells by-products such as prostaglandin E2, complement proteins and increased concentrations of pro-inflammatory cytokines (Maes 1995; Irwin, Mak et al. 1999; Maes 1999; Maes, Song et al. 1999; Nunes, Reiche et al. 2002; Zorrilla, Valdez et al. 2001; Tuglu, Kara et al. 2003; (Maes 1995; Zorrilla et al. 2001; O'Brien et al. 2004).

Another potential action of the pro-inflammatory cytokines that may contribute to depression is by an action on indoleamine 2,3-dioxygenase (IDO) (Wirleitner et al. 2003). IDO is an enzyme induced by pro-inflammatory cytokines (IL-1, IFN-γ and TNF-α) and that is involved in the catabolism of tryptophan, the precursor of serotonin (Russo et al. 2003; Wirleitner et al. 2003). The net result is a reduced synthesis and availability of serotonin in the brain, thus facilitating depression (Heyes et al. 1992; Wichers and Maes 2002).

Blocking cytokine synthesis with PTX (Wann et al. 2006) or, more recently, with a TNF-α blocker (Kaloustian et al. 2009) significantly reduced apoptosis in the limbic system. The presence of pro-inflammatory cytokines at the limbic level can be explained by different mechanisms. The first possibility refers to modifications in endothelial permeability. Indeed, it has been reported that TNF-α disrupts endothelial cell lining integrity in various organs, including the anterior cingulate gyrus (Worrall et al. 1997). The pattern of selective plasma protein extravasation induced by TNF-α injection is similar to the pattern of MI-induced leakage (ter Horst et al. 1997). A second possibility is that circulating pro-inflammatory cytokines trigger the transcription of genes in cells of the blood-brain barrier, including NF-kB and cyclooxygenase-2 (COX-2), the limiting enzyme for the formation of prostaglandins (Laflamme and Rivest 1999). Prostaglandins, such as PGE_2, can diffuse across the brain parenchyma and stimulate the hypothalamic-pituitary-adrenal axis and corticotropin-releasing-factor activity (Rivest 2001; Banan et al. 2002). Moreover, it has been reported that COX-2 expression is associated with increased PGE_2 tissue levels and neuronal apoptosis (Li et al. 2003; Sasaki et al. 2004). In another study, PGE_2 induced caspase-dependent apoptosis in rat cortical cells (Takadera et al. 2002). Our results (Wann et al. 2006) show biochemical changes in the hippocampus and amygdala, limbic regions that express high levels of PGE_2 receptors. This suggested that COX-2 inhibition can be a significant element in our model (Zhang and Rivest 1999). A third possibility is the presence of a carrier that mediates the transport of cytokines into the brain across the blood-brain barrier (Banks et al. 1995; Kronfol and Remick 2000; Banks 2001). The fourth possibility refers to "central cytokines induced by peripheral cytokines" via afferent nerves activated by myocardial ischemia (Francis et al. 2004). It was derived from the fact that cytokines are relatively large protein molecules ($\approx$15 kDa for interleukin-1 (IL-1) and TNF-α), the hydrophilic nature of which does not allow crossing of the blood-brain barrier. According to these authors, transmission of the cytokine signal to the brain could be due to epicardial afferences, since destruction of these nerves by phenol prevents the induction of brain cytokine expression in the hypothalamus and hippocampus (Layé et al. 1995; Hansen et al. 1998; Francis et al. 2004). Among these different hypotheses, we believe that neurotransmission, via afferent nerves, is probably the more interesting: 1. we observed apoptosis, via activation of the caspase-8 pathway (extrinsic pathway) as early as after 15 min of reperfusion in some specific regions of the limbic system (dentate gyrus); 2. pro-inflammatory cytokines increased in the brain as early as 30 min after the onset of myocardial ischemia, but could be blocked by the destruction of afferent epicardial nerves with phenol (Francis et al. 2004).

2.5 Hypothalamic-pituitary adrenal axis-dependent mechanism

The regulation of the hypothalamic-pituitary adrenal (HPA) axis plays a major role in metabolic homeostasis and its overactivation by stress is associated with deleterious effects to the brain (Bluthe et al. 1999; Bluthe et al. 2006). Dysregulation of the HPA axis is part of the pathophysiology of depression.

The classic description of the HPA axis includes 3 main components (Bao et al. 2008): 1) The hypothalamus, that secretes the corticotropin-releasing hormone (CRH) upon a stressful situation; 2) the pituitary gland that reacts to CRH by producing growth hormone, prolactin and the adrenocorticotropic hormone (ACTH); 3) the adrenal glands (also named suprarenal glands), that react to ACTH by producing and releasing glucocorticoid (GC), mainly cortisol in humans and corticosterone in rodents (Carvalho and Pariante 2008), epinephrine and norepinephrine. A feedback loop makes the hypothalamus capable of monitoring cortisol blood levels and inhibits the release of CRH when cortisol levels are too high; in depression, this feedback mechanism may be altered so that CRH is still released despite high amounts of circulating cortisol (Pariante and Lightman 2008). Cortisol activates two types of receptors, the high-affinity mineralocorticoid receptors (MRs) and the low affinity glucocorticoid receptors (GRs); MRs are thus activated by low (basal) levels of GC while GRs are activated as GC concentrations increase, i.e. after stress. MRs and GRs apparently activate different genes and elicit different, sometimes opposing, actions: high levels of corticosterone induce apoptosis through the activation of GRs via the direct regulation of the extrinsic and intrinsic apoptosis pathways while low doses of corticosterone can prevent cell death through MRs activation, conferring a neuroprotective role for these receptors (Crochemore et al. 2005; Herr et al. 2007; Krugers et al. 2007; Yu et al. 2008). More specifically, studies revealed that activation of the GRs mediates hippocampus neuron- and volume-reducing actions of GC whereas stimulation of the MRs abrogates the neurodegenerative actions of the GRs agonists (Yu et al. 2008). High levels of GC can affect the survival of immature neurons, decreasing neurogenesis in the dentate gyrus (Wong and Herbert 2004).

Hyperactivity of the HPA leads to depression because dysregulation of GC can affect brain regions involved in the physiopathology of depression (Herbert et al. 2006). Activation of GRs by the agonist dexamethasone induces apoptotic death of neurons, while activation of MRs would tend to induce neuronal survival (Crochemore et al. 2005). The hypotheses to explain the effect of antidepressants on the HPA is that such treatment could increase the expression and the function of GRs, and promote its nuclear translocation (Pariante 2006). No effects of antidepressants on MRs are noted (Lai et al. 2003). The administration of tricyclic antidepressants or serotonin reuptake inhibitors (SSRIs) are accompanied by an increase in mRNA of GRs in various tissues and neurons (Pepin et al. 1989). Desipramine (a tricyclic antidepressant) showed an increase in function and nuclear translocation of GRs (Pariante et al. 1997). The tricyclic antidepressant imipramine and the SSRI fluoxetine inhibit the CRH gene promoter (Budziszewska et al. 2002). With effective antidepressant treatment, 75% of patients who did not respond to the dexamethasone suppression test now do (Heuser et al. 1996), while remaining unresponsive often suffer a relapse (Zobel et al. 2001).

We now know that growth hormone and prolactin stimulate the immune response while cortisol inhibits the immune response, the inflammatory response and natural killer cells (NKC). Depression is associated with an increase of secretion of IL-1β, TNF-α and IFN-α (Smith 1991; Maes et al. 1993; Maes 1995). Hyperactivity of the HPA axis accompanies this phenomenon (Connor and Leonard 1998) and, in turn, IL-1, IL-6, interferon and TNF activate the HPA axis (Turnbull and Rivier 1995).

Cytokines are also released following MI and they will reach the paraventricular nucleus of the hypothalamus, stimulating the synthesis and secretion of stress-related glucocorticoids (Turnbull and Rivier 1995). Increased plasma levels of pro-inflammatory cytokines such as IL-1 and IL-6 in patients with depression are correlated with hyperactivity of the HPA axis and the severity of symptoms (Maes 1995; Maes 1999).

The immune system can also influence the HPA axis response through various mechanisms involving pro-inflammatory cytokines: for example they may contribute to resistance to GC (cortisol unable to induce the negative feedback loop) by a decrease in GR function or sensitivity to GC (Miller et al. 1999) or inhibit GR translocation to the nucleus and decreases the transcription of genes induced by GR (Pariante et al. 1999). GC resistance following exposure to cytokines can be induced via the MAP kinase pathway: 1) ERK and JNK can inhibit GR function directly, by phosphorylation, or indirectly, through cofactors (Rogatsky et al. 1998); 2) NF-kB can directly interact with GR at the nuclear level or may decrease its function indirectly by competing for the same coactivators (McKay and Cidlowski 1999). Cytokines also activate the JAK-STAT pathway, which can GR functions by a direct protein-protein interaction (Rogatsky and Ivashkiv 2006; Pace and Miller 2009).

We have measured the level of corticosterone in our model, 2 weeks post-MI and we have observed that myocardial infarction induces an increase in plasmatic concentrations of corticosterone. However, the contribution of HPA axis in our model seems to be modest since attenuation of the depressive behavior has been observed with Escitalopram whereas no significant effect was detected in the plasmatic concentration of corticosterone (Bah et al. 2011).

2.6 Neurotrophic factors in depression

The reduction of hippocampal volume in depression is related to a dysregulation of neurogenic and neurotrophic factors (Duman and Monteggia 2006). The chronic administration of antidepressants increases neurotrophic factors and facilitates neurogenesis in the hippocampus, thus reducing the damage described above (Dranovsky and Hen 2006). The brain-derived neurotrophic factor (BDNF) is more particularly frequently cited as playing a significant role in that respect.

BDNF belongs to the family of Nerve Growth Factors (NGF). Physiologically, neurotrophins are initially synthesized as precursor protein (or pro-neurotrophin) and transformed into mature proteins (Mowla et al. 2001). All neurotrophins have a common structure and a structure variable that determines their specific receptors and their biological action arising (Heumann 1994).

BDNF mRNA is expressed in the hippocampus, septum, hypothalamus, cortex and noradrenergic brainstem nuclei (Castren et al. 1995; Katoh-Semba et al. 1997). This distribution overlaps with immunohistochemical localization of BDNF itself in the rat cerebral cortex, hippocampus, basal forebrain, striatum, hypothalamus, cerebellum (Kawamoto et al. 1996) as well as in the parietal and entorhinal cortices, amygdala and in the somatic nuclei (Wetmore et al. 1991).

BDNF is decreased in patients with depression (Karege et al. 2002) and antidepressants regulate the transcription of its mRNA (Dias et al. 2003). Moreover, the chronic administration of antidepressants increases BDNF in the limbic system, including the hippocampus (Nibuya et al. 1999). The mRNA expression of TrkB, the BDNF receptor, is altered in the rat hippocampus or cortex after repeated stress (Nibuya et al. 1999) and after treatment with antidepressants (Saarelainen et al. 2003). Impaired BDNF or TrkB signaling in rats does not lead to behavioral signs of depression, but lessened the behavioral response to antidepressants (Saarelainen et al. 2003). In addition, increased neurogenesis in the hippocampus is required to find behavioral effects of antidepressants in animal models of depression (Santarelli et al. 2003).

In our rat model of post-MI depression, BDNF levels were found to be increased in the dentate gyrus of the hippocampus 2 days post-MI and in the medial amygdala 7 days post-MI, suggesting a potential role of BDNF in this model (Kaloustian et al. 2008).

3. Behavior observed in experimental model of post-MI depression

One of the major challenges in developing a model of a mental health disorder is at the behavioral level, trying to establish variables that mimic the clinical picture found in humans. In the particular case of post-MI depression, the challenge is increased by the fact that physical fitness should not interfere with the behavioral dependant variables. The major concern is that the damage induced to the heart by the ischemia may affect the performance of the animals and, with these constraints in mind, we elected to use an acute model of heart infarct, thus by-passing the physical impact of chronic heart failure. Moreover, since experimental acute MI involves thoracotomy, sham operated rats are used as controls and tasks involving physical fitness are tested. In our model, reperfusion is rapidly reinstated and the surgical procedure can be summarized as follows. A left thoracotomy is performed and the left anterior descending coronary artery is occluded. Ischemia is confirmed by ST segment alterations and ventricular subepicardial cyanosis. After 40 min of occlusion, the ligature is loosened so that the myocardial tissue can be reperfused. Reperfusion is confirmed by the disappearance of cyanosis. This procedure induces an infarct size that routinely approximates 25% of the left ventricle. A control (sham-operated) group of rats is submitted to the same thoracotomy protocol but without actual coronary artery occlusion.

Behavioral tests that we have chosen were selected on the basis of face validity with regards to the human clinical picture and proven to be reliable and sensitive to antidepressant treatments as shown by previously published results from other groups using different models of depression. In the present model, this is a rather long process that has started less than 10 years ago and will obviously need a few more years before it is firmly established. Nonetheless, we believe we have accumulated enough converging evidence to suggest that our model replicates a significant portion of the human post-MI depressive syndrome. In the following paragraphs we will describe behavioral tasks that are commonly used in behavioral models of depression and that were included in the test battery for our own post-MI depression model. Like most models of depression, the post-MI syndrome appears 2-3 weeks after the experimental procedure aimed at inducing depression and tests are now routinely administered in that interval following reperfusion.

3.1 Forced swim test

This test was first developed by Porsolt (Porsolt et al. 1977; Porsolt et al. 1978a; Porsolt et al. 1978b) as a procedure for validating antidepressant efficacy. It models behavioral despair and learned helplessness, as rats are natural swimmer. In our experiments, rats are individually placed in a clear plastic cylindrical pool (45 cm tall x 25 cm diameter) filled with 30 cm of water maintained at 22-25°C. Rats are tested for two consecutive days (15 min. on the first day and 5 min. on second day). Time spent swimming, trying to escape and being immobile on day 15 post surgery are the dependant variables. During the initial period of this test, rats will usually present an intense activity followed by a characteristic immobile posture, moving occasionally to keep at least their nose above the waterline. Depression has been positively correlated with the length of immobility during the second trial on the test. The Forced swim test has a good predictive validity to detect antidepressant-like activity (Arunrut et al. 2009). Antidepressants usually decrease immobility.

In our model, we observe that 14 days after the onset of reperfusion, the animals with MI present more immobility than the group of sham-operated control animals (figure 3A). This effect can be reversed by different interventions, as we will discuss later. We also determined if the myocardial infarct size influenced the behavioral results. Plotting swimming time against MI size, expressed as percent of the left ventricle, showed no relation between the two variables (figure 3B). This is further evidence that infarct size observed in our model had no influence on motor performance in the Forced Swim test.

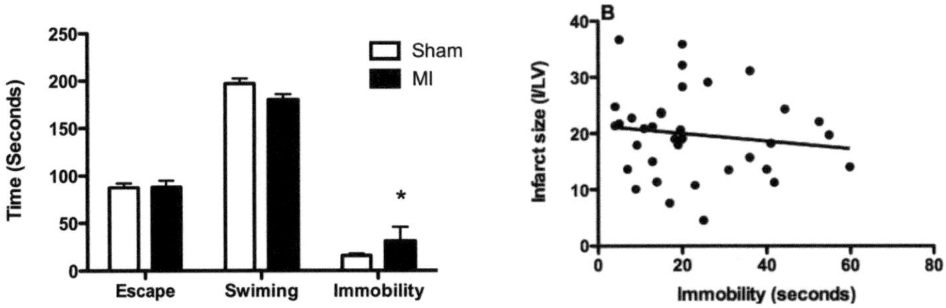

Fig. 3. A: Performance of rats in the forced swim test. Escape and swimming time is similar between groups whereas the time of immobility is significantly higher in the MI group. * indicates $p < 0.05$. n=16-18 per group. B: Relationship between infarct size (expressed as the proportion of infarcted tissue in the left ventricle) and immobility time in the forced swim test. The slope of the relationship is non-significant, $p = 0.44$ with a $r^2 = 0.02$.

3.2 Morris water maze

This is a test of motor performance and spatial memory requiring an intact hippocampus (Morris 1984). Rats are placed in a pool (150 cm diameter, 50 cm deep) filled to 25 cm with water maintained at 22°C–25°C and made opaque with powder milk. A submerged platform is placed just below the surface of the water. The rats are tested on 4 trials each day, 5 minutes apart, for 6 consecutive days (i.e., 14–19 days after surgery). The number of quadrants crossed, the number of successful trials and the time taken to reach the platform are recorded. Our results indicate no significant difference between MI and sham group, suggesting that MI: a) has no effects on hippocampus-dependant spatial memory; b) has no effects on the swimming capacity of experimental rats (Wann et al. 2007).

3.3 Sucrose preference

The sucrose preference test is classically used to define anhedonia in rat models of depression (Willner et al. 1987; Stock et al. 2000; Redei et al. 2001). For this test, rats have free access to two

250 ml bottles for five consecutive days (i.e., 14-18 days postsurgery): one containing tap water and the other containing a 1% sucrose solution. The position of the bottles is alternated each day. Volume intake (in ml) is estimated by weighing bottles each morning, at light onset. Contrary to most publication, rats are not deprived of water before running the test because we fear it might interfere with bodily functions. Anhedonia is operationally defined as a reduction in sucrose intake compared to a control group and untreated MI rats are found to take less sucrose solution than sham animals. In this case, it can be assumed that the physical condition of the animal has no significant effects on the results.

3.4 Social interaction test

It is known that depressed individuals have fewer interactions with congeners. In this test, two rats are placed together in a new, clean shoebox for 10 min. During this period, the following measures are taken for each of the two rats: duration and number of interactions with the other rat, number of grooming events and number of rearings. Sham rats are found to interact more with congeners than MI rats (figure 4).

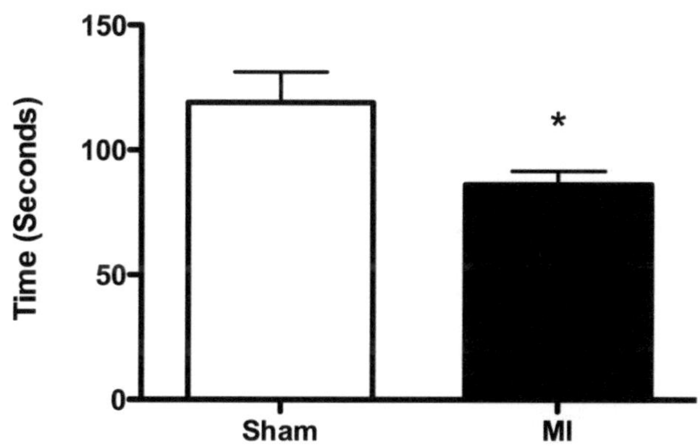

Fig. 4. Social interaction test. The data indicate that MI rats interact less than the sham group with their congeners. Time is expressed in seconds. n = 16 per group. *indicates $p < 0.05$ for Sham vs MI.

3.5 Passive avoidance step-down foot shock

This test is based on contextual memory and emotional memory, and depressed rats are known to show a decreased efficiency in response to a repeated aversive stimulus. It is a reliable behavioral indicator of depression in rats and it is also sensitive to the therapeutic action of antidepressants (Joly and Sanger 1986; van Riezen and Leonard 1991). For this test, the rat is placed on a plexiglass platform (14 X 19 cm). An electrifiable grid (14 X 14 cm) is alongside and 2.5 cm lower than the plexiglass platform. Initially, both sham and MI rats begin to wander around immediately, exploring the platform and the grid. When the animal places four feet on the electrifiable grid, it receives a mild, brief shock (5 mA for 1 sec) and is removed from the test box. After 30 sec, the rat is placed again on the platform. If the rat remains on the platform without going onto the grid for one minute, it is removed from the test box for 30 sec. Criterion is reached when the rat avoids going onto the grid for three consecutive trials. We have found that the number of trials and the time to succeed the test is significant higher in the MI rats compared to sham animals (figure 5).

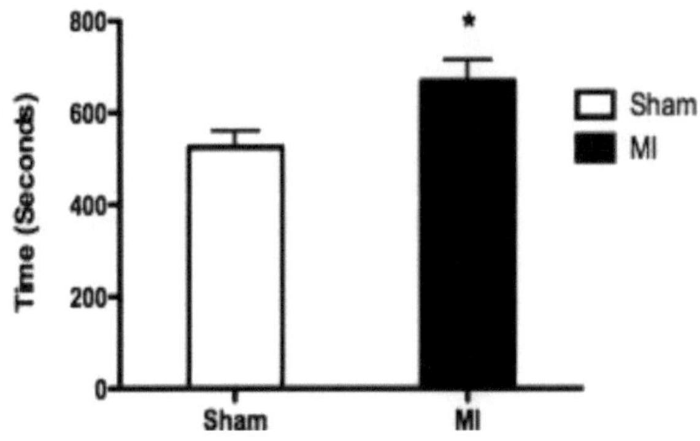

Fig. 5. Passive avoidance step-down foot shock test. In the passive avoidance step-down foot shock test, MI rats take more time to succeed in the test than the sham group (*p < 0.05). n = 16 per group.

3.6 Voluntary exercise-training cage

As an additional test to determine if MI affects the physical condition of experimental animals at baseline, we used a voluntary exercise-training cage (threadmills), using the distance travelled by 24 hours as the dependent variable. Measures were taken before and 2 weeks post-MI and the results indicate no differences between tests, i.e., more than 2 km/day (figure 6). Moreover the distance travelled at different moments of the day is similar between the two conditions. These results suggest that: 1) MI does not interfere with total spontaneous locomotion per 24 hour; 2) that circadian patterns may not be affected either.

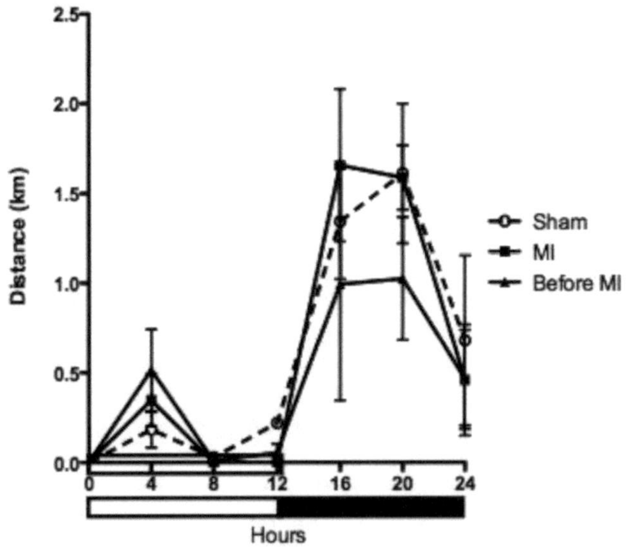

Fig. 6. Distance in km travelled by rats during a day in voluntary exercise-training cage. Open circles represented the distance travelled by the rats 2 weeks after the thoracotomy but without myocardial ischemia. The square represents the distance travelled by MI rats, 2 weeks post-MI whereas the triangle represented the same MI rats but before any manipulations. No significant difference are observed between conditions.

3.7 Sleep

In humans, depression is accompanied by sleep disorders, including difficulties initiating and maintaining sleep, less slow-wave sleep (SWS) together with a facilitation of rapid eye movement (REM) sleep, also known as paradoxical sleep (PS) (Benca et al. 1992). These sleep disorders have also been documented in rat models of depression, such as learned helplessness (Adrien et al. 1991), chronic, mild stress (Willner 2005), olfactory bulbectomy (Song and Leonard 2005), Flinders Sensitive Line (Overstreet et al. 2005), and the neonatal clomipramine model of endogenous depression (Vogel et al. 1990). Compared to sham rats, MI rats displayed a longer latency to sleep onset and to PS and fewer minutes in PS. The number of cholinergic neurons in the pedunculo-pontine tegmentum (PPT) area of MI rats, an area known to control PS, was decreased by 20% compared to sham rats while the number of latero-dorsal tegmentum (LDT) cholinergic neurons was not different (Bah et al. 2010).

These results partially replicate the sleep disorders observed in clinical depression and reveal that acute MI is accompanied, within 2 weeks, by PS-specific insomnia.

4. Treatment of post-MI depression

The pathophysiology of depression has been classically associated with monoamines, with more emphasis on serotonin (Leonard 2000; Delgado 2004): impaired serotoninergic neurotransmission is thought to be a major element in the pathophysiology of depression and SSRI antidepressants restore central serotoninergic neurotransmission. Monoaminergic theories of depression appear today, however, to be only one part of the story. It is known, for example, that pro-inflammatory cytokines influence serotonin metabolism in the central nervous system (Dunn 1992; Palazzolo and Quadri 1992; Cho et al. 1999) and studies have shown that antidepressants suppress the action of pro-inflammatory cytokines (Bengtsson et al. 1992; Xia et al. 1996). Moreover, pro-inflammatory cytokines such as IL-1, IFN-α, IFN-γ and TNF-α upregulate the serotonin transporter, thus causing a depletion of extracellular serotonin (Ramamoorthy et al. 1995; Morikawa et al. 1998; Mossner et al. 1998; Wichers and Maes 2002), whereas IL-4 (an anti-inflammatory cytokine) induces a reduction of serotonin reuptake like antidepressants do (Mossner et al. 2001; O'Brien et al. 2004). It is therefore not surprising that inhibition of pro-inflammatory cytokines is not only beneficial for the remission of depressive symptoms, but also to reduce the inflammation caused by myocardial infarction (Frangogiannis et al. 2002).

In animal models, administration of cytokines or cytokine inducers is associated with depressive symptoms (Dunn et al. 2005). Conversely, the administration of anti-inflammatory cytokines such as IGF-1 or IL-10 antagonizes the effects of cytokine inducers and lowers the symptoms of depression (Bluthe et al. 1999; Bluthe et al. 2006). Patients with depression have high levels of circulating inflammatory cytokines, including IL-1, IL-6 and TNF-α (Dowlati et al. 2009), and low levels of anti-inflammatory cytokines (Sutcigil et al. 2007). Despite the fact that small amounts of peripherally-released pro-inflammatory cytokines make it to the brain, it seems sufficient to induce depression in humans (Wilson and Warise 2008). It has been shown in patients with Cushing's syndrome that infliximab, a TNF-α inhibitor, reduces symptoms of depression before improving disease-specific symptoms (Lichtenstein et al. 2002).

The following paragraphs will review therapeutic strategies we have used in order to control for symptoms of depression in our animal model.

4.1.1 Tricyclic antidepressant (desipramine)

Desipramine is a tricyclic molecule that inhibits norepinephrine and serotonin reuptake, together with antidepressant properties (Katz et al. 2004). In our model, desipramine also reduces depressive-like symptoms such as behavioral despair as assessed by the Forced swim test as well as anhedonia as assessed by the Sucrose preference test. Interestingly, desipramine reduces apoptosis in models of stress-induced depressive disorders (Bachis et al. 2008) and we have found a significant negative correlation between swimming time on the Forced swim test and the Bax/Bcl2 ratio, a pro-apoptotic index, in the prefrontal cortex of MI depressed rats, suggesting again a link between apoptosis and depressive behavior (Wann et al. 2007).

4.1.2 Selective serotonin reuptake inhibitors (SSRIs)

4.1.2.1 Sertraline

The antidepressant SSRI fluoxetine inhibits apoptosis by blocking mitochondrial permeability transition pores (Nahon, et al., 2005) in vitro and we have shown that sertraline blocks post-MI apoptosis in vivo at three days post-MI, in different regions of the limbic system (Wann et al. 2009). At the behavioral level, MI rats showing signs of anhedonia (i.e., decreased sucrose intake) and despair (decreased swimming, increased immobility) improved with sertraline as they do in other models like chronic mild stress (Grippo, et al., 2006), social defeat or subordination (Rygula, et al., 2005).

4.1.2.2 Escitalopram

Escitalopram, an enantiomer of citalopram, is another SSRI antidepressant (Wu et al. 2009; Pan et al. 2011). In our model, we observed that escitalopram reduces the levels of pro-inflammatory cytokines (see above) and attenuates depressive-like behavior in MI rats without modifying their sleep (Bah et al., 2011).

These results with antidepressants together with the evidence cited in the previous sections suggest that cytokines and apoptosis could involve in the pathophysiology of depression, including after a MI.

4.2 Pentoxifylline

Pentoxifylline (PTX), a methylxantine-derivative and non-specific phosphodiesterase inhibitor with combined anti-inflammatory and anti-fibrogenic properties (Gutierrez-Reyes et al. 2006; Danjo et al. 2008), lowers circulating pro-inflammatory cytokines such as TNF-α, IL-1β and IL-6 (Raetsch et al. 2002), via a cyclic adenosine monophosphate (cAMP)-dependent mechanism. Systemically administered PTX in MI rats reduce apoptosis in the limbic system at three days post-MI (Wann et al. 2006) and attenuates depressive-like behavior at 14 day, indicating the importance of pro-inflammatory cytokines in both events (Bah et al., 2011b).

4.3 Nutritional interventions

A loss of equilibrium between pro-and anti-inflammatory proteins could be involved in the pathophysiology of depression (Szelenyi and Vizi 2007). Our previous work has shown that a reduction of circulating pro-inflammatory cytokines attenuates post-MI depressive-like behavior. Since diet can be used to modify the balance between pro- and anti-inflammatory cytokines, we hypothesized that targeted diets could attenuate post-MI depression.

4.3.1 Probiotics

The probiotics *Lactobacillus helveticus and Bifidobacterium longum* can reverse MI-induced apoptosis in the limbic system (Girard et al. 2009) by a mechanism that could include a reduction of pro-inflammatory cytokines. It has been observed that of *L. helveticus R0052* reduces IL-1β, IL-6 but not significantly TNF-α (Cazzola et al. 2010) whereas *B. longum R0175* can reduce IL-8 and TNF-α (Wagar et al. 2009) indicating that each strain has a specific effect on pro-inflammatory cytokines synthesis while they possibly are ineffective against stress (Diop et al. 2008; Girard et al. 2009; Messaoudi et al.). We combined both strains and found significant therapeutic effects on post-MI behavior, including behavioral despair (Forced swim test), passive avoidance and socialization Arseneault-Bréard et al. 2011).

4.3.2 Polyunsaturated fatty acids omega-3

Polyunsaturated fatty acids (PUFA) omega-3 are found mostly in the retinal and neuronal membranes. The lack of adequate levels of PUFA omega-3, and more particularly DHA, during brain development results into cognitive deficits (McNamara and Carlson 2006). Altered membrane concentration of PUFA omega-3 is also observed in depression (Peet et al. 1998; Mamalakis et al. 2006). Moreover, a recent study by Lespérance et al (2011) observed a clear benefit of PUFA omega-3 supplementation among patients with a major depressive episode but without comorbid anxiety disorders. Another study found that PUFA omega-3 had a similar effect on depression as the SSRI antidepressant fluoxetine, while the combination (EPA and fluoxetine) resulted in a superior effect than either of them alone (Jazayeri et al. 2008). The influence of PUFA omega-3 on psychiatric disorders has yielded mechanistic hypotheses, one of which involves the anti-inflammatory properties of fatty acids, in accordance with the fact that increased cytokine levels are associated with depression (Orr and Bazinet 2008; Kiecolt-Glaser 2010). A second hypothesis, based on PUFA omega-3 depletion studies, involves a modulation of monoaminergic neurotransmission (Chalon 2006) since a profound PUFA omega-3 deficiency is able to alter several neurotransmission systems such as dopaminergic and serotonergic. PUFA omega-3 may also improve depression via an anti-apoptotic neuroprotective mechanism. Indeed, DHA facilitates the activation and translocation of Akt, an anti-apoptotic protein (Akbar et al. 2005). Moreover, PUFA omega-3 induces the expression of the Bcl-2 anti-apoptotic protein and reduces the activation of caspase-3 (Bazan 2009; Sinha et al. 2009). In the more specific case of post-MI depression, it can be mentioned that omega-3 fatty acid levels were found to be lower in plasma and red blood cell membrane of depressed patients with acute coronary syndromes than non-depressed patients (Schins et al. 2007; Amin et al. 2008). Our own results show that an PUFA omega-3-rich diet reduces post-MI apoptosis in the limbic system (Rondeau et al. 2011) and depressive behavior (unpublished observations).

5. Conclusions

The data obtained over the last few years indicate that post-MI apoptosis occurs in the limbic system rapidly after the onset of reperfusion and our working hypothesis is that increased cytokines levels in the CNS are involved. Whether neurogenesis or HPA axis plays a significant role in the picture of post-MI depression is not yet clearly established and needs to be further investigated. In Figure 7 we propose a model to explain the etiology and consequences of post-MI depression. It is our hope that converging evidence will eventually lead to a better knowledge of how the heart and brain connection operates to allow post-MI occurring and possibly show the way for effective treatment strategies.

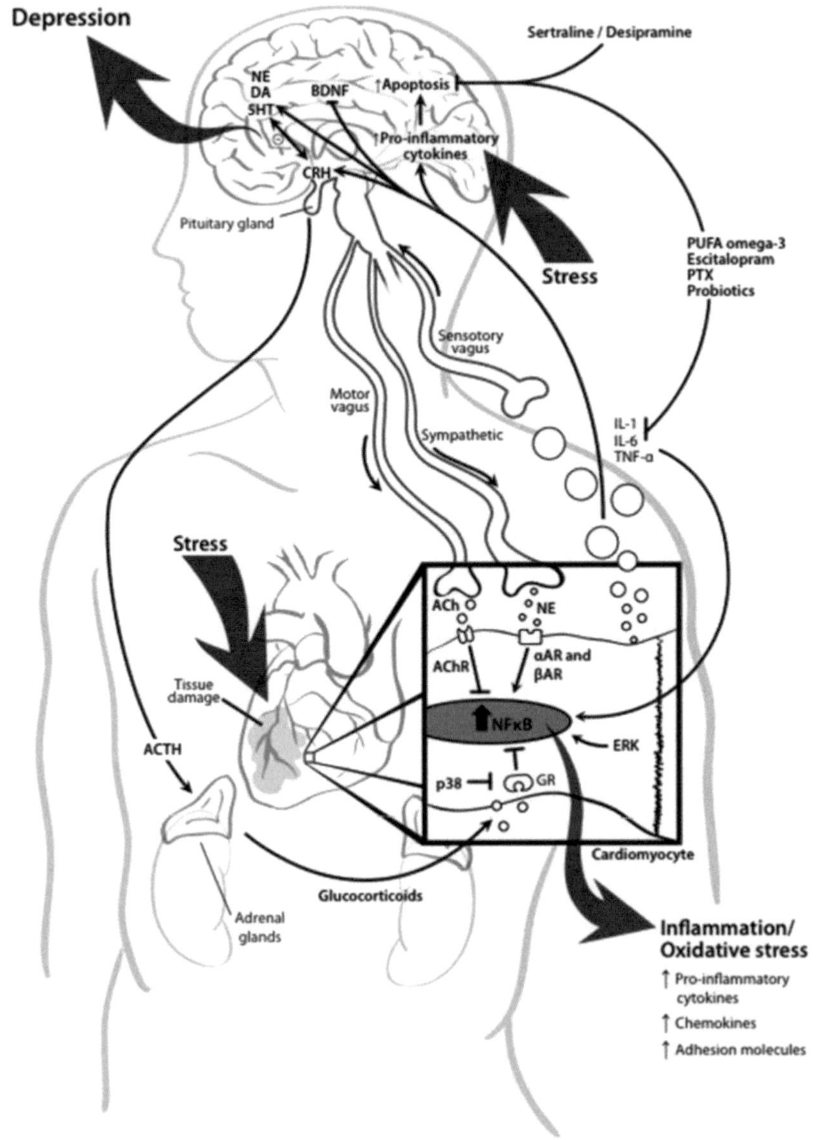

Fig. 7. Myocardial ischemia induces an increase in pro-inflammatory cytokines in the circulation and the limbic system. These cytokines may have access to brain via several routes (see text). Pro-inflammatory cytokines modulate different signaling pathways known to be involved in the development of depression including:

1. Presence of apoptosis and degenerating neurons;
2. Altered metabolism of neurotransmitters;
3. Reduction of neurogenesis by an action on BDNF.

Stress acting on heart, intestine or brain tissue contributes to the augmentation of pro-inflammatory cytokines by the activation of the NF-kB or the increase of the release norepinephrine.

Activation of different kinases such as P38 or MAP kinase inhibit the function of glucocorticoid receptor, releasing NF-kB from negative regulation by glucocorticoids released as a result of the HPA axis in response to stress.

PUFA-omega-3, PTX, escitalopram, probiotics reduce the circulating level of pro-inflammatory cytokines and apoptosis in the limbic system. These treatments as well as sertraline and desipramine could also attenuate the depressive-like behavior observed after myocardial infarction.

NE: Norepinephrine; DA: Dopamine; 5HT: Serotonin; BDNF: Brain-derived NEurotrophic Factor; CRH: corticotropin-releasing hormone; ACTH: adrenocorticotropic hormone; GR: Glucocorticoids receptor; AchR: Aceylcholine receptor, αAR; A-adrenergic receptor; βAR: b-adrenergic receptor, PTX: Pentoxifylline

6. References

Adams, J. M. (2003). "Ways of dying: multiple pathways to apoptosis." Genes Dev 17(20): 2481-2495.

Adrien, J., C. Dugovic, et al. (1991). "Sleep-wakefulness patterns in the helpless rat." Physiol Behav 49(2): 257-262.

Ahern, D. K., L. Gorkin, et al. (1990). "Biobehavioral variables and mortality or cardiac arrest in the Cardiac Arrhythmia Pilot Study (CAPS)." Am J Cardiol 66(1): 59-62.

Akbar, M., F. Calderon, et al. (2005). "Docosahexaenoic acid: a positive modulator of Akt signaling in neuronal survival." Proc Natl Acad Sci U S A 102(31): 10858-10863.

Amin, A. A., R. A. Menon, et al. (2008). "Acute coronary syndrome patients with depression have low blood cell membrane omega-3 fatty acid levels." Psychosom Med 70(8): 856-862.

Anda, R., D. Williamson, et al. (1993). "Depressed affect, hopelessness, and the risk of ischemic heart disease in a cohort of U.S. adults." Epidemiology 4(4): 285-294.

Arseneault-Bréard, J., I. Rondeau, et al. (2011). "Combination of Lactobacillus helveticus R0052 and Bifidobacterium longum R0175 reduces post-myocardial infarction depression symptoms and restores intestinal permeability in a rat model." Br J Nutr: 1-7.

Arunrut, T., H. Alejandre, et al. (2009). "Differential behavioral and neurochemical effects of exercise, reboxetine and citalopram with the forced swim test." Life Sci.

Bachis, A., M. I. Cruz, et al. (2008). "Chronic unpredictable stress promotes neuronal apoptosis in the cerebral cortex." Neurosci Lett 442(2): 104-108.

Bachis, A., A. Mallei, et al. (2008). "Chronic antidepressant treatments increase basic fibroblast growth factor and fibroblast growth factor-binding protein in neurons." Neuropharmacology.

Bah, T. M., M. Benderdour, et al. (2011). "Escitalopram reduces circulating pro-inflammatory cytokines and improves depressive behavior without affecting sleep in a rat model of post-cardiac infarct depression." Behav Brain Res 225(1): 243-251.

Bah, T.M., F. Laplante, B.P. Wann, R. Sullivan, G. Rousseau, R. Godbout (2010). "Paradoxical sleep insomnia and decreased cholinergic neurons after myocardial infarction in rats." Sleep 33(12): 1703-1710.

Bah, T.M., S. Kaloustian, R. Godbout, G. Rousseau.(2011b). ″Pretreatment with pentoxifylline has antidepressant-like effects in a rat model of acute myocardial infarction″. Behavioral Pharmacology 22(8): 779-784.

Banan, A., L. Zhang, et al. (2002). "PKC-zeta prevents oxidant-induced iNOS upregulation and protects the microtubules and gut barrier integrity." Am J Physiol Gastrointest Liver Physiol 283(4): G909-922.

Banks, W. A. (2001). "Anorectic effects of circulating cytokines: role of the vascular blood-brain barrier." Nutrition 17(5): 434-437.

Banks, W. A., A. J. Kastin, et al. (1995). "Passage of cytokines across the blood-brain barrier." Neuroimmunomodulation 2(4): 241-248.

Bao, A. M., G. Meynen, et al. (2008). "The stress system in depression and neurodegeneration: focus on the human hypothalamus." Brain Res Rev 57(2): 531-553.

Barefoot, J. C. and M. Schroll (1996). "Symptoms of depression, acute myocardial infarction, and total mortality in a community sample." Circulation 93(11): 1976-1980.

Bazan, N. G. (2009). "Cellular and molecular events mediated by docosahexaenoic acid-derived neuroprotectin D1 signaling in photoreceptor cell survival and brain protection." Prostaglandins Leukot Essent Fatty Acids 81(2-3): 205-211.

Benca, R. M., W. H. Obermeyer, et al. (1992). "Sleep and psychiatric disorders: A meta-analysis." Arch. Gen. Psychiatry 49: 651-668.

Bengtsson, B. O., J. Zhu, et al. (1992). "Effects of zimeldine and its metabolites, clomipramine, imipramine and maprotiline in experimental allergic neuritis in Lewis rats." J Neuroimmunol 39(1-2): 109-122.

Bluthe, R. M., N. Castanon, et al. (1999). "Central injection of IL-10 antagonizes the behavioural effects of lipopolysaccharide in rats." Psychoneuroendocrinology 24(3): 301-311.

Bluthe, R. M., K. W. Kelley, et al. (2006). "Effects of insulin-like growth factor-I on cytokine-induced sickness behavior in mice." Brain Behav Immun 20(1): 57-63.

Bras, M., B. Queenan, et al. (2005). "Programmed cell death via mitochondria: different modes of dying." Biochemistry (Mosc) 70(2): 231-239.

Budziszewska, B., L. Jaworska-Feil, et al. (2002). "Effect of antidepressant drugs on the human corticotropin-releasing-hormone gene promoter activity in neuro-2A cells." Pol J Pharmacol 54(6): 711-716.

Bürger, A., M. Benicke, et al. (2001). "Catecholamines stimulate IL-6 synthesis in rat cardiac fibroblasts." Am. J. Physiol. 281: H14-H21.

Bush, D. E., R. C. Ziegelstein, et al. (2001). "Even minimal symptoms of depression increase mortality risk after acute myocardial infarction." Am J Cardiol 88(4): 337-341.

Carvalho, L. A. and C. M. Pariante (2008). "In vitro modulation of the glucocorticoid receptor by antidepressants." Stress 11(6): 411-424.

Castren, E., H. Thoenen, et al. (1995). "Brain-derived neurotrophic factor messenger RNA is expressed in the septum, hypothalamus and in adrenergic brain stem nuclei of adult rat brain and is increased by osmotic stimulation in the paraventricular nucleus." Neuroscience 64(1): 71-80.

Cazzola, M., T. A. Tompkins, et al. (2010). "Immunomodulatory impact of a synbiotic in T(h)1 and T(h)2 models of infection." Ther Adv Respir Dis 4(5): 259-270.

Chalon, S. (2006). "Omega-3 fatty acids and monoamine neurotransmission." Prostaglandins Leukot Essent Fatty Acids 75(4-5): 259-269.

Chatelain, P., J. Latour, et al. (1987). "Neutrophil accumulation in experimental myocardial infarcts: relation with extent of injury and effect of reperfusion." Circulation 75: 1083-1090.

Chinnaiyan, A. M., K. Orth, et al. (1996). "Molecular ordering of the cell death pathway: Bcl-2 and Bcl-xL function upstream of the Ced-3 like apoptotic proteases." J. Biol. Chem. 271: 4573-4576.

Cho, L., M. Tsunoda, et al. (1999). "Effects of endotoxin and tumor necrosis factor alpha on regional brain neurotransmitters in mice." Nat Toxins 7(5): 187-195.

Connor, T. J. and B. E. Leonard (1998). "Depression, stress and immunological activation: the role of cytokines in depressive disorders." Life Sci 62(7): 583-606.

Crochemore, C., J. Lu, et al. (2005). "Direct targeting of hippocampal neurons for apoptosis by glucocorticoids is reversible by mineralocorticoid receptor activation." Mol Psychiatry 10(8): 790-798.

Cunningham, E. T., Jr. and E. B. De Souza (1993). "Interleukin 1 receptors in the brain and endocrine tissues." Immunol Today 14(4): 171-176.

Czeh, B., T. Michaelis, et al. (2001). "Stress-induced changes in cerebral metabolites, hippocampal volume, and cell proliferation are prevented by antidepressant treatment with tianeptine." Proc Natl Acad Sci U S A 98(22): 12796-12801.

Danjo, W., N. Fujimura, et al. (2008). "Effect of pentoxifylline on diaphragmatic contractility in septic rats." Acta Med Okayama 62(2): 101-107.

Dantzer, R. (2001). "Cytokine-induced sickness behavior: mechanisms and implications." Ann. NY Acad. Sci 933: 222-234.

de Lorgeril, M., G. Rousseau, et al. (1990). "Spacial and temporal profiles of neutrophil accumulation in the reperfused ischemic myocardium." Am J Cardiovasc Pathol 3(2): 143-154.

Delgado, P. L. (2004). "How antidepressants help depression: mechanisms of action and clinical response." J Clin Psychiatry 65 Suppl 4: 25-30.

Deten, A., H. C. Volz, et al. (2003). "Effect of propanolol on cardiac cytokine expression after myocardial infarction in rats." Mol. Cell. Biochem. 251: 127-137.

Deten, A. and H.-G. Zimmer (2002). "Heart function and cytokine expression is similar in mice and rats after myocardial infarction but differences occur in TNFα expression." Pflugers Arch - Eur. J. Physiol. 445: 289-296.

Dias, B. G., S. B. Banerjee, et al. (2003). "Differential regulation of brain derived neurotrophic factor transcripts by antidepressant treatments in the adult rat brain." Neuropharmacology 45(4): 553-563.

Diop, L., S. Guillou, et al. (2008). "Probiotic food supplement reduces stress-induced gastrointestinal symptoms in volunteers: a double-blind, placebo-controlled, randomized trial." Nutrition Research 28: 1-5.

Dowlati, Y., N. Herrmann, et al. (2009). "A Meta-Analysis of Cytokines in Major Depression." Biol Psychiatry.

Dranovsky, A. and R. Hen (2006). "Hippocampal neurogenesis: regulation by stress and antidepressants." Biol Psychiatry 59(12): 1136-1143.

Drevets, W. C. (2000). "Neuroimaging studies of mood disorders: implication for a neural model of major depression." Biol. Psychiatry 48: 813-829.

Duman, R. S. and L. M. Monteggia (2006). "A neurotrophic model for stress-related mood disorders." Biol Psychiatry 59(12): 1116-1127.

Dunn, A. J. (1992). "Endotoxin-induced activation of cerebral catecholamine and serotonin metabolism: comparison with interleukin-1." J Pharmacol Exp Ther 261(3): 964-969.

Dunn, A. J., A. H. Swiergiel, et al. (2005). "Cytokines as mediators of depression: what can we learn from animal studies?" Neurosci Biobehav Rev 29(4-5): 891-909.

Ferketich, A. K., J. A. Schwartzbaum, et al. (2000). "Depression as an antecedent to heart disease among women and men in the NHANES I study. National Health and Nutrition Examination Survey." Arch Intern Med 160(9): 1261-1268.

Fielding, R. (1991). "Depression and acute myocardial infarction: a review and reinterpretation." Soc Sci Med 32(9): 1017-1028.

Forrester, A. W., J. R. Lipsey, et al. (1992). "Depression following myocardial infarction." Int J Psychiatry Med 22(1): 33-46.

Francis, J., Y. Chu, et al. (2004). "Acute myocardial infarction induces hypothalamic cytokine synthesis." Am. J. Physiol. 286: H2264-H2271.

Francis, J., Z.-H. Zhang, et al. (2004). "Neural regulation of the proinflammatory cytokine response to acute myocardial infarction." Am. J. Physiol. 287: H791-H797.

Frangogiannis, N. G., C. W. Smith, et al. (2002). "The inflammatory response in myocardial infarction." Cardiovasc Res 53(1): 31-47.

Frasure-Smith, N., F. Lespérance, et al. (1993). "Depression following myocardial infarction. Impact on 6-month survival." JAMA 270(15): 1819-1825.

Frasure-Smith, N., F. Lespérance, et al. (1995). "The impact of negative emotions on prognosis following myocardial infarction: is it more than depression?" Health Psychol 14(5): 388-398.

Freedland, K. E., P. J. Lustman, et al. (1992). "Underdiagnosis of depression in patients with coronary artery disease: the role of nonspecific symptoms." Int J Psychiatry Med 22(3): 221-229.

Girard, S. A., T. M. Bah, et al. (2009). "Lactobacillus helveticus and Bifidobacterium longum taken in combination reduce the apoptosis propensity in the limbic system after myocardial infarction in a rat model." Br J Nutr 102(10): 1420-1425.

Glassman, A. H., S. P. Roose, et al. (1993). "The safety of tricyclic antidepressants in cardiac patients. Risk-benefit reconsidered." JAMA 269(20): 2673-2675.

Gould, E. and P. Tanapat (1999). "Stress and hippocampal neurogenesis." Biol Psychiatry 46(11): 1472-1479.

Grippo, A. J. and A. K. Johnson (2002). "Biological mechanisms in the relationship between depression and heart disease." Neurosci Biobehav Rev 26(8): 941-962.

Guck, T. P., M. G. Kavan, et al. (2001). "Assessment and treatment of depression following myocardial infarction." Am Fam Physician 64(4): 641-648.

Gutierrez-Reyes, G., P. Lopez-Ortal, et al. (2006). "Effect of pentoxifylline on levels of pro-inflammatory cytokines during chronic hepatitis C." Scand J Immunol 63(6): 461-467.

Gwechenberger, M., L. H. Mendoza, et al. (1999). "Cardiac myocytes produce interleukin-6 in culture and in viable border zone of reperfused infarctions." Circulation 99: 546-551.

Hansen, M. K., P. Taishi, et al. (1998). "Vagotomy blocks the induction of interleukin-1ß (IL-1ß) mRNA in the brain of rats in response to systemic IL-1ß." J. Neuroscience 18: 2247-2253.
Herbert, J., I. M. Goodyer, et al. (2006). "Do corticosteroids damage the brain?" J Neuroendocrinol 18(6): 393-411.
Herr, I., N. Gassler, et al. (2007). "Regulation of differential pro- and anti-apoptotic signaling by glucocorticoids." Apoptosis 12(2): 271-291.
Heumann, R. (1994). "Neurotrophin signalling." Curr Opin Neurobiol 4(5): 668-679.
Heuser, I. J., U. Schweiger, et al. (1996). "Pituitary-adrenal-system regulation and psychopathology during amitriptyline treatment in elderly depressed patients and normal comparison subjects." Am J Psychiatry 153(1): 93-99.
Heyes, M. P., K. Saito, et al. (1992). "Quinolinic acid and kynurenine pathway metabolism in inflammatory and non-inflammatory neurological disease." Brain 115 (Pt 5): 1249-1273.
Hillis, G. S., C. A. Terregino, et al. (2003). "Inflammatory cytokines provide limited early prognostic information in emergency department patients with suspected myocardial infarction." Ann. Emerg. Med. 42: 337-342.
Hirano, T. (1999). "Molecular basis underlying functional pleiotropy of cytokines and growth factors." Biochem Biophys Res Commun 260(2): 303-308.
Honig, A., R. Lousberg, et al. (1997). "[Depression following a first heart infarct; similarities with and differences from 'ordinary' depression]." Ned Tijdschr Geneeskd 141(4): 196-199.
Honig, A. and M. Maes (2000). "Psychoimmunology as a common pathogenic pathway in myocardial infarction, depression and cardiac death." Curr Opin Psychiatry 13: 661-664.
Huang, Y. Y., C. H. Peng, et al. (2007). "Desipramine activated Bcl-2 expression and inhibited lipopolysaccharide-induced apoptosis in hippocampus-derived adult neural stem cells." J Pharmacol Sci 104(1): 61-72.
Irwin, M. W., S. Mak, et al. (1999). "Tissue expression and immunolocalization of tumor necrosis factor-alpha in postinfarction dysfunctional myocardium." Circulation 99: 1492-1498.
Ivanova, S. A., V. Y. Semke, et al. (2007). "Signs of apoptosis of immunocompetent cells in patients with depression." Neurosci Behav Physiol 37(5): 527-530.
Jacobson, M. D., M. Weil, et al. (1997). "Programmed cell death in animal development." Cell 88(3): 347-354.
Jazayeri, S., M. Tehrani-Doost, et al. (2008). "Comparison of therapeutic effects of omega-3 fatty acid eicosapentaenoic acid and fluoxetine, separately and in combination, in major depressive disorder." Aust N Z J Psychiatry 42(3): 192-198.
Jeong, S. Y. and D. W. Seol (2008). "The role of mitochondria in apoptosis." BMB Rep 41(1): 11-22.
Joly, D. and D. J. Sanger (1986). "The effects of fluoxetine and zimeldine on the behavior of olfactory bulbectomized rats." Pharmacol Biochem Behav 24(2): 199-204.
Kaloustian, S., T. M. Bah, et al. (2009). "Tumor necrosis factor-alpha participates in apoptosis in the limbic system after myocardial infarction." Apoptosis 14(11): 1308-1316.
Kaloustian, S., B. P. Wann, et al. (2008). "Apoptosis time course in the limbic system after myocardial infarction in the rat." Brain Res 1216: 87-91.

Karege, F., G. Perret, et al. (2002). "Decreased serum brain-derived neurotrophic factor levels in major depressed patients." Psychiatry Res 109(2): 143-148.

Kato, K., T. Matsubara, et al. (1999). "Elevated levels of proinflammatory cytokines in coronary artery thrombi.." Int. J. Cardiol. 70: 267-273.

Katoh-Semba, R., I. K. Takeuchi, et al. (1997). "Distribution of brain-derived neurotrophic factor in rats and its changes with development in the brain." J Neurochem 69(1): 34-42.

Katon, W. and M. D. Sullivan (1990). "Depression and chronic medical illness." J Clin Psychiatry 51 Suppl: 3-11; discussion 12-14.

Katz, M. M., J. L. Tekell, et al. (2004). "Onset and early behavioral effects of pharmacologically different antidepressants and placebo in depression." Neuropsychopharmacology 29(3): 566-579.

Kawamoto, Y., S. Nakamura, et al. (1996). "Immunohistochemical localization of brain-derived neurotrophic factor in adult rat brain." Neuroscience 74(4): 1209-1226.

Kerr, J. F., A. H. Wyllie, et al. (1972). "Apoptosis: a basic biological phenomenon with wide-ranging implications in tissue kinetics." Br J Cancer 26(4): 239-257.

Kiecolt-Glaser, J. K. (2010). "Stress, food, and inflammation: psychoneuroimmunology and nutrition at the cutting edge." Psychosom Med 72(4): 365-369.

Kronfol, Z. and D. G. Remick (2000). "Cytokines and the brain: implications for clinical psychiatry." Am J Psychiatry 157(5): 683-694.

Krueger, J. M., M. L. Karnovsky, et al. (1984). "Peptidoglycans as promoters of slow-wave sleep. II. Somnogenic and pyrogenic activities of some naturally occurring muramyl peptides; correlations with mass spectrometric structure determination." J Biol Chem 259(20): 12659-12662.

Krugers, H. J., S. van der Linden, et al. (2007). "Dissociation between apoptosis, neurogenesis, and synaptic potentiation in the dentate gyrus of adrenalectomized rats." Synapse 61(4): 221-230.

Laflamme, N. and S. Rivest (1999). "An essential role of interleukin-1ß in mediatong NF-KB activity and COX-2 transcription in cells of the blood-brain barrier in response to a systemic and localized inflammation but not during endotoxemia." J. Neuroscience 19: 10923-10930.

Laghrissi-Thode, F., W. R. Wagner, et al. (1997). "Elevated platelet factor 4 and beta-thromboglobulin plasma levels in depressed patients with ischemic heart disease." Biol Psychiatry 42(4): 290-295.

Lai, M., J. A. McCormick, et al. (2003). "Differential regulation of corticosteroid receptors by monoamine neurotransmitters and antidepressant drugs in primary hippocampal culture." Neuroscience 118(4): 975-984.

Layé, S., R. M. Bluthé, et al. (1995). "Subdiaphramagtic vagotomy blocks induction of IL-1ß mRNA in mice brain in response to peripheral LPS." Am. J. Physiol. 268: R1327-R1331.

Leonard, B. E. (2000). "Evidence for a biochemical lesion in depression." J Clin Psychiatry 61 Suppl 6: 12-17.

Lespérance, F., N. Frasure-Smith, et al. (2011). "The efficacy of omega-3 supplementation for major depression: a randomized controlled trial." J Clin Psychiatry 72(8): 1054-1062.

Lespérance, F., N. Frasure-Smith, et al. (1996). "Major depression before and after myocardial infarction: its nature and consequences." Psychosom Med 58(2): 99-110.

Lespérance, F., N. Frasure-Smith, et al. (2002). "Five-year risk of cardiac mortality in relation to initial severity and one-year changes in depression symptoms after myocardial infarction." Circulation 105(9): 1049-1053.

Li, L. Y., X. Luo, et al. (2001). "Endonuclease G is an apoptotic DNase when released from mitochondria." Nature 412(6842): 95-99.

Li, R. C., B. W. Row, et al. (2003). "Cyclooxygenase 2 and intermittent hypoxia-induced spatial deficits in the rats." Am. J. Respir Crit. Care Med. 168: 469-475.

Lichtenstein, G. R., M. Bala, et al. (2002). "Infliximab improves quality of life in patients with Crohn's disease." Inflamm Bowel Dis 8(4): 237-243.

Littman, A. B. (1993). "Review of psychosomatic aspects of cardiovascular disease." Psychother Psychosom 60(3-4): 148-167.

Lorenzo, H. K. and S. A. Susin (2004). "Mitochondrial effectors in caspase-independent cell death." FEBS Lett 557(1-3): 14-20.

Lucassen, P. J., E. Fuchs, et al. (2004). "Antidepressant treatment with tianeptine reduces apoptosis in the hippocampal dentate gyrus and temporal cortex." Biol. Psych. 55: 789-796.

Lucassen, P. J., V. M. Heine, et al. (2006). "Stress, depression and hippocampal apoptosis." CNS Neurol Disord Drug Targets 5(5): 531-546.

Lucassen, P. J., M. B. Müller, et al. (2001). "Hippocampal apoptosis in major depression is a minor event and absent from subareas at risk for glucocorticoid overexposure." Am. J. Pathol. 158: 453-468.

Luo, X., I. Budihardjo, et al. (1998). "Bid, a Bcl2 interacting protein, mediates cytochrome c release from mitochondria in response to activation of cell surface death receptors." Cell 94(4): 481-490.

MacFarlane, M. and A. C. Williams (2004). "Apoptosis and disease: a life or death decision." EMBO Rep 5(7): 674-678.

Maes, M. (1995). "Evidence for an immune response in major depression: a review and hypothesis." Prog Neuropsychopharmacol Biol Psychiatry 19(1): 11-38.

Maes, M. (1999). "Major depression and activation of the inflammatory response system." Adv Exp Med Biol 461: 25-46.

Maes, M., E. Bosmans, et al. (1993). "Interleukin-1 beta: a putative mediator of HPA axis hyperactivity in major depression?" Am J Psychiatry 150(8): 1189-1193.

Malberg, J. E., A. J. Eisch, et al. (2000). "Chronic antidepressant treatment increases neurogenesis in adult rat hippocampus." J. Neuroscience 20: 9104-9110.

Mamalakis, G., M. Kiriakakis, et al. (2006). "Depression and serum adiponectin and adipose omega-3 and omega-6 fatty acids in adolescents." Pharmacol Biochem Behav 85(2): 474-479.

Marx, N., F. J. Neumann, et al. (1997). "Induction of cytokine expression in leukocytes in acute myocardial infarction." J. Am. Coll. Cardiol. 30: 165-170.

McKay, L. I. and J. A. Cidlowski (1999). "Molecular control of immune/inflammatory responses: interactions between nuclear factor-kappa B and steroid receptor-signaling pathways." Endocr Rev 20(4): 435-459.

McNamara, R. K. and S. E. Carlson (2006). "Role of omega-3 fatty acids in brain development and function: potential implications for the pathogenesis and prevention of psychopathology." Prostaglandins Leukot Essent Fatty Acids 75(4-5): 329-349.

Meneses, R., M. C. Almeida, et al. (2007). "Depression in patients with myocardial infarction." Rev Port Cardiol 26(11): 1143-1165.

Messaoudi, M., R. Lalonde, et al. (2011). "Assessment of psychotropic-like properties of a probiotic formulation (Lactobacillus helveticus R0052 and Bifidobacterium longum R0175) in rats and human subjects." Br J Nutr 105(5): 755-764.

Miller, A. H., C. M. Pariante, et al. (1999). "Effects of cytokines on glucocorticoid receptor expression and function. Glucocorticoid resistance and relevance to depression." Adv Exp Med Biol 461: 107-116.

Morikawa, O., N. Sakai, et al. (1998). "Effects of interferon-alpha, interferon-gamma and cAMP on the transcriptional regulation of the serotonin transporter." Eur J Pharmacol 349(2-3): 317-324.

Morris, R. (1984). "Developments of a water-maze procedure for studying spatial learning in the rat." J. Neuroscience Methods 11: 47-60.

Mossner, R., S. Daniel, et al. (2001). "Modulation of serotonin transporter function by interleukin-4." Life Sci 68(8): 873-880.

Mossner, R., A. Heils, et al. (1998). "Enhancement of serotonin transporter function by tumor necrosis factor alpha but not by interleukin-6." Neurochem Int 33(3): 251-254.

Mowla, S. J., H. F. Farhadi, et al. (2001). "Biosynthesis and post-translational processing of the precursor to brain-derived neurotrophic factor." J Biol Chem 276(16): 12660-12666.

Nahon, E., A. Israelson, et al. (2005). "Fluoxetine (Prozac) interaction with the mitochondrial voltage-dependent anion channel and protection against apoptotic cell death." FEBS Lett 579(22): 5105-5110.

Nibuya, M., M. Takahashi, et al. (1999). "Repeated stress increases catalytic TrkB mRNA in rat hippocampus." Neurosci Lett 267(2): 81-84.

Niiranen, A., R. Laaksonen, et al. (1988). "Behavioral assessment of patients treated with alpha-interferon." Acta Psychiatr Scand 78(5): 622-626.

O'Brien, S. M., L. V. Scott, et al. (2004). "Cytokines: abnormalities in major depression and implications for pharmacological treatment." Hum Psychopharmacol 19(6): 397-403.

Oprica, M., S. Zhu, et al. (2005). "Transgenic overexpression of interleukin-1 receptor antagonist in the CNS influences behaviour, serum corticosterone and brain monoamines." Brain Behav Immun 19(3): 223-234.

Orr, S. K. and R. P. Bazinet (2008). "The emerging role of docosahexaenoic acid in neuroinflammation." Curr Opin Investig Drugs 9(7): 735-743.

Overstreet, D. H., E. Friedman, et al. (2005). "The Flinders Sensitive Line rat: a selectively bred putative animal model of depression." Neurosci Biobehav Rev 29(4-5): 739-759.

Ozaki, K. and W. J. Leonard (2002). "Cytokine and cytokine receptor pleiotropy and redundancy." J Biol Chem 277(33): 29355-29358.

Pace, T. W. and A. H. Miller (2009). "Cytokines and glucocorticoid receptor signaling. Relevance to major depression." Ann N Y Acad Sci 1179: 86-105.

Palazzolo, D. L. and S. K. Quadri (1992). "Interleukin-1 inhibits serotonin release from the hypothalamus in vitro." Life Sci 51(23): 1797-1802.

Pan, Y. J., M. Knapp, et al. (2011). "Cost-effectiveness comparisons between antidepressant treatments in depression: Evidence from database analyses and prospective studies." J Affect Disord.

Pariante, C. M. (2006). "The glucocorticoid receptor: part of the solution or part of the problem?" J Psychopharmacol 20(4 Suppl): 79-84.

Pariante, C. M. and S. L. Lightman (2008). "The HPA axis in major depression: classical theories and new developments." Trends Neurosci 31(9): 464-468.

Pariante, C. M., B. D. Pearce, et al. (1997). "Steroid-independent translocation of the glucocorticoid receptor by the antidepressant desipramine." Mol Pharmacol 52(4): 571-581.

Pariante, C. M., B. D. Pearce, et al. (1999). "The proinflammatory cytokine, interleukin-1alpha, reduces glucocorticoid receptor translocation and function." Endocrinology 140(9): 4359-4366.

Peet, M., B. Murphy, et al. (1998). "Depletion of omega-3 fatty acid levels in red blood cell membranes of depressive patients." Biol Psychiatry 43(5): 315-319.

Penninx, B. W., A. T. Beekman, et al. (2001). "Depression and cardiac mortality: results from a community-based longitudinal study." Arch Gen Psychiatry 58(3): 221-227.

Pepin, M. C., S. Beaulieu, et al. (1989). "Antidepressants regulate glucocorticoid receptor messenger RNA concentrations in primary neuronal cultures." Brain Res Mol Brain Res 6(1): 77-83.

Politi, P., N. Brondino, et al. (2008). "Increased proapoptotic serum activity in patients with chronic mood disorders." Arch Med Res 39(2): 242-245.

Porsolt, R. D., G. Anton, et al. (1978a). "Behavioural despair in rats: a new model sensitive to antidepressant treatments." Eur J Pharmacol 47(4): 379-391.

Porsolt, R. D., A. Bertin, et al. (1978b). "Behavioural despair" in rats and mice: strain differences and the effects of imipramine." Eur J Pharmacol 51(3): 291-294.

Porsolt, R. D., M. le Pichon, et al. (1977). "Depression: a new animal model sensitive to antidepressant treatments." Nature 266: 730-732.

Pudil, R., V. Pidrman, et al. (1999). "Cytokines and adhesion molecules in the course of acute myocardial infarction." Clin Chim Acta 280(1-2): 127-134.

Raetsch, C., J. D. Jia, et al. (2002). "Pentoxifylline downregulates profibrogenic cytokines and procollagen I expression in rat secondary biliary fibrosis." Gut 50(2): 241-247.

Ramamoorthy, S., J. D. Ramamoorthy, et al. (1995). "Regulation of the human serotonin transporter by interleukin-1 beta." Biochem Biophys Res Commun 216(2): 560-567.

Redei, E. E., N. Ahmadiyeh, et al. (2001). "Novel animal models of affective disorders." Semin. Clin. Neuropsychiat 6: 43-67.

Reichenberg, A., R. Yirmiya, et al. (2001). "Cytokine-associated emotional and cognitive disturbances in humans." Arch Gen Psychiatry 58(5): 445-452.

Reyland, M. E. (2007). Protein kinase C and apoptosis. Apoptosis, Cell signaling , and human Diseases. R. Srivastava. Totowa, NJ, Humana Press. 2: 31-55.

Rivest, S. (2001). "How circulating cytokines trigger the neural circuits that control the hypothalamic-pituitary-adrenal axis." Psychoneuroendo 26: 761-788.

Rogatsky, I. and L. B. Ivashkiv (2006). "Glucocorticoid modulation of cytokine signaling." Tissue Antigens 68(1): 1-12.

Rogatsky, I., S. K. Logan, et al. (1998). "Antagonism of glucocorticoid receptor transcriptional activation by the c-Jun N-terminal kinase." Proc Natl Acad Sci U S A 95(5): 2050-2055.

Rondeau, I., S. Picard, et al. (2011). "Effects of different dietary omega-6/3 polyunsaturated fatty acids ratios on infarct size and the limbic system after myocardial infarction." Can J Physiol Pharmacol 89(3): 169-176.

Russo, S., I. P. Kema, et al. (2003). "Tryptophan as a link between psychopathology and somatic states." Psychosom Med 65(4): 665-671.

Saarelainen, T., P. Hendolin, et al. (2003). "Activation of the TrkB neurotrophin receptor is induced by antidepressant drugs and is required for antidepressant-induced behavioral effects." J Neurosci 23(1): 349-357.

Salvesen, G. S. and C. S. Duckett (2002). "IAP proteins: blocking the road to death's door." Nat Rev Mol Cell Biol 3(6): 401-410.

Santarelli, L., M. Saxe, et al. (2003). "Requirement of hippocampal neurogenesis for the behavioral effects of antidepressants." Science 301: 805-809.

Sapolsky, R. (1996). "Why stress is bad for your brain." Science 273: 749-750.

Sasaki, T., K. Kitagawa, et al. (2004). "Amelioration ofhippocampal neuronal damage after transient forebrain ischemia in cyclooxygenase-2-deficient mice." J. Cereb Blood Flow Metab. 24: 107-113.

Schins, A., H. J. Crijns, et al. (2007). "Altered omega-3 polyunsaturated fatty acid status in depressed post-myocardial infarction patients." Acta Psychiatr Scand 115(1): 35-40.

Schleifer, S. J., M. M. Macari-Hinson, et al. (1989). "The nature and course of depression following myocardial infarction." Arch Intern Med 149(8): 1785-1789.

Shi, Y. (2002). "Mechanisms of caspase activation and inhibition during apoptosis." Mol Cell 9(3): 459-470.

Sinha, R. A., P. Khare, et al. (2009). "Anti-apoptotic role of omega-3-fatty acids in developing brain: perinatal hypothyroid rat cerebellum as apoptotic model." Int J Dev Neurosci 27(4): 377-383.

Smith, R. S. (1991). "The macrophage theory of depression." Med Hypotheses 35(4): 298-306.

Song, C. and B. E. Leonard (2005). "The olfactory bulbectomised rat as a model of depression." Neurosci Biobehav Rev 29(4-5): 627-647.

Sprague, A. H. and R. A. Khalil (2009). "Inflammatory cytokines in vascular dysfunction and vascular disease." Biochem Pharmacol 78(6): 539-552.

Spriggs, D. R., M. L. Sherman, et al. (1988). "Recombinant human tumor necrosis factor administered as a 24-hour intravenous infusion. A phase I and pharmacologic study." J Natl Cancer Inst 80(13): 1039-1044.

Stock, H. S., K. Ford, et al. (2000). "Gender and gonadal hormone effects in the olfactory bulbectomy animal model of depression." Pharmacol. Biochem. Behav. 67: 183-191.

Strakowski, S. M., C. M. Adler, et al. (2002). "Volumetric MRI studies of mood disorders: do they distinguish unipolar and bipolar disorder?" Bipolar Disorders. 4: 80-88.

Sugawara, T., M. Fujimura, et al. (1999). "Mitochondrial release of cytochrome c corresponds to the selective vulnerability of hippocampal CA1 neurons in rats after transient global cerebral ischemia." J Neurosci 19(22): RC39.

Sutcigil, L., C. Oktenli, et al. (2007). "Pro- and anti-inflammatory cytokine balance in major depression: effect of sertraline therapy." Clin Dev Immunol 2007: 76396.

Szelenyi, J. and E. S. Vizi (2007). "The catecholamine cytokine balance: interaction between the brain and the immune system." Ann N Y Acad Sci 1113: 311-324.

Szuster-Ciesielska, A., M. Slotwinska, et al. (2008). "Accelerated apoptosis of blood leukocytes and oxidative stress in blood of patients with major depression." Prog Neuropsychopharmacol Biol Psychiatry 32(3): 686-694.

Takadera, T., H. Yumoto, et al. (2002). "Prostaglandin E2 induces caspase-dependent apoptosis in rat cortical cells." Neurosciences Letters 317: 61-64.

Tchelingerian, J. L., M. Monge, et al. (1995). "Differential oligodendroglial expression of the tumor necrosis factor receptors in vivo and in vitro." J Neurochem 65(5): 2377-2380.

ter Horst, G. J., G. J. Nagel, et al. (1997). Selective blood brain barrier dysfunction after intravenous injection of rTNFα in the rat. Neurochemistry; Cellular, molecular and clinical aspects. A. Teelken and J. Korf. New York, Plenum Press.

Thorburn, A. (2004). "Death receptor-induced cell killing." Cell Signal 16(2): 139-144.

Turnbull, A. V. and C. Rivier (1995). "Regulation of the HPA axis by cytokines." Brain Behav Immun 9(4): 253-275.

Tziakas, D. N., G. K. Chalikias, et al. (2003). "Anti-inflammatory cytokine profile in acute coronary syndromes: behavior of interleukin-10 in association with serum metalloproteinases and proinflammatory cytokines." Inter. J. Cardiol. 92: 169-175.

van Riezen, H. and B. E. Leonard (1991). Effect of psychotropic drugs on the behavior and neurochemistry of olfactory bulbectomized rats. Psychopharmacology of anxiolytics and antidepressants. F. E. New York, Pergamon: 231-250.

Vitkovic, L., J. Bockaert, et al. (2000). ""Inflammatory" cytokines: neuromodulators in normal brain?" J Neurochem 74(2): 457-471.

Vogel, G., D. Neill, et al. (1990). "A new animal model of endogenous depression: a summary of present findings." Neurosci Biobehav Rev 14(1): 85-91.

Wagar, L. E., C. P. Champagne, et al. (2009). "Immunomodulatory properties of fermented soy and dairy milks prepared with lactic acid bacteria." J Food Sci 74(8): M423-430.

Wang, S. and W. S. El-Deiry (2003). "TRAIL and apoptosis induction by TNF-family death receptors." Oncogene 22(53): 8628-8633.

Wann, B. P., T. M. Bah, et al. (2007). "Vulnerability for apoptosis in the limbic system after myocardial infarction in rats: a possible model for human postinfarct major depression." J Psychiatry Neurosci 32(1): 11-16.

Wann, B. P., T. M. Bah, et al. (2009). "Behavioural signs of depression and apoptosis in the limbic system following myocardial infarction: effects of sertraline." J Psychopharmacol 23(4): 451-459.

Wann, B. P., S. G. Béland, et al. (2004). "Permeability in the limbic system following myocardial infarction in the rat." Society for Neuroscience 34th Annual meeting: #568.564.

Wann, B. P., M. Boucher, et al. (2006). "Apoptosis detected in the amygdala following myocardial infarction in the rat." Biol Psychiatry 59(5): 430-433.

Wetmore, C., Y. H. Cao, et al. (1991). "Brain-derived neurotrophic factor: subcellular compartmentalization and interneuronal transfer as visualized with anti-peptide antibodies." Proc Natl Acad Sci U S A 88(21): 9843-9847.

Wichers, M. and M. Maes (2002). "The psychoneuroimmuno-pathophysiology of cytokine-induced depression in humans." Int J Neuropsychopharmacol 5(4): 375-388.

Willner, P. (2005). "Chronic mild stress (CMS) revisited: consistency and behavioural-neurobiological concordance in the effects of CMS." Neuropsychobiology 52(2): 90-110.

Willner, P., A. Towell, et al. (1987). "Reduction of sucrose preference by chronic unpredictable mild stress, and its restoration by tricyclic antidepressant." Psychopharmacology 93: 358-364.

Wilson, D. R. and L. Warise (2008). "Cytokines and their role in depression." Perspect Psychiatr Care 44(4): 285-289.

Wirleitner, B., G. Neurauter, et al. (2003). "Interferon-gamma-induced conversion of tryptophan: immunologic and neuropsychiatric aspects." Curr Med Chem 10(16): 1581-1591.

Wong, E. Y. and J. Herbert (2004). "The corticoid environment: a determining factor for neural progenitors' survival in the adult hippocampus." Eur J Neurosci 20(10): 2491-2498.

Worrall, N. K., K. Chang, et al. (1997). "TNF-α causes reversible in vivo systemic vascular barrier dysfunction via NO-dependent and -independent mechanisms." Am. J. Physiol. 273: H2565-H2574.

Wu, E. Q., P. E. Greenberg, et al. (2009). "Treatment persistence, healthcare utilisation and costs in adult patients with major depressive disorder: a comparison between escitalopram and other SSRI/SNRIs." J Med Econ 12(2): 124-135.

Wyllie, A. H., J. F. Kerr, et al. (1980). "Cell death: the significance of apoptosis." Int Rev Cytol 68: 251-306.

Xia, Z., J. W. DePierre, et al. (1996). "Tricyclic antidepressants inhibit IL-6, IL-1 beta and TNF-alpha release in human blood monocytes and IL-2 and interferon-gamma in T cells." Immunopharmacology 34(1): 27-37.

Yirmiya, R., Y. Pollak, et al. (2000). "Illness, Cytokines, and depression." Ann. NY Acad. Sci USA 917: 478-487.

Yu, C.-M., K. W.-H. Lai, et al. (2003). "Expression of macrophage migration inhibitory factor in acute ischemic myocardial injury." J. Histochem. Cytochem. 51: 625-631.

Yu, S., F. Holsboer, et al. (2008). "Neuronal actions of glucocorticoids: focus on depression." J Steroid Biochem Mol Biol 108(3-5): 300-309.

Yuan, J. and B. A. Yankner (2000). "Apoptosis in the nervous system." Nature 407(6805): 802-809.

Zhang, J. and S. Rivest (1999). "Distribution, regulation and colocalization of the genes encoding the EP2- and EP4-PGE2 receptors in the rat brain and neuronal responses to systemic inflammation." Eur J Neurosci 11(8): 2651-2668.

Zobel, A. W., T. Nickel, et al. (2001). "Cortisol response in the combined dexamethasone/CRH test as predictor of relapse in patients with remitted depression. a prospective study." J Psychiatr Res 35(2): 83-94.

Zorrilla, E. P., G. R. Valdez, et al. (2001). "Changes in levels of regional CRF-like-immunoreactivity and plasma corticosterone during protracted drug withdrawal in dependent rats." Psychopharmacology (Berl) 158(4): 374-381.

20

Cytochrome P450 Epoxygenase *CYP2J2* G-50T Polymorphism is an Independent Genetic Prognostic Risk Factor and Interacts with Smoking Cessation After Index Premature Myocardial Infarction

Ping-Yen Liu[1,2], Yi-Heng Li[1] and Jyh-Hong Chen[1]
[1]*Division of Cardiology, Departments of Internal Medicine,*
[2]*Institute of Clinical Medicine, National Cheng Kung University Hospital, Tainan*
Taiwan

1. Introduction

Cytochrome P450 epoxygenases metabolize arachidonic acid to epoxyeicosatrienoic acids (EETs). One human cytochrome P450 enzyme, *CYP2J2*, is abundantly expressed in coronary artery endothelial and smooth muscle cells, and in cardiac myocytes (Wu et al., 1996; Imig, 2000). One of the primary products of the NADPH-dependent epoxidation of arachidonic acid by CYP2J2 is the production of 11, 12-EET. This eicosanoid has potential anti-inflammatory effects by inhibiting endothelial nuclear factor- B, a transcription factor associated with the induction of many pro-inflammatory gene products in the vasculature (Imig, 2000; Node et al., 1999). Other EETs, including 5,6-, 8,9-, 11,12-, and 14,15-EETs have important vasodilatation properties via mechanism of smooth muscle cells relaxation (Fang et al., 2002; Pinto et al., 1987; Spieker & Liao, 2005; Liu et al., 2006). More recently, the additional vascular protective effects of EETs, including anti-thrombotic, antimigratory, antioxidant, and antiapoptotic effects, have also been observed (Gauthier et al., 2004; Sun et al., 2002).

Recently, a novel genetic variant G-50T of this novel gene *CYP2J2* was found to be associated with coronary artery disease (CAD) (Spieker et al., 2004). This mutation could functionally result in the loss of binding of the Sp1 transcription factor to the *CYP2J2* promoter and a decreased activity in *CYP2J2* promoter. The plasma concentrations of stable EETs metabolites were also lower in individuals with the G-50T polymorphism. However, the role of this novel gene variant in myocardial infarction (MI), especially premature MI, is still not well investigated.

Of the common environmental factors known to be associated with risk of acute MI, smoking is widely acknowledged to make a major contribution (Manson et al., 1992; Teng et al., 1994). Smoking can disturb lipoprotein metabolism by increasing insulin resistance and lipid intolerance, and is implicated in the production of small dense low-density lipoprotein (Craig et al., 1989; Eliasson et al., 1997; Barua et al., 2002). The smoking-associated risk of MI has been reported to be greater in subgrouping subjects with several genetic variants background (Li et al., 2002; Liu et al., 2005; Humphries et al., 2002).

We thus hypothesized that those who with the T allele may have higher inflammatory status, and thus have higher risk for plaque rupture or occurrence of MI, especially at a younger age. We also speculated that there should be an additive interaction between the effect of smoking behavior and the genetic variation for the onset of premature MI.

Smoking cessation could gradually improve the endothelial function and fibrinolytic status (Tsiara et al., 2003). However, successful cessation of smoking after MI and its interaction with this candidate gene for the subsequent events after index MI was still undefined. Thus, we hypothesized that premature MI patients carrying genetic polymorphism, especially genetic variant G-50T of this novel gene *CYP2J2*, might have a higher risk for subsequent coronary events. In addition, smoking cessation might interact with these gene variations for the prognosis after patients' index MI in Taiwan.

2. Methods

2.1 Study subjects

2.1.1 Study population

We enrolled 200 patients (mean age 42.2±2.5 years; 84% men) with documented MI onset prior to age of 45 years. The patients were recruited after their first MI. Diagnosis of MI was based on ischemic chest symptoms, typical electrocardiographic changes and elevation of serum creatine kinase and its MB isoenzyme, when more than twice the upper level of normal. Coronary angiography was performed using the Judkin's method within 2 weeks after the onset of symptoms. Coronary stenosis is defined as ≥ 50% diameter narrowing.

2.1.2 Control population

The control group was recruited by sex-matched 200 patients (mean age 42.5±2.1 years) from consecutive subjects admitted to our hospital for routine health examinations. They did not show any clinical or electrocardiographic evidence of MI or CAD. They also had no history of cerebrovascular disease or peripheral arterial disease. Written informed consents were obtained from all patients and this study was in agreement with guidelines approved by the research committee of National Cheng-Kung University Hospital.

2.1.3 Background of population

All patients and controls included in this study are Han Chinese/Taiwanese from the same geographic area. The demographic data and the presence of traditional coronary risk factors, including hypertension, diabetes mellitus, smoking and serum cholesterol, were collected from all study participants.

2.1.4 Data collection & history recording

For patients with MI, these data were taken from the medical records at the time of admission for acute MI; for control subjects, they were collected at the time of hospital admission for routine health examinations. They were considered to have hypertension if elevated blood pressure (>140/90 mmHg) were measured on 3 occasions or if they were already being treated with anti-hypertensive agents. They were defined as having diabetes mellitus (DM) if they had a fasting blood glucose level > 110 mg/dl or were already being treated for DM. All study participants were classified as either smokers (including current or ex-smokers) or non-smokers. The total cholesterol level was determined at the beginning of the study.

2.1.5 Blood collection

The blood sampling time in the study group was at least 2 weeks after the onset of acute MI. In the control group, the blood samples were taken during coronary angiography study. All patients with impaired renal function, malignancy, connective tissue disease or chronic inflammatory disease were excluded. The blood samples were drawn into a 5-ml EDTA glass tube and centrifuged at 2200 g for 15 minutes to separate the plasma contents. The buffy coat after centrifugation was obtained and deoxyribonucleic acid (DNA) in each sample was isolated by the method we used before (Liu et al., 2007). The DNA samples were stored at -70 degree C until use.

2.1.6 Genomic amplification by PCR

Patient's DNA was isolated from the whole-blood samples by the phenol-chloroform extraction method. A 273-bp promoter region proximal to the transcriptional start site was amplified with primers described previously (King et al., 2002). The sequence products were resolved on an ABI 377 automated sequencer. The promoter polymorphism G-50T was verified by direct sequencing. The numbering of the polymorphisms refers to the GenBank sequence AF272142 (accession number).

2.1.7 Functional EET analysis

Eicosanoids were extracted from plasma samples 3 times with ethyl acetate after acidification with acetic acid. After evaporation, saponification with 0.4*N* KOH in methanol, and re-extraction, concentrations of the stable EETs metabolite 14,15-dihydroxyeicosatrienoic acid (DHET) were determined by an ELISA kit (Detroit R&D) (Liu et al., 2007; Spieker et al., 2004).

2.1.8 Smoking habits definition

Individuals were classified according to their smoking status; a current smoker was defined as any person who smoked regularly (at least one cigarette per day and/or one cigar or one pipe per week). Subjects who had smoked at least one cigarette per day and/or one cigar or one pipe per week in the past were classified as former smokers. Never smokers were those who had never smoked any tobacco product regularly. Subjects were considered to have achieved smoking cessation if they were reported non-smoking from the quitting day until the end of the 6-month period.

2.1.9 Follow-up study

Patients received regular follow-up care in our cardiology ward or clinics for at least 6 months with a maximum of 13 years or until occurrence of one of the following coronary events: recurrent angina pectoris, non-fatal MI, or cardiac death. Recurrent angina pectoris was defined as recurrent chest pain with ischemic ECG changes lasting >10 min despite antiangina therapy. Diagnosis of recurrent MI was the same as for index MI (see Study population). Cause of death was determined from hospital records. In this study, the follow-up data were available for a total of 162 (95.3%) premature MI patients. Eight patients (4.7%) were not available for follow-up. The reasons included: 3 (1.8%) patients moved back to their primary residency region and we were unable to follow-up; 3 (1.8%) patients died of non-cardiovascular events, including two (1.2%) in traffic accidents and one (0.6%) by suicide; two (1.2%) patients were lost or changed their telephone numbers without detailed medical records. Those event-free patients who we were unable to follow-up completely were included in the event-free group. Their follow-up periods were defined between the index MI and their last clinic visit.

2.1.10 Statistical analysis

Data on age and cholesterol levels were presented as mean value ± standard deviation (SD). The values of DHET were presented as median ± SD. The difference between the groups was analyzed by the unpaired Student's t test. The differences in the frequencies of smoking, hypertension, hyperlipidemia, diabetes mellitus, and *CYP2J2* G-50T genotypes were analyzed by Fisher's exact test. χ^2 analyses were used to test deviations of genotype distribution from Hardy-Weinberg equilibrium and to determine allele or genotype frequencies between patients and control groups. The risk factors that appear to be possible significant predictors ($p<0.05$) in the single-variant analyses were included in the multiple logistic regression analyses. Multivariate analyses were conducted with multiple logistic regression methods, and adjusted estimations of conditioned relative risk and 95% confidence intervals (CIs) were done. The Kaplan–Meier method (log-rank test) was applied in subsequent event-free analysis. All statistical analyses were performed using SPSS Advanced Statistics 13.0 for Window. In this study, a value of $p<0.05$ was taken to be statistical significance.

3. Results

3.1 Comparison of traditional CAD risk factors between MI and control groups

We compared the control and premature MI group for traditional CAD risk factors, including hypertension, diabetes mellitus, smoking and serum cholesterol levels (Table 1).

Characteristics	Control (n=200)	Premature MI (n=200)
Age (yrs)	42.5±2.1	42.2±2.1
Men/Women	167/33	168/32
Systemic hypertension (%)	46 (23.0)	60 (30.0) †
Diabetes mellitus (%)	9 (4.5)	26 (13.0)*
Smoker (%)	89 (44.5)	154 (77.0)*
Total cholesterol (mg/dL)	182±37.5	210±34.5
Triglycerides (mg/dL)	135±32.1	136±30.8
HDL cholesterol (mg/dL)	46±10.5	41±10.1
LDL cholesterol (mg/dL)	120±29.3	128±21.5

Data are presented as number (%) of patients or mean ± standard deviation. HDL = high-density lipoprotein; LDL = low-density lipoprotein; MI = myocardial infarction. *: $p<0.001$; †: $p<0.01$.

Table 1. Clinical characteristics of study subjects

There were no significant differences in the age between these 2 groups (p = 0.890). The frequency of smoking (p <0.001), diabetes mellitus (p <0.001) and hypertension (p <0.01) were significantly higher in premature MI patients. However, the traditional CAD risk factor such as total cholesterol level was similar between 2 groups.

3.2 Distribution of CYP2J2 G-50T genotypes

Table 2 shows the distribution of *CYP2J2* G-50T genotype in both premature MI patients and control subjects. The frequency of the T allele was significantly higher in the premature MI than the control group (16.0% vs. 12.0%, p<0.01; odds ratio (OR) 2.15, 95% [CI] 1.30 to 6.80). There was a significantly higher prevalence of the T allele genotype (GT+TT) among patients with premature MI in comparison to the control subjects (28.0% vs. 22.0%; OR 2.0, 95% [CI] 1.3 to 6.8, p = 0.01). The distributions of genotype in both the premature MI group and control group were compatible with the Hardy-Weinberg equilibrium.

	Control (n=200)	Premature MI (n=200)	OR (95% CI)	P value
TT	4 (2.0)	8 (4.0)		
GT	40 (20.0)	48 (24.0)		
TT+GT	44 (22.0)	56 (28.0)	2.0 (1.3-6.8)	0.01
GG	156 (78.0)	144 (72.0)		
T allele frequency	0.12	0.16		0.01

Data are presented as number (%) of patients. CI = confidence interval; GG = homozygous G allele of *CYP2J2* G-50T gene; GT = heterozygous allele of *CYP2J2* G-50T gene; MI = myocardial infarction; TT = homozygous T allele of *CYP2J2* G-50T gene; OR = odds ratio.

Table 2. Frequency of genotypes of *CYP2J2* G-50T gene in control subjects and patients with premature myocardial infarction

3.3 Identification of independent risk factors of MI

Table 3 shows the results of multiple logistic regression analysis for identifying the independent risk factors of premature MI. Hypertension, DM, smoking and *CYP2J2* genotype were all used as independent variables. Multiple logistic regression analysis showed that the T allele was an independent risk factor (OR 1.78, 95% CI 1.12 to 6.40, p = 0.02), as well as smoking (OR 3.05, 95% CI 1.55 to 7.25, p<0.01), diabetes mellitus (OR 3.24, 95% CI 1.22 to 6.55, p<0.01) and hypertension (OR 1.95, 95% CI 1.13 to 5.73, p<0.01) for the premature onset of MI.

	OR for MI	95% CI	P value
Smoking	3.05	1.55-7.25	<0.01
Diabetes mellitus	3.24	1.22-6.55	<0.01
Hypertension	1.95	1.13-5.73	<0.01
CYP2J2 G-50T polymorphism	1.78	1.12-6.40	0.02

CI = confidence interval; GG = homozygous G allele of *CYP2J2* G-50T gene; GT = heterozygous allele of *CYP2J2* G-50T gene; MI = myocardial infarction; TT = homozygous T allele of *CYP2J2* G-50T gene; OR = odds ratio.

Table 3. Risk factors of premature myocardial infarction identified by multiple logistic regression analysis

Moreover, there was a synergistic effect between smoking and T allele of *CYP2J2* genotype on the occurrence of MI. (Table 4.) Among patients who did not smoke, the T allele was associated with a higher risk of young MI (OR 1.43, 95% CI 1.2 to 6.2). Smoking carrier with the G allele was associated with a 3-fold higher risk for premature MI (OR 3.78, 95% CI 3.3 to 10.6). Furthermore, smoking carriers of the T allele of *CYP2J2* allele had a significantly 5.6-fold higher risk of premature MI (OR 5.55, 95% CI 4.3 to 13.7) when compared with non-smoking and G allele genotype carriers.

Smoking	*CYP2J2* G-50T genotype	Control (n=200)	Premature MI (n=200)	OR	95% CI
No	GG	87	36	1	
No	GT+TT	24	10	1.43	1.2-6.2
Yes	GG	69	108	3.78	3.3-10.6
Yes	GT+TT	20	46	5.55	4.3-13.7

Data are presented as number of patients. CI = confidence interval; GG = homozygous G allele of *CYP2J2* G-50T gene; GT = heterozygous allele of *CYP2J2* G-50T gene; MI = myocardial infarction; TT = homozygous T allele of *CYP2J2* G-50T gene; OR = odds ratio

Table 4. Association between smoking and *CYP2J2* G-50T genotype on premature myocardial infarction

3.4 Functional analysis of EET metabolites

To further investigate the functional role of the G-50T polymorphism, we measured the plasma concentrations of the major *CYP2J2*-dependent epoxidation product from arachidonic acid. Given the instability of the primary products, EETs, concentration of the stable metabolite 14,15-DHET was determined after extraction from plasma samples. Median DHET plasma concentrations were significantly lower in samples from premature MI subjects with the G-50T polymorphism when compared with G allele individuals (6.2 ± 1.2 ng/mL vs. 10.8 ± 2.5 ng/mL; p = 0.025). Among premature MI subjects, the median DHET plasma concentrations were significantly lower among smoking carriers with the G-50T polymorphism (3.3 ± 1.0 ng/mL vs. 6.8 ± 1.3 ng/mL; p = 0.001). However, this effect was not significant for subjects without gene variation (G allele carriers) (10.2 ± 1.3 ng/mL vs. 10.8 ± 2.4 ng/mL; p = 0.18). (Fig 1)

Median DHET plasma concentrations were significantly lower in samples from premature MI subjects with the G-50T polymorphism when compared with G allele individuals. Among premature MI subjects, the median DHET plasma concentrations were significantly lower among smoking carriers with the G-50T polymorphism. However, this effect was not significant for subjects without gene variation (G allele carriers). Median DHET levels were significantly lower among *CYP2J2* G-50T polymorphism compared with G allele individuals. The median DEHT levels were significantly lower among smoking carriers with T allele subjects, but not among G allele ones. DHET = dihydroxyeicosatrienoic acid; MI = myocardial infarction.

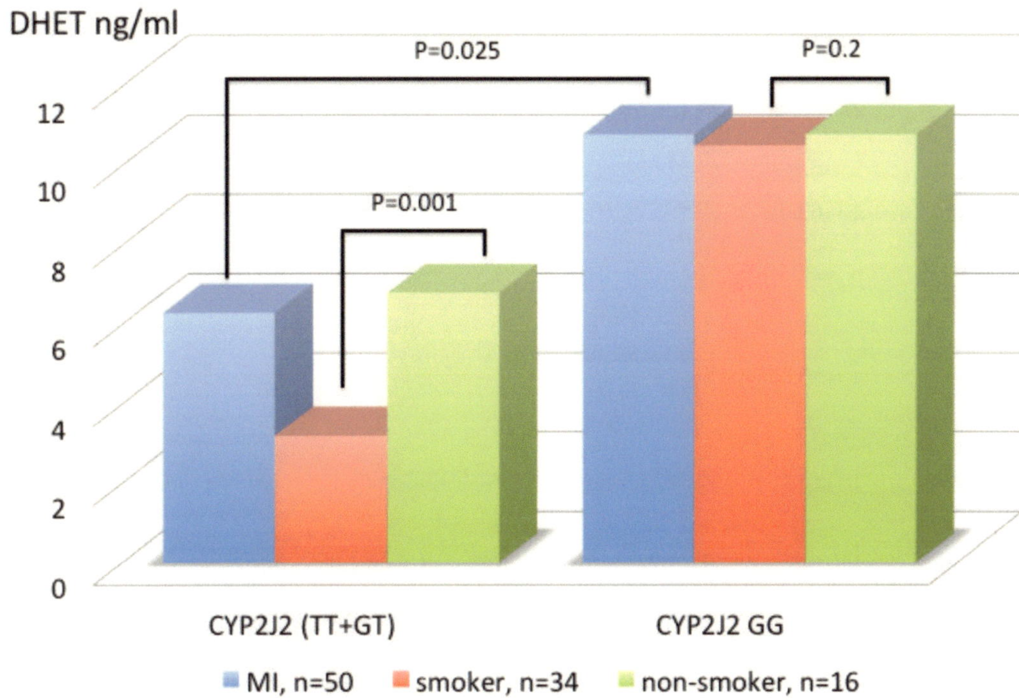

Fig. 1. Plasma concentrations of the 14, 15-dihydroxyeicosatrienoic acid (DHET), a major *CYP2J2*-dependent epoxidation product from arachidonic acid among premature myocardial infarction subjects.

3.5 The follow-up clinical and angiographic characteristics analyses

During a mean period of 4.43 years (from 0.5 to 13 years) follow-up, cardiac events occurred in 48 (28.2%) patients, including four (2.4%) with cardiac death, 24 (14.1%) with recurrent MI, and 20 (11.7%) with recurrent angina pectoris. The baseline and the available follow-up clinical and angiographic characteristics are shown in Table 5.

With similar mean follow-up periods, most of the clinical manifestations and treatment regimens were no different before and after follow-up in both groups that with-event and without-event, except that usage frequencies of both angiotensin-converting enzyme inhibitors (ACEI) and statin were higher after follow-up in both groups ($P < 0.05$, compared with their baseline data). Under these therapeutic profiles, patients' blood pressures and fasting sugar levels were also similar in both groups after follow-up. Almost 92% of our follow-up subjects received catheterization study. The prevalence distribution of the culprit coronary artery lesion changed among patients receiving follow-up coronary angiography (Table 5).

During the first catheterization study, most (48/84, 57.1%) patients had the culprit lesion located in the left anterior descending artery, followed by a right coronary artery lesion. However, during the late angiographic study, 31.3% of the initial culprit lesions regressed, while 33.8% of the new *De novo* lesions became culprit ones.

	With cardiac events (n=48, 30.0%)			Without cardiac events (n=114, 70.0%)		
	Initial treatment	Final treatment	P value	Initial treatment	Final treatment	P value
Hypertension	29 (60.4)	31 (64.5)	0.14	36 (31.5)	38 (33.3)	0.15
Diabetes mellitus	19 (39.5)	21 (43.8)	0.08	20 (17.5)	28 (24.5)	0.06
Smoking	40 (83.3)	32 (66.7)	0.04	100 (87.7)	43 (37.7)	0.01
Total cholesterol, mg/dL	204±33.5	208±32.7	0.24	207±36.1	207±40.7	0.36
HDL-cholesterol, mg/dL	42±10	44±11	0.38	43±9	44±12	0.33
LDL-cholesterol, mg/dL	135±32	137±40	0.28	136±29	137±39	0.54
Triglycerides, mg/dL	132±36	137±56	0.42	135±43	136±56	0.77
LVEF (%)	58.8±9.8	57.9±10.1	0.35	60.1±13.5	59.1±11.5	0.40
Angiography	43 (89.9)	44 (91.6)	0.67	100 (87.7)	94 (82.4)	0.58
PCI	25 (52.0)	29 (60.4)	0.44	60 (52.6)	59 (51.7)	0.38
CABG	6 (12.5)	8 (16.7)	0.40	18 (15.8)	19 (16.7)	0.28
CAD						
Single-vessel	24 (50.0)	26 (54.1)	0.32	64 (56.1)	60 (52.6)	0.85
LAD	16	10		34	26	
LCX	3	7		9	15	
RCA	5	9		21	19	
Double-vessel	13 (27.1)	13 (27.1)	1.00	30 (26.3)	32 (28.0)	0.61
Triple-vessel	10 (20.8)	8 (16.7)	0.44	22 (19.2)	23 (20.1)	0.22
Medications						
β-blocker	19 (39.5)	24 (50.0)	0.06	91 (79.8)	97 (85.0)	0.10
ACEI	10 (20.8)	20 (41.6)	0.04	69 (60.5)	80 (70.1)	0.06
Statin	10 (20.8)	18 (37.5)	0.03	42 (36.8)	60 (52.6)	0.04

With similar mean follow-up periods, most of the clinical manifestations and treatment regimens were no different before and after follow-up in both groups that with-event and without-event, except that usage frequencies of both angiotensin-converting enzyme inhibitors and statin were higher after follow-up in both groups. Under these therapeutic profiles, patients' blood pressures and fasting sugar levels were also similar in both groups after follow-up. Values are expressed as number (%) or mean ± SD. ACEI = angiotensin-converting enzyme inhibitor; CABG = coronary artery bypass graft surgery; CAD = coronary artery disease; CI = confidence intervals; ECG = electrocardiograms; HDL = high density lipoproteins; LAD = left anterior descending artery; LCX = left circumflex artery; LDL = low density lipoproteins; LVEF = left ventricular ejection fraction; MI = myocardial infarction; PCI = percutaneous coronary interventions; RCA = right coronary artery.

Table 5. The initial and follow-up clinical and angiographic characteristics of patients with premature myocardial infarction

Compared with event-free group, subjects with event during the follow-up period had significantly higher genetic prevalence rate of T allele (TT+GT) (Event vs. event-free subjects: 58.3% vs. 42.1%, p=0.02) as well as the whole T allele frequency (Event vs. event-free: 42.7% vs. 29.8%, p=0.02).

CYP2J2 genotypes	With event (n=48)	Event-free (n=114)	P value
TT+GT	11+17 (58.3)	16+30 (42.1)	0.02
GG	20 (41.6)	68 (60.0)	
T allele relative frequency	41/96 (42.7)	68/228 (29.8)	0.02

Compared with event-free group, subjects with event during the follow-up period had significantly higher genetic prevalence rate of T allele (TT+GT) as well as the whole T allele frequency. Values are expressed as n (%).

Table 6. Frequencies of *CYP2J2* G-50T genotypes in groups with or without cardiac events after index myocardial infarction

Kaplan–Meier analysis demonstrated a significantly lower probability (23.5% vs. 34.6%, log-rank P=0.04) of developing clinical coronary events among patients with the polymorphism of *CYP2J2* promoter G-50T genotype (Fig. 2).

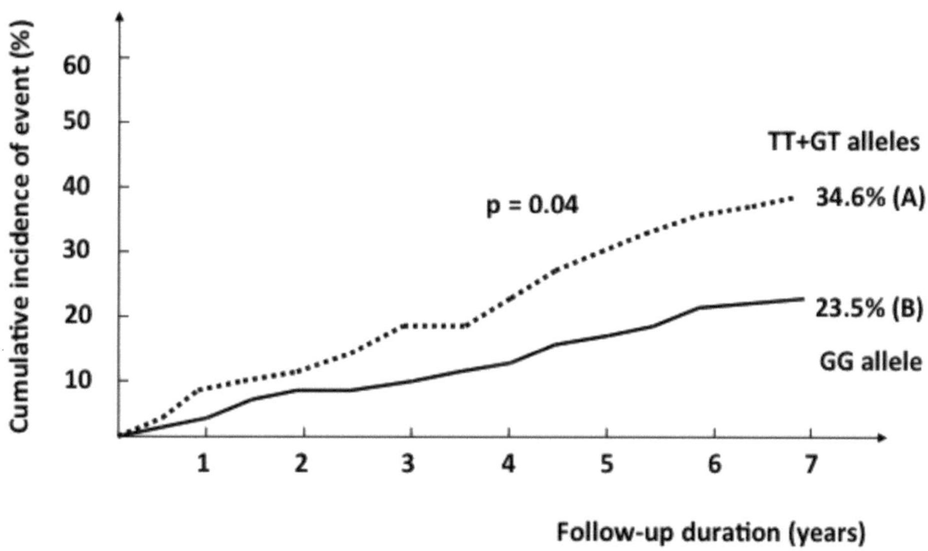

Fig. 2. Kaplan-Meier survival curve for subsequent coronary events after index acute myocardial infarction for the patients carrying TT or GT allele (A) (or GG allele for (B)) at their *CYP2J2* gene (after modified risk with age, diabetes mellitus, smoking, hypertension, and medication usage with ACEI or β-blockers).

For traditional risk factors, patients in event groups had significantly higher prevalence rates of DM, hypertension and initial severe Killip's status (>II) (all P < 0.05, see Table 7). The mean cholesterol level was also higher in the event group. Compared with the event group, patients without events received more medications such as ACEI, β-blocker and statin. The success rate of smoking cessation was higher in the event-free group (52.0% vs. 19.5%).

However, the event-free group patients received more frequent procedures of coronary bypass surgery in our MI group.

	Without cardiac events (n=114, 70.0%)	With cardiac events (n=48, 30%)	p value
Age (years)	40.3 ± 4.8	39.7 ± 4.4	0.43
Sex (male)	91 (79.8)	42 (87.5)	0.50
Family history	23 (20.1)	10 (20.8)	0.73
Hypertension	36 (28.9)	29 (60.4)	<0.01
Diabetes mellitus	20 (17.5)	19 (39.5)	<0.01
Smoking	100 (87.7)	42 (87.5)	0.77
Total cholesterol, mg/dL	191.4 ± 33.2	209.0 ± 35.3	<0.01
HDL-cholesterol, mg/dL	42 ± 11	44 ± 9	0.22
LDL-cholesterol, mg/dL	133 ± 32	136 ± 30	0.34
Triglycerides, mg/dL	135 ± 37	138 ± 44	0.25
Status of MI			
Q wave in EKG	98 (85.9)	36 (75.0)	0.47
Peak CK level (U/L)	2845 ± 1988	2975 ± 2354	0.38
LVEF (%)	55.4 ± 11.5	54.8 ± 12.3	0.64
LVEF <45%	26 (22.8)	14 (29.1)	0.06
Thrombolytic therapy	89 (78.0)	36 (75.0)	1.00
Primary PTCA	19 (16.6)	8 (16.7)	1.00
Coronary angiography	107 (93.8)	44 (91.6)	1.00
PCI	61 (53.5)	25 (52.0)	0.89
CABG	18 (15.8)	6 (12.5)	0.81
VT/Vf at MI	9 (7.8)	4 (8.3)	0.91
Killip's classification ≥ II	26 (22.8)	23 (47.9)	<0.01
Medication usage after MI			
β-blocker	91 (79.8)	19 (39.5)	<0.01
ACEI	69 (60.5)	10 (20.8)	<0.01
Statin	42 (36.8)	10 (20.8)	0.03

Patients in event groups had significantly higher prevalence rates of DM, hypertension and initial severe Killip's status (>II). The mean cholesterol level was also higher in the event group. Compared with the event group, patients without events received more medications such as ACEI, β-blocker and statin. The success rate of smoking cessation was higher in the event-free group. The event-free group patients received more frequent procedures of coronary bypass surgery in our MI group. Values are expressed as number (%) or mean ± SD. CK = creatine kinase; Vf = ventricular fibrillation; VT = ventricular tachycardia.

Table 7. Comparison between patient groups with- or without- subsequent cardiac events during follow-up period after index myocardial infarction

Univariate Cox regression analyses of the clinical characteristics and genetic backgrounds of premature MI patients are shown in Table 8. Finally, we included the variables as DM, hypertension, smoking cessation after MI, multiple (>2-vessel) coronary disease, medical therapies with β-blockers, ACEI, or statins in traditional risk factors; and the polymorphism of *CYP2J2* promoter G-50T genotype in genetic factors in the multiple logistic regression analysis. For clinical consideration, we also included factors such as treatment by thrombolysis or primary angioplasty or none into this survival analyses. That analysis showed that the polymorphism of *CYP2J2* promoter G-50T genotype, DM, smoking cessation and use of ACEI were independent survival predictors (Table 9).

	Hazard ratios (95% CI)	p value
Genetic variables		
CYP2J2 G-50T	2.78 (1.50-5.00)	<0.01
Traditional variables		
Age (>40 years-old)	1.59 (0.94-3.08)	0.07
Sex (male)	0.66 (0.18-2.18)	0.51
Family history vs. non-history	0.72 (0.35-1.55)	0.38
Systemic hypertension	2.09 (1.39-5.05)	<0.01
Diabetes mellitus	2.71 (1.46-4.89)	<0.01
Smoking behavior before MI	1.89 (0.82-3.01)	0.55
Smoking cessation after MI	0.21 (0.11-0.40)	<0.01
Total cholesterol > 200mg/dL	1.41 (0.50-1.98)	0.22
Anterior MI vs. other wall	1.47 (0.81-1.95)	0.25
LVEF (<45%)	0.68 (0.36-1.30)	0.25
Thrombolytic therapy	1.42 (0.62-6.39)	0.57
Primary PTCA	1.17 (0.93-8.78)	0.10
Coronary angiography	0.46 (0.78-4.76)	0.88
PCI procedure	0.53 (0.39-2.54)	0.70
CABG	0.87 (0.72-1.32)	0.89
VT/Vf at MI	0.77 (0.79-2.69)	0.72
Killip's classification ≥ II	1.88 (1.33-6.62)	<0.01
Multiple (>2-vessel) disease	2.96 (0.84-7.25)	0.42
Medication usage after MI		
Not-using β-blocker	2.34 (1.51-3.17)	0.01
Not-using ACEI	7.19 (2.84-10.2)	<0.01
Not-using statin	1.65 (1.02-2.93)	0.01

Table 8. Univariate analyses of traditional and genetic risk factors with Cox proportional hazards models for subsequent cardiac events. Values are expressed as number (%) or mean ± SD.

	Hazard ratios (95% CI)	p value
Not-using ACEI	10.5 (2.08-14.18)	<0.01
Diabetes mellitus	2.41 (1.23-6.95)	0.01
Smoking cessation after MI	0.33 (0.15-0.81)	0.01
Not-using statin	1.45 (1.02-2.95)	0.04
CYP2J2 G-50T	2.51 (1.09-5.78)	0.03
Not-using β-blocker	1.46 (0.99-3.29)	0.06
Multiple vessel disease	1.76 (0.88-7.56)	0.26
Systemic hypertension	1.57 (0.84-3.57)	0.32
Thrombolytic therapy	1.52 (0.25-8.40)	0.50
LVEF <45%	1.34 (0.87-10.56)	0.55
Primary PTCA	1.08 (0.80-10.12)	0.43
Killip's classification ≥ II	1.48 (0.59-8.76)	0.34
Age (>40 years-old)	1.32 (0.50-2.22)	0.65

The variables as DM, hypertension, smoking cessation after MI, multiple (>2-vessel) coronary disease, medical therapies with β-blockers, ACEI, or statins in traditional risk factors; and the polymorphism of *CYP2J2* promoter G-50T genotype in genetic factors were put in the multiple logistic regression analysis. That analysis showed that the polymorphism of *CYP2J2* promoter G-50T genotype, DM, smoking cessation and use of ACEI were independent survival predictors. Values are expressed as number (%) or mean ± SD.

Table 9. Multivariate analysis with Cox regression method assessing both traditional and genetic risk factors for subsequent cardiac events

3.6 The modification effect and gene–environment interaction of smoking cessation

We also analyzed the effect of smoking cessation after the smoker's index MI. We divided the smoking patients into two groups, based on their successful smoking cessation or not after the index MI and found that successful smoking cessation could improve the outcome (successful smoking cessation: event vs. event-free, 25% vs. 46.3%, HR 0.26, 95% CI 0.11 to 0.42; current smoking after index MI: event vs. event-free, 60% vs. 28.4%, HR 3.91, 95% CI 2.37 to 8.86; P=0.003 for HR difference). Gene–environment interactions were analyzed for the polymorphism of *CYP2J2* promoter G-50T genotype. Among the successful smoking cessation subjects, the risk of subsequent cardiovascular events was 1.6-fold higher among the G allele subgroup when compared with the T allele carrying subjects. With the same genetic background as T genotype, their risk was also 2.1-fold higher among current smokers. However, among patients who carried the G allele, the current smoking behavior increased the risk to 7.2-fold higher (Fig. 3). It seems that the risk could be lower after smoking cessation, even among high-risk gene carrying patients.

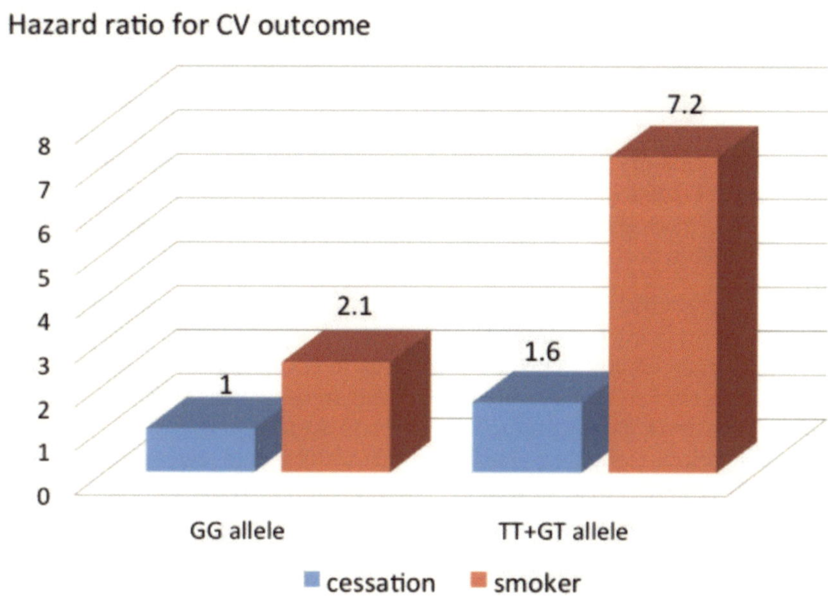

Fig. 3. Modification and interaction effects of the *CYP2J2* G-50T gene polymorphism and the cessation of smoking for the risk of subsequent cardiac events

4. Discussion

The present study investigates the association between the polymorphism of *CYP2J2* promoter G-50T genotype and the onset of premature MI in Taiwanese population. We found a higher frequency of T allele in patients with premature MI than in control subjects. There was a significant synergistic interaction between this polymorphism and the smoking behavior for the onset of MI at younger age in Taiwan.

4.1 Mechanism of the association between the polymorphism of the *CYP2J2* promoter G-50T genotype and premature MI

The polymorphism of *CYP2J2* promoter G-50T gene has been described among different disease status groups, including hypertension and CAD (Spieker et al., 2004; King et al., 2005). Spieker et al had demonstrated a functional relevance of this genetic variant by the method of electrophoretic mobility shift assays in human umbilical vein endothelial cells (Spieker et al., 2004). They found a functional consequence of reduced Sp1-DNA binding on transcriptional activation of the *CYP2J2* gene by using transfection studies *in vitro*. The construction containing the wild type promoter induced a 2-fold higher promoter activity compared with the mutant G-50T construct cells. In subjects of documented CAD, the frequency of the G-50T polymorphism was much higher. In our study, we also demonstrate that patients with *CYP2J2* G-50T allele have higher possibility of premature MI. In addition, the T allele in the promoter region of *CYP2J2* gene may functionally reduce EETs activities in the atherosclerotic vasculature, which was supported by the evidence of relationship between the genotype G-50T and the reduced EETs activities in these MI patients. This gene-phenotype association of the G-50T mutation in this promoter region could be considered as one of the possible causes to enhance the vulnerability of the atherosclerotic plaque under stimulation.

4.2 The synergistic effects of the *CYP2J2* G-50T genotype and smoking behavior

In our subgroup analysis, we also demonstrate this gene-environment interaction between smoking behavior and the *CYP2J2* G-50T polymorphism. Among non-smoker groups, the risk of MI in patients with T allele (*CYP2J2* GT+TT) is significantly higher when compared with the *CYP2J2* GG genotype patients (OR 1.43 and 1.0, respectively). The smoking behavior alone can increase 3-fold risk of MI in patients with lower activity of *CYP2J2* GG genotype at the promoter region. However, those smokers carrying the T allele polymorphism had a 5.6-fold higher risk of young MI when compared with non-smoking non-carriers.

Arachidonic acid metabolites contribute to the regulation of vascular tone and therefore tissue blood flow (Imig 2000; Gauthier et al., 2004). The vascular endothelium metabolizes arachidonic acid by cytochrome P450 epoxygenases to epoxyeicosatrienoic acids or EETs. In the vasculature, EETs are key components of cellular signaling cascades that cumulate in the activation of smooth muscle potassium channels to induce membrane hyperpolarization and vascular relaxation. Smoking habit might induce the hypercoagulable state by increasing platelet aggregability and had been recognized as a potent risk factor for premature MI (Teng et al., 1994).

In current gene-phenotype functional study, we successfully demonstrated that this genetic variant could influence the active EETs metabolites concentrations among premature MI subjects. Patients carrying T allele at promoter region of *CYP2J2* gene thus had lower median value of 14,15 EETs concentrations, which might protect their coronary vasculatures. In addition, smoking could alter the metabolites of arachidonic acid (Ye et al., 2004). This effect was observed, in our study, more significantly among *CYP2J2* G-50T polymorphism carriers whom probably were more prone to the oxidative stress damage due to their impaired EETs functions. These combination effects might explain the possible mechanism for the synergistic effect of smoking behavior and the functional change of EETs activities by polymorphism with different genotypes in its promoter gene.

4.3 Modification effects of smoking cessation and its association with gene variation on prognosis

Smokers have twice the risk of dying of coronary heart disease or stroke, and the risk diminishes by half in the first year after cessation. After 5–15 years of smoking cessation, the risk of both stroke and heart disease drops to the level of never-smokers. Previous studies usually used the history of smoking rather than current status of smoking for analysis (Li et al., 2002; Sacks et al., 1996). Our study analyzed the influence of smoking cessation on the prognosis following MI and found that those who kept on smoking could have a higher risk for subsequent coronary events when compared with those who stopped smoking. Moreover, among patients carrying higher risk genetic background, which indicated the T allele gene, the benefit was even greater from smoking cessation. It seems that a gene–environment modification relationship exists between smoking behavior and the *CYP2J2* gene variation.

In fact, the smoking behavior alone is a potent risk factor for MI at a young age (Teng et al., 1994; Liu et al., 2003). Smoking, in supporting of our current *in vitro* and *in vivo* findings, can also reduce the activities of DHET and may explain partially the possible mechanism for the smoking behavior alone or its interaction with gene variation to change the *CYP2J2* gene activity. Our findings also suggest that successful smoking cessation is very important and can improve the cardiovascular outcome, especially among those patients carrying high-risk genes.

5. Conclusion

There was a significant association between the polymorphism of G-50T genotype in the promoter region of *CYP2J2* gene and premature MI in Taiwan. Both the *CYP2J2* G-50T genotype and smoking were independent risk factors for young MI population. A synergistic effect between these two risk factors for the premature onset of MI had been shown in subgroup analyses. In addition, there was a significant association between the *CYP2J2* G-50T genotype and the prognosis after index premature MI. Successful smoking cessation after MI also could reduce the incidence of recurrent coronary events, especially among high-risk genetic background populations. Such findings lend credence to the concept that genetics and environment should not be viewed as independent risk factors for a particular disease; rather, environment and genetics interact with each to determine overall health.

6. Acknowledgement

This study was supported in part by the Multidisciplinary Center of Excellence for Clinical Trial and Research (DOH100-TD-B-111-002), Department of Health, Executive Yuan, Taiwan and by the Grant 98-2314-B-006-047-MY3 from National Science Council, Executive Yuan, Taipei, Taiwan

7. References

Barua, R.; Ambrose, J.; Saha, D. & Eales-Reynolds L. (2002). Smoking is associated with altered endothelial-derived fibrinolytic and antithrombotic factors, an in vitro demonstration. *Circulation*, Vol. 106, pp. 905-908.

Craig, M.; Palomaki, G. & Haddow, J. (1989). Cigarette smoking and serum lipid and lipoprotein concentrations: an analysis of published data. *Br Med J*, Vol. 298, pp. 784-788.

Eliasson, B.; Mero, N.; Taskinen M.; & Smith U. (1997). The insulin resistance syndrome and postprandial lipid intolerance in smokers. *Atherosclerosis*, Vol. 129, pp. 79-88.

Fang, X.; Weintraub, N.; Oltman, C.; Stoll, L.; Kaduce, T.; Harmon, S.; Dellsperger, K.; Morisseau, C.; Hammock, B. & Spector, A. (2002). Human coronary endothelial cells convert 14,15-EET to a biologically active chain-shortened epoxide. *Am J Physiol Heart Circ Physiol*, Vol. 283, pp. H2306-H2314.

Gauthier, K.; Falck, J.; Reddy, L. & Campbell, W. (2004). 14,15-EET analogs: characterization of structural requirements for agonist and antagonist activity in bovine coronary arteries. *Pharmacol Res;* Vol. 49, pp. 515-524.

Humphries, S.; Marin, S.; Cooper, J. & Miller, G. (2002). Interaction between smoking and the stromelysi-1 (MMP3) gene 5A/6A promoter polymorphism and risk of coronary heart disease in healthy men. *Ann Hum Genet*, Vol. 66, pp. 343-352.

Imig, J. (2000). Epoxygenase metabolites. Epithelial and vascular actions. *Mol Biotechnol*, Vol. 16, pp. 233-251. Review.

King, L.; Gainer, J.; David, G.; Dai, D.; Goldstein, J.; Brown, N. & Zeldin, D. (2005). Single nucleotide polymorphisms in the CYP2J2 and CYP2C8 genes and the risk of hypertension. *Pharmacogenet Genomics*, Vol. 15, pp 7-13.

King, L.; Ma, J.; Srettabunjong, S.; Graves, J.; Bradbury, J.; Li, L.; Spiecker, M.; Liao, J.; Mohrenweiser, H. & Zeldin, D. (2002). Cloning of CYP2J2 gene and identification of functional polymorphisms. *Mol Pharmacol*, Vol. 61, pp. 840-852.

Li, Y.; Chen, J.; Tsai, W.; Chao, T.; Guo, H.; Tsai, L.; Wu, H. & Shi, G. (2002). Synergistic effect of thrombomodulin promoter -33G/A polymorphism and smoking on the onset of acute myocardial infarction. *Thromb Haemost*, Vol. 87, pp. 86-91.

Liu, P.; Li, Y.; Chao, T.; Wu, H.; Lin, L.; Tsai, L. & Chen, J. (2007). Synergistic effect of cytochrome P450 epoxygenase CYP2J2*7 polymorphism with smoking on the onset of premature myocardial infarction. *Atherosclerosis*, Vol. 195, pp. 199-206.

Liu, P.; Li, Y.; Tsai, W.; Tsai, L.; Chao, T.; Wu, H. & Chen, J. (2005). Stromelysin-1 promoter 5A/6A polymorphism is an independent genetic prognostic risk factor and interacts with smoking cessation after index premature myocardial infarction. *J Thromb Haemost*, Vol. 3, pp. 1998-2005.

Liu, P.; Tsai, W.; Lin, L.; Li, Y.; Chao, T.; Tsai, L. & Chen, J. (2003). Time domain heart rate variability as a predictor of long-term prognosis after acute myocardial infarction. *J Formos Med Assoc*, Vol. 102, pp. 474-479.

Manson, J.; Tosteson, H.; Ridker, P.; Satterfield, S.; Hebert, P.; O'Connor, G.; Buring, J. & Hennekens, C. (1992). The primary prevention of myocardial infarction. *N Engl J Med*, Vol. 326, pp. 1406-1416.

Node, K.; Huo, Y.; Ruan, X.; Yang, B.; Spiecker, M.; Ley, K.; Zeldin, D. & Liao, J. (1999). Anti-inflammatory properties of cytochrome P450 epoxygenase-derived eicosanoids. *Science*, Vol. 285, pp. 1276-1279.

Pinto, A.; Abraham, N. & Mullane, K. (1987). Arachidonic acid-induced endothelial-dependent relaxations of canine coronary arteries: contribution of a cytochrome P-450-dependent pathway. *J Pharmacol Exp Ther*, Vol. 240, pp. 856-863.

Sacks, F.; Pfeffer, M.; Moye, L.; Rouleau, J.; Rutherford, J.; Cole, T.; Brown, L.; Warnica, J.; Arnold, J.; Wun, C.; Davis, B. & Braunwald, E. (1996). The effect of pravastatin on coronary events after myocardial infarction in patients with average cholesterol levels. Cholesterol and Recurrent Events Trial investigators. *N Engl J Med*, Vol. 335, pp. 1001-1009.

Sun, J.; Sui, X.; Bradbury, J.; Zeldin, D.; Conte, M. & Liao, J. (2002). Inhibition of vascular smooth muscle cell migration by cytochrome p450 epoxygenase-derived eicosanoids. *Circ Res*, Vol. 90, pp. 1020-1027.

Spiecker, M.; Darius, H.; Hankeln, T.; Soufi, M.; Sattler, A.; Schaefer, J.; Node, K.; Borgel, J.; Mugge, A.; Lindpaintner, K.; Huesing, A.; Maisch, B.; Zeldin, D. & Liao, J. (2004). Risk of coronary artery disease associated with polymorphism of the cytochrome P450 epoxygenase CYP2J2. *Circulation*, Vol. 110, pp. 2132-2136.

Spiecker, M. & Liao, J. (2005). Vascular protective effects of cytochrome p450 epoxygenase-derived eicosanoids. *Arch Biochem Biophys*, Vol.433, pp. 413-420. Review.

Teng, J.; Lin, L.; Tsai, L.; Kwan, C. & Chen, J. (1994). Acute myocardial infarction in young and very old Chinese adults: clinical and therapeutic implications. *Int J Cardiol*, Vol. 44, pp. 29-36.

Tsiara, S.; Elisaf, M. & Mikhailidis, D. (2003). Influence of smoking on predictors of vascular disease. *Angiology*, Vol. 54, pp. 507-530.

Wu, S.; Moomaw, C.; Tomer, K.; Falck, J. & Zeldin, D. (1996). Molecular cloning and expression of CYP2J2, a human cytochrome P450 arachidonic acid epoxygenase highly expressed in heart. *J Biol Chem*, Vol. 271, pp. 3460-3468.

Ye, Y.; Liu, E.; Shin, V.; Wu, W.; Luo, J. & Cho, C. (2004). Nicotine promoted colon cancer growth via epidermal growth factor receptor, c-Src, and 5-lipoxygenase-mediated signal pathway. *J Pharmacol Exp Ther*, Vol. 308, pp. 66–72.

Part 6

Miscellaneous

21

Coronary Artery Aneurysms: An Update

Karina M. Mata, Cleverson R. Fernandes,
Elaine M. Floriano, Antonio P. Martins,
Marcos A. Rossi and Simone G. Ramos
*Department of Pathology, Faculty of Medicine of Ribeirão Preto,
Ribeirão Preto, University of São Paulo,
Brazil*

1. Introduction

Coronary artery aneurysm (CAA) is a neglected topic in the pathology literature; most descriptions of CAAs have been limited to reports of single cases and some reviews. Because CAAs are usually found incidentally during cardiac examinations, most of the reported cases have been diagnosed by coronary angiography, intravascular ultrasound and, on rare occasions, during autopsy (Ramos et al., 2008). Although they are rare, CAAs can be potentially fatal if they are not managed in a judicious and timely manner.

The first description of a CAA has been attributed to Morgagni, an Italian anatomopathologist of the mid-18th century. However, the first CAA in a living patient was diagnosed by coronary angiography (Munkner et al., 1958). Since then, many studies have been conducted on the pathology of abnormal dilatations of the coronary arteries; however, attempts at defining and classifying these abnormalities still create problems for researchers and physicians who work in this area. The major problem is differentiating between aneurysms and ectasias. Currently, CAA is defined as a localized, irreversible dilatation of the blood vessel lumen that exceeds the diameter of the adjacent normal segment by more than 1.5-fold (Falsett & Carrol, 1978; Swaye et al. 1983; Syed & Lesch, 1997). In contrast, ectasia is used to describe a diffuse dilatation of coronary arteries that involves 50% or more of the length of the artery; this classification is made according to the appearance and number of vessels involved (Markis et al, 1976). Ectasia has been subcategorized based on the topographical extent in the major epicardial coronary arteries into the following 4 types: type I, diffuse ectasia of two or three arteries; type II, diffuse ectasia in one artery and localized in another; type III, diffuse ectasia of one artery only; and type IV, localized and segmental ecstatic lesions (Markis et al., 1976). The existence of the last type causes confusion in separating aneurysms from ectasias; therefore, additional efforts to define specific anatomic substrates will help to standardize the reporting of this disease and minimize discrepancies in the literature regarding management.

On rare occasions, a CAA grows large enough to be called a giant CAA, for which a precise definition is still lacking. Some authors consider coronary aneurysms to be giants when the CAA is greater than 2 cm (Mora et al., 2011), whereas the Committee of the American Heart

Association has defined giant aneurysms as those greater than 8 mm. In the literature, most of the reported maximum diameters of giant CAAs in adults have varied from 5 to 16 cm. Recently, cases of right giant CAAs have been recorded in MEDLINE and selected English-language articles describing CAAs with diameters exceeding 5 cm over a 10–year period (1998-2008; Ramos et al., 2008). A male predilection (63%) and a mean age of 58 years were observed. The most frequent cause was atherosclerosis (37%), especially in older patients. The symptoms of the CAAs varied, and only four patients were asymptomatic. Surgical resection was the treatment of choice (74%), and most patients underwent coronary artery bypass grafting (59%) or coronary artery reconstruction (7%). The majority of the patients had an uneventful recovery. Only 7% (2/27) of the patients died from cardiac causes related to the CAA (Ramos et al., 2008).

2. Incidence and anatomic distribution

A wide variation exists in the incidence of CAA. This variation can be attributed to the conceptual differences in the definition of coronary aneurysms and ectasia. In the literature, the incidence of coronary artery disease has been predominantly in men with an average age of 63.5 years (Befeler et al., 1977; Daoud et al., 1983). In the order of frequency, the following are the most affected coronaries: right coronary artery (RCA; 40.4%), left anterior descending artery (32.3%), left circumflex artery (23.4%), and rarely, left main coronary artery (3.5%); (Syed & Lesh, 1997). Atherosclerotic or inflammatory coronary aneurysms are usually multiple and involve more than one coronary artery. In contrast, congenital, traumatic, or dissecting aneurysms are usually single. Although coronary aneurysms are seen at any age, those related to atherosclerosis usually appear later in life than those associated with a congenital or inflammatory nature (Daoud et al., 1983).

3. Classification

CAAs have been classified in different ways based on the composition of the vessel wall and the morphological structure (Table 1). Aneurysms are often classified by macroscopic shape and size, according to the transversal and longitudinal size. Saccular aneurysms are spherical and show a transverse diameter greater than the longitudinal diameter, whereas fusiform aneurysms are characterized by a gradual and progressive dilatation that involves the complete circumference of the artery and have a transverse diameter that is smaller than the longitudinal diameter (Williams & Stewart et al., 1994). Moreover, CAAs may be true or false (pseudoaneurysms) depending on the composition of the aneurysmal wall. True aneurysms contain all normal vascular layers, and the blood remains within the confines of the circulatory system. False, or pseudoaneurysms, are extravascular hematomas that communicate with the intravascular space. Normal vascular integrity is usually lost, resulting in the formation of thin-walled structures that lack normal arterial wall layers. Pseudoaneurysms typically occur after disruption of the external elastic membrane and frequently result from blunt chest trauma or catheter-based coronary interventions (Aqel et al., 2004). Furthermore, pseudoaneurysms usually affect only a portion of the artery wall and are more vulnerable to thrombosis and rupture (Williams & Stewart, 1994).

Classification of CAAs		
Characteristics	**Categories**	**Luminal diameter of the aneurysm**
Shape	Saccular Fusiform	Maximum transverse diameter > longitudinal dimension Longitudinal dimension > maximum transverse diameter
Vascular wall integrity	True aneurysm Pseudoaneurysm	All vascular layers present Loss of the vascular wall integrity
Topographical extent	Type I Type II Type III Type IV	Diffuse dilatation of two or three vessels Diffuse dilatation in one vessel and localized in another Diffuse dilatation of one vessel only Localized or segmental dilatation

Modified from Antoniadis et al., 2008; Díaz-Zamudio et al., 2009.

Table 1. Morphologic and topographical classification of aneurysms and ectasias observed in coronary arteries.

4. Epidemiology

The prevalence of coronary artery disease in angiographic series has been documented to vary between 0.2 and 10%, but these studies have included both aneurysmal coronary disease and ectasias (Antoniadis et al., 2008). Because each angiographic diagnosis is operator-dependent, inter-observer variability may be responsible for the prevalence of discrepancies in different cohorts. Therefore, the documented frequencies may not represent the actual prevalence of coronary aneurysms in the general population. Moreover, one should not forget that a selection bias exists in patients referred for diagnostic coronary angiography. Table 2 shows exclusively the CAA prevalence in the most recent epidemiologic studies.

Undoubtedly, important genetic and environmental influences affect incidence, and the CAA incidence has been shown to be lower in Asia than in North America and Europe. In contrast, a study of 302 patients with Kawasaki disease showed an incidence of coronary aneurysms of 10.3% in patients of Asian ethnicity compared with 6.9% in those of Caucasian ethnicity and 1.2% in those of African ethnicity (Porcella et al., 2005).

Source	Diagnosis	Population	Prevalence (%)
Falsetti & Carrol, 1976	Angiography	742	1.5
Daoud et al., 1983	Autopsy	694	1.4
Tunick et al.,1990	Angiography	8,422	0.2
Wang et al., 1999	Angiography	10,120	0.1
Harikrishnan et al., 2000	Angiography	3,200	0.7
Groenke et al., 2005	Angiography	7,101	1.4
Rozenberg & Nepomnyashchikh, 2005	Autopsy	1,000	1.5

Table 2. Prevalence of coronary artery aneurysms in angiographic and autopsy studies.

5. Etiology

Coronary atherosclerosis and Kawasaki disease are the principal causes of CAAs. Atherosclerosis is the most common etiology in the U.S., and Kawasaki disease is the most common etiology in the Far East (Cohen & Ogara, 2008). Atherosclerosis is responsible for more than 50% of CAAs in adults in the Western world, whereas Kawasaki disease, which is characterized by an acute, self-limited vasculitis occurring in childhood, may lead to the development of CAAs in 15 to 25% of untreated children (Falsetti & Carrol, 1976; Pahlavan & Niroomand, 2006). Other causes of CAAs include inflammatory arterial diseases (polyarteritis nodosa, syphilis, Takayasu arteritis, Behçet´s disease), connective tissue disorders (systemic lupus erythematosus, rheumatoid arthritis, ankylosing spondylitis, scleroderma), hereditary collagen defects (Marfan syndrome, Ehlers-Danlos syndrome), coronary artery revascularization procedures (balloon angioplasty and laser atherectomy), candidiasis, chest traumas, and primary hyperaldosteronism (Alford et al., 1976; Antoniadis et al., 2008). CAA have also been noted in conjunction with infection, drug use, trauma, and percutaneous coronary intervention (Pahlavan & Niroomand, 2006). Therefore, many inflammatory disorders and infectious etiologies have been associated with CAAs. The etiologies usually vary according to the geographic location and age of the patient (Díaz-Zamudio et al., 2009).

Atherosclerosis
Kawasaki disease
Congenital
Arteritis (polyarteriritis nodosa, syphilis, systemic lupus erythematous, Takayasu arteritis disease, Behçet´s disease)
Mycotic
Dissection
Chest trauma
Drugs
Connective tissue disorders (SLE, rheumatoid arthritis, ankylosing spondylitis, scleroderma)
Hereditary collagen defects (Marfan and Ehlers-Danlos syndromes)
Metastatic tumor
Coronary angioplasty (balloon, laser atherectomy, stent implantation, directional coronary atherectomy, pulsed laser coronary angioplasty and brachytherapy)*

Modified from Syed & Lesch, 1997. SLE: systemic lupus erythematosus. *Mostly pseudoaneurysms.

Table 3. Etiology of Coronary Artery Aneurysms.

The following sections describe the primary causes of CAA.

5.1 Atherosclerosis

Atherosclerosis is the most common cause of morbidity and mortality worldwide. This disease is characterized by chronic inflammatory and intimal lesions, called atheromas or fibrofatty plaques, which protrude into the lumen, weaken the underlying media and undergo a series of complications affecting primarily elastic arteries and larger and medium sized muscular arteries, such as coronary arteries (Libby, 2002). Dauod et al. (1963) believed that aneurysms are formed as a result of poststenotic transformation of kinetic energy to potential energy and pressure abnormalities in the vessel. Moreover, Siouffi et al. (1984) have explained that the elevated velocity of blood flow, which results in increased shear stress at the stenotic site, can promote endothelial injury and poststenotic vasodilation. In contrast, atherosclerotic plaque borders have been suggested to be potential foci of plaque disruption and thrombus formation, which cause microcirculation impairment and clinical symptoms of ischemia. The atherosclerotic material located at the injured site presumably can act as the point of aneurysm formation (Berkoff & Rowe, 1975; Befeler et al., 1977). However, a theory from Markis et al. (1976) has suggested that the formation of the atherosclerotic aneurysm occurs as a result of an imbalance between the intravascular pressure and the elasticity of the vascular wall. In atherosclerosis, the vascular inflammation and plaques are distributed at near side branches or arterial stenosis (where blood flow is nonuniform) and at the lesser curvature of bends (where the blood flow rate is relatively low). Blood flow exerts shear stress on the vessel wall by altering cell physiology via several mechanisms. Shear stress also arises at the interplay between blood and the endothelial layer, where it induces a shearing deformation of the endothelial cells. Regions of the arterial tree with uniform geometry exert a physiologic shear stress, whereas arches and branches are exposed to a disturbed, oscillatory flow, which exerts low shear. Atherosclerotic lesions occur predominantly at sites of low shear, whereas regions of the vasculature exposed to a physiologic shear are protected (Koskinas et al, 2009). The occurrence of atherosclerotic lesions in the human carotid bifurcation, abdominal aorta and coronary artery strongly correlates with low shear regions experiencing an almost purely oscillatory flow (Moore et al., 1994). Atherosclerotic lesions are more frequent in the proximal portions of the three major coronary arteries (mainly the RCA). These data confirm that the coronary bifurcation pattern predisposes to the development of atherosclerotic lesions due to low endothelial shear stress. These atherosclerotic plaques develop in areas in which low endothelial shear stress occurs, inducing aneurysm formation as a result of endothelial damage (Chatzizisis et al., 2008). Inflammatory cells residing in the plaque (lymphocytes, macrophages, and foam cells) play an important role in the evolution and complication of atherosclerosis. These cells secrete cytokines that further amplify inflammation and produce proteases, such as metalloproteinase (MMPs) that destabilize the plaque by damaging the extracellular matrix (elastin) and thinning the fibrous cap (Libby, 2002). The result of elastin degradation is increased wall stiffness, elongation, and tortuosity of the vessel leading to areas of turbulent flow, which in combination with endothelial injury, favors the thrombus formation that is seen in most aneurysms (Hans et al., 2005).

Microscopic evaluation of the atherosclerotic aneurysmal wall usually demonstrates typical components of atherosclerotic plaques, such as mononuclear cells infiltrates, lipid deposits, cholesterol crystals, destruction of the intima and media, diffuse hyalinization, focal fibrosis, calcification of the media, intramural hemorrhage and sometimes a foreign-body giant cell reaction (Markis et al., 1976). A representative autopsy case is shown in the Figure 1.

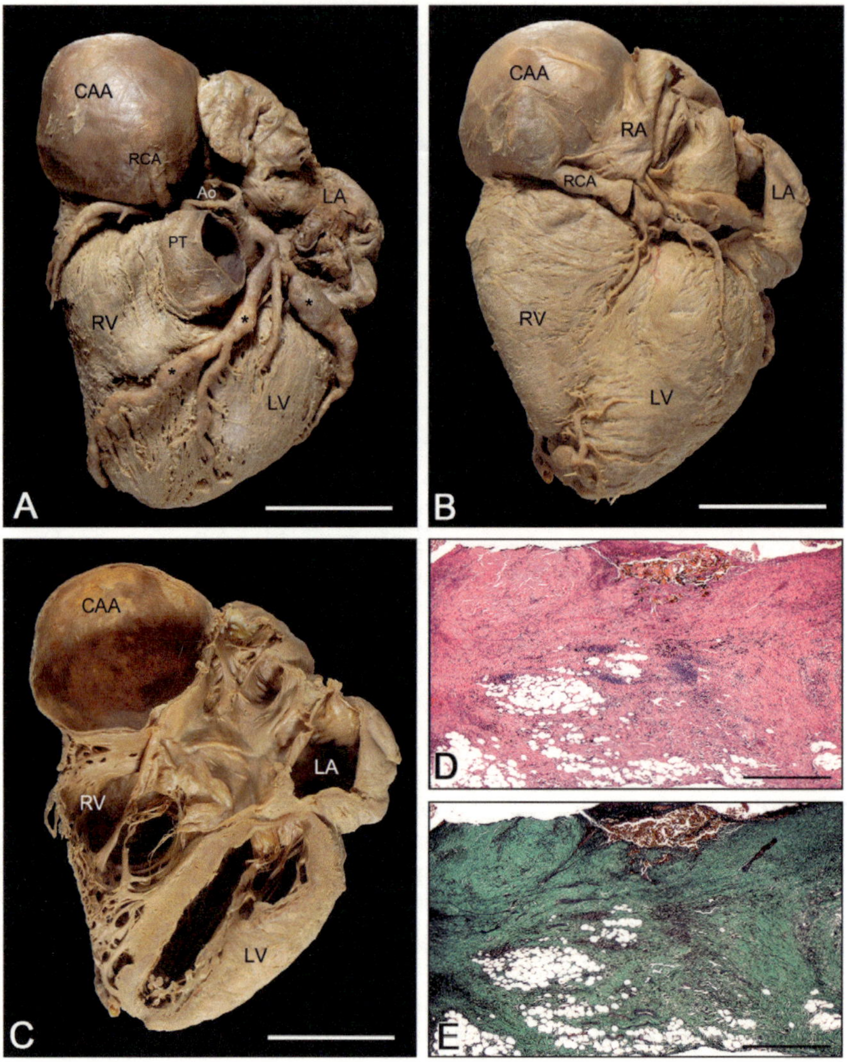

Fig. 1. **(A)** Anterior view of the heart. Note a giant CAA (6x6.2x7.5 cm) starting after a 10-mm-long segment of normal-sized RCA giving off the aorta and pushing back the right atrium. (B) Posterior view of the heart. The coronary aneurysm finishes as a 5-cm-long ecstasic arterial segment of the RCA along the atrioventricular groove to give off the posterior descending artery in the interventricular groove. In (A) and (B), the epicardium was removed to better show the diffuse atherosclerotic coronary artery disease (*). (C) Coronal section of the heart. The coronary aneurysm was empty and the wall was thickened with lipid deposits. Bar = 5cm. Microscopic section of the CAA wall. Note the dense fibrocollagenous thickening, extracellular lipids, mononuclear cells, and lymphocytic inflammatory infiltrates in the aneurysmal wall (D; Hematoxylin–eosin) and (E; Masson´s trichrome). Bar = 1mm. Ao: Aorta; CAA: coronary artery aneurysm; LA: left atrium; LV: left ventricle; PT: pulmonary trunk; RA: right atrium; RCA: right coronary artery, and RV: right ventricle.

5.2 Coronary vasculitis

Systemic vasculitis represents a large group of diseases that are defined as inflammatory lesions of blood vessels (Lightfoot et al., 1990). Inflammatory thickening of the coronary arteries may lead to their occlusion, weakness of the wall, and in some cases, the development of aneurysms.

5.2.1 Kawasaki Disease (KD)

KD or mucocutaneous lymph node syndrome, is the most common cause of CAA in children and the second most common in adults. KD is a multisystem inflammatory illness that predominately affects children 6 months to 5 years of age, although younger infants and older children can also develop the illness (Amano et al., 1979). KD can result in acute vasculitis, most strikingly of the coronary arteries (Newburger et al., 1986). Important complications include coronary artery dilation and aneurysm formation, which occurs in 10–15% of patients during the acute stage. The incidence of KD is at least ten times higher in Japan than in Western populations (Nakamura et al., 2008). Siblings of children with KD have a tenfold higher risk of developing the illness than the general population, and children whose parents had KD have a twofold increased incidence (Uehara et al., 2003).

The etiology of KD remains a major pediatric enigma, despite efforts to identify the cause over the last four decades. Many proposed etiologies of KD have been suggested since Dr. Tomisaku Kawasaki's initial description of the illness in Japan in the 1960s (Kawasaki, 1967). The most widely proposed theories have fallen under the categories of environmental toxin exposure, autoimmune pathogenesis, and infectious diseases. Because the clinical and epidemiologic features of KD support an infectious cause, one speculation is that the infectious agent travels from its portal of entry through the bloodstream and infects many organs and tissues; the immune response then targets these sites of infection. The theory of KD etiology that best fits the available data is that a ubiquitous infectious agent results in asymptomatic infection in most individuals but causes KD in a subset of genetically predisposed individuals (Rowley et al., 2008). Up to 25% of untreated children will develop persistent abnormalities in the coronary arteries; however, therapy with intravenous gammaglobulin and aspirin within the first ten days of fever onset reduces the prevalence of coronary artery abnormalities to approximately 5% (Newburger et al., 1986).

Inflamed tissues in acute KD show inflammatory cell infiltration of the arterial wall (mononuclear cells, lymphocytes, and macrophages), destruction of the internal elastic lamina, necrosis of smooth muscle cells, myointimal proliferation and subsequent occurrence of dilations or aneurysms (Burgner et al., 2009). Histopathological findings have indicated destruction of coronary artery walls with diffuse vasculitis, raising the possibility that MMPs are also involved in coronary arterial wall destruction and the formation of CAAs (Amano et al., 1979). Among patients with KD, those with coronary artery lesions have higher plasma levels of both MMP 3 and MMP 9. Within the arterial wall, the production of MMPs and other enzymes by macrophages results in the destruction of collagen and elastin fibers. The wall can lose its structural integrity and dilate or balloon, forming an aneurysm. The immune response is ultimately successful in controlling the pathogen, but damage to the coronary arteries may have already occurred (Yilmazet al., 2007).

The diagnosis of KD is clinical and is based on the major clinical features of the acute phase. Undoubtedly, many asymptomatic adult patients with coronary arterial lesions caused by

KD remain undiagnosed, forming a hidden cohort with this disease (Tsuda et al., 2007). Even once acute KD was recognized, the diagnosis of complicating coronary artery lesions was more difficult in the sixties and seventies. Symptoms are rare in this population until the onset of acute coronary syndrome; consequently, the presence of coronary artery disease is unsuspected in most patients. Only recently have technical developments allowed the detailed examination of coronary artery morphology.

Although the precise etiology and pathogenesis of KD are not completely understood, the current management of acute KD is based upon prospective, controlled, multicenter treatment trials that have clearly demonstrated the efficacy of intravenous immunoglobulin (IVIG) and high-dose aspirin to halt inflammation and reduce the likelihood of the development of coronary abnormalities when administered by the tenth day of illness (Newburger et al., 1991). Whether or not to continue antithrombotic therapy in patients with regressed giant aneurysms is an important problem to resolve in the future (Tsuda et al., 2010).

5.2.2 Polyarteritis nodosa (PAN)

For decades, most forms of vasculitis were termed periarteritis nodosa. Newly recognized types of this disease were characterized and classified according to features that were similar to or distinct from those of PAN (Klinger, 1931; Churg & Strauss, 1951). In the early 1900s, Ferrari (1903) and Dickson (1908) proposed the name polyarteritis nodosa, partly to distinguish the disorder described by Kussmaul & Maier (1866) from the vascular lesion of tertiary syphilis. Furthermore, the term polyarteritis nodosa emphasizes the panarteritic nature of this disease and underscores the fact that multiple arteries are affected by the process (Arkin, 1930). PAN is one of a spectrum of diseases that belong to the pathologic category of necrotizing vasculitis. The classic form of PAN was described by Kussmaul & Maier in 1866 as consisting of focal panmural, necrotizing inflammatory lesions in small- and medium-sized arteries and characterized by fibrinoid necrosis and infiltration of predominantly polymorphonuclear leukocytes. PAN is a multiple organ disorder with characteristic involvement of the renal and other visceral arteries. Coronary artery involvement (76%) ranks second in frequency behind the renal arteries (85%) (Lypsky et al., 1994). Thrombosis, aneurysms, and arteritis of the coronary vessels are known complications of the disease. PAN affects 2 to 6 people per 100,000 per year and can be seen in all ethnic groups. Any age group can be affected, but the disease occurs more commonly in men than in women (2:1) and is seen in people between the ages of 40 and 60 years. The cause of PAN is unknown for most patients. For years, an infectious etiology for PAN has been considered. Early observers considered streptococci or *Staphylococcus aureus* to be likely candidates (David et al., 1993). Hepatitis B surface antigenemia (with immune complex formation) has been reported to be associated with approximately 20% of patients with PAN (Trepo et al., 1974). The incidence is higher in areas where hepatitis B is endemic. In studies from France, the percentage of cases of PAN attributed to hepatitis B viral infection decreased from 36% to 7% during the past decade after the development of vaccines against viral hepatitis (Guillevin et al., 1996).

Aneurysms often form at the branching points of small- and medium-sized arteries and occur in 9% of patients with PAN (Kastner et al., 2000). The rupture of aneurysms may result in spontaneous hemorrhage in approximately 6% of cases (Zizic et al., 1982). Acute lesions in PAN swiftly evolve into a panarteritis with degeneration of the arterial wall, destruction of the external and internal elastic lamina, and fibrinoid necrosis. The cellular infiltrate is pleomorphic, with both polymorphonuclear cells and lymphocytes present to various degrees at different stages. Degranulation of neutrophils within and around the arterial wall leads to leukocytoclasis. In time, this inflammation leads to transmural necrosis and a homogeneous, eosinophilic appearance of the blood vessel wall (fibrinoid necrosis). The vascular wall inflammation in PAN may be strikingly segmental, affecting only part of the circumference of a given artery. Segmental necrosis, in turn, leads to aneurysm formation. During later stages, complete occlusion may occur secondary to endothelial proliferation and thrombosis. Throughout involved tissues, the coexistence of acute and healed lesions is typical. Features of granulomatous vasculitis are absent. Acute PAN evolves into a sclerotic process with fibrosis of the damaged arterial wall and mesenchymal organization. In some cases, there is also recanalization of thrombi. Chronic arterial narrowing may result (Stone, 2002).

The identification of PAN can be a clinical challenge given its varied spectrum of organ involvement, wide range of clinical symptoms, and variations in severity. The clinical course can last from months to years, and relapse occurs in 40% of treated patients with a median interval of 33 months (Gordon et al., 1993). If untreated, the disease may have a fulminant course; the 5-year survival is less than 15%. However, survival increases to 80% with steroid treatment, with or without cytotoxic drugs (Guillevin et al., 1996). Symptoms, such as fever, malaise, and weight loss, are common, and up to 70% of patients have abdominal pain, nausea, vomiting, and infarction are uncommon, occurring in 1% of cases (Zizic et al., 1982). A combination of corticosteroids and immunosuppressants is a highly effective therapy for progressive PAN. Therefore, early diagnosis, which is usually based on clinical signs and symptoms and laboratory and angiographic findings, is crucial for the prognosis of the patient (Parangui et al., 1991). Arterial angiography is still an important measure in cases suggestive of PAN when other noninvasive tests do not allow diagnosis. The diagnosis of PAN is strongly indicated by the finding of aneurysms within the vasculature during angiography (Holzknecht et al., 1997). Early diagnosis and treatment of PAN are necessary to prevent serious organ damage and should be suspected in patients with febrile disease, weight loss, and evidence of multiple organ involvement. The diagnostic criteria have been classified by the American College of Rheumatology (Ewald et al., 1987). Three of 10 criteria must be present for the diagnosis of PAN, and positive angiography is one of the criteria. In symptomatic patients (with primarily abdominal complaints, nephropathy, hypertension, or generalized malaise), angiography is a valuable diagnostic tool that can lead to the diagnosis in occult cases. Angiographic findings, including aneurysms, ectasia, or occlusive disease, are present in approximately 40%–90% of patients at the time clinical symptoms appear (Hekali et al., 1991).

Some case reports of coronary angiograms performed in patients with PAN have been published. Przybojewski (1981) has described a 29-year-old man for whom the coronary angiography revealed a diffusely aneurysmal RCA with severe obstructive lesions in the left circumflex and left anterior descending arteries. PAN was subsequently diagnosed by a skeletal muscle biopsy. The biopsy showed fibrinoid necrosis affecting connective tissue and blood vessels in the muscle epimysium and adjacent fascia, which are features that are characteristic of a collagen vascular disease such as PAN. Pick et al. (1982) have reported a 26-year-old woman who, during cardiac catheterization, revealed numerous aneurysms involving all three coronary vessels that were particularly worse in the distal RCA. Cassling et al. (1985) have described a 30-year-old female smoker who presented with intermittent chest pain and a strongly positive stress test. Coronary angiography revealed severe luminal narrowing of several coronary arteries without aneurysm formation. The clinical diagnosis was occlusive atherosclerotic coronary artery disease. The patient died intraoperatively after the anastomosis of coronary artery bypass grafts. Subsequent autopsy revealed an unexpected coronary adventitial thickening and a polymorphous lymphocytic infiltrate consistent with PAN. An autopsy case of PAN is shown in the Figure 2.

For cases of idiopathic PAN, corticosteroids and cytotoxic agents remain the cornerstones of treatment (Guillevin et al., 1996). Approximately half of patients with PAN achieve remissions or cures with high doses of corticosteroids alone (Lam et al., 1981). Fortunately, the availability of effective antiviral agents has revolutionized the treatment of hepatitis B virus (HBV) infection-associated cases in recent years (Guillevin et al., 1996). Prophylactic treatment of large aneurysms by means of catheter embolization should be considered in anticipation of the risk of rupture. Aortography may not adequately substitute for selective injections of the viscera, but the retroperitoneal branches are depicted, and they can also be involved with aneurysms that may rupture in rare cases. In a small percentage of patients with PAN, aneurysm rupture in an organ or retroperitoneal branch may be the first clinical evidence of the disease. Embolization therapy is often the treatment of choice (Hachulla et al., 1993). The presence of aneurysms may relate to the phase of the disease or its severity. Arterial segments of ectasia may be either a precursor to a fully expanded aneurysm or a phase in the healing process. Aneurysms of PAN may resolve over time as remission occurs (Guillevin et al., 1996).

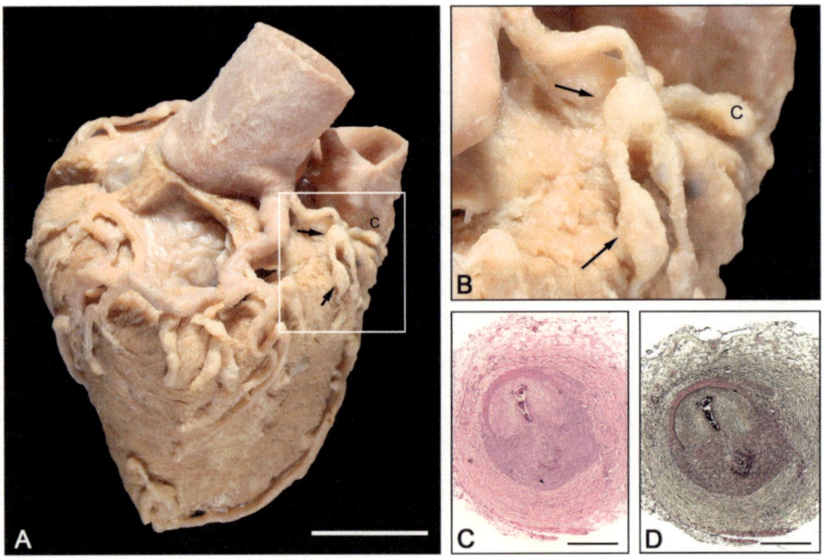

Fig. 2. (A) Right posterolateral view of the heart of a 56-year-old woman with systemic PAN. Note the multiple aneurysms in coronary arterial tree. (B) Detail of aneurysmal nodules in the right marginal artery (arrows). Histopathology of the coronary artery (C), showing an important luminal occlusion by intimal proliferation, partial disruption of the internal elastic laminae and tunica media, intense inflammatory infiltrate and remarkable adventitial fibrotic thickening (C; Hematoxylin–eosin and D; Masson´s trichrome). Bar = 1mm. PAN: Polyarteritis Nodosa.

5.2.3 Takayasu arteritis

Takayasu arteritis (TA) was first described in 1908 by the Japanese ophthalmologist Takayasu, who reported ocular changes, such as aneurysms and arteriovenous anastomoses, in patients with this disease. This primary systemic vasculitis is a group of autoimmune syndromes characterized by stenosis, occlusion, or aneurysmal dilation that involves the large cardiac vessels, chiefly the aorta and its main branches. Epidemiological data have demonstrated that TA is more common in Asian countries than in other parts of the world. The incidence of aneurysms in patients with TA has been reported to be approximately 18% and 24%, and approximately 150 new cases per year have been estimated in Japan. However, the disease may be found worldwide, including occidental countries (Subramanyan et al., 1989). TA primarily affects females, and the female to male ratio can reach up to 8:1 in adulthood (age ≤40 yr); in childhood, the ratio is significantly lower at 2:1 (Sharma et al., 1996; Mesquita et al., 1998). The etiology of TA remains unknown, although autoimmune mechanisms and infections are factors that have been reported to be associated with the disease. Genetic aspects also appear to contribute to the pathogenesis of TA (Buzaid et al., 1995).

The clinical progression of TA can be divided into acute and chronic phases. The acute phase comprises signs and symptoms of a systemic inflammatory process, such as fever, weight loss, anorexia, fainting, dizziness, nocturnal sweating, myalgia, arthralgia/arthritis, exanthema, abdominal pain, vomiting and anemia. The chronic phase is characterized by symptomatology of vascular occlusion with the appearance of hypertension and changes in peripheral pulses (Morales et al., 1991). However, these phases are not always distinct and may occur simultaneously (Kerr, 1995). Most of the lesions cause luminal narrowing, which can lead to occlusion; however, coronary aneurysms are extremely rare. CAA can develop as vascular walls weaken because of arterial hypertension and the extensive destruction of elastic fibers in the media. CAA often cause stasis of blood flow and result in mural thrombus (Lie, 1998). The histological changes are characterized by marked thickening of the adventitia, media, and intima (Subramanyan et al., 1989). The inflammatory process involves the coronary arteries in less than 10% of patients, mostly in the form of stenotic lesions (Sharma et al., 1995), and can be divided into 3 distinct morphologic types: stenosis or occlusion of the coronary ostia, diffuse or focal coronary arteritis, and coronary aneurysm formation (Panja et al., 1998). Rarely, the inflamed aorta of TA can be a source of dissection, but the various symptoms and signs more commonly mimic an aortic dissection (Reichman & Weber, 2004).

Diagnosis is difficult because the initial stage of the disease may be asymptomatic or may be characterized by the presence of signs and symptoms of the acute phase. The latter may lead to an erroneous diagnosis, such as rheumatic fever, juvenile rheumatoid arthritis or systemic lupus erythematosus (Kerr, 1995). Angiography and clinical examination remain the cornerstones for the diagnosis of TA. While arteriographic studies of the aortic and pulmonary territories are necessary to obtain a complete sense of the extent of the disease, these invasive techniques cannot be frequently repeated (Hata et al., 1996). Echocardiography has become a valuable noninvasive diagnostic technique for the detection of cardiovascular complications in patients with TA (Soto et al., 1996).The use of drug-eluting stents for the effective treatment of coronary lesions associated with TA (Kang et al., 2006). However, surgical treatment of TA poses many difficulties related to the timing of the operation, the techniques and materials used, and postoperative management. Even though TA is considered a severe disease, it rarely causes death (Kerr, 1995). Nevertheless, the outcome depends on the medical and surgical treatment and on the cardiac involvement, severity, type of arterial hypertension and distribution of the vascular lesions (Mesquita et al., 1998). Currently, all treatment remains symptomatic because the etiology and pathogenesis of the disease are as yet unknown (Buzaid et al., 1985). Corticosteroids are the most widely employed drugs for the treatment of TA, and because they suppress the inflammatory manifestations and are helpful in the reversal of arterial stenosis, they are administered at high doses during the initial stage of the disease. Other drugs, such as cyclophosphamide, methotrexate and cyclosporin have been indicated for patients who do not respond to corticotherapy (Mesquita et al., 1998). An autopsy case is demonstrated in the Figure 3.

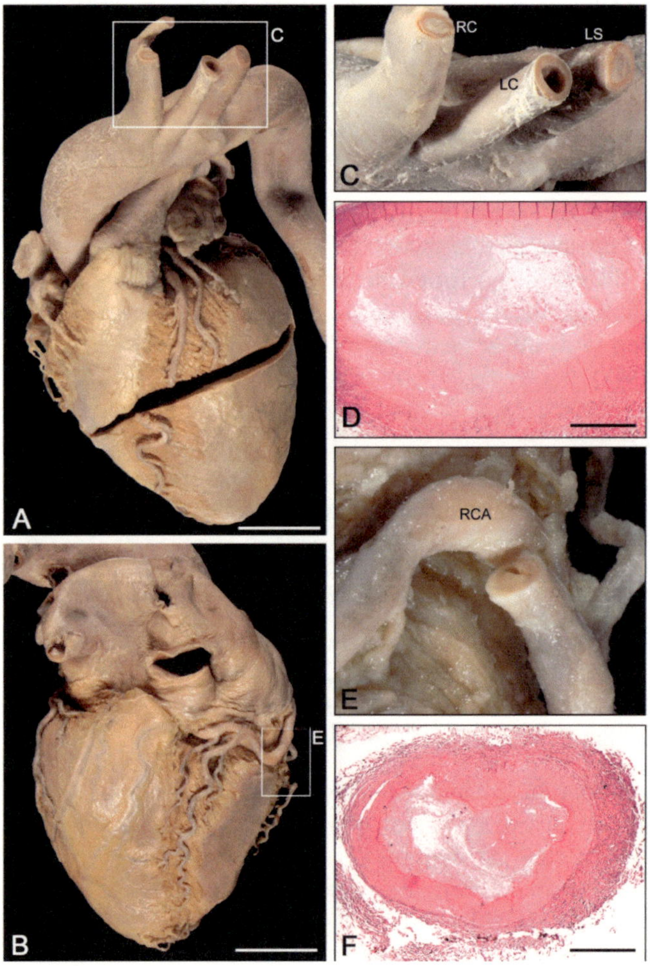

Fig. 3. (A) Anterior and (B) posterior view of the heart, aorta and the major thoracic branches of a 17-year-old female diagnosed with Takayasu arteritis. Bar = 2.5cm. (C) Detail of the important luminal occlusion of the major thoracic arteries. (D) Histopathological view of the right carotid showing intimal thickening and partially recanalized thrombus. Hematoxylin-eosin; Bar = 1 mm. (E) RCA transversely sectioned to show the stenotic lumen. (F) Histopathological view of the RCA showing intimal thickening, partially recanalized thrombus and prominent adventitial involvement. Hematoxylin-eosin; Bar = 1 mm.

5.3 Miscellaneous

In addition to those described above, some other diseases are also involved in the formation of CAA. Connective tissue diseases, such as Marfan syndrome, can cause aneurysms without atherosclerosis. Marfan syndrome is associated with mutations in the gene for fibrillin that is homologous to the family of latent TGF-β binding proteins, which hold TGF-β in an inactive complex (Gelb, 2006). Cystic medial degeneration is a common feature of the aneurysms in Marfan syndrome, so its presence in a CAA may be indicative of a congenital genetic defect that causes an excess of active TGF-β. However, cystic medial degeneration is also commonly seen in the aortic aneurysms of late middle-aged and elderly patients without Marfan syndrome, but this degeneration could be indicative of excess active TGF-β in these patients as well. TGF-β can be inhibited by angiotensin II type 1-receptor antagonists, such as losartan, which can prevent aortic aneurysms in a mouse model of Marfan syndrome (Habashi et al., 2006).

Systemic lupus erythematosus commonly causes arteritis, are rare and is most common in women of African descent who are of childbearing age (Matayoshi et al., 1999). Generally, these aneurysms are large and proximal and are in the setting of other obvious clinical markers of systemic disease. Clinical signs may include serositis, hematologic abnormalities, renal disease, dermatologic findings, abdominal angina, and neurologic findings, such as weakness, central nervous system vasculitis, and radiculopathy. In mycotic aneurysms, the injury and destruction of the tunica media may be due to microembolization to the vasa vasorum, direct pathogen invasion of the arterial wall, or immune complex deposition (Ford et al., 2007). Traumatic and iatrogenic aneurysms are frequently pseudoaneurysms. The pathogenesis of aneurysm formation after catheter-based interventions is not fully understood (Bjorn-Hansen et al., 1989). This consequence has been attributed to the use of an oversized balloon, high inflation pressures, coronary dissection, interventions in the setting of acute myocardial infarction, and inadequate healing due to antiproliferative treatment with cortisone, colchicine, and anti-inflammatory drugs (Vassanelli et al., 1989).

Recently, with the advent of implantation of drug-eluting stents, increasing numbers of reports have suggested that stents can cause CAA months or years after the procedure (Pahlavan & Niroomand, 2006; Nichols et al., 2008). The drug-eluting stent contains an immunosuppressant, such as Sirolimus, which inhibits inflammation, or chemotherapeutic agents, such as Paclitaxel, which is an anti-inflammatory agent that inhibits cell proliferation. In due course, once the drug is eluted, the polymer in which the drug is embedded may elicit a hypersensitivity reaction and vasculitis and result in weakening of the vessel wall and subsequent dilatation (Manghat et al., 2006). Mechanical damage to the arterial wall during balloon angioplasty and stent placement or turbulent blood flow may be an added factor for the development of an aneurysm (Nichols et al., 2008). This concept is supported by the finding of an eosinophilic infiltrate in the few cases of such post-stent CAA that have been examined histologically (Virmani et al. 2004). Patients with a history of cocaine abuse have an increased prevalence of CAA (30.4%). These patients appear to be at increased risk of acute myocardial infarction. Several mechanisms have been proposed for the development of aneurysms related to cocaine abuse. These include *(a)* direct endothelial damage caused by severe episodic hypertension and vasoconstriction and *(b)* underlying atherosclerosis (Satran et al., 2005).

6. Pathogenesis

The pathogenesis of CAA is not completely understood but is likely to involve the destruction of the arterial media, thinning of the arterial wall, increased wall stress, and progressive dilatation of the coronary artery segment (Hirsch et al., 2000). Inflammation spilling over into the tunica media from the tunica intima has been hypothesized to link atherosclerosis to aneurysm formation in susceptible individuals. One could hypothesize that the giant cells that are sometimes present in CAA are merely reacting to cholesterol from atheroma and erythrocyte breakdown in the adjacent tunica intima. The lymphohistiocytic inflammation is merely spillover from the atherosclerosis in the adjacent tunica media. The cystic medial degeneration and aneurysm formation may be merely side effects of this spillover inflammation. Alternatively, one could hypothesize that the inflammation is sometimes due to autoimmune vasculitis coexisting with the atherosclerosis (Nichols et al., 2008).

Aneurysm development can be a systemic or local disorder characterized by the overexpression of pro-inflammatory cytokines and enzymes that are capable of degrading elastin and other components of the vascular wall. The pathophysiology is focal destruction of the internal elastic lamina with early neutrophil infiltration followed by macrophages and cytotoxic T lymphocytes (Takahashi et al., 2005). Increased proteolysis of extracellular matrix proteins is probably a mechanism of CAA formation (Mata et al., 2011). MMPs (1, 2, 3, 9 and 12) are capable of degrading essentially all components of the arterial wall matrix (elastin, collagen, proteoglycans, laminin, fibronectin, etc.) and are present at elevated concentrations in aneurysms, while decreased levels of tissue inhibitors of MMPs are present. The MMP-3, 5A allele is associated with higher promoter activity for transcription of the gene, and this allele is more common in patients with CAA plus atherosclerosis than patients with only coronary atherosclerosis (Lamblin et al., 2005). CAAs have destruction of the tunica media, which is thinned, sometimes markedly, sometimes to the point of no longer being identifiable between the tunica intima and tunica adventitia. The normal smooth muscle cells and elastic fibers are replaced by hyalinized connective tissue. Destruction of the internal elastic lamina sometimes obscures the border between diseased tunica media and tunica intima diseased with atherosclerosis. Lipid deposits, foam cells, cholesterol clefts, eosinophilic debris, calcifications, neovascularization, inflammatory reactions, and sometimes hemorrhages can be seen and are sometimes limited to the tunica intima with atherosclerosis, sometimes extend into the tunica media and sometimes spread into the indistinct border zone. The inflammatory reaction chiefly consists of lymphocytes but can also include macrophages and sometimes foreign body giant cell formation around cholesterol clefts. Neutrophils, eosinophils, and plasma cells can be part of the inflammation. This inflammatory reaction is sometimes present in multiple arterial tunica and is sometimes transmural, involving all 3 layers of the artery. Thrombus formation is invariably present on the luminal surface of coronary aneurysms (Daoud et al., 1963).

Cause	Age	Description	Pathogenetic Mechanism
Atherosclerosis	Adults	Most common cause of CAA, clinical importance depends on association with significant coronary artery stenosis	Local mechanical stress from stenosis, atherosclerotic pathologic findings extending into tunica media
Vasculitis *Kawasaki disease*	Childhood	Most common cause of CAA in childhood in Japan, spontaneous resolution occurs in 50%	Autoimmune, vasculitis
Takayasu	Young adults	Common cause of CAA in young Asian females in Japan	Cellular immunity associated with chronic infection
Polyateritis Nodosa	Young adults	Necrotizing inflammatory lesions in small- and medium-sized arteries	Characterized by fibrinoid necrosis and infiltration by predominantly polymorphonuclear leukocytes
Connective tissue disorders	Young adults	Ehlers-Danlos syndrome, Marfan syndrome, cystic medial necrosis	IL-6, TGF-β, C-reactive protein, MMP-2, MMP-9
Mycotic	Any age	Infection with *Staphylococcus aureus* or *Pseudomonas aeruginosa*, syphilis, Lyme disease	Microembolization to vasa vasorum, direct pathogen invasion of arterial wall, immune complex deposition
Trauma/ iatrogenic	Adults	Clinical history helps establish diagnosis healing because of antiproliferative treatment with cortisone, colchicine, and anti-inflammatory drugs	Trauma from oversized balloon or high inflation pressures, coronary dissection, interventions in the setting of acute myocardial infarction, inadequate

Modified from Diaz-Zamudio et al., 2009.

Table 4. Cause, Age, Summary Description and Principal Pathogenetic Mechanisms of Coronary Artery Aneurysms

7. Clinical manifestations and complications

In most cases, CAAs are asymptomatic; then when symptomatic, the clinical manifestations depend on the underlying cause. Although CAA can be seen at any age, those that were related to atherosclerosis usually appear later in life than those of a congenital or inflammatory nature.

No clinical feature characteristics exist for atherosclerotic CAAs. The clinical manifestations are similar to those seen in coronary artery disease (Tunick et al., 1990), and the patients may have angina pectoris, dyspnea, edema, myocardial infarction and sudden death (Pappy et al., 2011). Occasionally, a systolic murmur is heard over the precordium. An association with an abdominal aortic aneurysm and hypertension can occur. Large aneurysms, particularly those that are partially or completely filled with mural thrombi, may create diagnostic challenges by masquerading as cardiac masses (Ramos et al., 2008). The main differential diagnoses include pericardial cysts and primary and metastatic tumors (Tunick et al., 1990). Transesophageal echocardiography and magnetic resonance imaging can add valuable diagnostic information; however, in many cases, diagnosis is not achieved until open-heart surgery.

Factors that can contribute to development of complications are: distal embolization with myocardial ischemia, rupture with associated fistula, cardiac tamponade or hemopericardium, thrombosis, dissection, vasospasm and vessel compression (Syed & Lesch, 1997; Díaz-Zamudio et al., 2009).

8. Diagnosis

CAA may be detected by non-invasive tools, including echocardiography, computed tomography, and magnetic resonance imaging, but coronary angiography remains the best method for the assessment of coronary anatomy and pathology (Pahlavan & Niroomand, 2006). Coronary angiography provides additional information regarding the size, shape, location and the number of existing anomalies and show an image of the coronary artery status (Gziut & Gil, 2008), determining the extent and severity of the coronary lumen obstruction in coronary artery disease (Scanlon et al., 1999). Multidetector row computed tomography (MDCT) technology, have led to widespread enthusiasm for the use of noninvasive coronary angiography (Hendel et al., 2006). The three dimensional evaluation helps to provide an easy understanding of complex anatomic structures and allows the analysis of the lumen and the vessel wall and the identification of thrombi and associated plaque formation. Other non-invasive methods can be also helpful in the diagnosis of aneurysms, including bidimensional transthoracic echocardiography, transesophageal echocardiography (Gziut & Gil, 2008) and electrocardiographic-gated scans, which is a dose modulation technique. These methods are recommended to minimize radiation dose and represent promising tools for the evaluation of children (Goz & Cakir, 2007), particularly children with Kawasaki disease (Beiser et al., 1998). Magnetic resonance (MR) angiography is an alternative for patients for whom exposure to repetitive radiation from multidetector CT is not wanted and for whom other noninvasive modalities are not suitable (Mavrogeni et al., 2004). However, these methods allow the investigation of only the proximal segments of the coronary arteries. Other modalities (such as intravascular ultrasound, Doppler flow wire, and pressure with for calculation of fractional flow reserve) can be incorporated into the invasive evaluation (e.g., angiography), and the pathology can often be treated during the same procedure. Multidetector-row computed tomography (MDCT), a technology that allows good noninvasive imaging of the coronary arteries, has been used despite of its indications and a still-to-be-defined role in the management of patients with cardiovascular symptoms (Zimmet & Miller., 2006).

Undoubtedly, invasive coronary angiography remains the "gold standard" for the evaluation of CAA for a number of reasons. Only blood flow within the lumen can be evaluated, and conventional invasive coronary angiography provides no information about the vessel wall. Thus, with conventional coronary angiography, the true size of the aneurysm may be underestimated or the aneurysm may not even be seen when it is occluded or contains substantial thrombi or plaque (LaMotte & Mathur, 2000).

9. Treatment

CAA treatment consists of medical management, surgical resection, and stent placement; however, the appropriate treatment for CAAs is controversial and depends on the particular clinical situation. The recently available results have been based primarily on case reports and not on controlled studies, which continue to cause a therapeutic dilemma. The medically conservative therapy generally consists of attempts to prevent thromboembolic complications in patients with aneurysmal arteries who are at increased thrombotic risk through administration of antiplatelet and anticoagulant medication (Demopoulos et al., 1997). The use of anticoagulants is based on the observations of thrombus formation in association with CAA and its distal embolization. Surgical management is appropriate in symptomatic patients who have obstructive coronary artery disease or evidence of embolization leading to myocardial ischemia and in patients with CAAs with a risk of rupture (LaMotte & Mathur, 2000). Recently, percutaneous application of polytetrafluoroethylene (PTFE)-covered stents has gained popularity due their ability to effectively limit the expansion of CAAs by reducing blood flow within the aneurysm, thereby preventing their rupture. Some authors have suggested that PTFE-covered stents should be limited to patients whose aneurysms are < 10 mm in diameter (Cohen & O'Gara, 2008). Percutaneous strategies also include coil embolization, autologous saphenous vein-covered stent grafting, and one case report of DES implantation superimposed on a PTFE-covered stent graft (Ghanta et al., 2007).

Surgical strategies that have been described include aneurysm ligation, resection, marsupialization with interposition graft, and coronary artery bypass surgery. The majority of the experience regarding the aforementioned strategies stem from atherosclerosis-induced CAAs (Antelmi et al., 1993). Some surgeons believe that surgical repair is mandatory when a coronary aneurysm is 3 times larger than the original vessel diameter. A complete surgical resection or stent placement may be performed, depending on the presence or absence of coexisting obstructive coronary artery disease. Another surgical option that is frequently used is coronary artery bypass graft (CABG) followed by the ligation or resection of the aneurysm. This approach is indicated in patients who have larger aneurysms that are at higher risk of rupture (Myler et al., 1991).

However, special consideration must be taken when an immunoinflammatory condition is involved. Treatment strategies to improve outcomes in vasculitis-induced CAA involve the use of immunosuppressive therapy to abate the underlying inflammatory process. The role of catheter-based intervention needs to be further explored in this particular patient population. It must be emphasized that there is no consensus regarding how coronary lesions related to systemic inflammatory diseases should be treated (Pappy et al., 2011). Currently, no treatment of CAAs has been universally accepted due to their low incidence and the lack of controlled clinical trials.

10. Conclusion

CAA is an uncommon and often accidental finding. CAAs are usually associated with atherosclerosis in adults in Western countries, while Kawasaki disease is the most common cause of CAA in Japan and in children or young adults. Nevertheless, the exact mechanisms leading to CAA formation are still unclear. Unfortunately, the lack of specific prodromal symptoms or factors predisposing to the formation of CAAs significantly limits the diagnostic possibilities, and consequently, the therapeutic modalities. One way to improve the understanding of the pathogenesis of aneurysms can be through the development of experimental models, such as those that are used for studying abdominal aortic aneurysms (Mata et al., 2011). Thus, this review aimed to provide an update on the pathogenesis and treatment of CAAs to highlight for physicians and thoracic surgeons the practical management of patients with this disease and to help avoid major complications, such as death.

11. Acknowledgments

We wish to thank Julio Matos and Marcela S. Oliveira for the photography assistance.

Financial support: This study was supported by FAPESP (Fundação de Amparo à Pesquisa do Estado de São Paulo) and CNPq (Conselho Nacional de Desenvolvimento Científico e Tecnológico). Karina M. Mata is supported by a scholarship through CNPq. Simone G. Ramos and Marcos A. Rossi are investigators at CNPq.

12. References

Alford, W.J., Stoney, W.S., & Burrus, G.T. (1976). Recognition and operative management of patients with arteriosclerotic coronary artery aneurysms. *Ann Thorac Surg*, Vol. 22, pp. 317-321, ISSN 1552-6259

Amano, S., Hazama, F., & Hamashima, Y. (1979). Pathology of Kawasaki disease: I. Pathology and morphogenesis of the vascular changes. *Jpn Circ J*, Vol.43, pp. 633–43, ISSN 0047-1828

Antelmi, I., Magalhaes, L., Caramelli, B. et al. (1993). Rescue PTCA in a 16 year old boy with Takayasu's disease and evolving myocardial infarciton. *Arquivos Brasileiros de Cardiologia*, Vol. 60, pp. 37–38, ISSN 0066-782X

Antoniadis, A.P., Chatzizisis, Y.S., & Giannoglou, G.D. (2008). Pathogenetic mechanisms of coronary ectasia. *Int J Cardiol*. Vol.130, No.3 (Nov), pp. 335-43, ISSN 0167-5273

Aqel, R.A., Zoghbi, G.J., & Iskandrian, A. (2004). Spontaneous coronary artery dissection, aneurysms, and pseudoaneurysms:a review. *Echocardiography*, Vol.21, No.2, pp. 175–182, ISSN 07422822

Arkin, A. (1930). A clinical and pathological study of periarteritis nodosa. *Am J Pathol*. Vol.6, pp.401-431.

Befeler, B., Aranda, J.M., Embi, A., et al. (1977). Coronary artery aneurysms. Study of their ethiology, clinical course and effect on left ventricular function and prognosis. *Am J Med*. Vol.62, pp.597-607, ISSN 0002-9343

Beiser, A.S., Takahashi, M., Baker, A.L, Sundel, R.P., & Newburger, J.W. (1998). A predictive instrument for coronary artery aneurysms in Kawasaki disease: US Multicenter Kawasaki Disease Study Group. *Am J Cardiol*, Vol.81, No.9, pp.1116–1120, ISSN0002-9343

Berkoff, H.A., & Rowe, G.G. (1975). Atherosclerotic ulcerative disease and associated aneurysms of the coronary arteries. *Am Heart J*, Vol. 90, pp.153-158, ISSN 0002-8703

Bjorn-Hansen, L.S., Thomassen, A.R., & Nielsen, T.T. (1989). Aneurysm of the left anterior descending coronary artery after chest trauma. *Eur Heart J*, Vol.10, No.2, pp.177–179, ISSN 0002-8703

Burgner, D., Davila, S., Breunis, W.B., Ng, SB., Li, Y., Bonnard, C., Ling, L., Wright, W.J., Thalamuthu, A., Odam, M., Shimizu, C., Burns, J.C., Levin, M., Kuijpers, T.W., & Hibberd, M.L. (2009). International Kawasaki Disease Genetics Consortium: A genome-wide association study identifies novel and functionally related susceptibility loci for Kawasaki disease. *PLoS Genet,* Vol.5, No.1 (Jan), e1000319, ISSN 1553-7390

Buzaid, A.C., Milani Júnior, R., Calich, I., & Gonçalves, V. (1985). Arterite de Takayasu: estudo de 16 casos, aspectos clínicos, laboratoriais e revisão da literatura. *AMB Revista Da Associação Médica Brasileira.* Vol.31, pp.85–90, ISSN 0102-843X

Cassling, R., Lortz, J., Olson, D., Hubbard, T., & McMannus, B. (1985). Fatal vasculitis (Polyarteritis nodosa) of the coronary arteries: Angiographic ambiguities and absence of aneurysm at autopsy. *J Am Coll Cardiol,* Vol.6, pp.707–714, ISSN 0735-1097

Chatzizisis, Y.S., Jonas, M., Coskun, A.U., et al. (2008). Prediction of the localization of high-risk coronary atherosclerotic plaques on the basis of low endothelial shear stress: an intravascular ultrasound and histopathology natural history study. *Circulation,* Vol. 117, pp.993–1002, ISSN 0009-7322

Churg, J., & Strauss, L. (1951). Allergic granulomatosis, allergic angiitis, and periarteritis nodosa. *Am J Pathol,* Vol.27, pp.277-301, ISSN 0002-9440

Cohen, P. & Ogara, P.T. (2008). Coronary artery aneurysms: a review of the natural history, pathophysiology, and management. *Cardiology in Review,* Vol. 16, No. 6, pp. 301–304, ISSN 1061-5377

Daoud, A.S., Pankin, D., Tulgan, H., Florentin, R.A. (1963). Aneurysms of the coronary artery: report of ten cases and review of literature. *Am J Cardiol,* Vol. 11, pp. 228–237, *ISSN:* 0002-9149

David, J., Ansell, B.M., & Woo, P. (1993). Polyarteritis nodosa associated with streptococcus. *Arch Dis Child,* Vol.69, pp.685–8, ISSN 0003-9888

Demopoulos, V.P., Olympios, C.D., Fakiolas, C.N., et al. (1997). The natural history of aneurysmal coronary artery disease. *Heart,* Vol.78, No.2, pp.136–141, ISSN 1355-6037

Díaz-Zamudio, M., Bacilio-Pérez, U., Herrera-Zarza, M.C., Meave-González, A., Alexanderson-Rosas, E., Zambrana-Balta, G.F., & Kimura-Hayama, E.T. (2009). Coronary artery aneurysms and ectasia: role of coronary CT angiography. *Radiographics,* Vol. 29, No. 7, pp. 1939-54, ISSN 0271-5333

Dickson, W. (1908). Polyarteritis acuta nodosa and periarteritis nodosa. *J Pathol Bacteriol.* Vol.12, pp.31-57, ISSN 0368-3494

Ewald, E.A., Griffin, D., McCune, W.J. (1987). Correlation of angiographic abnormalities with disease manifestations and disease severity in polyarteritis nodosa. *J Rheumatol,* Vol.14, pp.952–956, ISSN 0315-162X

Falsetti, H.L.& Carrol, R.J. (1976). Coronary artery aneurysm: a review of the literature with a report of 11 new cases. *Chest,* vol.69, No.5, pp. 630–636, ISSN 0012-3692

Ferrari, E. (1903). Ueber Polyarteritis acuta nodosa (sogenannte Periarteritis nodosa), und ihre Beziehungen zur Polymyositis und Polyneuritis acuta. *Beitr Pathol Anat,* Vol.34, pp.350-386, ISSN 0366-2446

Ford, S.R., Rao, A., & Kochilas, L. (2007). Giant coronary artery aneurysm formation following meningococcal septicaemia. *Pediatr Cardiol*. Vol.28, No.4, pp.300–302, ISSN 1432-1971

Gelb, B.D. (2006). Marfan's syndrome and related disorders: more tightly connected than we thought. *N Engl J Med*, Vol.355, pp.841–844, ISSN 0028-4793

Ghanta, R.K.., Paul, S., & Couper, G.S. (2007). Successful revascularization of multiple coronary artery aneurysms using a combination of surgical strategies. *Annals of Thoracic Surgery*, Vol. 84, no. 2, pp. e10–e11, ISSN 1552-6259

Gordon, M., Luqmani, R.A., Adu, D., et al. (1993). Relapses in patients with a systemic vasculitis. *Q J Med*, Vol. 86, pp.779–789, ISSN 0033-5622

Goz, M., & Cakir, O. (2007). Multiple coronary artery aneurysms that cause thrombosis: 22-month follow-up results with multi-slice spiral computerized tomography without surgery. *Int J Cardiol*, Vol.119, No.2, pp.e48–e50, ISSN 0167-5273

Groenke, S., Diet, F., Kilter, H., Boehm, M., & Erdmann, E. (2005) Charakterisierung der dilatativen Koronaropathie bei Patienten mit und ohne stenosierende koronare Herzkrankheit. *Dtsch Med Wochenschr*, Vol.130, pp. 2375–2379, ISSN 0012-0472

Guillevin, L., Lhote F, Gayraud M, et al. (1996). Prognostic factors in polyarteritis nodosa and Churg-Strauss syndrome: a prospective study in 342 patients. *Medicine*,Vol. 75:17-28, ISSN 0025-7974

Gziut, A.I., Gil, R.J. (2008). Coronary aneurysms. *Pol Arch Med Wewn*, Vol.118, No.12 (Dec), pp.741-6, ISSN 0032-3772

Habashi, J.P., Judge, D.P., Holm, T.M., et al. (2006). Losartan, an AT1 antagonist, prevents aortic aneurysm in a mouse model of Marfan syndrome. *Science*, Vol.312, pp.117–121, ISSN 0036-8075

Hachulla, E., Bourdon, F., Taieb, S., et al. (1993). Embolization of two bleeding aneurysms with platinum coils in a patient with polyarteritis nodosa. *J Rheumatol*, Vol.20, pp.158–161, ISSN 0315-162X

Hans, S.S., Jareunpoon, O., Balasubramaniam, M., & Zelenock, G.B. (2005). Size and location of thrombus in intact and ruptured abdominal aortic aneurysms. *J Vasc Surg*, Vol.41, pp.584–8, ISSN 0950-821X

Harikrishnan, S., Sunder, K.R., Tharakan, J.M., et al. (2000). Saccular coronary aneurysms: angiographic and clinical profile and follow-up of 22 cases. *Indian Heart J*, Vol. 52, pp.178–182, ISSN 0019-4832

Hata, A., Noda, M., Moriwaki, R., et al., (1996). Angiographic findings of Takayasu arteritis: new classification. *Int J Cardiol*, Vol.54,(Suppl):S155–S163, ISSN 0167-5273

Hekali, P., Kajander, H., Pajari, R., Stenman, S., & Somer, T. (1991). Diagnostic significance of angiographically observed visceral aneurysms with regard to polyarteritis nodosa. *Acta Radiol*. Vol.32, pp.143–148, ISSN 0284-1851

Hirsch, G.M., Casey, P.J., Raza-Ahmad, A., et al. (2006). Thrombosed giant coronary artery aneurysm presenting as an intracardiac mass. *Ann Thorac Surg*, Vol.69, pp.611-6137, ISSN 1552-6259

Holzknecht, N., Gauger, J., Helmberger, T., Stäbler, A., & Reiser, M. (1997). Cross-sectional imaging findings in a case of polyarteritis nodosa with a ruptured hepatic artery aneurysm. *AJR Am J Roentgenol*, Vol.169, No.5 (Nov), pp.1317-9, ISSN 0361-803X

Kang, W.C., Han, S.H., Oh, K.J., et al. (2006). Implantation of a drugeluting stent for the coronary artery stenosis of Takayasu arteritis. *Circulation*, Vol.113, pp.e735–7, ISSN 0009-7322

Kastner, D., Gaffney, M., Tak, T. (2000). Polyarteritis nodosa and myocardial infarction. *Can J Cardiol*, Vol.16, pp.515–518, ISSN 0828-282X

Kawasaki T. (1967). Acute febrile mucocutaneous syndrome with lymphoid involvement with specific desquamation of the fingers and toes in children. *Arerugi*, Vol.16, pp.178–222, ISSN 0021-4884

Kerr, G.S. (1995). Takayasu's arteritis. *Rheumatic Disease Clinics of North America*. Vol.21, pp.1041–1059, ISSN 0889-857X

Klinger, H. (1931). Grenzformen der Periarteritis nodosa. *Frankfurter Zeitschrift Pathol*, Vol.42, pp.455-480, ISSN 0367-3480

Koskinas, K.C., Chatzizisis, Y.S., Baker, A.B., Edelman, E.R., Stone, P.H., & Feldman, C.L. (2009). The role of low endothelial shear stress in the conversion of atherosclerotic lesions from stable to unstable plaque. *Curr Opin Cardiol*, Vol.24 (November), pp.580–90, ISSN 0268-4705

Kussmaul, A. & Maier, K. (1886). Uber cine bischer nicht beschreibene eigen thumchche arteriener krankung die mit morbus brightii und rapid forts chreitender allgemeiner muskellahmung embergent. *Dtsch Arch Klin Med*, Vol.1, pp.484-494, ISSN 0366-8576

Lam, K.C., Lai, C.L., Trepo, C., & Wu, P.C. (1981). Deleterious effects of prednisolone in hepatitis B surface antigenpositive chronic active hepatitis. *N Engl J Med*, Vol.304, pp.380-386, ISSN 0028-4793

Lamblin, N., Bauters, C., Hermant, X., Lablanche, J-M., Helbecque, N., & Amouyel, P. (2002). Polymorphisms in the promoter regions of MMP-2, MMP-3, MMP-9 and MMP-12 genes as determinants of aneurysmal coronary artery disease. *J Am Coll Cardiol*, Vol.40:43–48, ISSN 0735-1097

LaMotte, L.C., & Mathur, V.S. (2000). Atherosclerotic coronary artery aneurysms: 8-year angiographic follow-up. *Tex Heart Inst J*, Vol.27, No.1, pp.72–73, ISSN 1355-6037

Libby, P. (2002). Inflammation in atherosclerosis. *Nature*, Vol. 420, pp. 868–74, ISSN 0028-0836

Lie, J.T. (1998) Pathology of isolated nonclassical and catastrophic manifestations of Takayasu arteritis. *Int J Cardiol*, Vol.66, Suppl 1, pp.S11-21, ISSN 0167-5273

Lightfoot Jr., R.W., Michel, B.A., Bloch, D.A., et al. (1990). The American College of Rheumatology 1990 criteria for the classification of polyarteritis nodosa. Arthritis Rheum. Vol.33, pp.1088–93, ISSN 0004-3591

Lypsky, P.E. (1994). Rheumatoid arthritis. *Harrison´principles of internals medicine*, In: Isselbacher, K.J., Braunwald, E., Wilson J.D., et al. pp.1648-1653, Mc-Graw-Hill, ISBN 10: 0071466339, New York

Manghat, N.E., Hughes, G.J.M., Cox, I.D., & Roobottom, C.A. (2006). Giant coronary artery aneurysm secondary to Kawasaki disease: diagnosis in an adult by multi-detector row CT coronary angiography. *BJR*, Vol.79, pp.e133-136, ISSN 0482-5004

Markis, J.E., Joffe, C.D., & Cohn, P.F. (1976): Clinical significance of coronary arterial ectasia. *Am J Cardiol*, Vol. 37, pp. 217-222, ISSN 0002-9149

Mata, K.M., Prudente, P.S., Rocha, F.S., Prado, C.M., Floriano, E.M., Elias, J. Jr., Rizzi, E.,Gerlach, R.F., Rossi, M.A., & Ramos, S.G. (2011). Combining two potential causes of metalloproteinase secretion causes abdominal aortic aneurysms in rats: a newexperimental model. *Int J Exp Pathol*,Vol.92, No.1, (Feb.), pp.26-39, ISSN 1936-2625

Matayoshi, A.H., Dhond, M.R., Laslett, L.J. (1999). Multiple coronary aneurysms in a case of systemic lupus erythematosus. *Chest,* Vol116, pp.1116–1118, ISSN 0012-3692

Mavrogeni, S., Papadopoulos, G., Douskou, M., et al. (2004). Magnetic resonance angiography is equivalent tox-ray coronary angiography for the evaluation of coronary arteries in Kawasaki disease. *J Am Coll Cardiol,* Vol.43, No.4, pp.649–652, ISSN 0735-1097

Mesquita, Z.B., Sacchetti, S., Andrade, O.V., et al. (1998). Arterite de Takayasu na infância: revisão de literatura a propósito de 6 casos. *Journal Brasileiro de Nefrologia,*Vol.20, pp.263–275, INSS 0101-2800

Moore, Jr. J.E., Xu, C., Glagov, S., Zarins, C.K., Ku, D.N. (1994). Fluid wall shear stress measurements in a model of the human abdominal aorta: oscillatory behavior and relationship to atherosclerosis. *Atherosclerosis,* Vol. 110, pp. 225–40, ISSN 0214-9168

Mora, B., Urbanek, B., Loewe, C., Grimm, M., & Dworschak, M. (2011). Position dependent right ventricular dysfunction caused by a giant right coronary artery aneurysm. *Wien Klin Wochenschr.* vol.123, No.1-2, (Jan), pp.58-60, ISSN 0043-5325.

Morales, E., Pineda, C., & Martínez-Lavín, M. (1991). Takayasu's arteritis in children. *Journal of Rheumatology,*Vol.18, pp.1081–1084, ISSN 0315-162X

Morgagni, J.B. (1761). De Sedibus et Causis morborum. *Venectus Tom I,* vol.27, pp.28, ISSN.

Munkner, T., Petersen, O., & Vesterdal, J. (1958). Congenital aneurysm of the coronary artery with an arteriovenous fistula. *Acta Radiol,* vol.50, No. 4, pp. 333–340, ISSN 0001-6926.

Myler, R.K., Scheshumann, N.S., Rosenblum, J., et al. (1991). Multiple coronary artery aneurysms in an adult associated with extensive thrombus formation resulting in myocardial infarction: successful treatment with intracoronary urokinase, intravenosus heparin and oral anticoagulant. *Cathet Cardiovasc Diagn,* Vol.24, pp.51-54, ISSN 0098-6569

Nakamura, Y., Yashiro, M., Uehara, R., et al. (2008). Epidemiologic features of Kawasaki disease in Japan: results from the nationwide survey in 2005–2006. *J. Epidemiol,* Vol.18, pp.167–72, ISSN 0917-5040

Newburger, J.W., Takahashi, M., Beiser, A.S., et al. (1991). A single intravenous infusion of γ globulin as compared with four infusions in the treatment of acute Kawasaki syndrome. *N Engl J Med,*Vol.324, No.23, pp.1633–1639, ISSN 0028-4793

Newburger, J.W., Takahashi, M., Burns, J.C., et al. (1986). The treatment of Kawasaki syndrome with intravenous γ globulin. *N Engl J Med,* Vol.315, No.6, pp.341–347, ISSN 0028-4793

Nichols, L., Lagana, S., & Parwani, A. (2008). Coronary artery aneurysm: a review and hypothesis regarding etiology. *Arch Pathol Lab Med,* Vol.132, No.5 (May), pp.823-8, ISSN 0003-9985

Pahlavan, P.S., & Niroomand, F. (2006) Coronary artery aneurysm: a review. *Clin Cardiol,* Vol.29, No 10, pp.439–443, ISSN 0160-9289

Panja, M., Sarkar, C., Kar, A.K., Kumar, S., Mazumder, B., Roy, S., et al. (1998). Coronary artery lesions in Takayasu's arteritis--clinical and angiographic study. *J Assoc Physicians India,* Vol.46, No.8, pp.678-81, ISSN 0004-5772

Pappy, R., Wayangankar, S., Kalapura, T., Abu-Fadel, M.S. (2011). Rapidly evolving coronary aneurysm in a patient with rheumatoid arthritis. *Cardiol Res Pract,* Vol.21 (Feb), pp.659439, ISSN 2090-0597

Parangi, S., Oz, M.C., Blume, R.S., Bixon, R., Laffey, K.J., Perzin, K.H., Buda, J.A., Markowitz,A.M., & Nowygrod, R.(1991).Hepatobiliary complications of polyarteritis nodosa. *Arch Surg.*Vol.126, No.7 (Jul), pp.909-12, ISSN 0272-5533

Pick, R., Glover, M., & Viewer, W. (1982). Myocardial infarction in a young women with isolated coronary arteritis. *Chest,* Vol. 82, pp.378–380, ISSN 0012-3692

Porcella, A.R., Sable, C.A., Patel, K.M., Martin, G.R., & Singh, N. (2005). The epidemiology of Kawasaki disease in an urban hospital: does African American race protect against coronary artery aneurysms? *Pediatr Cardiol,* Vol. 26, pp. 775–781, ISSN 0172-0643

Przybojewski, J. (1981). Polyarteritis nodosa in the adult. *S Afr Med J.* Vol.60, pp.512–518, ISSN0256-9574

Ramos, S.G., Mata, K.M., Martins, C.C., Martins, A.P., & Rossi, M.A.(2008). Giant right coronary artery aneurysm presenting as a paracardiac mass. *Cardiovasc Pathol,* vol.17, No.5, (Sep-Oct), pp. 329-33, ISSN 1054-8807

Reichman, E.F., & Weber, J.M. (2004). Undiagnosed Takayasu's arteritis mimicking an acute aortic dissection. *J Emerg Med,* Vol.27, pp.139–42, ISSN 0736-4679

Rowley, A.H., Baker, S.C., Orenstein, J.M., & Shulman, S.T. (2008). Searching for the cause of Kawasaki disease cytoplasmic inclusion bodies provide new insight. *Nat Rev Microbiol,* Vol.6, No.5, pp.394–401, ISSN 1740-1526

Rozenberg, V.D., & Nepomnyashchikh, L.M. (2005). Pathomorphology of atherosclerotic coronary artery aneurysms and heart architectonics. *Byull Eksp Biol Med,* Vol.139, pp. 629–633, ISSN 0365-9615

Satran, A., Bart, B.A., Henry, C.R., et al.(2005). Increased prevalence of coronary artery aneurysms among cocaine users. *Circulation,* Vol.111, No.19, pp.2424–2429, ISSN 0009-7322

Scanlon, P.J, Faxon, D.P., Audet, A.M., et al. (1999). ACC/AHA guidelines for coronary angiography. A report of the Americ. College of Cardiology/American Heart Association Task Force on practice guidelines (committee on coronary angiography) developed in collaboration with the Society for Cardiac Angiography and Interventions. *J Am Coll Cardiol,* Vol.33, pp.1756-1824, ISSN 0735-1097

Sharma, B.K., Jain, S., Suri, S., & Numano, F. (1996). Diagnostic criteria for Takayasu arteritis. *Int J Cardiol,* Vol.54, Suppl:S141-7, ISSN 0167-5273

Soto, M.E., Espinola-Zavaleta, N., Ramirez-Quito, O., & Reyes, P.A. (2006). Echocardiographic follow-up of patients with Takayasu's arteritis: five-year survival. *Echocardiography,* Vol.23, No.5 (May), pp.353-60, ISSN 07422822.

Stioufii, M., & Pelissier, R. (1984). The effect of unsteadiness on the flow through stenoses and bifurcations. *J Biomechanics,* Vol 17 pp. 299-303, ISSN 0021-9290

Stone, J.H. (2002). Polyarteritis nodosa. *JAMA,* Vol.288, No.13 (Oct), pp.1632-9, ISSN 0098-7484

Subramanyan, R., Joy, J., & Balakrishnan, K.G. (1989). Natural history of aortoarteritis. *Circulation.,*Vol.90, pp.429 –37, ISSN 0009-7322

Swaye, P.S., Fisher, L.D., Litwin, P., et al. (1983). Aneurysmal coronary artery disease. *Circulation,* Vol. 67, pp.134-138, ISSN 0009-7322

Syed, M., & Lesch, M. (1997).Coronary artery aneurysm: a review. *Prog Cardiovasc Dis*, Vol.40, No.1 (Jul-Aug), pp.77-84, ISSN 0033-0620

Takahashi, K., Oharaseki, T., Naoe, S., Wakayama, M., Yokouchi, Y. (2005). Neutrophilic involvement in the damage to coronary arteries in acute stage of Kawasaki disease. *Pediatr Int*, Vol.47, pp.305–310, ISSN 1442-200X

Takayasu, M. (1908). A case with peculiar changes of the retinal central vessels (in Japanese). *Acta Opthal Soc Jpn*, Vol.12, pp.554–555, ISSN

Trepo, C.G., Zucherman, A.J., Bird, R.C., Prince, A.M. (1974). The role of circulating hepatitis B antigen/antibody immune complexes in the pathogenesis of vascular and hepatic manifestations in polyarteritis nodosa. *J Clin Pathol*, Vol.27, pp.863–8, ISSN 0021-9746

Tsuda, E., Abe, T., & Tamaki, W. (2010). Acute coronary syndrome in adult patients with coronary artery lesions caused by Kawasaki disease: review of case reports. *Cardiol Young*, Vol.21, No.1 (Feb), pp.74-82, ISSN 1047-9511

Tsuda, E., Matsuo, M., Kurosaki, K., et al. (2007). Clinical features of patients diagnosed as coronary artery lesions caused by presumed Kawasaki disease in adult. *Cardiol young*, Vol.17, pp. 84–89, ISSN

Tunick, P.A., Slater, J., Kronzon, I., Glassman, E. (1990). Discrete atherosclerotic coronary artery aneurysms: A Study of 20 patients. *J Am Coll Cardiol*, Vol 15, pp.279-282, ISSN 0735-1097

Uehara, R., Yashiro, M., Nakamura, Y., & Yanagawa, H. (2003). Kawasaki disease in parents and children. *Acta Paediatr*, Vol.92, No.3 (Jun), pp.694–7, ISSN 0001-656X

Vassanelli, C., Turri, M., Morando, G., Menegatti, G., & Zardini, P. (1989). Coronary arterial aneurysms after percutaneous transluminal coronary angioplasty: a not uncommon finding at elective follow-up angiography. *Int J Cardiol*, Vol.22, No.2, pp.151–156, ISSN 0167-5273

Virmani, .R, Guagliumi, G., Farb, A., et al. (2004). Localized hypersensitivity and late coronary thrombosis secondary to a sirolimus-eluting stent. *Circulation*, Vol.109, pp.701–705, ISSN 0009-7322

Wang, K.Y., Ting, C.T., St John Sutton, M.,& Chen, Y.T. (1999). Coronary artery aneurysms: A 25-patient study. *Catheter Cardiovasc Interv*, Vol.48, No. 1 (Sep) pp.31-8, ISSN 0098-6569

Williams, M.J., & Stewart, R.A. (1994). Coronary artery ectasia: local pathology or diffuse disease? *Cathet Cardiovasc Diagn*, Vol. 33, No. 2, pp. 116–119, ISSN 0098-6569

Yilmaz, A., Rowley, A., Schulte, D.J., et al. (2007). Activated myeloid dendritic cells accumulate and co-localize with CD3+ T cells in coronary artery lesions in patients with Kawasaki disease. *Exp Mol Pathol*, Vol.83, No.1, pp.93–103, ISSN 0014-4800

Zimmet JM & Miller JM. (2006)Coronary artery CTA: imaging of atherosclerosis in the coronary arteries and reporting of coronary artery CTA findings. *Tech Vasc Interv Radiol*, Vol.9, No.4, (Dec), pp.218-26, ISSN 1089-2516

Zizic, T.M., Classen, J.N., & Stevens, M.B. (1982). Acute abdominal complications of systemic lupus erythematosus and polyarteritis nodosa. *Am J Med*, Vol.73, pp.525-533, ISSN 0002-9343

22

Cardiac Function and Organ Blood Flow at Early Stage Following Severe Burn

Rong Xiao and Yue-Sheng Huang*
Institute of Burn Research, State Key Laboratory of Trauma, Burns and Combined Injury, Southwest Hospital, Third Military Medical University, Chongqing
China

1. Introduction

Multiple organ dysfunction syndrome (MODS) has been the difficulty in clinical treatment of severe burns. In the 1990s, the incidence rate of MODS was 28.1% in severe burn patients, while the mortality rate was as high as 78%-98% (Huang et al., 1998). MODS was caused by two “attacks": the first attack was the early plasma leakage and the effective circulating blood volume reduction, as resulted in the systemic hypoxic-ischemic damage; the second attack was the invasion of consequent systemic inflammatory response and sepsis on the organs (Sheng, 2002). With enhancement of the clinical treatment of burns, the present point of view argues that the key to prevention of MODS is against the first "attack", ie, to control the burn shock, which can effectively prevent or mitigate the second "attack" to reduce the incidence of MODS (Sheng, 2002).

Previously, only hypovolemia was concerned in the patients with burn shock. However, it is found that simple increase of the blood volume can not effectively curb the incidence of burn shock in a large number of clinical treatments of severely burned patients. These group of patients are often accompanied by hypodynamic blood circulation, thus too much or fast fluid perfusion may easily induce heart failure. Therefore, we have shifted our attention to the heart, a motivator organ for blood circulation. We further found that the heart is not the sole organ injured early by serious burn, and this damage and reduced pump function occurred before the vascular permeability change and the blood volume decrease (Huang, Li, & Yang, 2003; Huang et al., 1999b). The immediate early myocardial damage and weakened pump function of the heart can not only cause heart failure, but also induce or aggravate shock and hence become one of the generators leading to severe burn shock and systematic hypoxic-ischemic damage. Based on above, we proposed the hypothesis of "shock heart" involving systematic hypoxic-ischemic damage early after burn injury (Huang, Zheng, Fan, & Zhang, 2007; Huang, 2009; Xiao et al., 2008b). In order to confirm this hypothesis, we have conducted a large number of animal experiments and clinical trials. On the one hand, we explored the effects of the early emergence of myocardial damage and cardiac dysfunction on the systemic organ perfusion and hypoxic-ischemic injury; on the other hand, an in depth study has been done on its development mechanism so as to find effective therapeutic targets for clinical use.

* Corresponding Author

2. Early changes of cardiac function after severe burns

In the early 1960s, Fozzard observed myocardial damage and cardiac output decrease in the burn patients and further found that this kind of heart failure was not due to pre-injury heart disease or excessive fluid infusion (Fozzard, 1961). Some scholars attributed the cardiac dysfunction to the vascular leakage of plasma into the injured area, causing decreased venous return and cardiac preload reduction (Evans, Purnell, Robinett, Batchelor, & Martin, 1952). Nonetheless, the subsequent experimental results differed from this view. The researchers found that before obvious extravasation of plasma, the cardiac output was significantly reduced and even a large volume of fluid resuscitation could not improve the cardiac output . (Moyer, Coller, Iob, Vaughan, & Marty, 1944) Therefore, it was considered that the microcirculatory disturbances, abnormal coagulation system (Brooks, Dragstedt, Warner, & Knisely, 1950) and peripheral vasoconstriction (Salzberg & Evans, 1950; Wolfe & Miller, 1976) after severe burn were key causes to the combined cardiac dysfunction. In 1984, Adams et al established a guinea pig burn model to study the systolic and diastolic function changes of the the left ventricle after the injury. They found that when the burn injury exceeded 47% of the total body surface area (TBSA), the ventricular compliance was reduced and the cardiac isovolumic relaxation period extended, accompanied by significant myocardial contractile dysfunction, based on which they viewed that inherent myocardial damage led to the decrease of the adverse cardiac filling and ejection fraction of the left ventricle (Adams, Baxter, & Izenberg, 1984).

Cardiac dysfunction after severe burns has been confirmed in many experimental studies. However, the myocardial systolic/diastolic dysfunction occurred in different time post-burn in different species animal models including mice, rats, hamsters, guinea pigs, rabbits, dogs, pigs and sheep (Adams, Baxter, & Parker, 1982; Baxter, Cook, & Shires, 1966; Elgjo et al., 1998; Ferrara et al., 1998; Fozzard, 1961; Horton, Garcia, White, & Keffer, 1995; Horton, Maass, White, Sanders, & Murphy, 2004; Horton, White, Maass, & Sanders, 1998; White, Maass, Giroir, & Horton, 2001). Horton et al studied time course of heart function of the rabbit and rat after burn by dissecting the heart for in vitro perfusion at each time point. The results showed a transient decrease of the cardiac function after burn, which first appeared at 2 hours, decreased continually within 24-30 hours and gradually recovered at 48-72 hours after burn injury (Horton et al., 1995; Maass, Hybki, White, & Horton, 2002; Sheeran et al., 1998). This short-term decreased heart function may be less risk for the otherwise healthy young adults with burn but may be so risky for the young, the elderly and the immunocompromised patients that they had to receive unaffordable fluid resuscitation. Recent studies also showed that the cardiac dysfunction after burn is an index for predicting the proneness to secondary infection, ie, it is closely related with morbidity and mortality of MODS in severely burned patients and can predict the long-term infection complications.

Over the past 10 years, our laboratory have carried out a series of burn research on the pig, dog, rabbit, rat and other animal models and particularly established a mature rat model with 30% TBSA 3rd degree burn. When the rats were under anesthesia, the cardiac function was detected by inserting the catheter from the carotid artery to the left ventricle, when the other end of the catheter was connected with pressure transducer and multi-channel physiological recorder. Number of myocardial mechanical indicators were recorded early after burn injury (24 hours) at several preset time points, which could help deeper understand the course of the cardiac function change in the early time after burns (Xiao, Lei,

Dang, & Huang, 2011). As shown in Figure 1, in rats with 30% TBSA 3rd degree scald injury, the maximal rate of the rise/drop of left ventricular pressure (± dp/dt max) was significantly reduced 1 hour post-burn, while the mean arterial pressure (MAP) was declined until 3 hours after injury, indicating that the cardiovascular system itself has a certain compensatory ability and a stable blood pressure can be maintained temporarily by increasing the peripheral resistance. Our results showed that the heart function reached a valley at 12 hours after burn injury, then recovered for some extent but still remained at a low level at 24 hours after injury, which differed from the aforementioned time course results (the valley emerged at 24-30 hours after injury) reported by Horton et al. This difference may be due to different cardiac function test methods, ie, in vitro heart perfusion and in vivo intubation. However, our results undoubtedly confirm that the cardiac function was weakened rapidly after burn (1-2 hours after injury), when there was no obvious plasma extravasation or reduction of effective circulating blood volume (Carvajal, Linares, & Brouhard, 1979; Salzberg & Evans, 1950). Therefore, we can be sure that the cardiac dysfunction soon after severe burns was caused by myocardial cell damage and myocardial systolic/diastolic dysfunction of the heart itself rather than the burn shock, as is worthy of further study and exploration on these endogenous mechanism.

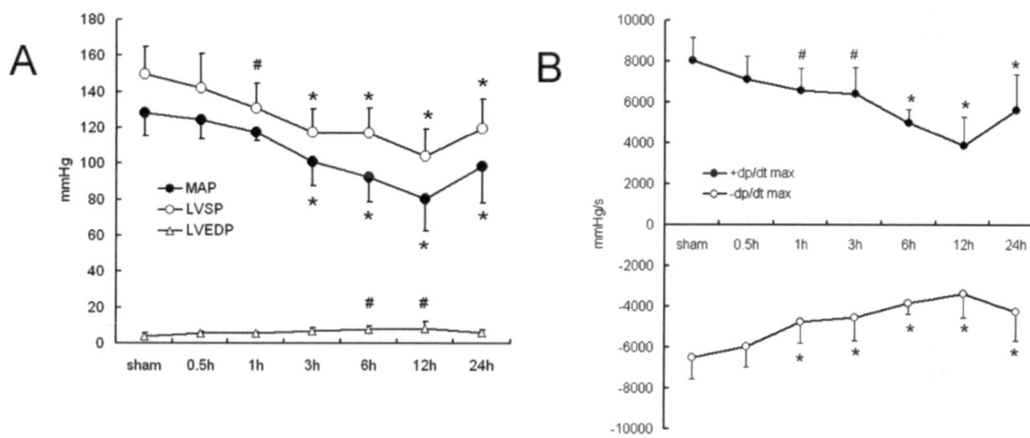

Fig. 1. Time course of heart function after 30%TBSA 3rd degree burns in rats in vivo. All values are mean ± SEM. MAP, mean arterial pressure; LVSP, left ventricular systolic pressure; LVEDP, left ventricular end-diastolic pressure; ± dp/dt max, maximal rate of the rise/drop of left ventricular pressure. * $p<0.05$ vs sham.

3. Organ perfusion at early stage following severe burns

Severe burns induce a strong stress response and high excitement of the sympathetic-adrenal medulla system. The catecholamines secreted by the sympathetic-adrenal medulla system can adjust the heart excitement, the peripheral vascular resistance and the capacitance vessels so that the blood supply to tissues and organs at the shock stage becomes more adequate and reasonable. However, the anatomy, physiology and tolerance to ischemia and compensatory ability differs in various organs, which leads to different blood supply of the main organs including heart, brain, liver, kidney and intestine after severe burns.

3.1 Heart

The traditional pathophysiological view was that under severe stress conditions, especially reduction of the effective circulating blood volume, the body reduced the blood supply of most abdominal organs and gave priority to ensuring the blood supply of the heart, brain and other vital organs. However, a lot of experiments conducted in our laboratory confirmed no effective protection of the myocardial blood supply after severe burns. Early in 1996, Yang et al (Yang, Yang, & Chen, 1996) used radioactive tracer ^{86}Rb uptake to detect the myocardial nutritional blood flow (NBF) changes of rats with 30% TBSA 3rd degree burn (Figure 2). The results showed that the myocardial nutritional blood flow was reduced by about 24% 1 hour after burn, then continued to decrease up to the valley at 12 hours and recovered mildly at 24 hours (but still lower than the sham group), which was similar to the trend of cardiac function change. Moreover, the earliest time point for determination of the myocardial blood flow was at 1 hour after injury, which was the same time that the cardiac function began to decline. Nonetheless, we are not sure about whether the myocardial ischemia damage resulted in decreased heart function or the reduced cardiac output led to the coronary flow decrease. Therefore, the myocardial blood flow was detected in the rats with 30% TBSA 3rd degree burns by using the fluorescent microspheres method at 10 min, 30 min, 1 hour, 3 hours and 6 hours post-burn (Figure 3). The results showed that the regional myocardial blood flow was decreased significantly at 10 minutes, recovered mildly at 30 minutes and 1 hour, and then continued to decline after burn (Yin, Huang, & Li, 2010). The myocardial blood flow was rapidly reduced 10 minutes after burn, which may be related to the contraction of the coronary caused by myocardial renin-angiotensin system (RAS) that was activated immediately after burn (Mackins et al., 2006). We used the enzyme linked immunosorbent assay (ELISA) method to detect the Ang II in the myocardial (Figure 4) and the results showed that the myocardial Ang II was increased from 10 minutes after injury. This is a very good explanation of the transient reduction of the myocardial blood flow at 10 minutes after burn. The subsequent rebound increase of the blood perfusion may be due to accumulation of hypoxic metabolites that offset or exceeded the vascular contraction effect of Ang II and finally caused vasodilation.

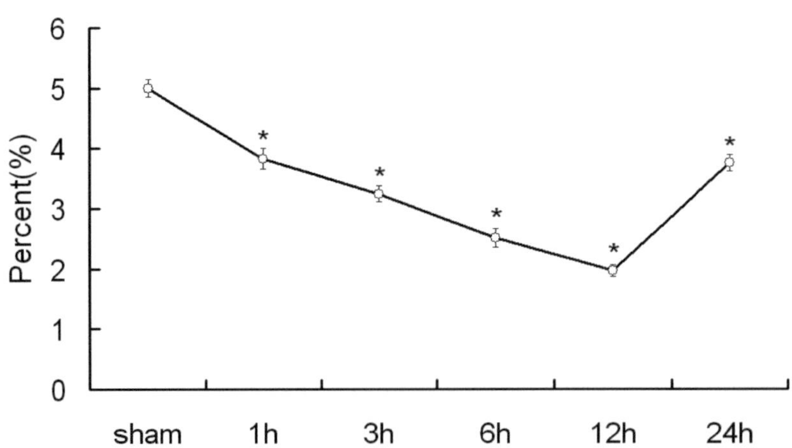

Fig. 2. Myocardial nutrition blood flow of the rats following 30%TBSA 3rd degree burns. All values are mean ± SEM. * $p<0.05$ vs sham.

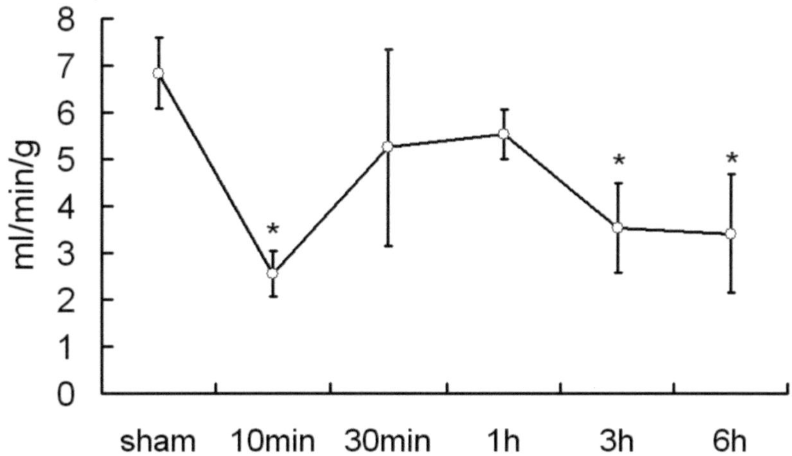

Fig. 3. Myocardial blood perfusion of the rats following 30%TBSA 3rd degree burns. All values are mean ± SEM. * $p<0.05$ vs sham.

In fact, under continuous increase of the Ang II, the compensatory mechanism of the heart itself was difficult to maintain too long and turned into decompensation about 3 hours post-burn, with continual decrease of the myocardial blood flow. Thus, the myocardial blood flow was reduced before cardiac dysfunction after severe burns, indicating that the myocardial ischemia and hypoxia was the main cause for the cardiac dysfunction (Huang et al., 2003).

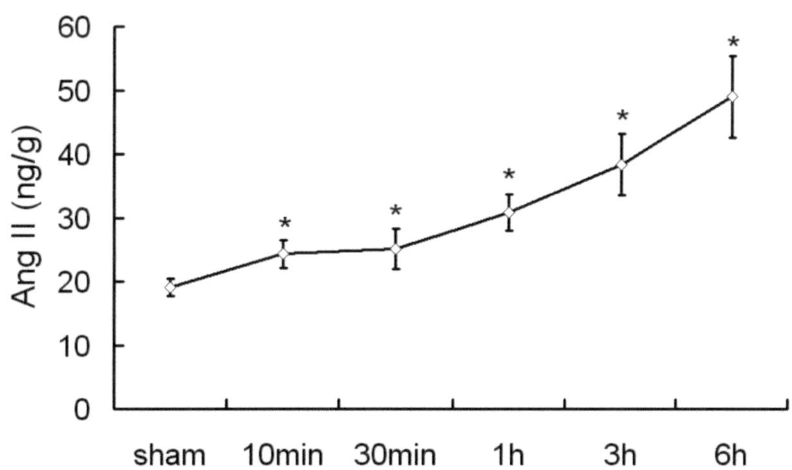

Fig. 4. Content of cardiac local angiotensin II in the rats following 30%TBSA 3rd degree burns. All values are mean ± SEM. * $p<0.05$ vs sham.

3.2 Brain

Currently, there has seldom reported the cerebral blood flow perfusion at early stage after severe burns. But the cerebral edema was often complicated clinically after burn, the pathological factors for which was different from brain trauma or brain damage simply caused by brain trauma or hypoxia. The complicated cerebral edema after burn is due to destructed microcirculation and blood-brain barrier function as well as increased permeability resulted from a variety of factors including ischemia and hypoxia, cell medium, endotoxin, electrolyte imbalance, acidosis and uncontrolled inflammation, which ultimately caused diffuse tissue edema. The vascular endothelial cells played a key role in the pathogenesis of brain edema after burn. On the one hand, the vascular endothelial cells had clear morphological changes, even formation of cracks and endothelial cell loss leading to the semi-permeable membrane barrier dysfunction and vascular permeability increase. On the other hand, the vascular endothelial cells could release a variety of media to further promote the microcirculation disorder, aggravate tissue ischemia and hypoxia and promote development of the tissue edema (Domres, Heller, & von Kothen, 1981; Li et al., 2001).

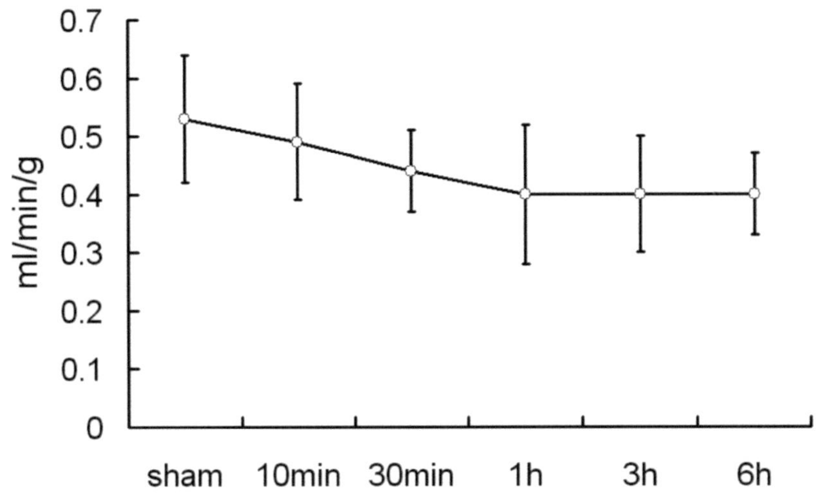

Fig. 5. Cerebullar blood perfusion of the rats following 30%TBSA 3rd degree burns. All values are mean ± SEM.

We have used the same fluorescent microspheres method to detect the brain blood flow in rats with 30% TBSA 3rd degree burns (Figure 5), which showed insignificant statistical difference upon the cerebral blood flow at all time points, indicating that the brain tissues still had a strong compensatory ability even after burn injury. Because the brain tissue has the minimum tolerance to the hypoxia out of all organs, the brain blood supply can still remain stable unless under a serious shortage of blood volume.

3.3 Reduced perfusion and hypoxic-ischemic injury of the liver, kidney and intestine

Catecholamines in the blood at early stage after burn was increased tens even hundreds times more than that in the normal time. The small blood vessels in the abdominal organs and kidney had rich sympathetic vasoconstrictor innervation, with dominant α-adrenergic receptors. With sympathetic excitement and catecholamine increase, the microvascular contraction of these organs significantly increased precapillary resistance and sharply decreased the microcirculation perfusion. While the β-adrenergic receptor stimulation opened the arterial-venous anastomosis, which resulted in increase of the microcirculation non-nutritive blood flow, decrease of the nutritional blood flow and severe tissue ischemia and hypoxia. In addition, a great deal of Ang II produced by the activated circulatory system RAS was also involved in the vasoconstriction (Dolecek, Zavada, Adamkova, & Leikep, 1973).

The laser Doppler flowmetry was employed to detect the blood flow of liver, kidney, and intestines of the rats with 30% 3rd degree burns, which showed that the hepatic, renal, and intestinal perfusion was significantly declined 1 hour post-burn and recovered for some extent at 24 hours (Figure 6). The blood flow changes differed significantly in different organs, ie, the blood flow was reduced the most significantly in the kidney, followed by the intestine and the liver the least. Despite obvious decrease, the hepatic blood flow remained stable overall. Judging from the recovery, the liver restored the blood flow better at 24 hours after burn, while the kidney and intestinal ischemia were still under serious condition, especially the intestines, which may be due to so-called "covert compensated shock", ie, the blood supply was difficult to recover even quite a long time after adequate systemic blood supply (Fiddian-Green, Haglund, Gutierrez, & Shoemaker, 1993).

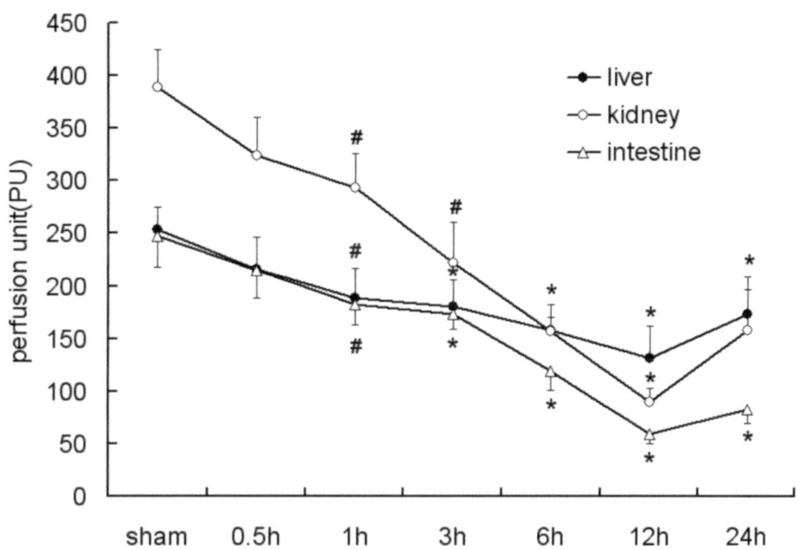

Fig. 6. Blood flow to liver, kidney, and intestine in the rats following 30%TBSA 3rd degree burns. All values are mean ± SEM. * $p<0.05$ vs sham.

Liver blood supply has its own peculiarities, the portal vein and hepatic artery converged in to the hepatic capillary network and subsequently returned to heat via the hepatic vein. Under the resting state, 20% of the cardiac output entered into the liver, of which 1/3 passed by the hepatic artery and 2/3 by the portal vein. Liver cells are extremely sensitive to the ischemia and hypoxia, easy inducing the liver cell damage. The central lobular hepatocytes received less blood flow than the peripheral cells of the lobule and it suffered the earliest and the most serious damage. Visceral injury was closely related to the circulatory state especially the micro-circulation after burn. After the ischemic phase, the substrate concentration of the intracellular xanthine oxidase was increased, which prompted the substrate transforming to the xanthine oxidase via proteolysis or histamine. During the course of reperfusion, a large number of free radicals were produced with the improvement of hypoxia and finally induced reperfusion injury (Horton, 2003). Toklu et al detected malondialdehyde (MDA), reduced glutathione (GSH) level and myeloperoxidase (MPO) activity of skin, lung, liver, ileum and kidneys in rats at 6 and 48 hours after burns and found significant increase of MDA level and MPO activity but decrease of antioxidant GSH content; hence they viewed that the oxygen free radicals and lipid peroxidation plays an important role in organ damage after burn injury (Toklu et al., 2006). Sakarcan et al carried out similar experiments to confirm the protective effect of antioxidant Ginkgo biloba extract (Egb) on the rat organs after burn injury and the results showed increase of MDA level and MPO activity but decrease of GSH in the liver and kidney, together with increase of AST, ALT, BUN, Cr and LDH, as suggested liver and kidney dysfunction (Sakarcan et al., 2005).

Zhou et al observed a series of liver changes 1 hour after burn in rats, mainly swelling, degeneration and necrosis of the hepatocytes, fatty degeneration or eosinophils detected by the light microscope, which resulted in point-like or small focal hepatocyte necrosis. In the meantime, the electron microscopy manifested different degrees of ultrastructure change of the hepatocytes and extensive damage to the nucleus and organelles. Their study also showed that ALT was increased at 1 hour and reached the peak at 12 hours after burn and that AST began to increase at 6 hours and continued to 48 hours after burn. The increase of blood AST and ALT was the inevitable result of serious liver parenchyma damage, indicating that burns can cause liver damage and progressive aggravation in a relatively short period of time. Especially the degeneration and necrosis of the hepatocytes, mitochondria degeneration and endoplasmic reticulum will undoubtedly and directly affect the normal function of the hepatocytes and weaken the detoxification function of the burn injury liver, when acute liver failure may occur in a few burn patients (Zhou, Huang, & Chen, 2002).

In the normal adult, the kidney is body organ with the largest blood flow, with 1000-1250ml/min, accounting for 20%-25% of cardiac output. The renal damage at burn shock stage is primarily due to sharp decline of the blood volume, reduction of the cardiac output and decrease of the renal blood flow. The heart failure induced by severe burns would directly result in of the effective circulating blood volume decrease, the sympathetic excitement and the redistribution of systemic blood, which affected the renal blood flow the most, with reduction of glomerular blood flow and filtration to 30%-50% or less of the normal (Figure 6). When the arterial pressure fell below 60 mmHg, the glomerular filtration would even stop and lead to anuria or oliguria. Sener et al found significant decrease of renal tissue GSH, increase of MDA, protein oxidation (PO) level and MPO activity and renal dysfunction (increase of BUN and local LDH) in rats at 6 hours post-burn and they argued that the kidney damage was mainly caused by lipid peroxidation and oxygen free radical damage and that the antioxidants Mesna exerted a protective effect on the kidneys (Sener et al., 2004). For oxygen free radical damage, Sener et al conducted a similar experiment in an attempt to prove the role of melatonin in preventing early kidney injury after burns (Sener, Sehirli, Satiroglu, Keyer-Uysal, & Yegen, 2002).

The nerve-humoral regulation early after burns induced redistribution of the blood and the gastrointestinal hypoperfusion lasted for the longest. The blood flow of intestinal mucosa and villi accounted for 80% and 60% of total gastrointestinal tract blood flow. A 10% decrease of systemic blood volume may lead to 40% decrease of the whole gastrointestinal tract blood flow. The vascular loop of the intestinal villi was with an extremely bent ring structure, which contributed to a short circuit exchange of the central villus arterioles with the venules and capillaries. Under shock and low perfusion state, the short circuit exchange increased to further reduce the oxygen supply of the villus top. The intestinal tissue had high metabolic rate and demanded great deal of the oxygen, indicating that the intestinal tissue was sensitive to ischemia and hypoxia and easy to be damaged, with slow recovery. Under stress state, the mucosal partial pressure of oxygen was decreased but the lactic acid levels significantly increased, the latter of which, during the ischemia-reperfusion process, released large amounts of oxygen free radicals that were the initiating factor for inflammatory mediators and cytokines cascade (Gianotti, Alexander, Pyles, James, & Babcock, 1993).

The burn resulted in up-regulation of a variety of proteins regulating the stress response, reduction of self-repair ability of the intestinal mucosa by free radical damage, energy metabolism disorder of the intestines, increase of cell apoptosis (Zhang et al., 2002), cytoskeletal damage of the intestinal smooth muscle and gastrointestinal motility disorders (Tong, Wang, & Guo, 2006). Reduction of the synthesis of secretory IgA and apoptosis of the intestinal lymph node cells destructed the intestinal immune barrier (Fan, Xie, Zhou, Chen, & Deng, 2006), which may cause damage to the intestinal bacterial translocation and even endotoxemia. The intestinal ischemia-reperfusion injury caused "waterfall-like" cascade of inflammatory mediators by the way of p38/mitogen activated protein kinase (MAPK) (Gan, Pasricha, & Chen, 2007), as made the intestines as the "source" of systemic inflammatory response syndrome (SIRS). The uncontrolled development of SIRS would inevitably lead to MODS or multiple organ failure (MOF), so Hassoun et al considered the intestines was the initiating organ for post-traumatic MOF (Hassoun et al., 2001). Extensive burns, shock and other factors induced potential intestinal hypotension, intestinal hypoperfusion or recessive intestinal shock that may cause intestinal mucos ischemia and hypoxia, intestinal barrier dysfunction, and intestinal SIRS and MODS, as was called "shock bowel" by some scholars (Tu & Xiao, 2002).

3.4 Effect of cardiac dysfunction on hepatic, renal, and intestinal blood flow

The heart is the power organ of the circulatory system. It still remains unclear whether the perfusion changes of the liver, kidney, intestines and other organs is induced by the weakened heart function after burn injury. In order to verify the effect of cardiac function on the liver, kidney and intestine perfusion after severe burns, we established the rat model with 30% 3rd degree burns and then the cardiac function of the rats was intervened with cedilanid, low-dose angiotensin-converting enzyme inhibitor (ACEI) enalaprilat and high-dose β-blocker propranolol. The cardiac function and the blood flow of liver, kidney and intestines were observed at 6 hours post-burn, which showed that cedilanid and low-dose enalaprilat could effectively enhance the heart function; ACEI action on the cardiac function indicated local RAS activation early after burn; Ang II increased the harmful effects of casoconstrictor on the myocardial (Figure 7A); and high-dose β-blocker propranolol could obviously inhibit the cardiac function. It was found that the liver, kidney and intestinal blood flow was significantly increased accordingly with cardiac function improvement and decreased with further suppression of the cardiac function (Figure 7B). With aim to clarify the effect of cardiac function changes on perfusion of various organs after burn, an analysis was done on the correlation between the mechanical index ± dp/dt max and the liver, kidney and intestinal blood flow, which showed a positive correlation of liver, kidney and intestinal perfusion with the cardiac function after burn (Table 1). The results indicated that immediate early cardiac dysfunction may be an important initiating factor for secondary ischemia and hypoxia damage of multiple organs after severe burn.

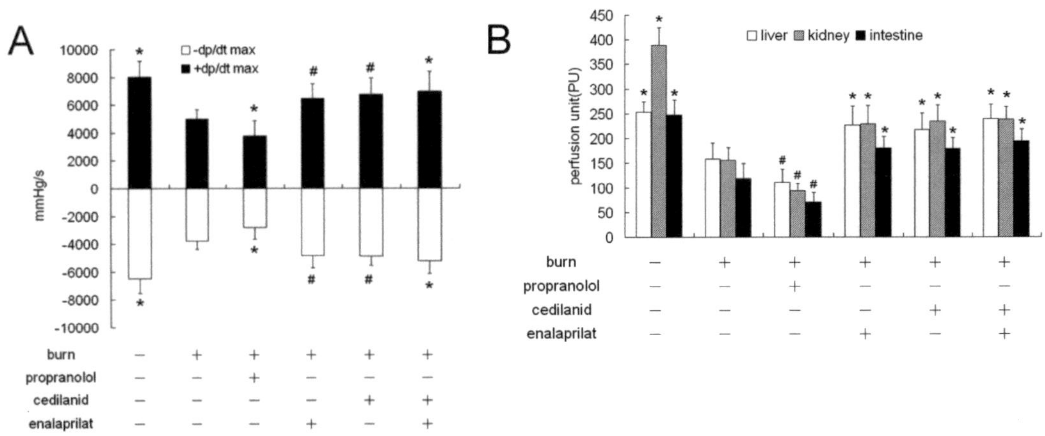

Fig. 7. Cardiac function and blood flow to liver, kidney, and intestine in the 30%TBSA 3rd degree burn rats treated with cedilanid, enalaprilat, and propranolol. All values are mean ± SEM. * p<0.05 vs simple burn.

	+dp/dt max		-dp/dt max	
Parameter tested	†PCC	P value (2-tailed)	PCC	P value (2-tailed)
Hepatic blood flow	0.956*	0.001	0.976*	0.000
Renal blood flow	0.985*	0.000	0.946*	0.001
Intestinal blood flow	0.964*	0.000	0.918*	0.003

Table 1. Summary table of correlation analysis between the maximal left ventricular pressure increase/decrease rate and organ blood flow in rats after a 3rd degree burn. Organ blood perfusion was significantly and positively correlated with heart systolic/diastolic function in rats after the burn (30% of body area) (* P < 0.01). †Pearson correlation coefficient.

4. Mechanism for cardiac damage / heart function depression at early post-burn stage

Undoubtedly, myocardial cell damage is the immediate cause of heart function depression in the early burn period. Back in 1961, Fozzard claimed that myocardial damage may be the reason of cardiac output decrease not matching the change of blood volume (Fozzard, 1961). In the 1990s, serum troponin I (cTnI) was proposed as a highly specific and sensitive indicator in detecting cardiomyocyte injury (Horton et al., 1995). Murphy et al (Murphy,

Horton, Purdue, & Hunt, 1998) randomly examined the level of serum cTnI in a large number of burn patients. They found the serum cTnI was negative in patients with less than 10% TBSA burns, while it continually rose in patients with more than 20% TBSA burns within 12 hours post-burn. It provided solid evidence for post-burn myocardial damage. By testing the serum cTnI in mature rat models of 30% TBSA 3rd degree burns at different time points, we found their serum cTnI levels increased at post-burn 30 minutes, reached the peak at 12 hours, but dropped at 24 hours. Nevertheless, their serum cTnI levels were still lower than the sham (non-burned) group (Xiao et al., 2008a). Bivariate correlation analysis indicated that serum cTnI levels were closely related with the post-burn change in heart function parameters (Xiao et al., 2008a). Other parameters of myocardial damage like myosin light chain 1 (CMLC1) and troponin T (cTnT) also increased evidently after burn (Huang et al., 2003; Huang et al., 1999b). Pathological observation found cloudy swelling of myocardial cells, interstitial vascular dilatation, congestion, edema, hemorrhage and inflammatory cell infiltration at 3 hours post-burn in scalded rats with 30% TBSA 3rd degree burns. At 12h hours post-burn, an irregular arrangement of cardiac muscle fibers (in the wavy-pattern) and sarcoplasm condensation were observed (Zhang et al., 2007a). All these facts implied that cardiac damage already existed in early severe burns, accompanied by decreased heart functions. Then what caused these cardiac damages?

Since the evidence of "burn toxin" presented (Allgower et al., 1968), Baxter and his colleagues attempted to seek myocardial depressant factors (MDF) in the plasma of burn patients. They infused the plasma of burn patients into the free hearts of normal guinea pigs and proved that such plasma was myocardial depressant (Baxter et al., 1966). To avoid species differences and immune reactions, Horton et al collected the serum of 40%TBSA burned rats to infuse the isolated hearts of homogeneous rats. The serum was also proved to be myocardial depressant (Horton et al., 2004). Ferrara et al found that lymph fluid from the posterior limbs of burned animals could reduce the regional myocardial blood flow, resulting in decreased coronary systolic and diastolic activity (Ferrara et al., 1998). Sambol et al found that pre-burn mesenteric lymph duct ligation could greatly improve the impaired cardiac contractile function, which suggested the existence of myocardial depressant factors in burned animals (Sambol, White, Horton, & Deitch, 2002). All these researches implied that burn injuries indeed stimulated the activation and release of certain protein factors which had a negative regulatory or damaging role on cardiac muscles.

Tumor necrosis factor (TNF-α) serum level were initially believed to be associated with the progression of infection (Marano et al., 1990; Marano et al., 1988). Some researchers also thought that the increase of TNF-α in post-burn plasma could be used as a measurement of the body's immune response, which indicated increased risks of secondary sepsis and death (Cannon et al., 1992; Yamada et al., 2000). Subsequent researchers assayed the post-burn TNF-α, IL-1β, IL-6 and other factors and suggested that taking multiple factors into consideration, rather than a single inflammatory factor TNF-α, could better predict the onset of sepsis (Drost et al., 1993a; Drost, Burleson, Cioffi, Mason, & Pruitt, 1993b; Zhang et al., 1998). However, Giroir and Beutler believed that the heart was an important source of TNF-α, although this inflammatory factor could be produced by many other cells and organs (Giroir, Johnson, Brown, Allen, & Beutler, 1992). Then Giroir and Horton studied the role of TNF-α in postburn myocardial dysfunction and found enhanced synthesis of TNF-α by myocardial cells with a more than 40% TBSA burns. The Anti-TNF-α strategy could prevent myocardial contractile dysfunction and elevate cardiac output (Giroir, Horton, White, McIntyre, & Lin, 1994). Substantial evidence has proved TNF-α to be one of the initial mediators in the "waterfall-like" inflammatory cascade response. In the animal models, intravenous injection of recombinated TNF-α could induce myocardial depression (Eichenholz et al., 1992; Pagani et al., 1992; Tracey et al., 1986). The administration of TNF-α to left ventricular myocardial cells cultured in vitro would produce a concentration-dependent negative inotropic effect (Heard, Perkins, & Fink, 1992; Horton, Maass, White, & Sanders, 2001a; Maass, White, & Horton, 2005; Yokoyama et al., 1993). Meanwhile, the fact that transgenic mice with myocardial overexpression of TNF-α all died of dilated cardiomyopathy and congestive cardiac failure demonstrated its negative effect on myocardial contraction (Bryant et al., 1998). It was also reported that the serum TNF-α increase in the burn patients was not accompanied by signs of infection (Cannon et al., 1992). The level of TNF-α produced by myocardial cells which were isolated from burned rats was 15 times that of the normal control rats (Williams, Bankey, Minei, McIntyre, & Turbeville, 1994). All these facts showed that TNF-α was a significant initiation factor in the postburn uncontrolled inflammatory cascade, as well as an important inflammatory factor in myocardial damage, playing an important role in MODS after sever burns.

In the case of severe burn, tissue ischemia and hypoxic metabolism still continues under large-volume fluid resuscitation (Demling, Ikegami, & Lalonde, 1995). When ischemia is improved in the tissues, re-exposure to molecular oxygen will generate a large number of oxygen free radicals, leading to tissue damage (Horton, 2003). Metabolism of xanthine oxidase (XO) is the major source of oxygen free radicals produced after burns. Allopurinol is a competitive antagonist of XO. Allopurinol-pretreatment can prevent oxyradical-induced myocardial damage and cardiac function depression in rats (Horton & White, 1993). The rise of myocardial lactic acid levels after burns suggests the existence of hypoxic metabolism. Rapid large-volume fluid replacement will remove lactic acid accumulation and improve the myocardial creatine phosphorylation level. The addition of allopurinol to the replacement fluid will remove depolarization in cardiac cell membrane and enhance myocardial contractile function (Horton & White, 1995). Other studies suggested that neutrophil adhesion and activation was another source of oxygen free radicals after burns. Neutrophils release a large number of oxygen free radicals explosively and strengthen the effect of xanthine oxidase, causing damage to tissues and organs (Horton, Mileski, White, & Lipsky, 1996). In addition, burns also destroy the body's antioxidant defense mechanism, so that the tissues are more vulnerable to oxygen free radicals. Further researches found that the rise of MDA in plasma and myocardial tissues led to increase in local concentrations of peroxidized lipid peroxide and conjugated diene. These experiment results all demonstrated the role of oxygen free radicals in postburn organ damage and dysfunction (Cetinkale et al., 1997; Cynober et al., 1985; Demling & LaLonde, 1990a, b; Takeda et al., 1984; Ward, Till, Hatherill, Annesley, & Kunkel, 1985).

Multiple cellular and molecular signal transduction pathways have been verified to cause myocardial damage and mechanical dysfunction. The p38/MAPK pathway, for instance, regulates the synthesis and secretion of cytokines and plays a significant role in many heart diseases like myocardial hypertrophy, ischemia/reperfusion injury, and myocardial cell apoptosis (Sugden & Clerk, 1998; Wang et al., 1998; Zhang et al., 2008b). Myocardial p38/MAPK activity was evidently elevated in cases of over 40% TBSA burns. This enhanced activity in the early postburn period (at 1 hour, 2 hours, and 4 hours post-burn) could be inhibited by its specific antagonist SB203580. Nevertheless, the activity of JNK was not interfered. The inhabitation of p38/MAPK activity decreased the production of myocardial TNF-α, improved postburn myocardial contractile function, as well as enhanced tolerance of vitro cultured myocardial cells to hypoxia and burn serum (Ballard-Croft, White, Maass, Hybki, & Horton, 2001; Zhang, Ying, Chen, Yang, & Huang, 2008a). Zhang et al also found that p38/MAPK involved in burn-induced degradation of myocardial cell membrane phospholipids, and revealed that it achieved such effects by adjusting cytosolic phospholipase A2 (cPLA2) (Zhang et al., 2007b). Moreover, hypoxia was recently found to cause myocardial cell microtubule depolymerization through activation of p38/MAPK and change of phosphorylation level of microtubule associated protein 4 (MAP4) and oncoprotein 18/stathmin (Op18) (Hu et al., 2009). Additionally, through F-actin cytoskeleton rearrangement and phosphorylation of L-caldesmon, p38/MAPK conducted an important role in endothelial barrier dysfunction induced by burn serum (Chu et al., 2010).

The Rho-kinase pathway has been proved by other researches to perform a critical role in the reconstruction of cardiac muscle fibers after burn injuries (Hoshijima, Sah, Wang, Chien, & Brown, 1998; Kobayashi et al., 2002). The activation and up-regulation of α-1-adrenergic pathway (Ballard-Croft, Maass, Sikes, White, & Horton, 2002) led to activation of RhoA/Rho-kinase (Suematsu et al., 2001). Evidence showed that the myocardial Rho-kinase expression was considerably enhanced at 1 hour, 2 hours, and 8 hours post-burn, and engaged in regulating the synthesis and release of inflammatory factors like TNF-α 、IL-1β and IL-6 by myocardial cells in rats with over 40% TBSA burns (Horton, Maass, & Ballard-Croft, 2005).

Protein kinase C (PKC) was also found by some researchers to engage in regulating myocardial inflammatory reaction and cardiac dysfunction. PKCε, a major PKC isoform in adult cardiomyocytes, presented up-regulated expression and increased activity after burn injury. The expression of PKCα was also up-regulated at early post-burn stage, while the PKCδ expression increased later (at 24 hours post-burn). Even though the impacts of each PKC isoform after burn injuries remain unclear, it has been confirmed that PKC pathway involved in the regulation of myocardial cytokine synthesis. The inhibitor of PKC, either calphostin or chelerythine, could significatly reduce inflammatory cytokines secretion by myocardial cells and improve the damaged myocardial contractile function (Horton, White, & Maass, 1998).

The transcription factor NF-κB, downstream of the PKC/p38/MAPK/JNK/Rho-kinase pathway, regulates a variety of genes of inflammatory cytokine, such as TNF-α and IL-1β, which are detrimental to cardiac function (Baeuerle & Baltimore, 1996). The level of myocardial NF-κB, according to Carlson et al's finding, continuously increased from 1 hour to 24 hours post-burn. The NF-κB activation started earlier than secretion of TNF-α and IL-1β by myocardial cells, which was again earlier than the occurrence of heart function impairment (Carlson et al., 2003). In further experiments, the NF-κB activity was inhibited by molecular or pharmacological approaches to explore its effect on myocardial inflammatory reaction and cardiac dysfunction. The NF-κB activity was elevated from 2 hours to 24 hours post-burn in wild-type mice. NF-κB nuclear translocation was not detected in burned mice with over-expression of IκB. In contrast with wild-type burned mice, burn mice overexpressing IκB presented decreased secretion of TNF-α and IL-1β and less heart function impairment. ALLN, the specific NF-κB antagonist agent, can also prevent NF-κB nuclear translocation, inhibit the secretion of TNF-α and IL-1β, and improve cardiac functions (Carlson et al., 2003). These facts imply that activation of NF-κB was upstream of signal transduction pathway, which performs a critical part in the pathological progression of burn-induced myocardial damage and cardiac dysfunction.

Reports from our laboratory showed that both energy dysmetabolism (Liang, Tang, Yang, & Huang, 2002) and apoptosis (Zhang et al., 2008c) of myocardial cells induced by mitochondrial Ca^{2+} disorder after burns directly led to myocardial damage. Activation of tumor necrosis factor receptor-associated protein (TRAP1) and adenosine A1 receptor, however, inhibited the mitochondrial permeability transition pores (MPTP) to open, so as to prevent apoptosis provoked by MPTP opening and to achieve myocardial protection (Xiang, Huang, Shi, & Zhang, 2010a; Xiang et al., 2010b). We examined the RAS active ingredients and endothelin in serum and myocardial tissues at 10 minutes, 30 minutes, 1 hour, 3 hours, and 6 hours post-burn and found that concentrations of myocardial Ang II and its convertase ACE rose significantly since 10 minutes, while serum Ang II concentration increased notably since 30 minutes postburn, a little later. It demonstrated that the rapid activation of local cardiac RAS occurred earlier than the activation of circulatory RAS. Myocardial endothelin levels also increased 10 minutes after burns, and then maintained at a relatively higher level all the time. Serum endothelin levels, however, did not change much. Simultaneous myocardial blood flow measured by fluorescent microspheres also dropped at the same time point, suggesting these two strong vaso-excitor materials both involved in coronary vasoconstriction, resulting in cardiac insufficiency. Either ACEI or endothelin receptor blocking pharmacon could greatly improve myocardial perfusion, indicating the two substances' crucial roles in myocardial impairment. The rapid activation of local cardiac RAS after burns increased the Ang II level in myocardial tissues within a short period. Vasoconstriction it induced then resulted in myocardial ischemia and damage, which might be the most immediate cause of myocardial impairment at the early post-burn stage (Yang, Yang, & Chen, 1999).

Although the mechanism of myocardial damage and cardiac function depression in the early post burn period has been explored and analyzed from various perspectives in multiple researches, it cannot be accurately explained only from a single aspect. The exact mechanism of myocardial damage may be the combined effects of multiple factors, or perhaps there are more convincing causes, which await our further investigation.

5. Prevention and therapy strategies of the burn-related myocardial damage/cardiac dysfunction

Based on the above-mentioned confirmed mechanisms of myocardial injury/decreased heart function, many scholars put forward the corresponding prevention and therapy strategies.

For the damage of inflammatory mediators to the myocardial function after burn injury, many studies have focused on limiting the adhesion and activation of the neutrophils. The monoclonal antibody specific for the intracellular adhesion molecule 1 and 2 (ICAM-1 and ICAM-2), P, L, E-selectin has been proved to be with hemodynamic and myocardial protection effect during the treatment of the burns (Flynn, Buda, Jeffords, & Lefer, 1996; Horton et al., 1996; Mileski, Winn, Harlan, & Rice, 1991). Some scholars even selected the ICAM-1 and P-selectin knockout mice to explore the role of the adhesion molecules and neutrophil activation in treatment of the organ damage, particularly the myocardial damage/decreased cardiac function after burn injury

The most widely recognized clinical prevention and therapy means is to curb the oxygen free radicals damaging the organs, including clinical use of a large dose of the anti-oxidants. After burn injury, vitamin C and N-acetylcysteine can effectively improve the tissue energy load, improve the level of vitamin C and E in the tissues, enhance the elastase activity, enhance the microvascular function and inhibit production of the free radicals. The enhanced antioxidant capacity is helpful for maintenance of the high-energy phosphate level in the tissues, improvement local micro-circulation and effective prevention of the burn edema (LaLonde, Nayak, Hennigan, & Demling, 1997; Lalonde, Picard, Campbell, & Demling, 1994; Matsuda et al., 1992; Matsuda et al., 1991). Antioxidant therapy can protect the mitochondrial membrane integrity and thereby prevent cardiac dysfunction after burns (Zang, Maass, White, & Horton, 2007). Matsuda et al even found that the antioxidant vitamin therapy could reduce the planned amount of resuscitation fluid with an adequate cardiac output (Matsuda et al., 1993). Other experiments showed that the left ventricular systolic dysfunction, the continual increase of the preload and the coronary blood flow decrease in the rats with lack of vitamin antioxidant therapy, which, however, could be improve with the antioxidant treatment (Horton, 2003).

Ulinastatin (UTI), the refined protease inhibitors extracted from the human urine, can not only inhibit the activities of many hydrolytic enzymes including trypsin, phospholipase A2, hyaluronidase and elastase, but also prevent the MDF production and ameliorate the circulatory state of shock. The experimental and clinical studies have proved that UTI exerted a significant effect on prevention and treatment of the myocardial damage, for it could regulate the inflammatory response balance, remove the oxygen free radicals, reduce the lipid peroxidation and inhibit the myocardial apoptosis (Huang, Xie, Zhang, Dang, & Qiong, 2008).

For the patients with total burn area over 35% TBSA (of which 3rd degree burn over 20% TBSA), surgical removal of the entire eschar early after burn can reduce SIRS and endothelial system damage and hence effectively prevent the MODS (Huang, Yang, Chen, Crowther, & Li, 1999a). The mitochondrial damage is a key factor to myocardial apoptosis, which can be alleviated by using the mitochondrial stabilizers ruthenium red after burns (Wan-Yi, Hui, Zong-Cheng, & Yue-Sheng, 2002). The other measures such as antisense c-jun and p38 gene transfection (Huang & Hu, 2004; Huang et al., 2007) and hypertonic saline dextran (Horton, Maass, White, & Sanders, 2001b) also have certain curative effect.

6. Conclusion

In brief, the cardiac local RAS which is activated immediately after severe burns causing vasoconstriction results in ischemic and hypoxic injury in myocardiums, which contributes mostly and initially to the post-burn myocardial damage and heart dysfunction. The uncontrolled cascade response of the inflammatory factors, cytoskeleton and mitochondria destruction in cardiomyocytes, apoptosis and necrosis following ischemia and hypoxia are directly responsible for the post-burn myocardial damage and cardiac dysfunction. And the cardaic pumping deficit with reduced output offers insufficient blood flow to the organs such as liver, kidney, and intestines, which induces and further aggravates the burn shock. In the pathophysiological course of severe burns, the myocardial damage/cardiac dysfunction and the burn shock (microcirculation disturbance and inadequate tissue and organ perfusion) are the two crossed main lines, the vicious circulation of which may lead the patients to MODS and even death. Can the originating factor for the myocardial damage be effectively blocked, the survival rate of the patients with extensive burns will be greatly improved. Thus, it is worthy of looking forward to a breakthrough in more in depth and effective endogenous protection mechanism of the myocardial damage.

7. Acknowledgment

This study was supported by a Key Grant from the State Key Laboratory of Trauma, Burns and Combined injury (SKLZZ200806), National Key Technology Research and Development Program (2009BAI87B03).

8. References

Adams, H. R.; Baxter, C. R. & Izenberg, S. D. (1984). Decreased contractility and compliance of the left ventricle as complications of thermal trauma. *American Heart Journal*, Vol.108, No.6, pp.1477-1487, ISSN.0002-8703

Adams, H. R.; Baxter, C. R. & Parker, J. L. (1982). Contractile function of heart muscle from burned guinea pigs. *Circulatory Shock*, Vol.9, No.1, pp.63-73, ISSN.0092-6213

Allgower, M.; Burri, C.; Cueni, L.; Engley, F.; Fleisch, H.; Gruber, U. F.; Harder, F. & Russell, R. G. (1968). Study of burn toxins. *Annals of the New York Academy of Sciences*, Vol.150, No.3, pp.807-815, ISSN.0077-8923

Baeuerle, P. A. & Baltimore, D. (1996). NF-kappa B: ten years after. *Cell*, Vol.87, No.1, pp.13-20, ISSN.0092-8674

Ballard-Croft, C.; Maass, D. L.; Sikes, P.; White, J. & Horton, J. (2002). Activation of stress-responsive pathways by the sympathetic nervous system in burn trauma. *Shock*, Vol.18, No.1, pp.38-45, ISSN.1073-2322

Ballard-Croft, C.; White, D. J.; Maass, D. L.; Hybki, D. P. & Horton, J. W. (2001). Role of p38 mitogen-activated protein kinase in cardiac myocyte secretion of the inflammatory cytokine TNF-alpha. *American Journal of Physiology. Heart and Circulatory Physiology*, Vol.280, No.5, pp.H1970-1981, ISSN.0363-6135

Baxter, C. R.; Cook, W. A. & Shires, G. T. (1966). Serum myocardial depressant factor of burn shock. *Surgical Forum*, Vol.17, pp.1-2, ISSN.0071-8041

Brooks, F.; Dragstedt, L. R.; Warner, L. & Knisely, M. H. (1950). Sludged blood following severe thermal burns. *Archives of Surgery*, Vol.61, No.3, pp.387-418, ISSN.0272-5533

Bryant, D.; Becker, L.; Richardson, J.; Shelton, J.; Franco, F.; Peshock, R.; Thompson, M. & Giroir, B. (1998). Cardiac failure in transgenic mice with myocardial expression of tumor necrosis factor-alpha. *Circulation*, Vol.97, No.14, pp.1375-1381, ISSN.0009-7322

Cannon, J. G.; Friedberg, J. S.; Gelfand, J. A.; Tompkins, R. G.; Burke, J. F. & Dinarello, C. A. (1992). Circulating interleukin-1 beta and tumor necrosis factor-alpha concentrations after burn injury in humans. *Critical Care Medicine*, Vol.20, No.10, pp.1414-1419, ISSN.0090-3493

Carlson, D. L.; White, D. J.; Maass, D. L.; Nguyen, R. C.; Giroir, B. & Horton, J. W. (2003). I kappa B overexpression in cardiomyocytes prevents NF-kappa B translocation and provides cardioprotection in trauma. *American Journal of Physiology. Heart and Circulatory Physiology*, Vol.284, No.3, pp.H804-814, ISSN.0363-6135

Carvajal, H. F.; Linares, H. A. & Brouhard, B. H. (1979). Relationship of burn size to vascular permeability changes in rats. *Surgery, Gynecology & Obstetrics*, Vol.149, No.2, pp.193-202, ISSN.0039-6087

Cetinkale, O.; Belce, A.; Konukoglu, D.; Senyuva, C.; Gumustas, M. K. & Tas, T. (1997). Evaluation of lipid peroxidation and total antioxidant status in plasma of rats following thermal injury. *Burns: Journal of the International Society for Burn Injuries*, Vol.23, No.2, pp.114-116, ISSN.0305-4179

Chu, Z. G.; Zhang, J. P.; Song, H. P.; Hu, J. Y.; Zhang, Q.; Xiang, F. & Huang, Y. S. (2010). p38 MAP kinase mediates burn serum-induced endothelial barrier dysfunction: involvement of F-actin rearrangement and L-caldesmon phosphorylation. *Shock*, Vol.34, No.3, pp.222-228, ISSN.1540-0514

Cynober, L.; Desmoulins, D.; Lioret, N.; Aussel, C.; Hirsch-Marie, H. & Saizy, R. (1985). Significance of vitamin A and retinol binding protein serum levels after burn injury. *Clinica Chimica Acta; International Journal of Clinical Chemistry*, Vol.148, No.3, pp.247-253, ISSN.0009-8981

Demling, R.; Ikegami, K. & Lalonde, C. (1995). Increased lipid peroxidation and decreased antioxidant activity correspond with death after smoke exposure in the rat. *The Journal of Burn Care & Rehabilitation*, Vol.16, No.2 Pt 1, pp.104-110, ISSN.0273-8481

Demling, R. H. & LaLonde, C. (1990a). Early postburn lipid peroxidation: effect of ibuprofen and allopurinol. *Surgery*, Vol.107, No.1, pp.85-93, ISSN.0039-6060

Demling, R. H. & Lalonde, C. (1990b). Systemic lipid peroxidation and inflammation induced by thermal injury persists into the post-resuscitation period. *The Journal of Trauma*, Vol.30, No.1, pp.69-74, ISSN.0022-5282

Dolecek, R.; Zavada, M.; Adamkova, M. & Leikep, K. (1973). Plasma renin like activity (RLA) and angiotensin II levels after major burns. A preliminary report. *Acta Chirurgiae Plasticae*, Vol.15, No.3, pp.166-169, ISSN.0001-5423

Domres, B.; Heller, W. & von Kothen, W. (1981). Brain edema and carbohydrate metabolism in the early stages of thermal injury and burn shock. *Acta Chirurgiae Plasticae*, Vol.23, No.2, pp.99-106, ISSN.0001-5423

Drost, A. C.; Burleson, D. G.; Cioffi, W. G., Jr.; Jordan, B. S.; Mason, A. D., Jr. & Pruitt, B. A., Jr. (1993a). Plasma cytokines following thermal injury and their relationship with patient mortality, burn size, and time postburn. *The Journal of Trauma*, Vol.35, No.3, pp.335-339, ISSN.0022-5282

Drost, A. C.; Burleson, D. G.; Cioffi, W. G., Jr.; Mason, A. D., Jr. & Pruitt, B. A., Jr. (1993b). Plasma cytokines after thermal injury and their relationship to infection. *Annals of Surgery*, Vol.218, No.1, pp.74-78, ISSN.0003-4932

Eichenholz, P. W.; Eichacker, P. Q.; Hoffman, W. D.; Banks, S. M.; Parrillo, J. E.; Danner, R. L. & Natanson, C. (1992). Tumor necrosis factor challenges in canines: patterns of cardiovascular dysfunction. *The American Journal of Physiology*, Vol.263, No.3 Pt 2, pp.H668-675, ISSN.0002-9513

Elgjo, G. I.; Mathew, B. P.; Poli de Figueriedo, L. F.; Schenarts, P. J.; Horton, J. W.; Dubick, M. A. & Kramer, G. C. (1998). Resuscitation with hypertonic saline dextran improves cardiac function in vivo and ex vivo after burn injury in sheep. *Shock*, Vol.9, No.5, pp.375-383, ISSN.1073-2322

Evans, E. I.; Purnell, O. J.; Robinett, P. W.; Batchelor, A. & Martin, M. (1952). Fluid and electrolyte requirements in severe burns. *Annals of Surgery*, Vol.135, No.6, pp.804-817, ISSN.0003-4932

Fan, J.; Xie, Y.; Zhou, N. J.; Chen, J. & Deng, Z. Y. (2006). The influence of apoptosis of lymphocytes of Peyer's patches on the pathogenesis of gut barrier damage in severely scalded mice. *Chinese Journal of Burns*, Vol.22, No.4, pp.254-257, ISSN.1009-2587

Ferrara, J. J.; Franklin, E. W.; Kukuy, E. L.; Flynn, D. M.; Gilman, D. A.; Keller, V. A.; Choe, E. U.; Flint, L. M. & Lefer, D. J. (1998). Lymph isolated from a regional scald injury produces a negative inotropic effect in dogs. *The Journal of Burn Care & Rehabilitation*, Vol.19, No.4, pp.296-304, ISSN.0273-8481

Fiddian-Green, R. G.; Haglund, U.; Gutierrez, G. & Shoemaker, W. C. (1993). Goals for the resuscitation of shock. *Critical Care Medicine*, Vol.21, No.2 Suppl, pp.S25-31, ISSN.0090-3493

Flynn, D. M.; Buda, A. J.; Jeffords, P. R. & Lefer, D. J. (1996). A sialyl Lewis(x)-containing carbohydrate reduces infarct size: role of selectins in myocardial reperfusion injury. *The American Journal of Physiology*, Vol.271, No.5 Pt 2, pp.H2086-2096, ISSN.0002-9513

Fozzard, H. A. (1961). Myocardial injury in burn shock. *Annals of Surgery*, Vol.154, pp.113-119, ISSN.0003-4932

Gan, H. T.; Pasricha, P. J. & Chen, J. D. (2007). Blockade of p38 mitogen-activated protein kinase pathway ameliorates delayed intestinal transit in burned rats. *American Journal of Surgery*, Vol.193, No.4, pp.530-537, ISSN.1879-1883

Gianotti, L.; Alexander, J. W.; Pyles, T.; James, L. & Babcock, G. F. (1993). Relationship between extent of burn injury and magnitude of microbial translocation from the intestine. *The Journal of Burn Care & Rehabilitation*, Vol.14, No.3, pp.336-342, ISSN.0273-8481

Giroir, B. P.; Horton, J. W.; White, D. J.; McIntyre, K. L. & Lin, C. Q. (1994). Inhibition of tumor necrosis factor prevents myocardial dysfunction during burn shock. *The American Journal of Physiology*, Vol.267, No.1 Pt 2, pp.H118-124, ISSN.0002-9513

Giroir, B. P.; Johnson, J. H.; Brown, T.; Allen, G. L. & Beutler, B. (1992). The tissue distribution of tumor necrosis factor biosynthesis during endotoxemia. *The Journal of Clinical Investigation*, Vol.90, No.3, pp.693-698, ISSN.0021-9738

Hassoun, H. T.; Kone, B. C.; Mercer, D. W.; Moody, F. G.; Weisbrodt, N. W. & Moore, F. A. (2001). Post-injury multiple organ failure: the role of the gut. *Shock*, Vol.15, No.1, pp.1-10, ISSN.1073-2322

Heard, S. O.; Perkins, M. W. & Fink, M. P. (1992). Tumor necrosis factor-alpha causes myocardial depression in guinea pigs. *Critical Care Medicine*, Vol.20, No.4, pp.523-527, ISSN.0090-3493

Horton, J. W. (2003). Free radicals and lipid peroxidation mediated injury in burn trauma: the role of antioxidant therapy. *Toxicology*, Vol.189, No.1-2, pp.75-88, ISSN.0300-483X

Horton, J. W.; Garcia, N. M.; White, D. J. & Keffer, J. (1995). Postburn cardiac contractile function and biochemical markers of postburn cardiac injury. *Journal of the American College of Surgeons*, Vol.181, No.4, pp.289-298, ISSN.1072-7515

Horton, J. W.; Maass, D. L. & Ballard-Croft, C. (2005). Rho-associated kinase modulates myocardial inflammatory cytokine responses. *Shock*, Vol.24, No.1, pp.53-58, ISSN.1073-2322

Horton, J. W.; Maass, D. L.; White, D. J.; Sanders, B. & Murphy, J. (2004). Effects of burn serum on myocardial inflammation and function. *Shock*, Vol.22, No.5, pp.438-445, ISSN.1073-2322

Horton, J. W.; Maass, D. L.; White, J. & Sanders, B. (2001a). Hypertonic saline-dextran suppresses burn-related cytokine secretion by cardiomyocytes. *American Journal of Physiology. Heart and Circulatory Physiology*, Vol.280, No.4, pp.H1591-1601, ISSN.0363-6135

Horton, J. W.; Maass, D. L.; White, J. & Sanders, B. (2001b). Hypertonic saline-dextran suppresses burn-related cytokine secretion by cardiomyocytes. *American Journal of Physiology. Heart and Circulatory Physiology*, Vol.280, No.4, pp.H1591-1601, ISSN.0363-6135

Horton, J. W.; Mileski, W. J.; White, D. J. & Lipsky, P. (1996). Monoclonal antibody to intercellular adhesion molecule-1 reduces cardiac contractile dysfunction after burn injury in rabbits. *The Journal of Surgical Research*, Vol.64, No.1, pp.49-56, ISSN.0022-4804

Horton, J. W. & White, D. J. (1993). Free radical scavengers prevent intestinal ischemia-reperfusion-mediated cardiac dysfunction. *The Journal of Surgical Research*, Vol.55, No.3, pp.282-289, ISSN.0022-4804

Horton, J. W. & White, D. J. (1995). Role of xanthine oxidase and leukocytes in postburn cardiac dysfunction. *Journal of the American College of Surgeons*, Vol.181, No.2, pp.129-137, ISSN.1072-7515

Horton, J. W.; White, J. & Maass, D. (1998). Protein kinase C inhibition improves ventricular function after thermal trauma. *The Journal of Trauma*, Vol.44, No.2, pp.254-264; discussion 264-255, ISSN.0022-5282

Horton, J. W.; White, J.; Maass, D. & Sanders, B. (1998). Arginine in burn injury improves cardiac performance and prevents bacterial translocation. *Journal of Applied Physiology*, Vol.84, No.2, pp.695-702, ISSN.8750-7587

Hoshijima, M.; Sah, V. P.; Wang, Y.; Chien, K. R. & Brown, J. H. (1998). The low molecular weight GTPase Rho regulates myofibril formation and organization in neonatal rat ventricular myocytes. Involvement of Rho kinase. *The Journal of Biological Chemistry*, Vol.273, No.13, pp.7725-7730, ISSN.0021-9258

Hu, J. Y.; Chu, Z. G.; Han, J.; Dang, Y. M.; Yan, H.; Zhang, Q.; Liang, G. P. & Huang, Y. S. (2009). The p38/MAPK pathway regulates microtubule polymerization through phosphorylation of MAP4 and Op18 in hypoxic cells. *Cellular and Molecular Life Sciences*, ISSN.1420-9071

Huang, Y. & Hu, A. (2004). Molecular mechanism of c-jun antisense gene transfection in alleviating injury of cardiomyocytes treated with burn serum and hypoxia. *World Journal of Surgery*, Vol.28, No.10, pp.951-957, ISSN.0364-2313

Huang, Y.; Li, Z. & Yang, Z. (2003). Roles of ischemia and hypoxia and the molecular pathogenesis of post-burn cardiac shock. *Burns: Journal of the International Society for Burn Injuries*, Vol.29, No.8, pp.828-833, ISSN.0305-4179

Huang, Y.; Xie, K.; Zhang, J.; Dang, Y. & Qiong, Z. (2008). Prospective clinical and experimental studies on the cardioprotective effect of ulinastatin following severe burns. *Burns: Journal of the International Society for Burn Injuries*, Vol.34, No.5, pp.674-680, ISSN.0305-4179

Huang, Y.; Yang, Z.; Chen, F.; Crowther, R. S. & Li, A. (1999a). Effects of early eschar excision en masse at one operation for prevention and treatment of organ dysfunction in severely burned patients. *World Journal of Surgery*, Vol.23, No.12, pp.1272-1278, ISSN.0364-2313

Huang, Y.; Zheng, J.; Fan, P. & Zhang, X. (2007). Transfection of antisense p38 alpha gene ameliorates myocardial cell injury mediated by hypoxia and burn serum. *Burns: Journal of the International Society for Burn Injuries*, Vol.33, No.5, pp.599-605, ISSN.0305-4179

Huang, Y. S. (2009). Further discussion on postburn "shock heart " and its clinical significance. *Chinese Journal of Burns*, Vol.25, No.3, pp.161-163, ISSN.1009-2587

Huang, Y. S.; Yang, Z. C.; Liu, X. S.; Chen, F. M.; He, B. B.; Li, A. & Crowther, R. S. (1998). Serial experimental and clinical studies on the pathogenesis of multiple organ dysfunction syndrome (MODS) in severe burns. *Burns: Journal of the International Society for Burn Injuries*, Vol.24, No.8, pp.706-716, ISSN.0305-4179

Huang, Y. S.; Yang, Z. C.; Yan, B. G.; Yang, J. M.; Chen, F. M.; Crowther, R. S. & Li, A. (1999b). Pathogenesis of early cardiac myocyte damage after severe burns. *The Journal of Trauma*, Vol.46, No.3, pp.428-432, ISSN.0022-5282

Kobayashi, N.; Horinaka, S.; Mita, S.; Nakano, S.; Honda, T.; Yoshida, K.; Kobayashi, T. & Matsuoka, H. (2002). Critical role of Rho-kinase pathway for cardiac performance and remodeling in failing rat hearts. *Cardiovascular Research*, Vol.55, No.4, pp.757-767, ISSN.0008-6363

LaLonde, C.; Nayak, U.; Hennigan, J. & Demling, R. H. (1997). Excessive liver oxidant stress causes mortality in response to burn injury combined with endotoxin and is prevented with antioxidants. *The Journal of Burn Care & Rehabilitation*, Vol.18, No.3, pp.187-192, ISSN.0273-8481

Lalonde, C.; Picard, L.; Campbell, C. & Demling, R. (1994). Lung and systemic oxidant and antioxidant activity after graded smoke exposure in the rat. *Circulatory Shock*, Vol.42, No.1, pp.7-13, ISSN.0092-6213

Li, H.; Ying, D.; Sun, J.; Bian, X.; Zhang, Y. & He, B. (2001). Comparative observation with MRI and pathology of brain edema at the early stage of severe burn. *Chinese Journal of Traumatology*, Vol.4, No.4, pp.226-230, ISSN.1008-1275

Liang, W. Y.; Tang, L. X.; Yang, Z. C. & Huang, Y. S. (2002). Calcium induced the damage of myocardial mitochondrial respiratory function in the early stage after severe burns. *Burns: Journal of the International Society for Burn Injuries*, Vol.28, No.2, pp.143-146, ISSN.0305-4179

Maass, D. L.; Hybki, D. P.; White, J. & Horton, J. W. (2002). The time course of cardiac NF-kappaB activation and TNF-alpha secretion by cardiac myocytes after burn injury: contribution to burn-related cardiac contractile dysfunction. *Shock*, Vol.17, No.4, pp.293-299, ISSN.1073-2322

Maass, D. L.; White, J. & Horton, J. W. (2005). Nitric oxide donors alter cardiomyocyte cytokine secretion and cardiac function. *Critical Care Medicine*, Vol.33, No.12, pp.2794-2803, ISSN.0090-3493

Mackins, C. J.; Kano, S.; Seyedi, N.; Schafer, U.; Reid, A. C.; Machida, T.; Silver, R. B. & Levi, R. (2006). Cardiac mast cell-derived renin promotes local angiotensin formation, norepinephrine release, and arrhythmias in ischemia/reperfusion. *The Journal of Clinical Investigation*, Vol.116, No.4, pp.1063-1070, ISSN.0021-9738

Marano, M. A.; Fong, Y.; Moldawer, L. L.; Wei, H.; Calvano, S. E.; Tracey, K. J.; Barie, P. S.; Manogue, K.; Cerami, A.; Shires, G. T. & et al. (1990). Serum cachectin/tumor necrosis factor in critically ill patients with burns correlates with infection and mortality. *Surgery, Gynecology & Obstetrics*, Vol.170, No.1, pp.32-38, ISSN.0039-6087

Marano, M. A.; Moldawer, L. L.; Fong, Y.; Wei, H.; Minei, J.; Yurt, R.; Cerami, A. & Lowry, S. F. (1988). Cachectin/TNF production in experimental burns and Pseudomonas infection. *Archives of Surgery*, Vol.123, No.11, pp.1383-1388, ISSN.0004-0010

Matsuda, T.; Tanaka, H.; Hanumadass, M.; Gayle, R.; Yuasa, H.; Abcarian, H.; Matsuda, H. & Reyes, H. (1992). Effects of high-dose vitamin C administration on postburn microvascular fluid and protein flux. *The Journal of Burn Care & Rehabilitation*, Vol.13, No.5, pp.560-566, ISSN.0273-8481

Matsuda, T.; Tanaka, H.; Williams, S.; Hanumadass, M.; Abcarian, H. & Reyes, H. (1991). Reduced fluid volume requirement for resuscitation of third-degree burns with high-dose vitamin C. *The Journal of Burn Care & Rehabilitation*, Vol.12, No.6, pp.525-532, ISSN.0273-8481

Matsuda, T.; Tanaka, H.; Yuasa, H.; Forrest, R.; Matsuda, H.; Hanumadass, M. & Reyes, H. (1993). The effects of high-dose vitamin C therapy on postburn lipid peroxidation. *The Journal of Burn Care & Rehabilitation*, Vol.14, No.6, pp.624-629, ISSN.0273-8481

Mileski, W. J.; Winn, R. K.; Harlan, J. M. & Rice, C. L. (1991). Transient inhibition of neutrophil adherence with the anti-CD18 monoclonal antibody 60.3 does not increase mortality rates in abdominal sepsis. *Surgery*, Vol.109, No.4, pp.497-501, ISSN.0039-6060

Moyer, C. A.; Coller, F. A.; Iob, V.; Vaughan, H. H. & Marty, D. (1944). A Study of the Interrelationship of Salt Solutions Serum and Defibrinated Blood in the Treatment of Severely Scalded, Anesthetized Dogs. *Annals of Surgery*, Vol.120, No.3, pp.367-376, ISSN.0003-4932

Murphy, J. T.; Horton, J. W.; Purdue, G. F. & Hunt, J. L. (1998). Evaluation of troponin-I as an indicator of cardiac dysfunction after thermal injury. *The Journal of Trauma*, Vol.45, No.4, pp.700-704, ISSN.0022-5282

Pagani, F. D.; Baker, L. S.; Hsi, C.; Knox, M.; Fink, M. P. & Visner, M. S. (1992). Left ventricular systolic and diastolic dysfunction after infusion of tumor necrosis factor-alpha in conscious dogs. *The Journal of Clinical Investigation*, Vol.90, No.2, pp.389-398, ISSN.0021-9738

Sakarcan, A.; Sehirli, O.; Velioglu-Ovunc, A.; Ercan, F.; Erkanl, G.; Gedik, N. & Sener, G. (2005). Ginkgo biloba extract improves oxidative organ damage in a rat model of thermal trauma. *The Journal of Burn Care & Rehabilitation*, Vol.26, No.6, pp.515-524, ISSN.0273-8481

Salzberg, A. M. & Evans, E. I. (1950). Blood volumes in normal and burned dogs; a comparative study with radioactive phosphorus tagged red cells and T-1824 dye. *Annals of Surgery*, Vol.132, No.4, pp.746-759, ISSN.0003-4932

Sambol, J. T.; White, J.; Horton, J. W. & Deitch, E. A. (2002). Burn-induced impairment of cardiac contractile function is due to gut-derived factors transported in mesenteric lymph. *Shock*, Vol.18, No.3, pp.272-276, ISSN.1073-2322

Sener, G.; Sehirli, A. O.; Satiroglu, H.; Keyer-Uysal, M. & Yegen, B. C. (2002). Melatonin prevents oxidative kidney damage in a rat model of thermal injury. *Life Sciences*, Vol.70, No.25, pp.2977-2985, ISSN.0024-3205

Sener, G.; Sehirli, O.; Erkanli, G.; Cetinel, S.; Gedik, N. & Yegen, B. (2004). 2-Mercaptoethane sulfonate (MESNA) protects against burn-induced renal injury in rats. *Burns:Journal of the International Society for Burn Injuries*, Vol.30, No.6, pp.557-564, ISSN.0305-4179

Sheeran, P. W.; Maass, D. L.; White, D. J.; Turbeville, T. D.; Giroir, B. P. & Horton, J. W. (1998). Aspiration pneumonia-induced sepsis increases cardiac dysfunction after burn trauma. *The Journal of Surgical Research*, Vol.76, No.2, pp.192-199, ISSN.0022-4804

Sheng, Z. (2002). Prevention of multiple organ dysfunction syndrome in patients with extensive deep burns. *Chinese Journal of Traumatology*, Vol.5, No.4, pp.195-199, ISSN.1008-1275

Suematsu, N.; Satoh, S.; Kinugawa, S.; Tsutsui, H.; Hayashidani, S.; Nakamura, R.; Egashira, K.; Makino, N. & Takeshita, A. (2001). Alpha1-adrenoceptor-Gq-RhoA signaling is upregulated to increase myofibrillar Ca^{2+} sensitivity in failing hearts. *American Journal of Physiology. Heart and Circulatory Physiology*, Vol.281, No.2, pp.H637-646, ISSN.0363-6135

Sugden, P. H. & Clerk, A. (1998). "Stress-responsive" mitogen-activated protein kinases (c-Jun N-terminal kinases and p38 mitogen-activated protein kinases) in the myocardium. *Circulation Research*, Vol.83, No.4, pp.345-352, ISSN.0009-7330

Takeda, K.; Shimada, Y.; Amano, M.; Sakai, T.; Okada, T. & Yoshiya, I. (1984). Plasma lipid peroxides and alpha-tocopherol in critically ill patients. *Critical Care Medicine*, Vol.12, No.11, pp.957-959, ISSN.0090-3493

Toklu, H. Z.; Sener, G.; Jahovic, N.; Uslu, B.; Arbak, S. & Yegen, B. C. (2006). beta-glucan protects against burn-induced oxidative organ damage in rats. *International Immunopharmacology*, Vol.6, No.2, pp.156-169, ISSN.1567-5769

Tong, T. H.; Wang, C. Y. & Guo, L. (2006). Influence of scald on the cytoskeleton of colonic smooth muscle cells of the rats. *Chinese Journal of Burns*, Vol.22, No.4, pp.273-276, ISSN.1009-2587

Tracey, K. J.; Beutler, B.; Lowry, S. F.; Merryweather, J.; Wolpe, S.; Milsark, I. W.; Hariri, R. J.; Fahey, T. J., 3rd; Zentella, A.; Albert, J. D. & et al. (1986). Shock and tissue injury induced by recombinant human cachectin. *Science*, Vol.234, No.4775, pp.470-474, ISSN.0036-8075

Tu, W. F. & Xiao, G. X. (2002). Shock gut and multiple organ dysfunction syndrome. *Chinese Journal of Anesthesiology*, Vol.22, No.2, pp.125-128

Wan-Yi, L.; Hui, T.; Zong-Cheng, Y. & Yue-Sheng, H. (2002). Ruthenium red attenuated cardiomyocyte and mitochondrial damage during the early stage after severe burn. *Burns:Journal of the International Society for Burn Injuries*, Vol.28, No.1, pp.35-38, ISSN.0305-4179

Wang, Y.; Huang, S.; Sah, V. P.; Ross, J., Jr.; Brown, J. H.; Han, J. & Chien, K. R. (1998). Cardiac muscle cell hypertrophy and apoptosis induced by distinct members of the p38 mitogen-activated protein kinase family. *The Journal of Biological Chemistry*, Vol.273, No.4, pp.2161-2168, ISSN.0021-9258

Ward, P. A.; Till, G. O.; Hatherill, J. R.; Annesley, T. M. & Kunkel, R. G. (1985). Systemic complement activation, lung injury, and products of lipid peroxidation. *The Journal of Clinical Investigation*, Vol.76, No.2, pp.517-527, ISSN.0021-9738

White, J.; Maass, D. L.; Giroir, B. & Horton, J. W. (2001). Development of an acute burn model in adult mice for studies of cardiac function and cardiomyocyte cellular function. *Shock*, Vol.16, No.2, pp.122-129, ISSN.1073-2322

Williams, J. G.; Bankey, P.; Minei, J. P.; McIntyre, K. & Turbeville, T. (1994). Burn injury enhances alveolar macrophage endotoxin sensitivity. *The Journal of Burn Care & Rehabilitation*, Vol.15, No.6, pp.493-498, ISSN.0273-8481

Wolfe, R. R. & Miller, H. I. (1976). Cardiovascular and metabolic responses during burn shock in the guinea pig. *American Journal of Physiology*, Vol.231, No.3, pp.892-897, ISSN.0002-9513

Xiang, F.; Huang, Y. S.; Shi, X. H. & Zhang, Q. (2010a). Mitochondrial chaperone tumour necrosis factor receptor-associated protein 1 protects cardiomyocytes from hypoxic injury by regulating mitochondrial permeability transition pore opening. *The FEBS Journal*, Vol.277, No.8, pp.1929-1938, ISSN.1742-4658

Xiang, F.; Huang, Y. S.; Zhang, D. X.; Chu, Z. G.; Zhang, J. P. & Zhang, Q. (2010b). Adenosine A1 receptor activation reduces opening of mitochondrial permeability transition pores in hypoxic cardiomyocytes. *Clinical and Experimental Pharmacology & Physiology*, Vol.37, No.3, pp.343-349, ISSN.1440-1681

Xiao, R.; Huang, Y. S.; Lei, Z. Y.; Ruan, J.; Zhang, B. Q.; Wang, G. & Zhang, Q. (2008a). Instigating effect of shock heart on the injury to the liver, kidney and intestine at early stage of severe burn in rat. *Chinese Journal of Burns*, Vol.24, No.3, pp.175-178, ISSN.1009-2587

Xiao, R.; Huang, Y. S.; Lei, Z. Y.; Ruan, J.; Zhang, B. Q.; Wang, G. & Zhang, Q. (2008b). Instigating effect of shock heart on the injury to the liver, kidney and intestine at early stage of severe burn in rat. *Chinese Journal of Burns*, Vol.24, No.3, pp.175-178, ISSN.1009-2587

Xiao, R.; Lei, Z. Y.; Dang, Y. M. & Huang, Y. S. (2011). Prompt myocardial damage contributes to hepatic, renal, and intestinal injuries soon after a severe burn in rats. *The Journal of Trauma*, Vol.71, No.3, pp.663-672, ISSN.1529-8809

Yamada, Y.; Endo, S.; Inada, K.; Nakae, H.; Nasu, W.; Taniguchi, S.; Ishikura, H.; Tanaka, T.; Wakabayashi, G.; Taki, K. & Sato, S. (2000). Tumor necrosis factor-alpha and tumor necrosis factor receptor I, II levels in patients with severe burns. *Burns: Journal of the International Society for Burn Injuries*, Vol.26, No.3, pp.239-244, ISSN.0305-4179

Yang, J.; Yang, Z. & Chen, F. (1999). Changes in cardiac renin-angiotensin system after severe burn injury in rats. *Chinese Journal of Burns and Plastic Surgery*, Vol.15, No.2, pp.102-104, ISSN.1000-7806

Yang, J. M.; Yang, Z. C. & Chen, F. M. (1996). Relationship between myocardial nutrition blood flow and energy charge in the early stage of severe burn injury in rats. *Chinese Critical Care Medicine*, Vol.8, No.9, pp.523-524

Yin, Z. G.; Huang, Y. S. & Li, B. X. (2010). Changes and relations between heart function and organ blood flow in rats at early stage of severe burn. *Chinese Journal of Burns*, Vol.26, No.1, pp.10-13, ISSN.1009-2587

Yokoyama, T.; Vaca, L.; Rossen, R. D.; Durante, W.; Hazarika, P. & Mann, D. L. (1993). Cellular basis for the negative inotropic effects of tumor necrosis factor-alpha in the adult mammalian heart. *The Journal of Clinical Investigation*, Vol.92, No.5, pp.2303-2312, ISSN.0021-9738

Zang, Q.; Maass, D. L.; White, J. & Horton, J. W. (2007). Cardiac mitochondrial damage and loss of ROS defense after burn injury: the beneficial effects of antioxidant therapy. *Journal of Applied Physiology*, Vol.102, No.1, pp.103-112, ISSN.8750-7587

Zhang, B.; Huang, Y. H.; Chen, Y.; Yang, Y.; Hao, Z. L. & Xie, S. L. (1998). Plasma tumor necrosis factor-alpha, its soluble receptors and interleukin-1beta levels in critically burned patients. *Burns: Journal of the International Society for Burn Injuries*, Vol.24, No.7, pp.599-603, ISSN.0305-4179

Zhang, B. Q.; Huang, Y. S.; Zhang, J. P.; Zhang, D. X.; Dang, Y. M.; Wang, G.; Hu, J. Y.; Lei, Z. Y. & Xiao, R. (2007a). Protective effects of administration of enalapril maleate on rat myocardial damage in early stage of burns. *Chinese Journal of Burns*, Vol.23, No.5, pp.335-338, ISSN.1009-2587

Zhang, C.; Sheng, Z. Y.; Hu, S.; Gao, J. C.; Yu, S. & Liu, Y. (2002). The influence of apoptosis of mucosal epithelial cells on intestinal barrier integrity after scald in rats. *Burns: Journal of the International Society for Burn Injuries*, Vol.28, No.8, pp.731-737, ISSN.0305-4179

Zhang, J. P.; Liang, W. Y.; Luo, Z. H.; Yang, Z. C.; Chan, H. C. & Huang, Y. S. (2007b). Involvement of p38 MAP kinase in burn-induced degradation of membrane phospholipids and upregulation of cPLA2 in cardiac myocytes. *Shock*, Vol.28, No.1, pp.86-93, ISSN.1073-2322

Zhang, J. P.; Ying, X.; Chen, Y.; Yang, Z. C. & Huang, Y. S. (2008a). Inhibition of p38 MAP kinase improves survival of cardiac myocytes with hypoxia and burn serum challenge. *Burns: Journal of the International Society for Burn Injuries*, Vol.34, No.2, pp.220-227, ISSN.0305-4179

Zhang, J. P.; Ying, X.; Liang, W. Y.; Luo, Z. H.; Yang, Z. C.; Huang, Y. S. & Wang, W. C. (2008b). Apoptosis in cardiac myocytes during the early stage after severe burn. *The Journal of Trauma*, Vol.65, No.2, pp.401-408, ISSN.1529-8809

Zhang, J. P.; Ying, X.; Liang, W. Y.; Luo, Z. H.; Yang, Z. C.; Huang, Y. S. & Wang, W. C. (2008c). Apoptosis in cardiac myocytes during the early stage after severe burn. *The Journal of Trauma*, Vol.65, No.2, pp.401-408, ISSN.1529-8809

Zhou, P.; Huang, H. & Chen, L. (2002). The relationship between liver function and pathological changes in burned rats. *Chinese Critical Care Medicine*, Vol.14, No.4, pp.201-203

23

Aging, Reactive Nitrogen Species and Myocardial Apoptosis Induced by Ischemia/Reperfusion Injury

Huirong Liu, Ke Wang, Xiaoliang Wang,
Jue Tian, Jianqin Jiao, Kehua Bai,
Jie Yang and Haibo Xu
Capital Medical University Beijing
P. R. China

1. Introduction

Globally, the proportion of elderly people is growing faster than any other age group. In 2000, one in ten, or about 600 million, people were 60 years or older. By 2025, it is expected to reach 1.2 billion people, and in 2050 around 1.9 billion (Hutton, 2008). Aging is a multifactorial process and has been defined as a time-dependent general decline in physiological function of an organism associated with a progressively increasing risk of morbidity and mortality. It is apparent that during aging different organs are losing their functional reserve and plasticity and become less able to fulfill their physiological function, especially under conditions of stress (Beneke & Bürkle, 2007).

Coronary heart disease is the leading cause of death worldwide, and 3.8 million men and 3.4 million women die of the disease each year (Yellon & Hausenloy, 2007). Heart aging is accompanied by changes that are progressive, pervasive, potentially deleterious, and, as far as is known, irreversible (Juhaszova et al., 2005). The incidence of heart disease begins to increase in men after the age of forty-five and in women after the age of fifty-five, and the rate for women tends to equal that of men after the age of seventy (MacDonald, 2002). Regardless of age, the heart's well-being is critically dependent on its blood supply, and vascular disease places this in jeopardy. With increasing age, narrowing may develop in the coronary arteries, which lead to the heart. Reduced blood supply causes ischemia (insufficient blood supply for the heart's work) and may produce chest pain or angina. If ischemia is prolonged, irreversible damage resulting in widespread cell death appears, leading to loss of contractility and impairment of cardiac pump function.

Several studies have identified age as a strong predictor of adverse events after acute coronary syndromes; as a result, elderly persons are a high-risk subgroup. Mortality due to ischemic cardiovascular diseases is significantly higher in the elderly than in young adults. The average age for a first MI is 66 years in men and 70 years in women, nearly 50% of hospital admissions for acute MI and 80% who die are age 65 years and over (Jugdutt et al., 2008, as cited in Ertl &Frantz, 2005; Cheitlin & Zipes, 2001; Thom et al., 2006). After an acute myocardial infarction, early and successful myocardial reperfusion with the use of thrombolytic therapy or primary percutaneous coronary intervention (PCI) is the most effective strategy for reducing the size of a myocardial infarct and improving the clinical outcome. The process of restoring blood flow to the ischemic myocardium, however, can induce injury. This phenomenon is termed myocardial ischemia/reperfusion (MI/R) injury. This form of myocardial injury, which by itself can induce cardiomyocyte death and increase infarct size, may in part explain why, despite optimal myocardial reperfusion, the rate of death after an acute myocardial infarction approaches 10% and the incidence of cardiac failure after an acute myocardial infarction is almost 25% (Yellon & Hausenloy, 2007, as cited in Keeley, 2003).

Cell death is a primary factor in the pathogenesis of infarction after I/R and, because survival is strongly correlated to the cardiac myocytes mass lost after I/R injury, can be induced by two different pathways, necrosis and apoptosis which coexist during I/R. Apoptosis is more prevalent than necrosis in senescent animals and humans and increased more significantly in old rats than in young adult ones after renal ischemia reperfusion. Different from necrosis, which is induced by injurious agents, apoptosis is an active programmed cell death characterized by a series of stereotypic morphological and biochemical features. Therefore, it is easier to inhibit apoptosis than to prohibit necrosis for the aging heart. Inhibition of apoptosis may confer protection. So, apoptosis would be one of the efficient targets to ameliorate more serious MI/R injury in aging. In this chapter we focus on aging-induced cardiac myocyte apoptosis and its potential mechanisms after I/R injury. The chapter is divided into 4 sections: (1)High sensitivity to ischemic heart disease in elderly people; (2) Aging increases myocardial apoptosis under basal and stressed conditions; (3) RNS signaling induced apoptosis contributes to increased susceptibility of aging hearts to myocardial ischemic injury; (4) A mitochondrial pro-apoptotic protein, HtrA2/Omi, is another reason for enhanced MI/R injury in the aging heart.

2. High sensitivity to ischemic heart disease in the elderly

2.1 Risk factors for ischemic heart disease

Ischemic heart disease (IHD), defined as the earliest manifestation of myocardial infarction, stable or unstable angina pectoris or sudden death, is a vital problem in our society and remains to be a major cause of morbidity and mortality in the elderly. Consequently, the identification of factors related to IHD and quantification of levels of risk is increasingly popular. There are many risk factors contributing to IHD, ranging from blood pressure, both systolic blood pressure (SBP) and diastolic blood pressure (DBP), to living habits like smoking and excessive fat in take. These are undoubtedly the predictors of long term coronary heart disease. IHD, or myocardial ischemic injury, results from severe impairment of the coronary blood supply usually produced by thrombosis or other acute alterations of coronary atherosclerotic plaques resulting from these risk factors.

Curiously, however, the question was raised if these risk factors for IHD found at a young age are still predictive at older ages because IHD may develop in men at a young, middle, or older age. Via long-term studies concerning changing effects of risk factors with age, it has been confirmed (Mathewson et al.,1960; Robert et al.,1998) that blood pressure up to age 65 years manifested itself as a significant factor for IHD—for one thing, the benefit of 10mmHg lower blood pressure was smaller in older compared to younger men; smoking relevance is higher for younger men than for older men; more interesting, the role of either BMI (Body Mass Index) or DM (Diabetes Mellitus) does not vary significantly with age, even though BMI has the largest relative risk in younger men. In 2003, Lakatta and his colleagues ascertained that the aging artery was a "set-up" for vascular diseases (Lakatta & Levy, 2003). In consideration of studies, both in aging animal models of IHD and censuses on clinical symptoms, it is now well acknowledged that age is a major independent risk factor for IHD although the mechanisms responsible for this age-related pathologic change remain implicit.

2.2 Aging and IHD

Aging, characterized by a progressive deterioration of organs and cells, play an imperative role in the manifestation of IHD. The incidence and prevalence of ischemic heart disease increases steeply with advancing age. Considerable evidence from animal studies and clinical observations indicates that aged hearts are more susceptible to I/R injury, suffer from greater infarct expansion, and exhibit poorer outcomes. It is also disappointing that therapies such as thrombolysis and preconditioning confer less benefit in the aged with myocardial infarction than in younger adults. With the "graying of the population," the morbidity and mortality attributable to cardiovascular diseases will likely continue to increase, resulting in a significant increase in the already huge economic health care burden. These factors call for a multitude of our efforts in uncovering the mechanisms responsible for MI/R in aging patients.

2.3 Possible mechanisms of high sensitivity to IHD in the elderly

Aging is a complex phenomenon associated with changed DNA transcription and RNA translation together with protein expression. Ischemic heart disease results from severe impairment of the coronary blood supply usually produced by thrombosis or other acute alterations of coronary atherosclerotic plaques. A crucial early step of atherosclerosis is the binding to endothelial cells and subsequent subendothelial migration of circulating monocytes and their transformation into foam cells by the uptake of lipids. Intercellular adhesion molecule-1(ICAM-1) and vascular cell adhesion molecule-1(VCAM-1) in endothelial cells, mediating the adhesion of leukocytes, are suspected of playing an important role in the formulation of early atherosclerotic lesions. Nobuhiro Morisaki (Morisaki et al., 1997) found, through determining the two molecules soluble in serum, that sICAM-1 was correlated only to the presence of IHD but not to age; yet sVCAM-1, not sICAM-1, was positively correlated to age. In other words, age was the most powerful independent predictor of the level of sVCAM-1 and increased susceptibility to ischemia in some sense.

What's more, aging is considered as an energy deficit implicated in myocardial weakness and reduced functions in humans' hearts. The deficit has been demonstrated to be related to the dysfunctional mitochondria that is responsible for the maximum output of ATP, working as a primary site of generation of Reactive Oxygen Species (ROS) and participating in the regulation of apoptosis. With growing age, in the cell and particularly in mitochondria, the defense capacities against ROS become insufficient. Excessive ROS attacks mRNA, DNA, and long-term proteins, which is especially obvious with aging.

A decrease in the total number of myocytes is associated with heart damage and an accelerated decline in cardiac functional capacity observed in aging hearts (Zhang et al.,

2003). It was commonly believed that cardiac myocytes had little ability to regenerate. Therefore, the cardiac function mainly relies on the survival of cardiomyocytes. Two of the most common forms of cell death are programmed cell death and accidental cell death. Programmed cell death is characterized by a series of stereotypic morphological and biochemical features, which is easier to manipulate. It is reported that compared with necrosis, apoptosis is one of the major factors contributing to cardiomyocyte loss. An abundance of evidences certify that cytosolic cytochrome c content is sharply elevated in aging rats (Sharon et al., 2002). Furthermore, Bcl-2, an antiapoptotic protein shows a strong tendency to decrease with age, while Bax, a proapoptotic protein, remains unchanged, so do apoptotic protease-activating factor 1 levels and caspase-3 activities, regarded as executor caspases following caspase-8 or caspase-9 activation. Additionally, chronic oxidative stress with age induces the increase of manganese superoxide dismutase, glutathione peroxidase activity and lipid peroxidation in aging heart mitochondria, which may contribute to IHD. Therefore, age was a major independent risk factor for IHD, and cardiomyocyte death with age may be the last and main event of high sensitivity to IHD.

3. Aging increases myocardial apoptosis under basal and stressed conditions

Nowadays, our population is aging at an unprecedented rate, and during 2000-2030, the worldwide population aged >65 years is projected to increase by approximately 550 million to 973 million (U.S. Census Bureau), increasing from 6.9% to 12.0% worldwide (Kinsella & Velkoff, 2001). Data from numerous animal researches and clinical studies support that aging is a major independent risk factor in the markedly enhanced risk of cardiovascular diseases in the elderly. There are marked changes related to age in myocardial structure and function in both animals and humans. Previous studies have demonstrated that both diastolic and systolic functions were aggravated in senescent hearts. As the basis of cardiac function, cardiac structure has incurred numerous changes, such as enlarged cardiac myocyte size and reduced myocyte numbers in elderly hearts.

3.1 Aging and myocardial apoptosis

Numerous studies have demonstrated that there was a significant loss of cardiac myocytes constituting an important determinant of the aging process, possibly mediating the aggravation of cardiac function. In animal research models, there was around a 32.5% reduction of myocytes in the left ventricles of rats during a period of 4 to 29 months (Anversa et al., 1990). The study carried out on aging human hearts by G. Olivetti displayed that there was around 35% aggregate loss of myocytes in both ventricles for 70 year-old healthy men compared to 25 year-old healthy young adults (Olivetti et al., 1991). The factors responsible for the abnormal loss of the cells in the ventricles remain unclear, and it will possibly open a new field to prevent or even reverse the disappearance of cardiac myocytes of aged hearts to reveal the potential mechanism for the aging associated cell loss.

Cell death may occur through active mechanisms like cellular suicide or active or programmed cell death, often referred to as apoptosis. Inactive mechanisms normally induced in acute situations by infarct, severe toxic chemicals and extreme thermal damage, normally conferred as necrosis. Many studies suggest that both apoptosis and necrosis are involved in the aging process (Ohshima, 2006). Apoptosis is more prevalent than necrosis in senescent animals and humans and increased more significantly in old rats than in young adult ones after myocardial ischemia reperfusion (Liu et al., 2002). Different from necrosis, which is induced by injurious agents, apoptosis is an active programmed cell death characterized by a series of stereotypic morphological and biochemical features. Therefore, it is easier to inhibit apoptosis than to prohibit necrosis for the aging heart.

3.2 Apoptosis with age and IHD

Accumulating studies indicate that aging is associated with an increase in myocardial susceptibility to ischemia and a decrease in postischemic recovery of cardiac function. Zhang et al. reported that in aging rats, myocardial ischemia and reperfusion-induced cardiac injury was enhanced in aging mice as evidenced by enlarged infarct size (38.5±2.7% vs 52.0±1.8%) (Zhang et al, 2007).

As stated above, myocardial apoptosis, a gene-regulated programmed cell death, markedly increases with aging. It has been determined that compared to young mice, myocardial ischemia and reperfusion in aging mice induced an increased apoptosis. Zhang investigated the detailed apoptotic cell death by TUNEL staining and caspase 3 activity assay, and found that TUNEL positive cells increased from 5.0±1.8% in young hearts to 8.8±0.9% in old ones, and that the caspase 3 activity increased from 18.0±0.9 nmol/h/mg protein to 27.4±1.9 nmol/h/mg protein (Zhang et al, 2007). However, the molecular mechanisms and signaling transduction pathways that are responsible for increased susceptibility of cardiomyocytes to apoptosis with aging remain largely unidentified.

3.3 Signal transduction pathways of apoptosis

Accumulating evidence indicates that apoptosis is an active, gene-directed process. One of the most widely recognized biochemical features of apoptosis is the activation of a class of cysteine proteases known as caspases. Cells possess multiple caspases that may work in a cascade fashion. The redundancy may serve to amplify and accelerate the response, as well as provide multiple mechanisms for success. Three pathways that activate caspases have been identified: the first one is activated through a cell surface signal leading to caspase 8 (and/or 10 in some cell types) activation; the second, more complicated pathway involves the mitochondria and results in caspase 9 activation; the third is activated via the endoplasmic reticulum and induces caspase 12 activation.

A variety of cellular stresses have been found to cause the disruption and collapse of the inner mitochondrial transmembrane potential, thus opening mitochondrial pores (termed "mitochondrial permeability transition" or MPT) and resulting in the release of cytochrome c. Cytochrome c released from the mitochondria activates caspase 9 in the presence of Apaf-1 (apoptosis protease activating factor-1) and ATP. In some cell types, activation of caspase 8 (and/or caspase 2) by the cell surface death receptor also increases mitochondrial cytochrome c release and subsequent caspase 9 activation by facilitating the translocation of full-length or truncated Bid (p15 Bid) from the cytosol to the mitochondrial membrane. As well known, caspase 9 can also be activated by caspase 12 released from the endoplasmic reticulum (ER) under stress. The activation of caspases 8 and 9 (initiator) followed by caspase 3 (executor)(6, and 7 in some cell types) with subsequent degradation of a variety of proteins results in irreversible damage of the cells (apoptotic cell death). Recent studies have demonstrated that formation of MPT also results in mitochondrial release of AIF (apoptosis-inducing factor), a molecule that directly results in apoptosis.

Under physiologic conditions, apoptosis is regulated by the balance of a variety of pro- and anti-apoptotic molecules. The disturbance of these balances contributes to well-known pathologies, such as neurodegenerative diseases, ischemia/reperfusion injury and cancer. Specifically, the formation of MPT and subsequent release of cytochrome c and AIF are controlled by the balance between anti-apoptotic (e.g., Bcl-2, Bcl-xl, Bcl-w, Bag-1 and BI-1) and pro-apoptotic (e.g., Bax, Bak, Bad, Bid and Bim) Bcl-2 family members, which themselves are regulated by the balance of upstream regulators, such as extracellular signal-regulated kinase 1/2 (ERK1/2) and Akt (anti-apoptotic), p38 mitogen-activated protein kinase (MAPK) and JNK (c-Jun N-terminal Kinase) (pro-apoptotic) at both transcriptional and post-transcriptional levels. In a recent study, Jiang and colleagues reported that activation of caspase 9 is positively regulated by tumor suppressor putative HLA-DR-associated proteins (PHAP) but inhibited by oncoprotein prothymosin-α (ProT)(Jiang et al, 2003). Finally, the activation of caspase 3 is inhibited by IAP (inhibitor of apoptosis protein) and αB-Crystallin, and promoted by Smac/DIABLO and Omi/HtrA2 (proteins that are also released from mitochondria under stress) by interaction with IAP. Given the extreme complexity of the apoptosis signal transduction and the exponentially-increasing number of pro- and anti-apoptotic molecules, it is highly unlikely that a specific cell type, i.e., cardiomyocytes, under specific stress, i.e., aging, will involve all of these apoptotic molecules and disturb every pro- and anti-apoptotic balance. Identifying the specific anti-/pro-apoptotic balance(s) that is (are) disturbed by aging, and uncovering the mechanisms responsible for the deregulation of apoptotic cell death in the aging heart will be the critical first step toward prevention and treatment of apoptotic cell death in patients with any heart disease. In the next section we will identify the reactive nitrogen species (RNS) signal and HtrA2/Omi related mitochondrial apoptotic pathway disturbed in the aging heart.

4. RNS signaling induced apoptosis contributes to increased susceptibility of aging hearts to myocardial ischemic Injury.

4.1 An overview of reactive nitrogen species and pathway

Considerable evidence suggests that reactive oxygen species (ROS) play critical roles in the aging process and post-ischemic myocardial apoptosis. However, the outcome of clinical trials with antioxidant treatment during MI/R has been rather disappointing, suggesting that other factors in addition to ROS exist. Most recent data have identified nitric oxide derived reactive nitrogen species (RNS) intermediates as critical contributors and cell injury.

RNS are produced by the reaction of NO with superoxide (Carr et al., 2000) and include NO and its derivatives (Wu et al., 2007). NO, as the most important mediator of RNS, has been identified as having three categories of signaling pathways in controlling cell death: (1) Classical signaling involves the selective activation of soluble guanylate cyclase (sGC) (cGMP-dependent protein kinases) (2) Less classical signaling: NO binds to cytochrome c oxidase (CcO) in the mitochondria and its functional consequences (3) Nonclassical signaling alludes to the formation of NO-induced posttranslational modifications (PTMs), especially S-nitrosylation, S-glutathionylation, and tyrosine nitration(Antonio et al., 2011).

4.1.1 Nitric oxide signaling pathway - Classical signaling pathways and apoptosis

In classical signaling pathways, NO induces the rupture of the His–Fe(II) bond within the heme of sGC, which catalyzes in the conversion of GTP to cGMP (Antonio et al., 2011). Effects of cGMP occur through three main groups of cellular targets: cGMP-dependent protein kinases (PKGs), cGMP-gated cation channels, and PDEs. cGMP binding activates PKG, which phosphorylates serines and threonines on many cellular proteins, frequently resulting in changes in activity or function, subcellular localization, or regulatory features (Francis et al., 2010). Accumulating data have showed NO could regulate apoptosis in classical signal pathways.

4.1.1.1 cGMP-Dependent inhibition of apoptotic signal transduction

Research has shown that NO protects against PC12 cell death by inhibiting the activation of caspase proteases through cGMP production and activation of protein kinase G (Kim et al., 1999). Another work further proves that the NO/cGMP pathway suppresses 6-OHDA-induced PC12 cell apoptosis by suppressing the mitochondrial apoptosis signal viaPKG/PI3K/Akt-dependent Bad phosphorylation (HA et al., 2003). NO has also been shown to inhibit TNF-a-induced TRADD recruitment and caspase 8 activity in a cGMP-dependent way (De Nadai et al., 2000). More direct data shows that over production of endogenous NO or supplementation with exogenous NO protects SK-N-BE human neuroblastoma againstapoptosis induced by serum deprivation by using cGMP as an intermediate effector (Ciani et al., 2002). The anti-apoptotic role of NO through cGMP is also revealed in hepatocytes (Calafell et al., 2009). In vivo data reveal that enhancing the NO/cGMP pathway reduces hypoxia-induced neuron apoptosis by upregulating the bcl-2/Bax ratio (Caretti et al., 2008). NO has also been shown to antagonize estrogen induced apoptosis in breast epithelial cells (Kastrati et al., 2010).

4.1.1.2 cGMP-Dependent induction of apoptotic signal transduction

Despite evidence that NO is anti-apoptotic, data also show that NO can induce apoptosis in a cGMP dependent manner in isolated adult cardiomyocytes. Induction of apoptosis by SNAP in cardiomyocytes was blocked by inhibitors of caspase-3, soluble guanylyl cyclase (sGC) or of cGMP dependent protein kinase (PKG) (Taimor et al., 2000). In vascular cells NO is shown to induce apoptosis through cGMP-dependent Protein Kinase (PKG) (Chiche et al., 1998).

4.1.2 Nitric oxide signaling pathway - Less classical signaling pathways and apoptosis

The critical mediator of NO regulating apoptosis in less classical signalling pathways is cytochrome c oxidase (CcO), which is located on the inner membrane of the mitochondrion and catalyzes the oxidation of cytochrome c and the reduction of oxygen to water (Taylor & Moncada, 2010). The enzyme belongs to the superfamily of heme-copper oxidases and contains a highly conserved bimetallic active site composed of the heme iron of cytochrome a3 and a copper ion, CuB. The binuclear center, in its reduced form, is the binding site of the physiological substrate, O2. NO closely resembles O2 and therefore can also bind to this site (Martinez-Ruiz et al., 2011). NO at low concentrations inhibits mitochondrial CcO, resulting in an increase in H2O2 in the mitochondria, and this excess of H2O2 activates the death signaling pathways (Yuyama et al., 2003). CcO potentially generates impairment of mitochondrial function, which in turn may potentiate apoptotic commitment. The NO toxicity can be indicated by the decrease of cytochrome c oxidase activity, which is paralleled the extent of apoptosis (Ciriolo et al., 2000).

4.1.3 Nitric oxide signaling pathway-nonclassical signaling pathways and apoptosis

Nitric oxide could exert part of its effects not only in a cGMP independent manner, but also without the need of binding to other metal centers, through covalent posttranslational modification (PTM) of target proteins. This mode of action is defined as denominate nonclassical signaling and affects mainly cysteine and tyrosine residues in proteins. The three best known NO-induced posttranslational modifications are S-nitrosylation, S-glutathionylation, and tyrosine nitration.

4.1.3.1 S-nitrosylation and apoptosis

S-nitrosylation is an important biological reaction of nitric oxide; it refers to the conversion of thiol groups, including cysteine residues in proteins, to form S-nitrosothiols. S-Nitrosylation is a mechanism for dynamic, post-translational regulation of most classes of protein. NO has been shown to regulate apoptosis through S-nitrosylation of protein.

Research hasrevealed that S-nitrosylation mainly antangonizes apoptosis by targeting many elements in both extrinsic and intrinsic pathways (Iyer et al., 2008). Fas, as a cell surface receptor, is a member of the tumor necrosis receptor superfamily that induces apoptosis when cross-linked by Fas ligand or by Fas agonist antibody (Park et al., 2006; Lavrik et al., 2005; Mannick & Schonhoff, 2004). Regulation of cell signaling by protein nitrosylation is well exemplified in the Fas signalling pathway (Mannick & Schonhoff, 2004). Consistent with receptor-mediated apoptosis, two main pathways of Fas-mediated apoptosis have been identified (Park et al., 2006). In type1 cells caspase-8 directly cleaves caspase-3, which starts the death cascade. In type2 cells the quantity of caspase-8 is insufficient to directly activate the executioner caspase-3. Instead, it involves (activates) tBid- mediated cytochrome c (Cyto-C) release from mitochondria followed by apoptosome formation (Park et al., 2006; Lavrik et al., 2005). In resting cells caspase-3 zymogens in mitochondria are kept inactive via S-nitrosylation of their catalytic site cysteine. Caspase-3 may be S-nitrosylated in mitochondria due to an association between S-nitrosylated caspase-3 and NOS. Moreover, S-nitrosylated but not denitrosylated caspase-3 associates with acid sphingomyelinase (ASM) in mitochondria. The association of S-nitrosylated caspase-3 with ASM provides another level of apoptosis regulation by inhibiting capase-3 cleavage and activation by initiator caspases. When cells are stimulated by Fas ligand, caspase-3 becomes denitrosylated. Denitrosylation stimulates caspase-3 activity by two mechanisms. First, denitrosylation allows the catalytic site of caspase-3 to function. In addition, denitrosylated caspase-3 presumably dissociates from ASM, allowing initiator caspases to cleave caspase-3 to its fully active form. Thus S-nitrosylation/denitrosylation serves as an off/on switch for caspase-3 function during apoptosis. Cyto-C activity is also regulated by nitrosylation during Fas-induced apoptosis. However, in contrast to caspase-3, Cyto-C is not nitrosylated in resting cells. Instead, when cells receive an apoptotic stimulus, Cyto-C is nitrosylated on its heme iron in mitochondria and then is rapidly released into the cytoplasm. In the cytoplasm, hemenitrosylated Cyto-C stimulates caspase-3 cleavage by the apoptosome. Thus, coordinated denitrosylation of caspase- 3 and hemenitrosylation of Cyto-C serves to enhance caspase activation and Fas-induced apoptosis. It remains to be determined if denitrosylation of caspase-3 is directly linked to nitrosylation of Cyto-C in mitochondria via a direct transfer of a NO+ group from the catalytic site cysteine of caspase-3 to the heme iron of Cyto-C (Mannick et al., 1997; Mannick & Schonhoff, 2004; Schonhoff et al., 2003; Stamler et al., 2001(Mannick et al., 1997; Mannick & Schonhoff, 2004; Schonhoff et al., 2003; Stamler et al., 2001). NO can also inhibit apoptosis by direct nitrosylation of caspase-9 (Török et al., 2002).

In intrinsic apoptosis pathways, Cyto-C is released from mitochondria into cytoplasm initiates the apoptotic signals (Brüne, 2003; Schonhoff et al., 2003) and has been suggested as the commitment step for apoptosis (Gaston et al., 2003). Previous studies suggest that nitrosylation of Cyto-C is a novel mechanism of apoptosis regulation in cells and a very early event in apoptotic signalling (Schonhoff et al., 2003). However, the critical commitment step in the mitochondrial pathway of apoptosis has not been firmly established. Several recent findings suggest that caspase-9 activation is essential for, and likely represents, the commitment step for the mitochondrial pathway of apoptosis. Nitrosylation of caspase-9 by induced (i) NOS generated NO inhibits apoptosis downstream of Cyto-C release and would appear to be another mechanism negatively regulating this pathway of apoptosis (Török et al., 2002). Besides nitrosylation of caspases, another mechanism underlying the anti-apoptotic effects of NO via S-nitrosylation includes stimulation of the anti-apoptotic activity (function) of thioredoxin (Trx), which depends on S-nitrosylation at Cys69 (Haendeler et al., 2002). S-nitrosylation and inhibition of Apoptosis signal regulating kinase (ASK1) (in L929 cells) at Cys869 also lead to anti-apoptosis (Park et al., 2004).

Although most of the reports have proven that S-nitrosylation mainly inhibits apoptosis, there are also data showing that S-nitrosylation could induce apoptosis as well. The mechanisms underlying the pro-apoptotic effects of NO via S-nitrosylation include inhibition of the anti-apoptotic transcription factor NF-κB through a variety of mechanisms, including S-nitrosylation of NF-κB (in A549 cells) or nitrosylation of the target cysteine in the IκB kinase complex (IKK) (in Jurkat cells) leading to decreased NF-κB–mediated transcription and decreased Bcl-2 expression (Marshall & Stamler, 2002; Schonhoff et al., 2006). p21ras, JNK kinase, and the p50 monomer (of p50-p65) have been identified as sites of S-nitrosylation that mediate the stimulation or inhibition of NF-κB by NO (Marshall and Stamler, 2002). Glyceraldehyde-3-phosphate dehydrogenase (GAPDH) is S-nitrosylated by NO, which initiates an interaction with the E3 ligase Siah1, leading to nuclear translocation and ubiquitin-mediated degradation of nuclear target proteins (Benhar & Stamler, 2005). Hara et al. has demonstrated that deprenyl and TCH346 are neuroprotective by preventing the S-nitrosylation of GAPDH and inhibiting GAPDH/Siah cell death cascade (Hara et al., 2006). NO can also enhance apoptosis by NO-induced persistent inhibition and nitrosylation of mitochondrial Cyto-C oxidase in lung endothelial cells (Zhang et al., 2005). The work done by Gu et al. has illustrated that S-Nitrosylation activated Matrix metalloproteinase-9 in vitro was implicated in the pathogenesis of neurodegenerative diseases, stroke, and induced neuronal apoptosis (Gu et al., 2002).

4.1.3.2 S-Glutathionylation and apoptosis

S-thiolation refers to the incorporation of a low-molecular-mass (LMM) thiol to a protein via formation of a mixed disulfide bridge between a cysteine residue and the LMM thiol. In the intracellular environment in which GSH is the major thiol present, its incorporation results in a PTM named S-glutathionylation or S-glutathiolation, or more commonly S-thiolation

(Martinez-Ruiz et al., 2011). Protein S-glutathiolation, the reversible covalent addition of glutathione to cysteine residues on target proteins, is emerging as a candidate mechanism by which both changes in the intracellular redox state and the generation of reactive oxygen and nitrogen species may be transduced into a functional response (Klatt & Lamas, 2000). S-glutathionylation is a redox signaling mechanism that can be produced without the concourse of NO. However, evidence for S-glutathionylation induced by NO and/or RNS has accumulated, linking this modification with NO signalling (Giustarini et al., 2004). At least two mechanisms explain the link between RNS production and S-glutathionylation. One is the observed glutathionylation induced by peroxynitrite. The other is a nitrosylated protein cysteine may react with GSH, or S-nitrosoglutathione can be formed and react with the cysteine thiol, both leading to S-glutathionylation (Martinez-Ruiz et al., 2011).

Vikas Anathy et al. demonstrated that stimulation with Fas ligand (FasL) induces S-glutathionylation of Fas at cysteine 294 independently of nicotinamide adenine dinucleotide phosphate reduced oxidase – induced ROS. Instead, Fas is S-glutathionylated after caspase-dependent degradation of Grx1, increasing subsequent caspase activation and apoptosis (Anathy et al., 2009). Suparna Qanungo et al. indicated S-glutathionylation of p65-NFκB as a major mechanism underlying the inhibition of the NF_B survival pathway and promotion of apoptosis after GSH supplementation in hypoxic pancreatic cancer cells (Qanungo et al., 2007). Therefore, RNS could regulate apoptosis through S-glutathionylation of protein

4.1.3.3 Tyrosine nitration and apoptosis

RNS-mediated nitration modifications include nitration of tyrosine, tryptophan, amine, carboxylic acid, and phenylalanine groups. However, nitration of tyrosine residues to produce nitrotyrosine has recently received much attention. Protein tyrosine nitration is a covalent protein modification resulting from the addition of a nitro (-NO2) group onto one of the two equivalent ortho carbons of the aromatic ring of tyrosine residues (Gow et al., 2004). Biological nitration of tyrosine depends largely on free radical chemistry. There are two main key nitration pathways that operate in vivo and involve peroxynitrite and hemoperoxidase-catalyzed nitration (Peluffo & Radi, 2007). Tyrosine nitration is a two-step process where the initial reaction is the oxidation of the aromatic ring of tyrosine to yield tyrosyl radical (Tyr•) (oxidation step), which in turn adds •NO2 (addition step) to yield 3-NO2-Tyr (Peluffo & Radi, 2007).

4.1.3.3.1 RNS-mediated Tyrosine nitration induction of Apoptotic Signal Transduction

Work by Hortelano et al. indicates that nitric oxide-dependent apoptosis in macrophages occurs in the presence of a sustained increase of the mitochondrial transmembrane potential, and that the chemical modification and release of cytochrome c from the mitochondria precedes the changes of the mitochondrial transmembrane potential. NO-dependent apoptosis in macrophages involves a chemical modification of cytochrome c that alters its structure and facilitates release from the mitochondria, regardless of the changes of the mitochondrial transmembrane potential (Hortelano et al., 1999). Cassina et al. has shown that Tyr-67 is a preferential site of nitration among the four conserved tyrosine residues in cytochrome c. Cytochrome c3+ was more extensively nitrated than cytochrome c2+ by mitochondrial but also cytosolic or extracellular derived ONOO- diffusing to the intermembrane space (Cassina et al., 2000). Tao et al. proved that nitrative inactivation of Trx plays a proapoptotic role in postischemic myocardium (Tao et al., 2006). Studies conducted by Li et al. demonstrated that there exists a TNF-α-initiated, cardiomyocyte iNOS/NADPH oxidase-dependent, peroxynitrite-mediated signaling pathway that contributes to posttraumatic myocardial apoptosis. In this paper nitrotyrosine content acted as a footprint of in vivo peroxynitrite formation (Li et al., 2007).

4.1.3.3.2 RNS-Mediated tyrosine nitration inhibition of apoptotic signal transduction

Although many studies have shown that RNS-mediated tyrosine nitration mainly induce apoptosis. Some research indicated that it also can inhibit apoptosis. Work by Sonsoles Reinehr et al. indicates that CD95 nitration as a novel mechanism for apoptosis inhibition by NO, which competes with pro-apoptotic CD95-tyrosine phosphorylation(Reinehr et al,2004). The study of Nakagawa et al determined that cytochrome c nitrated by continuous treatment with peroxynitrite lost its ability to cause caspase cascade activation in vitro, whereas cytochrome c nitrated by a bolus peroxynitrite treatment had preserved activity (Nakagawa et al, 2007).

Previous data have shown that Reactive Nitrogen Species can either stimulate (pro-apoptosis) or prevent apoptosis (anti-apoptosis) (Boyd & Cadenas, 2002; Brüne, 2003; Choi et al., 2002; Patel et al., 1999). The concentrations and local environments including cellular redox state and the presence of free radicals of NO and RNS play a key role in determining whether they stimulate or inhibit apoptosis (Brüne, 2003). Peroxynitrite(ONOO-), an important RNS, is formed by the reaction between high concentrations of NO and superoxide . High concentrations of NO or ONOO-can induce apoptosis (Choi et al., 2002). Liang et al. demonstrated for the first time that L-arginine administered at different time points during I/R exerted different effects on post-ischemic myocardial injury and suggests that stimulation of eNOS reduces nitrative stress and decreases apoptosis whereas stimulation of iNOS increases nitrative stress and enhances myocardial reperfusion injury (Liang et al., 2004). But, Rus et al.'s results demonstrated that inhibition of iNOS raises the peroxidative and apoptotic level in the hypoxic heart indicating that this isoform may have a protective effect on this organ against hypoxia/reoxygenation injuries, and this challenges the conventional wisdom that iNOS is deleterious under these conditions (Rus et al., 2010). So, the effect on apoptosis of RNS and its regulation need further clarification.

4.2 RNS signaling and aging myocardial ischemic injury

Accumulated data have shown that nitric oxide derived reactive nitrogen intermediates are critical contributors in controlling apoptosis which determine the susceptibility of aging hearts to myocardial ischemic Injury.

Gao et al's results showed that the protective effects of adenosine on myocardial I/R injury are markedly diminished in aged animals and that the loss in NO release in response to adenosine may be at least partially responsible for this age-related alteration (Gao et al., 2000). Studies also show that increased susceptibility of the type 2 diabetic GK rat heart to ischemic injury is not associated with impaired energy metabolism. Reduced coronary flow, upregulation of eNOS expression, and increased total NOx levels confirm NO pathway modifications in this model, presumably related to increased oxidative stress. Modifications in the NO pathway may play a major role in I/R injury of the type 2 diabetic GK rat heart (Desrois et al., 2010). Our results show that aging induces phenotypic upregulation of iNOS in the heart, in which β-AR stimulation interacts with ischemia and triggers a markedly increased NO production, which creates a nitrative stress, generates toxic peroxynitrite, activates apoptosis, and eventually causes cardiac dysfunction and myocardial injury. An iNOS inhibitor-1400W can markedly attenuate these adverse effects in the aging heart (Li, 2006).

4.3 Thioredoxin and aging-related myocardial apoptosis

Thioredoxin (Trx) is a 12-kDa protein ubiquitously expressed in all living cells that fulfils a variety of biological functions related to cell proliferation and apoptosis. It is involved not only in cytoprotective functions against oxidative stress but also in the regulation of cellular proliferation and the aging process. Clinical and experimental results have demonstrated that inhibition of Trx promotes apoptosis (Lincoln et al, 2003). Recent in vitro studies demonstrate that Trx interacts directly with, and inhibits, the activity of apoptosis-regulating kinase-1 (ASK1), a mitogen-activated protein (MAP) kinase that activates two proapoptotic kinases, p38 MAP kinase (MAPK) and c-Jun N-terminal kinase (JNK) (Liu & Min, 2002). In aged mouse livers, the ratio of ASK1/Trx–ASK1 (free ASK1/Trx-binding ASK1) increases and this correlates with the increased basal activity of the p38 MAPK pathway. These results suggest that Trx may play critical roles in cell proliferation and cell death in aging, and Trx activity/expression might be reduced in the aging heart, thus tilting the death/survival balance toward cell death and promoting ischemia/reperfusion injury.

Under physiologic conditions, ASK1 activity is inhibited by several cellular factors, including Trx, glutaredoxin, and phosphoserine-binding protein 14-3-3 (Bishopric & Webster, 2002). Previous studies have demonstrated that many cellular stresses and apoptotic stimuli activate mitochondrial-dependent apoptotic pathways by facilitating dissociation of ASK1 with its inhibitory protein. Trx is physically associated with ASK1 in cardiac tissues from young animals. However, Trx–ASK1 binding was reduced in cardiac tissue from aging animals. Therefore, it is likely that increased posttranslational Trx modification in aging hearts results in disassociation of Trx from ASK1, thus increasing postischemic myocardial apoptosis by increasing p38 MAPK activity.

Lots of studies have demonstrated that, in addition to upregulation or downregulation of Trx expression at the gene level, Trx activity is regulated by posttranslational modification. Three forms of posttranslational modification of Trx have been previously identified. These include oxidation, glutathionylation, and S-nitrosylation. Interestingly, all three forms of modification occur at cysteine residues but affect Trx function differently. Oxidation of the thiol groups of Cys-32 and-35 forms a disulfide bond which results in Trx inactivation. However, previous studies have demonstrated that administration of oxidized Trx-1 exerts significant antioxidant and cytoprotective effects unless intracellular Trx reductase is inhibited, indicating that oxidative Trx inhibition is reversible and this form of posttranslational modification may not be the major mechanism responsible for Trx inactivation in vivo (Andoh et al, 2003). Glutathionylation occurs at Cys-73, and this posttranslational modification significantly inhibits Trx activity (Casagrande et al, 2002). However, whether Trx glutathionylation may occur in vivo in diseased tissues remains completely unknown and the role of this form of posttranslational modification in regulating Trx function in vivo remains to be determined. S-nitrosylation has been reported to occur at either Cys-69 or Cys-73. In contrast to oxidation and glutathionylation, S-nitrosylation increases Trx activity and further enhances its antiapoptotic effect (Haendeler et al., 2004; Mitchell & Marletta, 2005).

In a recent study, it has been demonstrated that, in addition to three previously reported posttranslational Trx modifications which all occur at the cysteine residue, Trx can also be modified at the tyrosine residue (protein nitration) in a peroxynitrite-dependent fashion (Tao et al., 2006). More interestingly, in contrast to the reversible (by Trx reductase) oxidative Trx inactivation, nitrative modification of Trx results in an irreversible inactivation. Therefore, nitric oxide and its secondary reaction products, particularly peroxynitrite, exert opposite effects on Trx activity. Specifically, nitric oxide itself induces Trx S-nitrosylation and enhances its activity. In contrast, peroxynitrite results in Trx nitration and causes an irreversible inactivation. In Zhang et al.'s study, Trx activity was determined by using the insulin disulfide reduction assay. Compared with young animals, cardiac Trx activity is decreased in the aging heart before myocardial ischemia and reperfusion, and this difference can be further amplified after myocardial ischemia and reperfusion. However, Trx expression is slightly increased, rather than decreased, in aging hearts. These results indicate that it is posttranslational Trx modification rather than reduced protein expression that reduces Trx activity in the aging heart (Zhang et al., 2007).

5. A Mitochondrial pro-apoptotic protein, HtrA2/Omi, is another reason of enhanced MI/R injury in the aging heart

It is well known that apoptotic cell death is orchestrated by a family of caspases. X-chromosome linked inhibitor of apoptosis protein (XIAP), as a member of IAPs, was the most potent endogenous inhibitor of caspases in human beings. XIAP has three baculovirus IAP repeat (BIR1, BIR2, BIR3) domains and a really interesting new gene (RING) domain. Biochemical studies suggested BIR2 inhibits caspase-3 and caspase-7, whereas BIR3 inhibits caspase-9 (Deveraux et al., 1999). The RING domain is an E3 ligase that presumably directs targets to the ubiquitin-proteasome degradation system, such as caspase-3 (Salvesen & Duckett, 2002; Martin, 2002). The anti-apoptotic activity of XIAP is regulated by a group of proteins that bind to the BIR domains via N-terminal conserved 4-residue IAP-binding motif (Shi, 2002). Recently it has been shown that overexpression of XIAP via in vivo delivery in an adenovirus could reduce both myocardial apoptosis and infarction following I/R (Kim et al., 2011). Wang et al. the protein and mRNA content of XIAP in the heart after MI/R was decreased, while the protein content of XIAP showed positive correlation with cardiac function in 42 rats after MI/R(Wang et al., 2010). These findings suggested a link between myocardial apoptosis, and anti-apoptotic therapy was effective in reducing I/R injury. Meanwhile we found the degradation of XIAP in aging myocardium after MI/R was more than that in young myocardium after MI/R, which are consistent with previous results in which myocardial apoptosis was exaggerated with aging after MI/R. Additionally, the expression of XIAP was also significantly decreased than that in the young adult heart without the intervention of MI/R, which suggested that the decline of XIAP expression may be a major factor responsible for the increased susceptibility of the aging heart.

XIAP is regulated by two cellular proteins, Smac/DIABLO and HtrA2/Omi, which are nuclear-encoded mitochondrial proteins. The cleavage of their mitochondrial-targeting sequences inside mitochondria generates processed active Smac /DIABLO and HtrA2/Omi with new apoptotic N termini, named the IAP-binding motif (IBM) (Srinivasula et al., 2003). Stimulated by apoptotic triggers, Smac/DIABLO and HtrA2/Omi release into the cytosol and competitively bind to the BIR domains of IAPs via IBM, so that the BIR-bound caspases are released and reactivated, resulting in cell apoptosis (Wu et al., 2000, Suzuki et al., 2001). Unlike Smac/DIABLO, the pro-apoptotic activity of HtrA2/Omi involves not only IAP binding but also serine protease activity. Although Omi/HtrA2 and Smac/DIABLO both seem to target XIAP once released into the cytosol, increasing evidence suggests that Omi/HtrA2 may play a unique role in apoptosis. Several different Smac/DIABLO-deficient cells respond normally to various apoptotic stimuli, suggesting the existence of a redundant molecule or molecules compensating for a loss of Smac/DIABLO function (Okada et al., 2002). In contrast, Omi/HtrA2-knockdown cells have shown to be more resistant to apoptotic stimuli (Martins et al., 2002).

In addition, Liu et al. first provided direct evidence that a normal level of endogenously expressed HtrA2/Omi contributes to apoptosis after MI/R in vivo (Liu et al., 2005). Althaus et al. have also suggested that HtrA2/Omi plays a decisive role in apoptosis after MI/R in young rats (Althaus et al., 2007). Then Wang et al showed that the release of HtrA2/Omi from mitochondria to cytosol was significantly increased in the old MI/R rat heart compared with that in the young MI/R rats (Wang et al, 2006). Meanwhile, cytosol was markedly increased in the old sham group compared with that in the young sham group. Taken together, these results reveal that HtrA2/Omi plays a causative role in increased post-ischemic cardiomyocyte apoptosis in the aging heart (Okada et al., 2002). In order to investigate whether increased HtrA2/Omi plays an important role in aged myocardial apoptosis resulting in myocardial dysfunction and increased susceptibility to MI/R injury, Wang et al observed the effect of ucf-101, a highly selective Omi/HtrA2 inhibitor, on MI/R injury. They have provided direct evidence in the current study that treatment with ucf-101 in aging MI/R animals reduced the caspase-3 activity and improved the cardiac functions. Their results demonstrated that translocation of Omi/HtrA2 from the mitochondria to the cytosol enhanced MI/R injury in aging heart via promoting myocardial apoptosis. These studies may provide some therapies to prevent the over-release of HtrA2/Omi from mitochondria with aging and reduce the risk for MI/R in the elderly. This could help to explain the loss of ventricular function with age and may lead to discoveries of specific therapeutic interventions that can attenuate this type of cell loss (Wang et al., 2010).

6. Prospect

Aging has become a major health issue and socioeconomic burden worldwide. Coronary heart disease is the leading cause of death worldwide, for patients presented with an acute myocardial infarction, early and successful myocardial reperfusion is the most effective interventional strategy for reducing infarct size and improving clinical outcomes. The process of myocardial reperfusion itself, however, can induce injury to the myocardium, thereby reducing the beneficial effects of myocardial reperfusion. Aging renders the heart more susceptible to cell death from ischemia/reperfusion. In order to develop strategies aimed to limit reversible and irreversible myocardial damage in older patients, there is a need to better understand how aging increases myocardial apoptosis in myocardial ischaemia/reperfusion.

This chapter introduced that RNS signaling induced apoptosis contributes to increased susceptibility of aging hearts to myocardial ischemic injury, and the age-associated alterations in translocation of HtrA2/Omi from mitochondria to cytosol are implicated in the markedly increased risk for MI/R injury in old persons.

As mentioned above, three RNS signaling pathways have been recognized .On the one hand, many studies show that RNS can be pro-apoptotic; on the other hand, many studies show that RNS exert anti-apoptotic effects through the same signaling pathway. Further studies should continue to elucidate the many factors that determine how RNS promotes or inhibits apoptosis.

Wang et al. results provide strong evidence that HtrA2/Omi plays a causative role in increased post-ischemic cardiomyocyte apoptosis in the aging heart, but the mechanisms of age-associated alterations in translocation of HtrA2/Omi from mitochondria to cytosol need elucidation.

There is an urgent need for more research of myocardial ischemia/reperfusion conducted on senescent animals. Some researches about RNS signaling induced apoptosis contributes to increased susceptibility of aging hearts to myocardial ischemic injury have been performed in rats or mice. However, biological signaling pathways, proteolytic portfolios, and the overall response to myocardial injury can be quite different in these small rodents when compared to larger mammals. While these murine studies have provided invaluable insight and provoked new hypotheses, they must be carried forward using large animals that more closely recapitulate the clinically-relevant context and for carefully designed clinical trials involving aged human subjects. There also needs to be better coordinated efforts between basic science investigators, clinical trial managers and physicians. (Spinale, 2010, as cited in Bujak et al., 2008; Singh et al., 2010; Lindsey, 2005; Juhaszova et al. ,2005 as cited in Bolli et al., 2004).

Otherwise, most studies have been conducted on healthy aging animals. Ischemic heart disease develops as a consequence of a number of etiological risk factors and always coexists with other disease states. These include systemic arterial hypertension and related left ventricular hypertrophy, hyperlipidemia, and atherosclerosis, diabetes and insulin resistance, as well as heart failure. These systemic diseases with aging as a modifying condition exert multiple biochemical effects on the heart that can potentially affect the development of I/R injury and interfere with responses to cardioprotective interventions. Therefore, the development of rational therapeutic approaches to protect the ischemic heart requires preclinical studies that examine cardioprotection specifically in relation to complicating disease states and risk factors. Surprisingly, relatively little effort has been made to uncover the cellular mechanisms by which risk factors and systemic diseases such as hypertension, hyperlipidemia and atherosclerosis, diabetes, insulin resistance, and heart failure interfere with cardioprotective mechanisms of aging (Ferdinandy et al., 2007).

Although, as mentioned above, RNS and HtrA2/Omi may be critical contributors in controlling apoptosis which determine the susceptibility of aging hearts to myocardial ischemic injury.

7. References

Althaus, J., Siegelin, M.D., Dehghani, F., Cilenti, L., Zervos, A.S. & Rami A.(2007). The serine protease HtrA2/Omi is involved in XIAP cleavage and in neuronal cell death following focal cerebral ischemia/reperfusion. *Neurochem int* 50(1):172-180.

Anathy, V., Aesif, S.W., Guala, A.S., Havermans, M., Reynaert, N.L., Ho, Y.S., Budd, R.C., and Janssen-Heininger, Y.M.W. (2009). Redox amplification of apoptosis by caspase-dependent cleavage of glutaredoxin 1 and S-glutathionylation of Fas. *J Cell Biol* 184(2):241-252.

Andoh, T., Chiueh, C.C. & Chock, P. B.(2003). Cyclic GMP-dependent protein kinase regulates the expression of thioredoxin and thioredoxin peroxidase-1 during hormesis in response to oxidative stress-induced apoptosis. *J Biol Chem.* 278(2): 885-90.

Anversa, P., Palackal, T., Sonnenblick, E., Olivetti, G., Meggs, L., & Capasso, J.M. (1990). Myocyte cell loss and myocyte cellular hyperplasia in the hypertrophied aging rat heart. *Circulation Research* 67(4): 871-885.

Beneke, S. & Bürkle, A. (2007). Poly(ADP-ribosyl) ation in mammalian ageing, *Nucleic Acids Res* 35(22):7456-7465.

Benhar, M. & Stamler, J.S. (2005). A central role for S-nitrosylation in apoptosis. *Nat cell biol* 7(7) :645-646.

Bishopric, N.H. & Webster, K.A. (2002). Preventing apoptosis with thioredoxin: ASK me how. *Cir Res* 90(12): 1237-1239.

Boyd, C.S. & Cadenas, E. (2002). Nitric oxide and cell signaling pathways in mitochondrial-dependent apoptosis. *Biol chem* 383(3-4):411-423.

Brüne, B. (2003). Nitric oxide: NO apoptosis or turning it ON? *Cell Death Differ* 10(8), 864-869.

Calafell, R., Boada, J., Santidrian, A.F., Gil, J., Roig, T., Perales, J.C., and Bermudez, J. (2009). Fructose 1, 6-bisphosphate reduced TNF-[alpha]-induced apoptosis in galactosamine sensitized rat hepatocytes through activation of nitric oxide and cGMP production. *Eur j pharmacol* 610, 128-133.

Caretti, A., Bianciardi, P., Ronchi, R., Fantacci, M., Guazzi, M. & Samaja, M. (2008). Phosphodiesterase-5 inhibition abolishes neuron apoptosis induced by chronic hypoxia independently of hypoxia-inducible factor-1 {alpha} signaling. *Exp Biol Med* 233(10):1222-1230.

Carr, A.C., McCall, M.R. & Frei, B. (2000). Oxidation of LDL by myeloperoxidase and reactive nitrogen species: reaction pathways and antioxidant protection. *Arteriosclerosis, thrombosis, and vascular biology* 20:1716-1723.

Casagrande, S., Bonetto, V., Fratelli, M., Gianazza, E., Eberini, I., Massignan, T., Salmona, M., Chang, G., Holmgren, A. & Ghezzi, P. (2002). Glutathionylation of human thioredoxin: a possible crosstalk between the glutathione and thioredoxin systems. *Proc Natl Acad Sci USA* 99(15):9745-9749.

Cassina, A.M., Hodara, R., Souza, J.M., Thomson, L., Castro, L., Ischiropoulos, H., Freeman, B.A. & Radi, R. (2000). Cytochrome c nitration by peroxynitrite. *J Biol Chem* 275(28):21409-21415.

Chiche, J.D., Schlutsmeyer, S.M., Bloch, D.B., de la Monte, S.M., Roberts, J.D., Filippov, G., Janssens, S.P., Rosenzweig, A. & Bloch, K.D. (1998). Adenovirus-mediated gene transfer of cGMP-dependent protein kinase increases the sensitivity of cultured vascular smooth muscle cells to the antiproliferative and pro-apoptotic effects of nitric oxide/cGMP. *J Biol Chem* 273(51): 34263-34271.

Choi, B.M., Pae, H.O., Jang, S.I., Kim, Y.M. & Chung, H.T. (2002). Nitric oxide as a pro-apoptotic as well as anti-apoptotic modulator. *J biochem mol biol* 35(1):116-126.

Ciani, E., Guidi, S., Della Valle, G., Perini, G., Bartesaghi, R. & Contestabile, A. (2002). Nitric oxide protects neuroblastoma cells from apoptosis induced by serum deprivation through cAMP-response element-binding protein (CREB) activation. *J Biol Chem* 277(51), 49896-49902.

Ciriolo, M.R., De Martino, A., Lafavia, E., Rossi, L., Carr , M.T. & Rotilio, G. (2000). Cu, Zn-superoxide dismutase-dependent apoptosis induced by nitric oxide in neuronal cells. *J Biol Chemi* 275(7):5065-5072.

De Nadai, C., Sestili, P., Cantoni, O., Li¨¨vremont, J.P., Sciorati, C., Barsacchi, R., Moncada, S., Meldolesi, J. & Clementi, E. (2000). Nitric oxide inhibits tumor necrosis factor-alpha-induced apoptosis by reducing the generation of ceramide. *Proc Nati Acad Sci USA* 97(10), 5480-5485.

Desrois, M., Clarke, K., Lan, C., Dalmasso, C., Cole, M., Portha, B., Cozzone, P.J. & Bernard, M. (2010). Upregulation of eNOS and unchanged energy metabolism in increased susceptibility of the aging type 2 diabetic GK rat heart to ischemic injury. *Am J Physiol Heart Circ Physiol* 299(5) :H1679-H1686.

Deveraux, Q.L., Leo, E., Stennicke, H.R., Welsh, K., Salvesen, G.S. & Reed, J.C. (1999). Cleavage of human inhibitor of apoptosis protein XIAP results in fragments with distinct specificities for caspases. *EMBO J.* 18(19): 5242–5251.

Ferdinandy, P., Schulz, R. & Baxter, G.F.,(2007). Interaction of cardiovascular risk factors with myocardial ischemia/reperfusion injury, preconditioning, and postconditioning. *Pharmacol Rev* 59(4): 418-58.

Francis, S.H., Busch, J.L., Corbin, J.D. & Sibley, D. (2010). cGMP-dependent protein kinases and cGMP phosphodiesterases in nitric oxide and cGMP action. *Pharmacol rev* 62(3): 525-563.

Gao, F., Christopher, T.A., Lopez, B.L., Friedman, E., Cai, G. & Ma, X.L. (2000). Mechanism of decreased adenosine protection in reperfusion injury of aging rats. *Am J Physiol Heart Circ Physiol* 279(1):H329-H338.

Gaston, B.M., Carver, J., Doctor, A. & Palmer, L.A. (2003). S-nitrosylation signaling in cell biology. *Mol interv* 3(5): 253-263.

Giustarini, D., Rossi, R., Milzani, A., Colombo, R., and Dalle-Donne, I. (2004). S-Glutathionylation: from redox regulation of protein functions to human diseases. Journal of cellular and molecular medicine 8, 201-212.

Gow, A.J., Farkouh, C.R., Munson, D.A., Posencheg, M.A. & Ischiropoulos, H. (2004). Biological significance of nitric oxide-mediated protein modifications. *Am J Physiol Lung Cell Mol Physiol* 287(2): L262-L268.

Gu, Z., Kaul, M., Yan, B., Kridel, S.J., Cui, J., Strongin, A., Smith, J.W., Liddington, R.C. & Lipton, S.A. (2002). S-nitrosylation of matrix metalloproteinases: signaling pathway to neuronal cell death. *Science* 297(5584): 1186-1190.

HA, K.S.O.O., KIM, K.I.M.O., KWON, Y.G., BAI, S.E.K., NAM, W.O.O.D., YOO, Y.M.I.N., KIM, P.K.M., CHUNG, H.U.N.T., BILLIAR, T.R., and KIM, Y.M. (2003). Nitric oxide prevents 6-hydroxydopamine-induced apoptosis in PC12 cells through cGMP-dependent PI3 kinase/Akt activation. *The FASEB journal* 17, 1036.

Haendeler, J., Hoffmann, J., Tischler, V., Berk, B.C., Zeiher, A.M., & Dimmeler, S. (2002). Redox regulatory and anti-apoptotic functions of thioredoxin depend on S-nitrosylation at cysteine 69. *Nat cell biol* 4(10), 743-749.

Haendeler, J., Hoffmann, J., Zeiher, A.M. & Dimmeler, S. (2004). Antioxidant effects of Statins via S-nitrosylation and activation of thioredoxin in endothelial cells: a novel vasculoprotective function of Statins. *Circulation*. 110(7): 856-61.

Hara, M.R., Thomas, B., Cascio, M.B., Bae, B.I., Hester, L.D., Dawson, V.L., Dawson, T.M., Sawa, A. & Snyder, S.H. (2006). Neuroprotection by pharmacologic blockade of the GAPDH death cascade. *Proc Nati Acad Sci USA* 103(10):3887-3889.

Hortelano, S., Alvarez, A.M. & Boscá L. (1999). Nitric oxide induces tyrosine nitration and release of cytochrome c preceding an increase of mitochondrial transmembrane potential in macrophages. *The FASEB J* 13(15):2311-2317.

Hutton & David. (2008). Older people in emergencies: considerations for action and policy development, In:*World Health Organization. http://www.who.int/ageing/publications/Hutton_report_small.pdf*

Jiang X., Kim H., Shu H., Zhao Y., Zhang H., Kofron J., Donnelly J., Burns D., Ng SC., Rosenberg S., Wang X. (2003). Distinctive roles of PHAP proteins and prothymosin-alpha in a death regulatory pathway. *Science* 299(5604):223-226.

Jugdutt,B.I.&Jelani,A.(2008).Aging and defective healing,adverse remodeling, and blunted post-conditioning in the reperfused wounded heart, *J Am Coll Cardio* 51(14): 1399-1403.

Juhaszova, M., Rabuel ,C., Zorov, D.B., Lakatta, E.G. & Sollott ,SJ.(2005). Protection in the aged heart: preventing the heart-break of old age?, *Cardiovasc Res* 66(2): 233-244.

Kastrati, I., Edirisinghe, P.D., Wijewickrama, G.T. & Thatcher, G.R. (2010). Estrogen-induced apoptosis of breast epithelial cells Is blocked by NO/cGMP and mediated by extranuclear estrogen receptors. *Endocrinology* 151(12):5602-5616.

Kim, S.J., Kuklov, A. & Crystal, G.J. (2011) In vivo gene delivery of XIAP protects against myocardial apoptosis and infarction following ischemia/reperfusion in conscious rabbits. *Life Sci.* 88(13-14): 572-577.

Kim, Y.M., Chung, H.T., Kim, S.S., Han, J.A., Yoo, Y.M., Kim, K.M., Lee, G.H., Yun, H.Y., Green, A., Li, J., Simmons,R.L.& Billiar,T.R. (1999). Nitric oxide protects PC12 cells from serum deprivation-induced apoptosis by cGMP-dependent inhibition of caspase signaling. *J Neurosci* 19(16): 6740-6747.

Kinsella, K. & Velkoff, V. (2001). U.S. Census Bureau. An Aging World: 2001. U.S. Government Printing Office, Washington, DC.

Klatt, P. & Lamas, S. (2000). Regulation of protein function by S-glutathiolation in response to oxidative and nitrosative stress. *Eur J Biochem* 267(16), 4928-4944.

Lakatta, E. G. & Levy, D. (2003). Arterial and cardiac aging: major shareholders in cardiovascular disease enterprises: Part I: aging arteries: a "set up" for vascular disease. *Circulation* 107(1):139–146.

Lavrik, I.N., Golks, A. & Krammer, P.H. (2005). Caspases: pharmacological manipulation of cell death. *J Clin Invest* 115(10):2665-2672.

Li, D., Qu, Y., Tao, L., Liu, H., Hu, A., Gao, F., Sharifi-Azad, S., Grunwald, Z., Ma, XL.and Sun JZ.(2006). Inhibition of iNOS protects the aging heart against beta-adrenergic receptor stimulation-induced cardiac dysfunction and myocardial ischemic injury. *J Surg Res.* 131(1):64-72.

Li, S., Jiao, X., Tao, L., Liu, H., Cao, Y., Lopez, B.L., Christopher, T.A. & Ma, X.L. (2007). Tumor necrosis factor-alpha in mechanic trauma plasma mediates cardiomyocyte apoptosis. *Am JPhysiol Heart Circ Physiol* 293(3):H1847-H852.

Liang, F., Gao, E., Tao, L., Liu, H., Qu, Y., Christopher, T.A., Lopez, B.L. & Ma, X.L. (2004). Critical timing of L-arginine treatment in post-ischemic myocardial apoptosis-role of NOS isoforms. *Cardiovas res* 62(3): 568-577.

Lincoln, D.T, Ali Emadi, E.M., Tonissen, K.F. & Clarke, F.M.(2003). The thioredoxin-thioredoxin reductase system: over-expression in human cancer. *Anticancer Res* 23(3B): 2425-2433.

Liu, H.R., Gao, E., Hu, A., Tao, L., Qu, Y., Most, P., Koch, W.J., Christopher, T.A., Lopez, B.L., Alnemri, E.S., Zervos, A.S., Ma, X.L. (2005). Role of HtrA2/Omi in Apoptotic Cell Death after Myocardial Ischemia and Reperfusion. *Circulation* 111(1) :90-96.

Liu, P., Xu, B., Cavalieri, TA.& Hock CE. (2002). Age-related difference in myocardial function and inflammation in a rat model of myocardial ischemia-reperfusion. *Cardiovascular Research* 56(3): 443-453.

Liu, Y. & Min, W. (2002). Thioredoxin promotes ASK1 ubiquitination and degradation to inhibit ASK1-mediated apoptosis in a redox activity-independent manner. *Circ Res* 90(12): 1259-66.

MacDonald, Paul. (2002). Heart Disease, In: Encyclopedia.com, Encyclopedia of Aging, <http://www.encyclopedia.com/topic/Antilipemic_agents.aspx>

Mannick, J.B., Miao, X.Q. & Stamler, J.S. (1997). Nitric oxide inhibits Fas-induced apoptosis. *J Biol Chem* 272(39):24125-24128.

Mannick, J.B. & Schonhoff, C.M. (2004). NO means no and yes: regulation of cell signaling by protein nitrosylation. *Free radic res* 38(1):1-7.

Marshall, H.E. & Stamler, J.S. (2002). Nitrosative stress-induced apoptosis through inhibition of NF-kappa B. *J Biol Chem* 277(37), 34223-34228.

Martin, S.J. (2002). Destabilizing influences in apoptosis: sowing the seeds of IAP destruction. *Cell* 109(7): 793-796.

Martinez-Ruiz, A., Cadenas, S. & Lamas, S. (2011). Nitric oxide signaling: Classical, less classical, and nonclassical mechanisms. *Free radic biol med* 51(1):17-29.

Martins, L.M, Iaccarino, I., Tenev, T., Gschmeissner, S., Totty, N.F., Lemoine,N.R., Savopoulos, J., Gray, C.W., Creasy, C.L., Dingwall, C., Downward, J. The serine protease Omi/HtrA2 regulates apoptosis by binding XIAP through a reaper-like motif. *J Biol Chem* 277(1):439–444.

Mathewson, F. & Varnam, G. (1960). Abnormal electrocardiograms in apparently healthy people. I. Long term follow-up study. *Circulation* 21(2):196–203.

Mitchell, D.A. & Marletta, M. A.(2005). Thioredoxin catalyzes the S-nitrosation of the caspase-3 active site cysteine. *Nat Chem Biol* 1(3): 154-158.

Morisaki,N.,Saito,I.,Tamura, K.,Tashiro, J.,Masuda, M..,Kanzaki, T.,Watanabe, S., Masuda, Y., Saito, Y.(1997). New indices of ischemic heart disease and aging:studies on the serum levels of soluble intercellular adhesion molecule-1 (ICAM-1) and soluble vascular cell adhesion molecule-1 (VCAM-1) in patients with hypercholesterolemia and ischemic heart disease. *Atherosclerosis* 131(1) :43-48.

Nakagawa, H., Komai, N., Takusagawa, M., Miura, Y., Toda, T., Miyata, N., Ozawa, T., Ikota ,N.(2007). Nitration of specific tyrosine residues of cytochrome C is associated with caspase-cascade inactivation. *Biol Pharm Bull* 30(1):15-20.

Ohshima S. (2006). Apoptosis and necrosis in senescent human fibroblasts. *Annals of the New York Academy of Sciences* 1067:228-234.

Okada, H., Suh, W.K., Jin, J., Woo, M., Du, C., Elia, A., Duncan, G.S., Wakeham, A., Itie, A., Lowe, S.W., Wang, X. & Mak, T.W. (2002). Generation and characterization of Smac/DIABLO-deficient mice. *Mol Cell Biol* 22(10): 3509–3517.

Olivetti, G., Melissari, M., Capasso, J. & Anversa, P. (1991). Cardiomyopathy of the aging human heart. Myocyte loss and reactive cellular hypertrophy. *Circulation Research* 68(6): 1560-1568.

Park, H.S., Yu, J.W., Cho, J.H., Kim, M.S., Huh, S.H., Ryoo, K., & Choi, E.J. (2004). Inhibition of apoptosis signal-regulating kinase 1 by nitric oxide through a thiol redox mechanism. *J Biol Chem* 279(9), 7584-7590.

Park,J.B., Park,I.C., Park,S.J., Jin,H.O., Lee,J.K., & Riew, K.D.(2006). Anti-apoptotic effects of caspase inhibitors on rat intervertebral disc cells. *J Bone Joint Surg Am* 88(4):771-779.

Patel, R.P., McAndrew, J., Sellak, H., White, C.R., Jo, H., Freeman, B.A. & Darley-Usmar, V.M. (1999). Biological aspects of reactive nitrogen species. *Biochimica et Biophysica Acta (BBA)-Bioenergetics* 1411(2-3):385-400.

Peluffo, G. & Radi, R. (2007). Biochemistry of protein tyrosine nitration in cardiovascular pathology. *Cardiovas res* 75(2):291-302.

Phaneuf ,S. & Leeuwenburg, C. (2002). Cytochrome c release from mitochondria in the aging heart : a possible mechanism for apoptosis with age. *Am J Physiol Regulatory Integrative Comp Physiol* 282(2): R423–R430.

Qanungo, S., Starke, D.W., Pai, H.V., Mieyal, J.J. & Nieminen, A.L. (2007). Glutathione supplementation potentiates hypoxic apoptosis by S-glutathionylation of p65-NF-kappa B. *J Biol Chem* 282(25):18427-18436.

Reinehr R., Görg B., Höngen A., and Häussinger D. (2004). CD95-tyrosine nitration inhibits hyperosmotic and CD95 ligand-induced CD95 activation in rat hepatocytes. *J Biol Chem* 279(11): 10364-10373.

Rus, A., del Moral, M.L., Molina, F. & Peinado, M.A. (2010). Does inducible NOS have a protective role against hypoxia/reoxygenation injury in rat heart? *Cardiovas Pathol* 20(1):e17-25.

Salvesen, G. S. & Duckett, C. S. (2002). IAP proteins: blocking the road to death's door. *Nat. Rev. Mol. Cell Biol* 3:401–410.

Schonhoff, C.M., Gaston, B. & Mannick, J.B. (2003). Nitrosylation of cytochrome c during apoptosis. *J Biol Chem* 278(20), 18265-18270.

Schonhoff, C.M., Matsuoka, M., Tummala, H., Johnson, M.A., Estevéz A.G., Wu, R., Kamaid, A., Ricart, K.C., Hashimoto, Y., Gaston, B., Macdonald,T.L., Xu, Z. & Mannick, J.B. (2006). S-nitrosothiol depletion in amyotrophic lateral sclerosis. *Proc Nati Acad Sci USA* 103(7): 2404-2409.

Shi, Y. A conserved tetrapeptide motif: potentiating apoptosis through IAP-binding.(2002). *Cell Death Differ* 9(2), 93–95.

Spinale,F.G. (2010).Amplified bioactive signaling and proteolytic enzymes following ischemia reperfusion and aging: remodeling pathways that are not like a fine wine. *Circulation* 122(4):322-324.

Srinivasula, S.M., Gupta, S., Datta, P., Zhang, Z., Hegde, R., Cheong,N., Fernandes-Alnemri, T. & Alnemri,E.S. (2003). Inhibitor of Apoptosis Proteins Are Substrates for the Mitochondrial Serine Protease Omi/HtrA2. *J biol chem* 278(34): 31469–31472.

Stamler, J.S., Lamas, S. & Fang, F.C. (2001). Nitrosylation. the prototypic redox-based signaling mechanism. *Cell* 106(6): 675-683.

Suzuki Y, Lmai Y, Nakayama H, Takahashi K, Koji Takio, Ryosuke Takahashi. A serine protease, HtrA2, is released from the mitochondria and interacts with XIAP, inducing cell death. *Mol cell* 2001; 8:613-621.

Török, N.J., Higuchi, H., Bronk, S. & Gores, G.J. (2002). Nitric oxide inhibits apoptosis downstream of cytochrome C release by nitrosylating caspase 9. *Cancer res* 62(6), 1648-1653.

Taimor, G., Hofstaetter, B. & Piper, H. M.(2000). Apoptosis induction by nitric oxide in adult cardiomyocytes via cGMP-signaling and its impairment after simulated ischemia. *Cardiovasc res* 45(3):588-594.

Tao, L., Jiao, X., Gao, E., Lau, W., Yuan, Y., Lopez, B., Christopher, T., Ramachandrarao, S.P., Williams, W., Southan, G., Sharma, K., Koch, W. & Ma, X. (2006). Nitrative inactivation of thioredoxin-1 and its role in postischemic myocardial apoptosis. *Circulation.* 114(13): 1395-1402.

Taylor, C.T. & Moncada, S. (2010). Nitric oxide, cytochrome C oxidase, and the cellular response to hypoxia. *Arterioscler Thromb Vascular Biol* 30(4):643-647.

U.S. Census Bureau. International database. Table 094. Midyear population, by age and sex. Available at http://www.census.gov/population/www/projections/ natdet-D1A. html.

Vandervliet, A., Eiserich, J.P., O'Neill, C.A., Halliwell, B. & Cross, C.E. (1995). Tyrosine modification by reactive nitrogen species: a closer look. *Arch biochem biophys* 319(2):341-349.

Wang, K., Zhang, J, Tian., J, Liu, J., Wang, L., Ma, X., Guo, L., Yang, G., Liu, H. (2008). The pro-apoptotic effect of HtrA2/Omi in myocardial ischemia/ reperfusion injury in aged rats. *Acta Physiology Sinica.* 60 (Suppl.1):195-300.

Wang, K., Liu, J., Tian., J., Yan, Z., Zuo, L., Zheng, R. Liu, H. (2010). Time course of XIAP expression after myocardial ischemia/reperfusion in adult rats. *Chinese Journal of Cardiovascular Review* 8(5):376-379.

Wu, G., Chai, J., Suber, T.L.,Wu, J.W., Du ,C., Wang, X. & Shi, Y. (2000). Structural basis of IAP recognition by Smac/DIABLO. *Nature.* 408(6815): 1008–1012.

Wu, K., Jiang, L., Cao, J., Yang, G., Geng, C. & Zhong, L. (2007). Genotoxic effect and nitrative DNA damage in HepG2 cells exposed to aristolochic acid. *Mutation Research/Genetic Toxicology and Environmental Mutagenesis* 630(1-2):97-102.

Yellon, D.M. & Hausenloy, D.J.(2007). Myocardial reperfusion injury, *N Engl J Med* .357(11) :1121-1135.

Yuyama, K., Yamamoto, H., Nishizaki, I., Kato, T., Sora, I. & Yamamoto, T. (2003). Caspase-independent cell death by low concentrations of nitric oxide in PC12 cells: involvement of cytochrome C oxidase inhibition and the production of reactive oxygen species in mitochondria. *J neurosci res* 73,(3):351-363.

Zhang, J., Jin, B., Li, L., Block, E.R. & Patel, J.M. (2005). Nitric oxide-induced persistent inhibition and nitrosylation of active site cysteine residues of mitochondrial cytochrome-c oxidase in lung endothelial cells. *Am J Physiol Cell Physiol* 288(4):C840-C849.

Zhang, JH., Zhang,Y., Herman B.(2003). Caspases, apoptosis and aging. *Aging Research Review* 2(4):357-366.

Zhang, H., Tao, L., Jiao, X., Gao, E., Lopez, B. L., Christopher, T.A., Koch, W. & Ma ,X.L. (2007). Nitrative thioredoxin inactivation as a cause of enhanced myocardial ischemia/reperfusion injury in the aging heart. *Free Radical Biology and Medicine* 43(1):39-47.